6th Edition

Jonas and Kovner's
Health Care Delivery in the United States

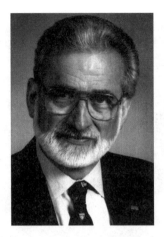

Steven Jonas, MD, MPH, MS, is Professor of Preventive Medicine, School of Medicine, State University of New York at Stony Brook. He received his B.A. from Columbia in 1958, his M.D. from the Harvard Medical School in 1962, his M.P.H. from the Yale School of Medicine in 1967, and his M.S. in Health Management from New York University in 1997. He has also studied at the London School of Economics and the Touro College School of Law (Huntington, NY). He interned at the Lenox Hill Hospital in New York City and took his residency in Preventive Medicine/Public Health in the New York City Department of Health. He is board certified in Preventive Medicine.

He is a Fellow of the American College of Preventive Medicine, the American Public Health Association, and the New York Academy of Medicine. He is Editor of the Springer (Publishing) *Series on Medical Education*, an Associate Editor of *Preventive Medicine*, a member of the Editorial Board of the *American Journal of Preventive Medicine*, and Continuing Medical Education Liaison between the American College of Preventive Medicine and the American Medical Athletics Association. He is a Past President of the Association of Teachers of Preventive Medicine and a past member of the New York State Board for Medicine.

On health policy, preventive medicine, and drug-abuse policy, Dr. Jonas has published over 100 professional articles and book reviews and delivered over 75 papers at conferences and seminars. He has also published numerous articles and given many talks on sport, exercise promotion, and weight management. He was a designated speaker on behalf of the National Health Care Campaign for the Clinton Health Plan in 1994.

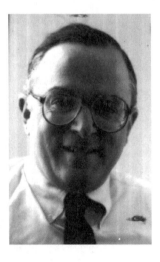

Anthony R. Kovner, Ph.D., is Professor of Health Policy and Management at the Robert F. Wagner Graduate School of Public Service at New York University, in New York City. He is trained in organizational behavior, health services management, and social and economic development. He received bachelor's and master's degrees from Cornell University, and his doctorate in public administration from the University of Pittsburgh. An award-winning author, Kovner has been at NYU since 1979. Prior to that he was on the Wharton School faculty. He is also an experienced health care manager having served as CEO of a community hospital, a senior health care consultant for United Autoworkers Union in Detroit, and manager of a group practice, a nursing home, and a large ambulatory care services program. He is a board member of the Lutheran Medical Center of Brooklyn, NY.

6th Edition

Jonas and Kovner's
Health Care Delivery
in the United States

Anthony R. Kovner, PhD
Steven Jonas MD, MPH, MS
Editors

Springer Publishing Company
New York

Springer Publishing Company, Inc.
536 Broadway
New York, NY 10012-3955

Cover design by Janet Joachim
Acquisitions Editor: Matt Fenton
Production Editor: Pamela Lankas

99 00 01 02 03/5 4 3 2 1

Library of Congress Cataloging-in-Publication Data

Jonas and Kovner's healthcare delivery in the US / edited by Anthony R. Kovner
  and Steven Jonas. — 6 ed.
     p. cm.
     Rev. ed. of: Jonas's health care delivery in the United States. 5th ed. c1995.
     Includes bibliographical references and index.
     ISBN 0-8261-2083-0. — ISBN 0-8261-2082-2
     1. Medical care—United States. I. Kovner, Anthony R.
  II. Jonas, Steven. III. Jonas's health care delivery in the United States.
     [DNLM: 1. Delivery of Health Care—United States. 2. Health Services—
  United States. W 84 AA1J68 1998]
  RA395.A3H395 1998
  362.1'0973—dc21
  DNLM/DLC
  for Library of Congress   98-27316
                                                                        CIP

Printed in the United States of America

To all those who have struggled to assure equitable insurance and access to health care for all Americans, and for all those who continue to so struggle.

Contents

III: System Performance

IV: Futures

Acknowledgments

The editors wish to acknowledge the wise counsel of Judith Haber, RN, PhD, and David A. Kindig, MD, PhD in revising the format and the topics of this sixth edition.

Organization of This Book

This book, *Health Care Delivery in the United States*, is organized into four parts: "Perspectives," "Settings," "System Performance," and "Futures" (see Figure 1). The titles of these four parts can be formulated as answers to the following questions: How do we assess and also understand the health care sector of our economy? Where is health care provided and what are the characteristics of those institutions that provide health care? What are some of the determinants of how well the system performs? Over the short term, where is the health care sector going in terms of the health of the people, the cost of care, access, and quality?

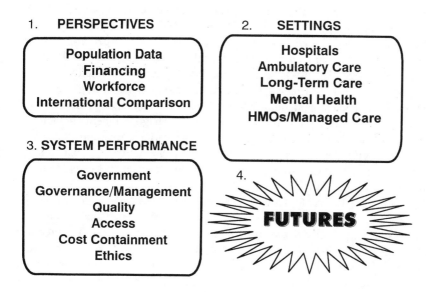

1. **PERSPECTIVES**

> **Population Data**
> **Financing**
> **Workforce**
> **International Comparison**

2. **SETTINGS**

> **Hospitals**
> **Ambulatory Care**
> **Long-Term Care**
> **Mental Health**
> **HMOs/Managed Care**

3. **SYSTEM PERFORMANCE**

> **Government**
> **Governance/Management**
> **Quality**
> **Access**
> **Cost Containment**
> **Ethics**

4. **FUTURES**

FIGURE 1   Health care delivery in the United States.

Part I, "Perspectives," is divided into an overview and chapters on population data, financial resources, workforce, and international comparisons. The overview answers some of the following questions: What is the state of health care delivery in the United States: what are we doing "right" and what are we doing "wrong"? Next, Thorpe and Knickman analyze health care costs and discuss where the money comes from that goes to pay for what kinds of health care expenses. Chris Kovner and Salsberg then examine what kinds of workers are employed to provide health care, how are they trained, and what is the impact of the changing health care system on the health care workforce. Rodwin then compares health care systems for various countries and answers how we can learn from each other?

Part II, "Settings," contains six chapters on hospitals, ambulatory care, nursing homes and home care, mental health, public health, and HMOs/managed care organizations. Part II answers some of the following questions. A. R. Kovner describes how hospitals are financed and organized and how they are changing in the face of managed care. Mezey examines the different ways of providing ambulatory care, how primary care differs from ambulatory care, and how primary and emergency care are organized in the United States. Richardson, Raphael, and Barton then describe how long-term care is organized and financed, and how nursing home and home care are changing in the managed care environment.

Further in Part II, Sharfstein, Stoline, and Koran examine how mental health care has evolved and how it is organized and financed. How is the mental health care system different from and similar to that for other kinds of health care? A. R. Kovner next examines HMOs and managed health care organizations (MCOs) and what purchasers expect from them. How are HMOs financed and organized? How are they changing? What kind of value does the public get from HMOs/MCOs as compared with other kinds of health care organizations? How are physicians organized in HMOs? How is the HMO premium divided?

Part III, "System Performance," is divided into six chapters, on government, governance and management, quality, access, cost containment, and ethics. Some of the questions Brecher answers in his chapter on government include the following: What is and should be the role of the various governmental levels (federal, state, city, county, and regional) in health care delivery? What changes should be made in Medicare so that the program "breaks even"? How is Medicaid changing as a result of managed care?

Further in Part III, A. R. Kovner examines what governance is, who owns health care organizations, and how they are managed. Weitzman analyzes indicators of health care quality based on structure, on process and on the outcomes of care, and what are the most critical factors to consider in designing a program for quality improvement. Billings presents the kinds of access various groups of Americans have to different kinds of health care. He then reviews the strengths and weaknesses of the American system with regard to providing all Americans with adequate access to health care. Thorpe, in reviewing cost containment in health care, explains the trends in the growth of health care expenditures and describes some of the efforts to control health care costs in this country. He answers questions about how successful they have been and what has been the impact of the managed care revolution on private and public health care spending.

Hofmann's chapter on ethical behavior examines how health care organizations can balance organizational and community priorities, how they can contend with managed care's conflicting incentives, and how they can confront the painful dimensions of downsizing. He also discusses how policymakers and providers can recognize the current and future dilemmas of medical rationing and how the various stakeholders in the health care sector can promote ethical behavior.

Finally, in Part IV, "Futures," Knickman attempts to specify what health care in the United States will look like over the near term. What are the key drivers of change in health care at the turn of the century? What are consumer preferences? How is the population changing in age and ethnic background? Knickman predicts the areas in which change will be most striking in coming years, such as providing service to the elderly and chronically ill, advances in molecular genetics and a range of technological innovations, market change, changes in Medicare, advances in medical information technology, and health promotion.

Each of these 17 chapters has learning objectives, a topical outline, a list of key terms, and several questions for further discussion, and most include a mini-case study. There is also a glossary and indices by author and by subject.

Contributors

Lynne Barton, a cum laude graduate of Bryn Mawr College, joined the Visiting Nurse Service of New York in 1994, and has been part of the Center for Home Care Policy and Research since February 1997. She is currently the Deputy Director of the Home Care Research Initiative (HCRI), a program of the Robert Wood Johnson Foundation. Under HCRI, The Foundation is funding policy-relevant research that aims to improve the knowledge base underlying home care policy and practice. Specifically, HCRI supports research that focuses on mechanisms for the allocation of long-term-care resources and the efficient delivery of home- and community-based services. Ms. Barton is responsible for the day-to-day management of the program, oversees all aspects of the grant process, and is the primary liaison among the grantees, the National Advisory Committee, and the Foundation. The HCRI is housed in the Center for Home Care Policy and Research of the Visiting Nurse Service of New York. As part of the Research Center, Ms. Barton is also the Project Manager for a primary research project concerning state options for allocating long-term care resources. In 1995, she received a Master of Public Health degree, with a concentration in Health Policy and Management, from the Columbia University School of Public Health.

John Billings is currently an associate professor at the Robert F. Wagner Graduate School of Public Service at New York University, and he is the director of the school's Health Research Program. Mr. Billings' recent work has involved analysis of patterns of hospital admission rates and emergency department utilization as tools to evaluate access barriers to outpatient care and to assess the performance of the ambulatory care delivery system. Mr. Billings is currently the principal investigator on a project funded by the Robert Wood Johnson Foundation to assess models for delivering primary care to low-income populations and is coprincipal investigator with Columbia University and the United Hospital Fund of New York to evaluate the impact of Medicaid managed care in New York City. Previously, Mr. Billings headed the Ambulatory Care Access Project, a 4-year effort to evaluate access barriers in New York City and urban areas in five other states. He has also worked extensively analyzing the problems of the medically indigent and developing solutions for coverage and provision of care for the uninsured in Florida, Virginia, North Carolina, Pennsylvania, Utah, and the District of Columbia. Mr. Billings' other health policy work has focused on issues related to quality of care, the management of quality in the inpatient and outpatient setting, and the physician decision-making process. Mr. Billings holds a law degree from the University of California at Berkeley.

Charles Brecher is a Professor of Public and Health Administration at the Robert F. Wagner Graduate School of Public Service, New York University. He has a PhD in political science from the City University of New York and serves as Research Director of the Citizens Budget Commission. He has published frequently in the fields of state and local politics and finance as well as health policy. His two most recent books, both published in 1993, are *Power Failure: New York City Politics and Policy since 1960* for Oxford University Press and *Managing Safety Net Hospitals: Cases for Executive Development* for the Health Administration Press.

Paul B. Hofmann is Senior Vice President with Aon Consulting's Healthcare Industry Practice in San Francisco. Dr. Hofmann previously served as Executive Vice President and Chief Operating Officer of the Alta Bates Corporation, a diversified nonprofit health care system in Northern California. He has served as the Executive Director of Emory University Hospital in Atlanta and Director of Stanford University Hospital and Clinics in Palo Alto, California. Dr. Hofmann is a fellow of the American College of Healthcare Executives, a member of its leadership Advisory Committee, and the College's consultant on healthcare management ethics. He has held a variety of appointments with the American Hospital Association, including chairman of both the Council on Research and Development and the Special Committee on Biomedical Ethics; he serves currently on its Organizational Ethics Task Force. Dr. Hofmann is also a member of the Ethics Task Force of the Society of Critical Care Medicine, the Ethics Committee of Alta Bates Medical Center, board chairman of the New Century Healthcare Institute, and he recently served as visiting scholar at Stanford University's Center for Biomedical Ethics. An author of over 100 publications, Dr. Hofmann has held faculty appointments at Harvard, UCLA, Stanford, Emory, and the University of California. His undergraduate, Masters of Public Health, and Doctor of Public Health degrees are from the University of California, Berkeley.

James R. Knickman is Vice President for Research and Evaluation at The Robert Wood Johnson Foundation. Prior to joining the Foundation in October 1992, Dr. Knickman was a Professor of Health Administration at New York University's Robert Wagner Graduate School of Public Service. Dr. Knickman has published extensively on a range of health care issues. He has done research on insurance markets and health care reimbursement systems with particular attention to long-term-care services. He also has written about methods for improving health services for urban, vulnerable populations such as the homeless, the frail elderly, and individuals with HIV illness. Dr. Knickman has served on a range of state government, local government, and health care sector advisory committees, and has offered consultation to a range of health sector organizations. Currently, he serves on the Board of Trustees of Robert Wood Johnson University Hospital. Dr. Knickman received his PhD in Public Policy Analysis from the University of Pennsylvania and did undergraduate work at Fordham University.

Lorrin M. Koran, Professor of Psychiatry at Stanford University Medical Center, is the Director of the Obsessive Compulsive Disorders Clinic and Chief of the Psychiatric Consultation Service. His research interests include new drug treatments for obsessive-compulsive and depressive disorders, and characteristics of the mental health services delivery system. Dr. Koran has served as Special Assistant to the Director of the National Institute of Mental Health. He received his MD from Harvard Medical School.

Christine Tassone Kovner is Associate Professor, Division of Nursing, School of Education at New York University. She has worked as a public health nurse, a home-care coordinator, and as a director of staff development at a small acute-care hospital. Her research interests are nursing resource use and the cost of nursing care. She earned her baccalaureate from Columbia University, her MSN from the University of Pennsylvania, and PhD in nursing from New York University.

Andrew P. Mezey is Chair of Pediatrics at Beth Israel Medical Center. He was formerly Associate Dean of Graduate Medical Education and Affiliations at Einstein. From 1989–1994 he was the Medical Director of the Jacobi Medical Center, a member hospital of the New York City Health and Hospitals Corporation. He received his MD degree from New York University in 1960 and an MS degree in management in 1992, also from NYU. He is coeditor of *Primary Care Pediatrics: A Sympomatic Approach*, is on the editorial board of the American Academy of Pediatrics book *Caring for Your Baby and Young Child: Birth to Age 5*, and the former coeditor of the journal *Emergency and Office Pediatrics*. He is a member of the New York State Board of Midwifery and the New York State Council on Graduate Medical Education.

Carol Raphael is President and Chief Executive Officer of the Visiting Nurse Service of New York and its subsidiaries, the largest nonprofit home health care agency in the United States with a budget of $550 million and over 6,000 employees. The organization provides care to 21,000 patients daily in their homes and communities. Ms. Raphael initiated an array of innovative acute, long-term and managed care programs to improve quality and contain costs. These programs include capitated managed care programs for the chronically ill elderly and people with HIV. Ms. Raphael developed the Health Connect network, a horizontally integrated network of 20 community care providers in the Greater New York area that provides comprehensive home care to eight health maintenance organizations and three million covered lives. She developed Centers of Excellence for chronic illnesses including diabetes, cardiac care, and wound care. She launched the Center for Home Care Policy and Research, a research center to advance knowledge about the needs, costs, and outcomes of home- and community-based care. Ms. Raphael holds a Master of Public Administration degree from Harvard University's Kennedy School of Government and completed the Kennedy School's Senior Executive Program.

Hila Richardson is Clinical Professor and Director for Practice Management in the Division of Nursing, School of Education at New York University. She is responsible for the development of nurse-managed practices in health care and community-based organizations throughout the New York City region. Previously, she was the Deputy Director of Medical Research and Practice Policy at the National Center on Addiction and Substance Abuse (CASA) at Columbia University, where she directed a cost study of the impact of substance abuse on New York City and was the project director for two national evaluations of substance-abuse treatment. Dr. Richardson was on the staff of the Institute of Medicine and has held several nursing positions. She held teaching positions at the University of Virginia School of Nursing, Columbia University School of Public Health, and New York University's Robert Wagner School of Public Service. She served on the Executive Board of the American Public Health Association and was President of the Public Health Association of New York City. Dr. Richardson received a BS in Nursing from the University of Virginia, an MPH from Johns Hopkins University, and a DrPH from Columbia University.

Victor G. Rodwin is Professor of Health Policy and Management at the Robert F. Wagner Graduate School of Public Service, New York University. Between 1986 and 1991, he was Director of the Advanced Management Program for Clinicians (AMPC), a program he designed with Professor Kovner under a grant from the W. K. Kellogg Foundation to enable physicians and other clinicians to obtain an Advanced Professional Certificate or a Master's degree in management. Professor Rodwin holds an MPH in health care administration and a PhD in city and regional planning from the University of California at Berkeley. He has taught at the University of California (Berkeley and San Francisco) and at the University of Paris IX (Dauphine). Professor Rodwin is a specialist in the comparative analysis of health care systems and policy. He is the author of numerous articles and books: *The Health Care Planning Predicament: France, Quebec, England and the United States* (University of California, 1984); *The End of An Illusion: The Future of Health Policy in Western Industrialized Nations* (with J. Kervasdoué and J. Kimberly, University of California Press, 1984); *Public Hospitals in New York and Paris* (with C. Brecher, D. Jolly, and R. Baxter, New York University Press, 1992); and *Japan's Universal and Affordable Health Care: Lessons for the U.S.?* (with the assistance of L. Kawasaki and J. Littlehales, Japan Society, 1994).

Edward S. Salsberg is the Director of the Bureau of Health Resources Development in the New York State Department of Health. The Bureau is responsible for health professions planning and policy development for the State Department of Health. Prior to his present position, he held a variety of positions with the New York City Health Services Administration and New York State Department of Health. Mr. Salsberg holds a Masters degree in Public Administration from New York University and a Bachelors degree in political science from the State University of New York at Stony Brook.

Steven S. Sharfstein is President, Medical Director, and Chief Executive Officer of Sheppard Pratt, a nonprofit behavioral health system in Baltimore; Clinical Professor of Psychiatry at the University of Maryland; and a practicing clinician for over 20 years, he specializes in psychotherapy and psychopharmacology for patients with long-term mental illness. He spent 13 years with the National Institute of Mental Health, where he was Director of Mental Health Service Programs and also held positions in consultation/liaison psychiatry and research in behavioral medicine on the campus of the National Institutes of Health. He has written on a wide variety of clinical and economic topics and has published more than 140 articles, 40 book chapters, and 10 books, including (as coauthor) *Madness and Government: Who Cares for the Mentally Ill?*, a history of the federal community mental health centers program. A graduate of Dartmouth College and the Albert Einstein College of Medicine, he trained in psychiatry at the Massachusetts Mental Health Center in Boston from 1969 to 1972. Dr. Sharfstein also received a Masters degree in Public Administration from the Kennedy School of Government in 1973 and a certificate from the Advanced Management Program at the Harvard Business School in 1991. He was Secretary of the American Psychiatric Association from 1991–95. Dr. Sharfstein is also a member of the Presidential Advisory Commission on Consumer Protection and Quality in the Health Care Industry.

Anne M. Stoline obtained her undergraduate degree from Kalamazoo College. She attended medical school and psychiatry residency at The Johns Hopkins

School of Medicine, where she coauthored *The New Medical Marketplace*. During several years as staff psychiatrist at the Sheppard and Enoch Pratt Hospital under the mentorship of Dr. Steven Sharfstein, she coauthored several chapters and articles about managed mental health care. She currently serves as Director of Women's Mental Health at Mercy Medical Center in Baltimore, Maryland.

Kenneth E. Thorpe is currently Director, Institute for Health Services Research, Department of Health Systems Management. He is also the Van Selow Professor of Health Policy at the School of Public Health and Tropical Medicine, Tulane University. He was formerly Deputy Assistant Secretary for Health Policy in the Department of Health and Human Services. He was an associate professor at the School of Public Health, University of North Carolina at Chapel Hill. He has served as consultant to the Rand Corporation and the Subcommittee on Health Insurance for the New York State Council on Health Care Financing, where he aided in the development of New York's new hospital payment system. His primary research interests include evaluations of the impact of public policies on hospital and nursing home behavior. Recent projects include an evaluation of the cost and access implications of alternative hospital payment methodologies in New York's (Medicare) waiver program and the impact of DRG payment on hospital readmission rates, as well as his ongoing research evaluating the RUG-II nursing home payment system in New York. Most recently, his research has focused on the effects of proposed employer health insurance mandates and expansions of Medicaid. He received his MA in public policy analysis from Duke University and his PhD from the Rand Graduate School.

Beth C. Weitzman is an Associate Professor at New York University's Robert F. Wagner Graduate School of Public Service, where she currently serves as director of the school's program in Health Policy and Management. Dr. Weitzman teaches courses on quantitative methods and on community health and medical care. Dr. Weitzman's research has focused on the health, social service, and educational needs of urban poor families; over the past 15 years she has evaluated a range of programs aimed at meeting these needs. She recently completed an NIMH-funded longitudinal study on the dynamics of homelessness and mental illness among families and is currently working with the Robert Wood Johnson Foundation to evaluate its Urban Health Initiative for child and youth. Dr. Weitzman has authored and coauthored a number of articles and book chapters on poor and vulnerable families including "Predictors of Shelter Use Among Low-Income Families: Psychiatric History, Substance Abuse, and Victimization" in the *American Journal of Public Health* and "Health Status and Health Care Utilization Among New York City Home Attendants: An Illustration of the Needs of Working Poor, Immigrant Women" in the journal *Women and Health*. She coedited a 1990 issue of the *Journal of Social Issues* entitled "Urban Homelessness."

I

PERSPECTIVES

Part I, "Perspectives," is divided into five chapters: Introduction, Population Data for Health and Health Care, Financing for Health Care, The Health Care Workforce, and Comparative Analysis of Health Systems: An International Perspective. Perspectives are ways to think about the whole health care system from different points of view, such as that of an ideal or standard health care system; the data used to measure the important aspects of the health care system, such as supply, utilization, access, quality, cost, and health of the population; the flows of money through the system—what it buys and where the financing comes from; who does the work of providing health care (some of which is provided by consumers themselves); and comparing the American health care system with health care systems in other countries most comparable to us in resources, health needs, and culture.

In chapter 1, an overview, A. R. Kovner and Steven Jonas try to assess the state of health care delivery in the United States, presenting problems and concerns about the present system and positing constraints and opportunities for improving the system. To those who say, "We don't have a health care *system* in the United States," a common response is "Well, try to change what we have and see how hard it is to change something"—such as Medicare, how specialist physicians get paid, or hospital information systems. The authors argue that Americans require a national (not a wholly public) system, can afford to have one, and can ill afford not to. Currently, there are "winners" (those who have adequate health insurance, public and private, and those employers who do not pay health insurance for their employees) and "losers" (who are the reverse of the winners). We believe that more public attention should be given to this inequality relative to a basic good such as health care and to ways that we as a nation can reduce some of the gaps between winners and losers. Kovner and Jonas indicate what is "right" and what is "wrong" about the American health care system, ask where do we go from here, and invite readers to join in thinking about what can be done to continually improve the health sector in which so many Americans work or will work.

In chapter 2, Jonas reviews population data for health and health care. Some believe that future purchasers of health care for a population will require from providers information as to how the providers will improve the health of that population (say for 100,000 people) over a period of time and what this will cost the purchaser. Jonas reviews the data that are (and could be) available for health and health services and the primary defining characteristics of the American population. He also presents the basic vital statistics and data on morbidity, health status, health related-behaviors, and the utilization of health services, as well as a description of the primary published sources of data.

In chapter 3, Thorpe and Knickman explain how the American health care financing system operates. They focus on what health resources buy, where resources come from, how health care providers are paid, and why health care expenditures have been increasing. Did you know that, in 1996, $3,759 was spent on health care for each American (dividing the total expenditures for health care by the number of Americans)? Do you think this is enough money to assure adequate health insurance for all Americans? If so, on what services should we as a nation be spending less money (or from whom should the government be raising additional revenues to pay for the extra expenditures)?

C. T. Kovner and Salsberg, in chapter 4, "The Health Care Workforce," describe the types of health care workers in the United States and the types of facilities in which they work. They describe as well the impact of the changing health care system on the health care workforce. They discuss professional licensure as a mechanism for health care worker quality assurance. They identify areas of work overlap among several health care professionals. Finally, they present and identify the difficulties in estimating the future demand and supply of health workers.

In chapter 5, Rodwin compares several different national health systems. He identifies some conceptual and methodological issues in the comparative study of health care systems and some common problems of health policy in diverse health systems. He presents key features of health care systems in France, Canada, and Great Britain. He concludes by suggesting how we can think about the uses of comparative analysis in learning from abroad, for example, by learning how other countries deal with the problems and issues we have identified concerning our own health care system.

1

Introduction: The State of Health Care Delivery in the United States

Anthony R. Kovner and Steven Jonas

In the third edition of this book, Jonas cited a study of medical care delivery made in 1932, which summarized its findings in these terms:

> The problem of providing satisfactory medical service to all the people of the United States at costs which they can meet is a pressing one. At the present time, many persons do not receive service which is adequate either in quantity or quality, and the costs of service are inequitably distributed. The result is a tremendous amount of preventable physical pain and mental anguish, needless deaths, economic inefficiency, and social waste. The United States has the economic resources, the organizing ability and the technical expertise to solve this problem. (Committee on the Costs of Medical Care, p. 2)

This statement is applicable to the health care delivery system in 1998. Based on this conclusion, the following questions, among others, can be raised about the American health care system: How does the performance of our system compare to that of other developed countries? Why does the U.S. health care delivery system perform as it does (and is such performance characteristic of other services systems in the USA)? Why haven't we done anything about the current situation and what should Americans consider doing about it? Do the problems lie primarily in the health system or the medical care system? Do the problems arise primarily from the subsystem for financing care or the way delivery of care is organized? Can we also differentiate the extent and

3

seriousness of issues as between the acute medical care system and the delivery system for chronic care, which includes nursing home and other care for the frail elderly, and care for those with chronic disease? What is the appropriate role of government and that of large, for-profit companies such as insurance companies and HMOs that have so recently become such a major factor in the operation of the health care enterprise?

Our book, as in the five previous editions, will attempt to frame these and other issues and help the reader to find answers to these and other questions. The approach taken here focuses on key elements of the health care delivery system, presents the facts and the issues, and makes references to leading authors and articles and books on each topic. One reader of the 5th edition has suggested that instead we present our own recommendations to solving the problems and taking advantage of the opportunities to improve health care delivery in the United States.

Coming up with the designs for change and assembling the information that enables one to advocate for them effectively is not the only task for an analyst of the health care delivery system. We shall resist taking this approach, as we wish readers to reach their own conclusions on the principles as well as the details, other than to assert the view that the time has come (has long since come) to establish a national system for organizing and paying for health services that would provide every American with some basic health benefits and access to care. In our view, health care should be as available to all Americans as is public education. Not every American attends public schools, goes to college or gets a PhD, but all can attend public elementary and high schools and are offered the availability of a decent basic education at public expense.

Reasonable persons can differ on what is basic health care, how providers should be paid, and how the system should be organized and financed precisely. But we do think (and certainly not all observers presently agree) that the Committee on the Costs of Medical Care was right in 1932: the nation needs a national (not a wholly public) system; can afford to have one; and in the present era, given the very high proportion of the gross national product devoted to paying for health services, can ill afford not to. Such a national system should therefore be designed and appropriately phased in, soon.

What Are We Doing Right?

The United States has a very large number of the best clinicians, hospitals, equipment, and medical care facilities in the world. We spend a great deal of money on acute medical care, and Americans with excellent insurance coverage or adequate finances have available to them a very wide range of choices as to providers and therapies. The United States has a very high average standard of living for its people and a high employment rate. Our medical care delivery system is characterized by a high degree of innovation and technological change. Our health care providers—some of them—probably have the best information systems, quality control systems, and cost accounting systems worldwide. We spend a great deal of money educating both clinicians and the workforce for support services, and we have very high employment in the health care enterprise. American products, such as drugs, medical equipment, and supplies, are a source of large export revenues. We spend more on research in health care delivery than do other countries. The United States ranks near the top worldwide in only one major health vital statistics category: life expectancy after age 80 (Rice, 1997).

What Are We Doing Wrong?

Even as we spend much more money on health care per capita than does any other country, our health care delivery system does not seem to be performing as well as that of other countries in terms of both the health status and insurance coverage of our population. Our systems of financing and governing medical care are complex and fragmented, resulting in large and unnecessary administrative costs. Most experts believe that, relative to total expenditures, we are spending too much money on acute medical care and not enough money on chronic health care. Although there is a lot of talk about it, we do not do nearly what we could do to promote health and prevent disease. We have serious problems in systems and institutions affecting both the demand for and provision of medical care, such as education and welfare. These problems seem to be worse than in other countries. Causes range from too many homicides (related to too many guns), to poor performance by the schools (millions of Americans cannot effectively read and write), to too many Americans, particularly Black males, in jail and too few two-parent families raising children.

So Where Do We Go from Here?

This book is written in the hope that with facts and evidence on the table the reader can see where the money for health care delivery goes now and what we get for the money spent. Then ask yourself: given these expenditures, how could we reallocate these funds so that the American people could get more of what we want and need from the health care delivery system and less of what we do not want or need. This effort should involve, first, developing a conception of what the health care delivery system should look like in 5 or 10 years. Following that, a plan or at least a set of guidelines for getting from here to there can be developed. Of course, expenditures equal incomes. Numerous individuals, groups, and economic entities benefit greatly from the way the system is presently organized (and if you think we don't have a system, just try changing it!) They fear that their interests would be negatively affected by changes in the reallocation of resources. They argue that what makes the United States a great country is our "free market" economy and that there is no difference between the health care system and the hotel system and the telephone and the banking systems in terms of how resources should be owned and services provided. There is great distrust of government and serious question about the value citizens get for the tax dollars that are paid to governments.

It's Up to You

We hope our text will provide you with data and views of the data so that you can form your own conclusions or develop future lines of inquiry so that you can ultimately get answers to presently unanswered questions. One of the great fascinations in teaching, learning, and undertaking research about the health care delivery system is the difficulty posed in finding satisfactory solutions. Humbling are the changes we have observed in our own views and conclusions in the face of the changing realities of new technologies, new demands and preferences, and new ways of organizing services and training clinicians.

We hope you will enjoy the journey!

References

Committee on the Costs of Medical Care, *Medical Care for the American People*. Chicago: University of Chicago Press, 1932; reprinted, Washington, DC: USDHEW, 1970.

Rice, T., "Can Markets Give Us the Health System We Want?" *Journal of Health Politics, Policy and Law, 22*, 400, April 1997.

2

Population Data for Health and Health Care

Steven Jonas

Learning Objectives

1. To be able to list and characterize the major categories of data used to describe the people served by the health care delivery system.
2. To be able to list and characterize the major categories of data used to describe the health care delivery system and its activities.
3. To be able to describe the principal sources of health and health services data and state how and where to find them (using Appendix II as well as this chapter).
4. To be able to define the list of "key words."

Topical Outline

Data for health and health services: What are they?
How are health and health services data commonly organized and presented?
What are the primary sources for the common data?
Numbers and rates.
The purposes of quantification.
The U.S. population: primary defining characteristics.
Vital statistics.
Morbidity and mortality.
Health status and health-related behaviors.
Utilization of health services.

Key Words: **Data, census, vital statistics, demographic characteristics, numbers, rates, numerator, denominator, morbidity (sickness), mortality (death),**

natality, infant mortality, crude and specific rates, incidence, prevalence, health status, provider- and patient-perspective utilization, ambulatory services, hospitalization, health services utilization, program planning.

Quantitative description and analysis provide the basic means for understanding the nature and health status of the population the health care delivery system serves and the system's operations. Because of the nature of most data gathering and reporting, on the one hand, and book writing and publishing on the other, most of the data presented in this chapter will be out of date by the time this book is published. Thus, the utility of the numbers presented is found not in their description of current reality at the time the book is being read. Rather, the data presented are to be viewed as examples of *how* numbers are and can be used to better comprehend the health care delivery system and those it serves.

Virtually all the numbers presented in this chapter are from sources that are published on a regular, usually annual, basis. (See Appendix II for descriptions of each of the principal data sources.) Thus, the diligent reader can fairly easily find the most recent numbers for the data category in question at the time they are needed. There is a relative torrent of data appearing in regularly recurring sources. Nonetheless, not all of the important data categories are regularly reported. For example, under "Mortality" (see below), the cause of death by diagnosis is regularly reported, but the cause of death by risk factor is not. Thus, on occasion nonrecurring data reports have to be paid attention to as well.

Little if any study of the question "why certain data categories and not others?" has been done, but some answers can be hazarded. Data that are easy or relatively easy to collect, like deaths by diagnosis, are much more likely to be regularly reported than data that are not so easy to collect, like death by risk factor. Data that have been routinely collected for decades, whether they are any longer important or not—like that for many of the reportable infectious diseases (see below)—are more likely to be regularly reported. Data that have some use for an important and powerful set of institutions, like hospital utilization figures (see below), are more likely to be regularly collected and reported than, say, use of certain hospital-based services stratified by geography, social class, ethnic group, and insurance status.

There are a number of important data-related questions with which this chapter does not deal. Among them are how changing technology affects data collection, publication, and analysis; confidentiality and its impact on data collection and use; how health data categories, counting, counts, frequency, availability, and use vary by country; the costs of obtaining and publishing data and data analyses; and the politics of health data collection, publication, and analysis.

The principal sources for the data presented in this chapter are the *Monthly Vital Statistics Report, Vital Statistics of the United States*, and special studies published in the NCHS publication *Vital and Health Statistics*, Series 20. Some of these data are also published regularly in the *Statistical Abstract of the United States* and the recurrent publication *Health United States*. (See Appendix II for descriptions of each of these sources.)

Quantitative Perspectives

Overview

There are three major quantitative perspectives from which a population's health status and the health care services provided for it can be viewed. First are the simple *numbers* of people and what are called their *demographic* characteristics (from the Greek for "describing the people"). Among the important demographic characteristics are age, sex, marital status, geographic location, and such social characteristics as ethnicity, income, education, employment, and measures of social class.

Second are the direct measures of health and sickness in a population. Given the current level of sophistication of data gathering and analysis, it is much easier to characterize the latter than the former. The ill-health status of the population is described by measures of mortality (death) and morbidity (sickness). Mortality and morbidity may be counted for the population as a whole. In this case the rates (see below) derived from the data are defined as *crude*. Alternatively, mortality and morbidity may be counted by cause or by demographic characteristics used in describing segments of the population (e.g., age, sex, ethnicity). As such, they are called *specific* rates (i.e., age-specific, disease-specific, etc.). *Health* status indicators have proved much more difficult to develop.

The third quantitative perspective for viewing a population in terms of health and sickness is that of its *utilization of health services*: who uses how many of what kinds of services, when, and where. Utilization can be measured from two points of view: that of the consumer and that of the provider. For example, physician/patient encounters can be reported in terms of how many visits the average patient makes to the physician each year (patient perspective). The same set of events can be reported in terms of how many patient visits the average physician provides each year (provider perspective).

When one knows how many and what kinds of people there are where, what their health and sickness status is, and their service utilization levels, one has fairly well characterized a population's health and health care status quantitatively.

The system's operations are fairly well quantified by the provider-perspective data recording of the same events.

Numbers and Rates

Population, health status, and utilization data all can be presented in two forms: numbers and rates. A *number* is simply a count of conditions, individuals, or events. A *rate* has two parts: a numerator and a denominator. The numerator is the number of conditions, individuals, or events counted. The denominator is a (usually) larger group of persons, conditions, or events from among which the subset described by the numerator data is drawn.

It is customary to present a rate as applying during a particular time period. For example, one could determine that 1,000 deaths occurred in a particular population during a year. This *number* of deaths becomes a *rate* if one counts the whole population, finds that number to be 100,000, and then says that the mortality *rate* is 1,000/100,000 per year. The rate can be expressed as a percentage (in this case, 1%) or as a rate per thousand (in this case, 10) per year or by any other formulation that is useful.

The magnitude of the denominator is usually chosen to make the rate a number of reasonable size. Thus, the less frequent the event being counted by the numerator, the larger the denominator. For example, crude death rates for a whole population, all causes, are usually given as per 1,000 population. Cause-specific mortality rates are usually presented as per 100,000 or even as per 1,000,000. This is done so that the rate's numerator will not be a fractional number.

Both denominators and numerators can be quite specific, and the units can be the same. For example, in describing deaths from lung cancer among cigarette smokers, an age/cause-specific rate would be the number of deaths per year from lung cancer in males over age 45 who have smoked two or more packs of cigarettes per day for 20 years or more (the numerator), divided by the number of *all* males over 45 who have smoked two or more packs of cigarettes per day for 20 years or more (the denominator). The units of the numerator and the denominator in health indices can also be different. For example, in cause-specific mortality rates, the unit for the numerator is deaths by cause, whereas the unit for the denominator is the total number of persons in the population counted.

Although rates are usually fractions, occasionally they will be whole numbers. For example, in measuring total morbidity in a population, one may find that the number of diagnosed disease conditions is greater than the number of people. The rate then is usually given with a denominator of 1. For example: "In the population of a central African city there are 2.5 diseases per person." This usage also occurs in utilization rates. For example: "The annual physician-visit rate in the United States is about 5.6 per person." Rates are especially useful for measuring and describing changes over time, in everything from deaths to per capita health care expenditures.

There is a special group of health service utilization rates, not usually presented in terms of numerators and denominators. For example, hospital-specific admission rates are commonly presented simply as a number per unit of time, as follows: "In 1997, the admission rate for hospital Y was 1,000 per month." One reason for using this formulation is that the sizes of the populations served by both institutional and individual providers are generally not known.

The Purposes of Quantification

Description. There are two major purposes for quantification of health care delivery system events. First, quantification _describes_ the population being served. Demographic characteristics such as geographic location (do many people live near marshes inhabited by malaria-carrying mosquitoes?) and age distribution (are there many infants and/or old people?) by themselves may well provide some indication of the population's relative disease risks.

2) Disease-specific mortality and morbidity rates highlight the major clinically apparent health and illness problems in the population. The infant mortality rate gives some indication of both general health levels and the availability of medical care. The distribution of crude and disease-specific mortality and morbidity rates by place, age, sex, ethnic group, and social class shows which population subgroups are being affected by what diseases.

Consumer-perspective utilization data can provide some idea about the possible differential use of health services by social class, ethnicity, and geography. Provider-perspective utilization data can tell us the average number of visits provided annually by physicians according to their age, practice location, and specialty.

In summary, health status and services quantification describes how many of what kind of people are at risk, what kinds of diseases and ill-health conditions they have, how those problems are distributed in the population, and who goes where for how many of what kinds of health services, delivered by which types of providers.

Program Planning. The second purpose of quantification in health care delivery is for *program planning*. It may be done, for example, by a hospital, a health services network, a city health services administration, a federal government agency, or a private physician. Descriptive data can reveal the existence of health or health services problems. Then, if there is the interest, the will, and the money to do something about them, data can also be used to help design solutions, in the first instance by clearly defining the unmet need that is to be met by the proposed new program. Among the other uses of data for health services program planning, data-based utilization projections are essential for estimating costs. Once new programs are under way, having data on them is necessary if their effects and effectiveness are to be evaluated.

However, it must be remembered that data in themselves are not sufficient for effective and useful planning. Before data have any real meaning for planning, the agencies and institutions in charge must first make a policy decision to actually engage in the process. They must also agree to make their planning data-based. (Too often in the real world, program planning, even if it is done, is not data-based.) Further, to make the planning process worth the candle, the policymakers who have authorized it must also have decided that, once arrived at, a suitable plan will be implemented. Data for planning mean nothing unless the planning is data-based and planned programs are implemented as indicated.

To illustrate the use of data for planning, let us take the hypothetical case of program and then physical planning for a medical school hospital located in a suburban/semirural area. The university trustees for the medical school have already decided that this hospital is to be designed so that it can help meet the health care needs of the community as well as serve the educational and research needs of the medical school. (The three functions of any medical school, in theory at least, are patient care, teaching, and research.) It is to be hoped, of course, that the subprograms for carrying out each of these three functions can be coordinated in a positive way so that all will be benefited.

The first step in rationally planning for a new medical school hospital is to delineate a proposed service area. One counts the population, determines population densities, examines modes of transportation, and evaluates existing health care resources, particularly the more complex and sophisticated ones already in place. Health and sickness status indicators for the proposed target population are assembled. Some of the data-based questions to be asked are listed in Table 2.1.

TABLE 2.1   Major Classes of Data Used for Health Services Planning

How many people live in the proposed service area, and where are they located?
What are the age, sex, and marital status distributions?
What are the social class and ethnic makeups?
What is the sickness and health profile?
How is the population size and composition changing over time?
What are the existing health care resources, and how are they used?
What do existing providers see as their needs?
How do they view the new facility, and how will they relate to it?

The answers to these questions and many similar ones define the health and health care needs of the population to be served. They also characterize the existing health care resources. These and other data are essential for identifying and quantifying both the met and unmet health and health care needs of the population.

The data thus afford the opportunity to make intelligent decisions on facility design, location, services and service priorities, space allocation, administrative structure, community relations, staffing and personnel policies, teaching and research programs, capital cost alternatives, expense budget, and the other myriad details that confront the health services program planner.

Amalgamating, classifying, and analyzing all these data provides the base for rational program planning. In general, one can say that intelligent decisions in health services planning depend on intelligent use of health and health care data. Unfortunately that does not always happen in the United States. Now let us turn to a consideration of certain classes of data in some detail.

Population

Number

The Constitution of the United States requires that a census of the nation be taken at least once every 10 years (U.S. Bureau of the Census [USBOC], 1996, p. 1). The original purpose of the census was to provide the basis for the apportionment among the states of seats in the House of Representatives of the U.S. Congress. A census has been carried out every 10 years since 1790. Although every effort is made for completeness, the Census Bureau has estimated that in 1990 it undercounted by between 1% and 2%, ranging from 5.0% for Hispanics through 4.4% for Blacks to 0.7% for non-Hispanic Whites (USBOC, 1996, p. 1).

The primary reasons for undercounting are thought to be fear of authority in general on the part of members of those population segments that are undercounted and fear in particular by certain persons of being reported for one reason or another to such agencies as those responsible for immigration, social services, or criminal justice, even though guarantees are made by the census takers that such reporting will not occur.

In addition to carrying out the decennial census, the Census Bureau makes interim population estimates on various parameters, based on information gathered from samples and a variety of other sources. The estimated U.S. resident population as of July 1, 1995, was 262,755,000 (USBOC, 1996, Table 2). In addition, there were about 280,000 U.S. citizens (including members of the military) living abroad.

Births, deaths, immigration, and emigration are the four factors producing change in population size. During the 1970s and 1980s, the population growth rate in the United States averaged about 1.0% per year (USBOC, 1996, Tables 2, 4). During the 1960s the population had grown at the rate of about 1.3% per year. The decline in rate of growth resulted primarily from a decrease in the birthrate. It is projected that population growth will likely decline further, to 0.6% per year by 2050. Nevertheless, the midrange U.S. population size projection for that year is still about 393 million, an increase of about 33% over the 1995 population. Even without taking into account the accompanying changes in the age composition of a population growing ever older as well as growing in size, the bearing on health services need and utilization of such factors as simple population size and growth rate is obvious.

Demographic Characteristics

In 1994, 79.8% of the U.S. population lived in what are called *metropolitan statistical areas* (MSAs, also referred to, with slightly different definitions, as standard metropolitan statistical areas [SMSAs] and consolidated metropolitan statistical areas [CMSAs]) (USBOC, 1996, Table 40). The figures for 1960 and 1980 were 63% and 78%, respectively.

The federal Office of Management and Budget, an agency of the executive branch, is charged with defining the term "metropolitan statistical area" (USBOC, 1996, p. 937). The definition has changed over time. As of 1990 an MSA included at least (1) one city with a population of 50,000 or more or (2) a Census Bureau–defined urbanized area of at least 50,000 inhabitants and a total MSA population of at least 100,000 (75,000 in New England). In addition, the county (or counties) containing the central city and adjacent counties that have at least 50% of their population in the urbanized area surrounding the city are included. Outlying "commuting counties" may be included as well if they meet certain requirements.

As of 1995 it was estimated that the U.S. population was 48.8% male and 87.4% non-Black, with a median age of 34.3 (33.1 for males, 35.4 for females) (USBOC, 1996, Tables 13, 14). The median age was up from 28 in 1970. In 1995, 28.9% of the population was under 20, and 12.7% was age 65 and over, up from 9.8% in 1970. In 1995, about 63% of males and 59% of females 18 and over were married, contrasting with 74% and 70%, respectively, in 1970 (USBOC, 1996, Table 59). In 1990, about 6.7 million Americans lived in "group quarters," including 1.8 million persons in nursing homes and 1.9 million in college dormitories (USBOC, 1996, Table 85). In 1994, over 1 million Americans were imprisoned (USBOC, 1996, Table 350). (See Table 2.2.)

Social class status is often thought to be a valuable parameter by which to cross-tabulate population, health/illness, and utilization data (Williams & Collins, 1996).[1] However, unlike the British government, for a variety of primarily political reasons the U.S. government has not developed a "social class" index by which it cross-tabulates its demographic data. Thus, we are forced to use ethnicity and income as rough indicators of social class. This is unfortunate, because social class is determined not simply by income but by a combination of several factors, including education, employment, and dwelling place. A great deal of such information is, in fact, collected by the government. Nevertheless, a social class index has never been created for the country.

(The information presented so far in this chapter comes primarily from the "Population" section of the *Statistical Abstract of the United States: 1996* (US-BOC, 1996). Additional information necessary to develop a comprehensive profile of the population is contained in the "Vital Statistics," "Education," "Social Insurance and Human Services," "Labor Force, Employment, and Earnings," and "Income Expenditures, and Wealth" sections of the same publication.)

Vital Statistics

How They Are Collected

In public health, the "vital statistics" are classically defined as data on births, deaths, marriages, and divorces (USBOC, 1996, p. 71). In the United States, primary responsibility for collecting these data lies with the states, usually through the State Department of Health or its equivalent. Not all states collect all categories of data (although all states have collected birth and death data since 1933). On a regular basis the states generally publish at least some of the data they collect. Where they exist, county and other-jurisdiction local health departments do the actual counting and then transmit the results to the state level. The states in turn send their results to the federal National Center for Health Statistics (NCHS). The District government for Washington, DC, carries out primary data collection for that city.

The first vital statistic to be collected in the United States on an annual basis was mortality. In 1900, 10 states and the District of Columbia became the first

---

[1] A classic study of this very important subject area, with an extensive bibliography, was presented in *The Health Gap*, edited by Robert Kane, MD (New York: Springer Publishing Co., 1975). See also Office of Health Resources Opportunity, *Health Status of Minorities and Low Income Groups* (DHEW Pub. No. HRA 79-627; Washington, DC: U.S. Government Printing Office, 1979), and for a more recent perspective, see V. Alcena, *The Status of Health of Blacks in the United States of America* (Dubuque, IA: Kendall/Hunt Publishing Co., 1992).

TABLE 2.2   Demographic Characteristics, U.S. Population, 1994–95, with Selected Comparisons for 1970

Characteristic	1994–95		1970
Number (millions)	263	(1995)	203
Percent population living in an MSA	80	(1994)	69
Percent female	51	(1995)	49
Percent White	83	(1995)	87
Median age	34.3	(1995)	28
Marriage rate (per thousand)	9.1	(1994)	10.6
Divorce rate (per thousand)	4.6	(1994)	3.5

Sources: USBOC, *Statistical Abstract of the United States: 1971*, Tables 14, 15, 21; *1996*, Tables 2, 13, 42, 146. Washington, DC: U.S. Government Printing Office, 1971, 1996.

"death registration states," carrying out that task and forwarding the results to the federal government (USBOC, 1996, p. 71). Until 1946 the Census Bureau assembled the vital statistics at the national level. From 1946 to 1960 the work was performed by the Bureau of State Services of the U.S. Public Health Service. Since 1960, the NCHS of the Department of Health and Human Services has carried out the function.

Beginning in 1915, 10 states and the District of Columbia formed a "birth registration area," collecting birth data on an annual basis. Fetal deaths have been counted annually since 1922. Since 1933 the birth and death registration area has included all of the states and the District of Columbia. A "marriage registration area" was first formed in 1957. By 1995 it included 42 states, the Virgin Islands, Puerto Rico, and the District of Columbia. The "divorce registration area" was established in 1958; by 1995 it covered 31 states and the Virgin Islands.

By implication the Constitution grants "police power" to the states as an element of their independent sovereignty. That power includes such responsibilities as collecting public health data. Thus, the federal government cannot require the states to become members of any national registration area. That is why not all states are members of either the marriage or divorce registration areas, although all have chosen to become part of the birth and death registration areas.

The NCHS determines the national vital statistics rates. They are based on the actual number of persons counted by the Census Bureau on April 1 of each decennial year, as well as on the midyear estimates made for other years. Cause-specific mortality data are classified according to the *International Classification of Diseases, Ninth Revision, Adapted for Use in the United States* (NCHS, 1979a), the so-called ICDA. The *ICDA-9-Clinical Modification* (ICDA-9-CM) is an extension of the ICDA-9 that all U.S. hospitals receiving federal funds are required to use.

Natality

In 1994 about 3.95 million babies were born in the United States, a decline of 5% from 1990 (*Monthly Vital Statistics Report* [MVSR], 1996, p. 1). The annual live birth rate was 15.2 per 1,000 population. That was higher than the lowest rate recorded in recent years, 14.6 in 1975–1976 (USBOC, 1996, Table 90) but still down by 2% from the rate for 1993. Until the turnaround that occurred in 1975–1976, the birthrate had been steadily dropping from a post–World War II high of 25, reached in 1955, the peak of the so-called baby boom.

The fertility rate is defined as the number of births per 1,000 women aged 15–44. For 1994 it was 66.7 (MVSR, 1996, p. 1). That was down from the post–World War II high of 123 reached in 1957, down 1% from 1993, 6% from 1990, and close to the low of 65 recorded in 1976. If the death rate were to remain stable over a long period and there were no immigration, with the current birthrate the U.S. population would gradually decrease over time.

Mortality

Crude Death Rates. Mortality data are reported rather neatly. Death is a well-defined event in the vast majority of cases (although with recent developments in medical technology, legal, ethical, religious, and biomedical disputes arise at the definitional margins as to just what "death" is [President's Commission, 1981; Wikler & Weisbard, 1989]). As noted, there is one primary reporting authority for deaths, usually the local health department or, where none exists, the state health department acting in its place. Because both hospitals and funeral directors are legally required to report all deaths, with rather serious penalties for failure to comply, we can assume that most deaths are reported.

For 1994 the crude death rate (total deaths per 1,000 population) in the United States was 8.8 (USBOC, 1996, Table 90). This compares with a rate of 9.6 for 1950, 9.5 for 1960, 9.5 for 1970, 8.8 for 1980, but 8.5 for 1992. Mortality is relatively high during the first year of life; it drops by increasing age group to a relatively low level until the mid-40s and then begins to climb again (USBOC, 1996, Tables 118–120).

Males have a higher mortality rate than females at all ages. Thus, as the average age of the population increases, the female/male ratio increases as well. Although the crude death rate for non-Whites is lower than for Whites, the age-specific death rates for non-Whites are higher than for Whites at all ages until

85. The crude death rate is lower for non-Whites because the non-White population has a lower average age.

Much data on differential death rates by the basic demographic variables of age, color, and sex can be found in the *Monthly Vital Statistics Report, Vital Statistics of the United States,* special studies published in the NCHS publication *Vital and Health Statistics,* Series 20, and the *Statistical Abstract* (again, refer to Appendix II).

Disease-Specific Mortality. From time to time, determination of the disease-specific cause of death in a given case presents some problems as noted. In most cases it is the responsibility of a physician to certify that a patient is dead. As well as the social issues concerning the definition of death noted above, physicians have varying diagnostic styles, perspectives, and abilities. Furthermore, there have been changes in the medical/technical definitions of causes of death over time.[2] As an example of the potential difficulty, consider the following question: if a patient dies from a heart attack that resulted from the complications of diabetes, is the cause of death diabetes or coronary artery disease? The reporting authorities do have rules covering most of these instances; most physicians follow them, but some do not.

In 1996 the 10 leading causes of death by disease-specific diagnostic category (excluding "symptoms and ill-defined conditions" and "all other diseases") were heart disease, cancer, stroke, chronic obstructive pulmonary disease, "accidents and adverse effects" (all leading to personal injury as the cause of death), pneumonia and influenza (primarily pneumonia), diabetes mellitus, all other infectious and parasitic diseases, human immunodeficiency virus infection, and suicide (MVSR, 1997).

By contrast, in 1980 the 10 leading causes of death by disease-specific diagnosis were heart disease, cancer, personal injury, stroke, chronic obstructive pulmonary disease, pneumonia and influenza, cirrhosis of the liver, suicide, diabetes mellitus, homicide, and "legal intervention" (execution) (USBOC, 1996, Table 128), with the rates for heart disease, stroke, and personal injury being considerably higher at that time and the rate for chronic obstructive pulmonary disease considerably lower. In certain categories we are making progress. In others we are not.

Risk-Factor-Specific Mortality. In the modern United States most deaths are caused by chronic diseases or conditions (such as personal injury) in which

---

[2]For a detailed discussion of this problem, see "Estimates of Selected Comparability Ratios Based on Dual Coding of 1976 Death Certificates by the Eighth and Ninth Revisions of the International Classification of Diseases," *MVSR, 28* (11) (Suppl.), February 1980).

environmental and personal risk factors play a major causative role. To make the mortality data picture more useful for understanding what is truly going on in matters of health status and for program planning, in 1993, McGinniss and Foege took a different approach to characterizing the causes of death in the United States.

They went beyond the classic lists of death-associated disease-specific diagnoses to the identification of the major external (nongenetic) factors known to be causally associated with death. After an exhaustive review of the literature covering the period 1977–1993, McGinniss and Foege (1993) were able to attribute approximately half of all deaths occurring in 1991 to the following 10 risk factors: tobacco use (400,000 deaths annually), diet and activity patterns (300,000), alcohol use (100,000), microbial agents (90,000), toxic agents (60,000), firearms (35,000), sexual behaviors (30,000), motor vehicle use (25,000), and use of the "illicit drugs," primarily heroin and cocaine (20,000).

The picture arising from the McGinniss/Foege analysis is particularly helpful in planning public health programs to prolong life, especially healthy life. Using it, one can focus on changeable/modifiable human behaviors (e.g., cigarette smoking, eating patterns, physical activity, and using machines) rather than on classic, diagnostically related, disease-specific prevention for such conditions as heart disease, cancer, and stroke. The former, focusing on the here and now, has much more relevance to the otherwise healthy patient than does the latter, concerning as it does an event that may or may not happen to any one individual in the future.

Infant Mortality. The infant mortality rate is the number of deaths before the age of 1 year among children born alive, divided by the number of live births. A nation's infant mortality rate appears to be related to a variety of socioeconomic, environmental, and health care factors. Some authorities (Morris, 1964, pp. 56ff., 267; Rosen, 1958, p. 342) have considered it to be a fairly sensitive indicator of general health levels in a population. In 1993 the infant mortality rate in the United States was 8.4 per 1,000 live births (USBOC, 1996, Table 124), the lowest ever recorded in the United States. The rate has been declining steadily since 1940, when it was 47 (Grove & Hetzel, 1968, Table 38). In fact, the infant mortality rate has been falling since it was first recorded in this country, at 99.9, in 1915.

The most striking feature of the U.S. infant mortality rate is that although it has consistently declined over the years, the rate for Blacks has just as consistently remained about double the White rate (USBOC, 1996, Table 124). Detailed examinations of the relationships among ethnicity, other factors, and infant mortality are contained in *Vital and Health Statistics* (NCHS, 1992) and in a publication of the Office of Health Services Opportunity (1979, pp. 35–39).

A classic study of factors related to infant mortality is the work of David Kessner and his colleagues (1973) sponsored by the National Academy of Sciences. It found that in 140,000 births in New York City, with the infectious diseases that formerly took the lives of many infants mainly under control, "generally, adequacy of [health] care . . . is strongly and consistently associated with infant birth weight . . . and survival" (Kessner, Singer, Kalk, & Schlessinger, 1973, p. 1). Kessner and his coauthors also concluded from their study that

> the survival of infants of different ethnic groups varies widely; . . . there is consistent association between social classes as measured by the educational attainment of the mothers and infant birth weight and survival; . . . within categories of mothers' educational attainment, there are consistent trends relating the adequacy of care . . . to infant survival; . . . there is a gross misallocation of services by ethnic group and care when the risks of the women are taken into account. (pp. 2–3)

Twenty-five years later, the results of this study appear to be valid still.

Marriage and Divorce

In 1994 the marriage rate stood at 9.1 per 1,000 population (USBOC, 1996, Table 146), down from 10.6 in 1970. The divorce rate, which had been 5.2 per 1,000 population in 1980 (USBOC, 1996, Table 153), was 4.6 in 1994, slightly over 50% of the marriage rate. Even as the marriage rate has dropped over time, the proportion ending in divorce has increased slightly. Detailed analyses of birth, marriage, and divorce statistics can be found in *Vital and Health Statistics*, Series 21, "Data on Natality, Marriage and Divorce," as well as in the publication *Monthly Vital Statistics Report*.

Morbidity

Definitions

Morbidity refers to sickness, illness, and disease. Like mortality, morbidity data can be expressed in both numbers and rates. Like other data classes, morbidity data can be cross-tabulated with the broad range of demographic characteristics. Morbidity data are extremely important in characterizing the health status of a population. Because many widely prevalent diseases and conditions of ill health do not appear in mortality figures, by themselves the latter are not adequate for health status characterization. This is particularly so in a country like the United

States, in which communicable disease, with a few notable exceptions such as AIDS, is not a major cause of death.

Morbidity data can be reported in terms of both incidence and prevalence. *Incidence* is the number of new cases of the disease in question occurring during a particular period, usually a year. *Prevalence* is the total number of cases existing in a population during a time period or at one point in time (in which case it is known as *point-prevalence*).

The list of significant nonfatal causes of ill health in the United States includes arthritis, low back pain, the common cold, influenza, nonfatal injuries, dermatitis, and mild emotional and sexual problems. There are other diseases that may kill but do so rarely in relation to their prevalence. Included in this category are sexually transmitted disease (STD) other than AIDS, duodenal ulcer, and gallbladder disease. Morbidity data not only highlight the important diseases and the patterns of their distribution in the population, they also illustrate disease-related limitations of activity.

Counting and reporting morbidity is not nearly as simple as reporting mortality, however. Consider the following questions. What is meant by the term "sickness," and just when is a person "sick"? Who decides? The physician? The patient? Furthermore, although the law requires that all deaths be reported, only certain categories of sickness, the infectious diseases, must be reported. The list appears in a weekly publication of the Centers for Disease Control of the U.S. Public Health Service called *Morbidity and Mortality Weekly Report.* Among the 24 such diseases only 5 are significant in the United States: AIDS, gonorrhea, viral hepatitis, syphilis, and tuberculosis. On the other hand, there are no mandatory reporting requirements for many disease categories that are important.

It is known that some physicians fail to report certain diseases even when legally required to do so. Some private physicians will not report venereal disease in private patients on the grounds of "avoiding embarrassment." Physicians may be inhibited in the reporting of tuberculosis because of possible economic consequences for the patient in terms of maintaining employment. (Although the disease is one of low infectivity, it is commonly thought to be highly contagious, even by some health professionals. Thus, for example, the automatic firing of persons with tuberculosis would technically be illegal, but it does happen.)

Many physicians fail to report cases of the common childhood viral infections because they consider them to be "inconsequential."[3] The reporting of both AIDS and seropositivity for the human immunodeficiency virus (HIV) is an extremely

---

[3]For example, we can estimate that, just before the introduction of the measles vaccine in the mid-1960s, the measles reporting rate was around 10%. Almost all children get measles before their fifth birthday. Although there were about 4 million births annually in the United States at that time, only 400,000 cases of measles were reported annually. Because close to 4 million children under the age of 5 were getting the disease each year, it can be concluded that the reporting rate was about 10%.

complex and controversial subject (Bayer, 1991; Dickens, 1988; Karon, Rosenberg, & McQuillan, 1996; Walters, 1988).

Data

Turning to the data itself, for mortality there is only one possible source—and it isn't the patient. For morbidity, it is obvious that both providers and patients can be data sources; as a result, quite different pictures of the same reality can be obtained. Providers can report morbidity by diagnostic categories and also by patient chief complaints (i.e., what the patient reports to the physician as being the problem).

However, patients don't usually come to a physician saying "I think I've got diabetes mellitus, Doc" but rather something like, "Doc, I've been feeling kind of weak; I'm drinking a great deal of water and urinating a lot. Do you think maybe something's wrong?" It is up to the physician to characterize the problem and make a diagnosis that he or she then can report. Patients can also report chief complaints directly to data gatherers, as in a population survey.

From a chief complaint profile for a population, obtained from either source, a partial picture of morbidity patterns can be drawn. One advantage of deriving information directly from a population sample is that certain people with certain types of illnesses will never come to medical attention. Thus, morbidity surveys that gather information only from providers will not give a complete picture.

In the United States, morbidity data are published on a regular basis by the NCHS and, as noted, for the reportable communicable diseases, by the Centers for Disease Control and Prevention (in the *Morbidity and Mortality Weekly Report*). The data sources of the NCHS include the Health and Nutrition Examination Survey (HANES), the Health Interview Survey (HIS), the Hospital Discharge Survey (HDS), and the National Ambulatory Medical Care Survey (NAMCS). The results of these surveys are published periodically in both *Vital and Health Statistics* and *Monthly Vital Statistics Report*. Together these activities constitute the National Health Survey (NCHS, 1963). Series 1 of *Vital and Health Statistics* contains the general methodological and historical accounts of the whole endeavor. Detailed descriptions of all the surveys can be found in Appendix I of *Health United States 1992* (NCHS, 1993).

Considering some examples of morbidity data, in 1994 the incidence of acute conditions was 172 per 100 persons per year, down from 190 per 100 in 1993 (NCHS, 1995, p. 4). Most common were respiratory conditions (including the common cold and influenza) (80.5 per 100), injuries (24 per 100), infective and parasitic diseases (21 per 100), and digestive system conditions (6.6 per 100).

Persons sought medical attention for these conditions about two thirds of the time. Acute conditions were associated with about 693 days of restricted activity per 100 persons per year, leading to approximately 288 days in bed due to illness and 331 school-loss days per 100 persons 5–17 years of age and about 312 workloss days per 100 for persons 18 and over.

Roughly 15% of the population experienced limitation in all activity due to chronic conditions (NCHS, 1995, p. 6). The major chronic conditions causing limitations in activity in 1991 were (in descending order of frequency) sinusitis, arthritis, deformity or orthopedic impairment, hypertension, and hay fever or allergic rhinitis, heart disease, and chronic bronchitis (NCHS, 1995, p. 5).

The HDS reports on morbidity and mortality occurring in hospitals. This is an example of provider-perspective data. It affords a rather accurate illness profile of those patients in hospitals. It must be remembered, however, that the overwhelming majority of ill persons do not require hospitalization. Thus, the morbidity profile of the population as a whole does not match that seen in hospitals. The results of the HDS are published in *Vital and Health Statistics*, Series 13, and in *Advance Data* from *Vital and Health Statistics*, published on an irregular basis. Selected results are also published periodically in *Health United States*.

The HDS is carried out on a sampling basis in nonfederal, short-stay hospitals (hospitals with six or more beds and an average length of stay of 30 days or less). In 1995 over one quarter of the 30.7 million discharges that occurred from those hospitals was accounted for by just two diagnostic groups: diseases of the heart, 14.2%, and female delivery, 12.2% (NCHS, 1997, Table 89). The five most common specific diagnoses were heart disease; females with deliveries; malignant neoplasm (cancer); pneumonia, all forms; and injuries and poisoning.

The NAMCS (NCHS, 1974a, 1974b) was developed in the 1970s as a component of the National Health Survey. It is a continuing survey of private, office-based federal physicians practicing in the United States (*Advance Data*, 1997). The data are collected by using a stratified random sample of all office-based physicians (both allopathic and osteopathic) in the contiguous United States, excluding anesthesiologists, pathologists, radiologists, and physicians engaged primarily in teaching, research, and administration. In the early 1990s the data were being reported primarily by specialty.

In the NAMCS, morbidity data are collected from both patient and physician perspectives. For example, in 1995 the five leading patients' reasons for coming to a physician's office (other than for a checkup or follow-up visit) were cough, symptoms referable to the throat, earache or ear infection, back symptoms, and fever (*Advance Data*, 1997, Table 5). The five leading physician's diagnoses were acute upper respiratory infections, excluding pharyngitis; essential hypertension; otitis media and eustachian tube disorders (both ear problems); arthropathies (joint problems) and related disorders; rheumatism, excluding back (*Advance Data*, 1997, Table 10).

Health Status and Health-Related Behaviors

In 1979 the Office of the Assistant Secretary for Health (OASH) of the U.S. Department of Health and Human Services published the first national health status report, *Healthy People: The Surgeon General's Report on Health Promotion and Disease Prevention*. Subsequently, the Office of Disease Prevention and Health Promotion (ODPHP), part of OASH, published *Promoting Health and Preventing Disease: Objectives for the Nation* (ODPHP, 1980). Two hundred sixteen objectives were established for dealing with 15 major diseases and conditions that can be prevented by using existing knowledge and techniques. The 15 were grouped into three sets of five: conditions such as high blood pressure and sexually transmitted disease, for which preventive health services could be effective; such problems as toxic agent control and occupational safety and health, for which health protective services could be useful; and such conditions as cigarette smoking and sedentary lifestyle, to which health promotion programs could be applied.

Implementation plans were published by ODPHP in 1983, 1984 (*Prospects for a Healthier America*), and 1986 (*A Midcourse Review*). In 1990, the U.S. Public Health Service published the next comprehensive update for the program, *Healthy People 2000* (USPHS, 1991). This document provided the public health planning guide for the 1990s. In 1995, *Healthy People 2000: Midcourse Review* was published (USDHHS, 1995).

In support of this effort, in 1985 the NCHS carried out a Health Promotion/ Disease Prevention (HPDP) Survey as part of the ongoing HIS (NCHS, 1988). The HPDP Survey was repeated in 1990. Results are published in *Vital and Health Statistics*, Series 10; *Advance Data*; and *Morbidity and Mortality Weekly Report* (reporting data from the related Behavioral Risk Factor Surveillance System).

Key findings include the following (NCHS, 1997, Tables 64–73): as of 1994, 25.5% of persons 18 or older regularly smoked cigarettes; about 19% of persons between 20 and 74 years of age had an elevated serum cholesterol; about 23% of persons had hypertension; close to 35% of the population between 20 and 74 could be classified as overweight; and (as of 1990) of the 72% of men and 51% of women who drank alcohol, 13.6% of the men and 3.4% of the women could be classified as "heavier" drinkers. As of 1993 over one quarter of adults engaged in no leisuretime physical activity whatsoever, over 62% wore an automobile seatbelt regularly, about 78% of women 40 and over had had at least one mammogram, and close to 94% of women 18 and over had had at least one uterine cervix Pap smear (CDCP, Tables 1–7). Note that this "risk factor" approach to morbidity has much in common with the McGinnis-Foege approach to classification of causes of death.

By 1995 the Healthy People project had expanded its scope to set national health promotion and disease prevention objectives for dealing with 22 diseases, conditions, and health-related behaviors (and the means for tracking them) (USDHHS, 1995, Appendix A): physical activity and fitness, nutrition, tobacco use, substance abuse (alcohol and other drugs), family planning, mental health and mental disorders, violent and abusive behavior, unintentional injuries, occupational safety and health, environmental health, food and drug safety, oral health, maternal and infant health, heart disease and stroke, cancer, diabetes and chronic disabling conditions, HIV infection, sexually transmitted diseases, and immunization and infectious diseases. Objectives were also established for educational and community-based programs, clinical preventive services, and surveillance and data systems. For the 22 designated areas a total of 520 objectives and subobjectives were established.

Utilization of Health Care Services

We come now to the third health data perspective: how the population utilizes the health care delivery system (see also Part Two). We have pointed out that in quantifying the utilization of health services, the same series of events can be counted from either the patient's or the provider's perspective. The results of the two types of counts are not always the same. Thus, when discussing utilization, one has to be careful to distinguish between the two approaches.

It should be noted that reliable utilization data are regularly reported primarily for services provided by licensed MDs and DOs (doctors of osteopathic medicine) in licensed allopathic (MD-staffed) and osteopathic hospitals and by licensed dentists. In the United States there is an unknown amount of "alternative therapy" provided by such healing disciplines as chiropractic, naturopathy, homeopathy, acupuncture/acupressure therapy and its variants, and by "holistic health practitioners," among many others. Practitioners of these disciplines do not report utilization, they are not surveyed, and payment for much of their service is only sporadically reimbursed by insurance companies.

Although regular utilization statistics are not collected, a one-time sampling survey estimated that about a third of all adults use at least one alternative therapy, with an average annual visit rate of 19 (Eisenberg et al., 1993). This means that (for 1990 at least) there were more visits made to alternative therapists (425 million) than to primary care physicians (388 million).

Ambulatory Services

As we have noted, the HIS provides patient-perspective data for the utilization of ambulatory services (see also chapters 7, 9, and 10). According to the HIS, in 1994 there were about 6.1 physician contacts per person (NCHS, 1995, Table 71). Of these, about 56% took place in a physician's office, 13% in a hospital (primarily in the outpatient department, including the emergency department), 18% on the telephone, 3% in the home, and 12% in other locations. Females averaged 7.6 visits per year; males averaged 5.2. Whites averaged 6.3 visits; Blacks averaged 5.4. Persons in families with an income of $10,000 or less averaged 8.1 visits per year. Persons in the western geographic region averaged the most visits, 6.5. All of these numbers were up somewhat from 1991.

There are several sources of provider data on the utilization of ambulatory services. The most comprehensive one is the NAMCS (described briefly above), reported on most commonly in *Advance Data*. In addition to morbidity data, the NAMCS provides data on visits by age, race, sex, geographic region, metropolitan/nonmetropolitan living area, type of physician, and duration of visit. The other major source of provider-perspective ambulatory service utilization data is the annual publication *Hospital Statistics*, published each summer by the American Hospital Association (AHA). It reports hospital clinic and emergency department visits by such variables as number of beds, ownership, type, geographical region, and medical school affiliation.

Utilization of Hospital Inpatient Services

Turning to utilization of hospital inpatient services, from the patient perspective the HIS reported that in 1994 there were about 27.4 million discharges from short-stay hospitals, including about 3.3 million deliveries (down from 31.1 million discharges in 1991). These patients used about 164 million inpatient days of care with an average length of stay of 5.9 days (down from 199 million days in 1991) (NCHS, 1995, Table 77). Other classes of data provided by the HIS are utilization according to various hospital characteristics, morbidity (discussed previously), and an analysis of surgery.

The NCHS also furnishes provider-perspective hospital utilization data through the HDS. The NCHS points out that, because of "differences in collection procedures, population sampled, and definitions," the results from the HIS and the HDS are not entirely consistent (NCHS, 1979b, p. 1 and footnotes; NCHS, 1997, Tables 85 and 86). For example, for 1994 the HIS reported significantly fewer discharges from short-stay hospitals than did the HDS: 87.5 per thousand population for the former, compared with 104.7 per thousand for the latter (NCHS, 1997, Tables 85 and 86).

Hospital utilization data also are published in the AHA's *Hospital Statistics*. For AHA-registered hospitals, it presents much data on bed size, admissions, occupancy rate, average daily census, and fiscal parameters, according to hospital type, size, ownership, geographical location, and the like (see also chapter 6,

"Hospitals"). Certain provider-perspective hospital utilization data also appear in *Health: U.S.*

Conclusions

In the United States much data concerning the population, its health, and how it uses the health care delivery system are collected and published. As noted previously, in the case of hospital utilization not all of these data are consistent, which may result in part from a lack of coordination of data-collection efforts. Furthermore, there is the obvious gap between the provider perspective and the patient perspective on the counts of events. One initiative of the proposed Clinton health plan of 1993 was to significantly improve health and health services data collection and analysis.

There have been criticisms of the federal statistical collection, reporting, and analysis system over a period of many years. A 1979 study by the Office of Technology Assessment (1979) found "federal data collection activities . . . to be overlapping, fragmented, and often duplicative" (p. iii).[4] In brief, the report recommended that a "strengthened coordinating and planning unit within [HHS]" be established that "would embody three basic characteristics: sufficient authority to impose decisions on agencies; the necessary statistical and analytical capabilities to conduct activities requiring technical expertise and judgement; and adequate resources to build a viable core effort" (p. 55). Apparently, this recommendation has yet to be followed.

Among the many policy issues concerning and involving data collection and use that are in need of a good deal of further examination are the utility and application of clinical trials evaluating what health professionals do; health services malpractice and malpractice litigation; technological and ethical matters arising from the use of electronic data collection and analysis; the relationship between data collected and data actually used; the decision-making process governing what is counted and what data are disseminated; cost/benefit analysis of health sciences interventions; government data-collection requirements and utilization; the impact of the Internet on health data requirements and availability; the costs of data collection, analysis, and application; what to do when we have too much or too little data; and what is changing and will change about health care data collection, publication, and analysis.

There are still many gaps in our knowledge of data collection, analysis, and use. Some would have been filled if the provisions of the National Health

---

[4]This report will still be valuable to students of the federal data system and its users. It not only described data collection activities and the way they were organized and supervised but also presented and analyzed all of the statutory authorities existing at the time that establish those activities (they happen to be almost all of those still in use.)

Resources Planning and Development Act (P.L. 93-641, Sec. 1513, b, 1, passed late in the Carter administration) relating to data had been carried out. They were not. These requirements called for the mandatory national collection of data on (1) population health status, (2) health care delivery system utilization, (3) effects of the health care delivery system on health, (4) health care delivery resources, and (5) environmental and occupational exposure factors relating to health. It may well be that these data reforms will be instituted as part of any national health care reform measure.

Regardless of the problems with the system, however, we do know a great deal about health, disease, and illness in the United States and about the functioning of the U.S. health care delivery system. Further, given whatever problems there may or may not be with the available health and health care data, we must remember, above all, that data mean little unless they are put to proper use.

Mini-Case: Data and Health Services Competitiveness

You are a health planning specialist attached to the Office of the Director of the Health Care Financing Administration of the federal department of Health and Human Services. You have been temporarily detailed to the Anti-Trust Division (ATD) of the Department of Justice. The ATD is reviewing a merger proposal by two major suburban hospitals located just outside the second-largest city in the country.

Under the law, ATD is charged with, among other things, examining the "threat to competitiveness" posed by mergers of large, presently competitive organizations providing essentially the same set of services in the same market. Traditionally, ATD has looked primarily at only financial data (prices, costs, revenues, profit/ loss statements) in cases of this kind. However, there is a brand-new director of ATD. She has determined that, as part of the review process for proposed hospital mergers, the review team is also to consider the profiles of the services the hospitals provide to those they serve.

The director has asked you to prepare a "quick and dirty" list of the data the hospitals will be asked to provide to develop their respective "profiles of service." When you ask the director what is meant by the term "profile of service," her reply indicates that she has not given much thought to this question. Thus, at this time your task is twofold. First, you must define precisely what the term should mean. Second, you will have to list the data categories and types that you will need to create the profiles, explaining why each is essential to the task at hand. The director has asked you to have your report on her desk in 1 week.

Discussion Questions

1. What are the uses of health data?
2. What are the uses of health services data?

3. How should data be used in the health and health services planning process?
4. How do health and health services data relate to each other?
5. What are the similarities and differences between disease-specific and risk-factor-specific health and illness data?
6. What are the uses of data for health program planning?
7. How should data collection, analysis, and utilization in the United States be reformed?

References

Advance Data, "1991 Summary: National Hospital Discharge Survey," no. 227, March 3, 1993a.

Advance Data, "Office Visits to General Surgeons 1989–90, National Ambulatory Medical Care Survey," no. 228, March 2, 1993b.

Advance Data, "National Ambulatory Medical Care Survey: 1995 Summary," no. 286, May 8, 1997.

Bayer, R., "AIDS: The Politics of Prevention and Neglect," *Health Affairs,* Spring 1991, p. 87.

Centers for Disease Control and Prevention, *CDC Surveillance Summaries,* Dec. 27, 1996, *MMWR* 1996, *45*(SS-6).

Dickens, B. M., "Legal Rights and Duties in the AIDS Epidemic." *Science, 239,* 580, 1988.

Eisenberg, D. M., Kessler, R. C., Foster, C., Norlock, F. F., Calkins, D. R., & DelBanco, T. L., "Unconventional Medicine in the United States," *New England Journal of Medicine, 328,* 246–52, 1993.

Grove, R. D., & Hetzel, A. M., *Vital Statistics Rates for the United States: 1940–1960.* Washington, DC: NCHS, 1968.

Karon, J. M., Rosenberg, P. S., & McQuillan, G., "Prevalence of HIV Infection in the United States, 1984 to 1992," *Journal of the American Medical Association, 276,* 126, 1996.

Kessner, D. M., Singer, J., Kalk, C. E., & Schlesinger, E. R., *Infant Death: An Analysis by Maternal Risk and Health Care.* Washington, DC: Institute of Medicine, National Academy of Sciences, 1973.

McGinniss, J. M., & Foege, W. H., "Actual Causes of Death in the United States," *Journal of the American Medical Association, 270,* 2207–2212, 1993.

Monthly Vital Statistics Report, "Advance Report of Final Natality Statistics, 1994," *44*(11; Suppl.), June 24, 1996.

Monthly Vital Statistics Report, "Births and Deaths: United States, 1996," *46*(1; Suppl. 2), September 11, 1997.

Morris, J. N., *Uses of Epidemiology.* Baltimore: Williams and Wilkins, 1964.

National Center for Health Statistics, "Origin, Program and Operation of the U.S. National Health Survey," *Vital and Health Statistics,* ser. 1, no. 1, August 1963.

National Center for Health Statistics, "National Ambulatory Medical Care Survey: Background and Methodology: United States, 1967–1972," *Vital and Health Statistics,* ser. 2, no. 61, 1974a.

National Center for Health Statistics, "The National Ambulatory Medical Care Survey: Symptom Classification," *Vital and Health Statistics*, ser. 2, no. 63, 1974b.

National Center for Health Statistics, *International Classification of Diseases, Ninth Revision, Adapted for Use in The United States.* Hyattsville, MD: USGPO, 1979a.

National Center for Health Statistics, *Health Resources Statistics: Health Manpower and Health Facilities, 1976–77,* (DHEW Pub. No. [PHS] 79-1509). Hyattsville, MD: USGPO, 1979b.

National Center for Health Statistics, "Health Promotion and Disease Prevention, U.S., 1985," *Vital and Health Statistics*, ser. 10, no. 163, 1988.

National Center for Health Statistics, "Infant Mortality Rates: Socioeconomic Factors," *Vital and Health Statistics*, ser. 22, no. 14, 1992.

National Center for Health Statistics, *Health United States 1992 and Healthy People 2000 Review* (DHHS Pub. No. [PHS] 93-1232). Hyattsville, MD: U.S. Public Health Service, 1993.

National Center for Health Statistics, "Current Estimates from the National Health Survey, 1994," *Vital and Health Statistics*, ser. 10, no. 193, 1995.

National Center for Health Statistics, *Health United States 1996–97 and Injury Chartbook* (DHHS Pub. No. [PHS] 97-1232). Hyattsville, MD: Centers for Disease Control and Prevention, 1997.

Office of the Assistant Secretary for Health, *Healthy People: The Surgeon General's Report on Health Promotion and Disease Prevention* (DHEW Pub. No. [PHS] 70-55071). Washington, DC: USGPO, 1979.

Office of Disease Prevention and Health Promotion, *Promoting Health/Preventing Disease: Objectives for the Nation.* Washington, DC: USGPO, 1980.

Office of Disease Prevention and Health Promotion, "Public Health Service Implementation Plans for Attaining the Objectives for the Nation," *Public Health Reports*, Sept.–Oct. 1983 (Suppl.).

Office of Disease Prevention and Health Promotion, *Prospects for a Healthier America.* Washington, DC: USGPO, 1984.

Office of Disease Prevention and Health Promotion, *The 1990 Health Objectives for the Nation.* Washington, DC: USGPO, 1986.

Office of Health Services Opportunity, *Health Status of Minorities and Low Income Groups* (DHEW Pub. No. HRA 79-627). Washington, DC: USGPO, 1979.

Office of Technology Assessment, *Selected Topics in Federal Health Statistics.* Washington, DC: USGPO, 1979.

President's Commission for the Study of Ethical Problems in Medicine and Biomedical and Behavioral Research, *Defining Death.* Washington, DC: USGPO, 1981.

Rosen, G., *A History of Public Health.* New York: MD Publication, 1958.

Siegel, P. Z., Frazier, E. L., Mariolis, P., Brachbill, R. M., & Smith, C., "Behavioral Risk Factor Surveillance, 1991: Monitoring Progress Toward the Nation's Year 2000 Health Objectives," *Morbidity and Mortality Weekly Report, 42*(SS-4) August 27, 1993.

U.S. Bureau of the Census, *Statistical Abstract of the United States: 1996* (116th ed.). Washington, DC: USGPO, 1996.

U.S. Department of Health and Human Services, *Healthy People 2000: Midcourse Review and 1995 Revisions.* Washington, DC: USGPO, 1995.

United States Public Health Service, *Healthy People 2000: National Health Promotion and Disease Prevention Objectives* (DHHS Pub. No. (PHS) 91-50213). Washington, DC: USGPO, 1991.

Walters, L., "Ethical Issues in the Prevention and Treatment of HIV Infection and AIDS," *Science, 239*, 537, 1988.

Wikler, D., & Weisbard, A. J., "Appropriate Confusion Over 'Brain Death,' " *Journal of the American Medical Association, 261*, 2246, 1989.

Williams, D. R., & Collins, C., "U.S. Socioeconomic and Racial Differences in Health: Patterns and Explanations," in P. Brown (ed.), *Perspectives in Medical Sociology* (2nd ed., chap. 1). Prospect Heights, IL: Waveland Press, 1996.

3

Financing for Health Care

Kenneth E. Thorpe and James R. Knickman

Learning Objectives

1. To understand the dollar magnitude of health care spending in the United States over time, both in the aggregate and how it is spent.
2. To develop an understanding of what services these dollars purchase and where the dollars come from to purchase them.
3. To develop an understanding of the types of health care spending financed by the public and private sectors.
4. To develop an understanding of the extent to which health care spending is rising and the factors that contribute to such growth.

Topical Outline

What the money buys
Where the money comes from
  Public outlays
    Medicare
    Medicaid
    Other public expenditures
  Private health care expenditures
    Structure of the private insurance industry
    Blue Cross and Blue Shield
    Commercial insurance
    HMOs
    PPOs
    Extent of private health insurance coverage in the United States
How the money is paid out
  Paying physicians

Key Words: Prospective payment, capitation, managed care, uninsured, sources and uses of funds.

A key factor that shapes the delivery of health care in the United States is the evolving system for financing services. The types of services delivered and the organizational approaches to delivering services are heavily influenced by how health care is paid for and the aggregate resources available for health care.

The financing system that has evolved over the past 30 years in the United States involves a complex blend of public and private responsibilities. This system varies substantially from the largely public financing systems that exist in many European countries. An understanding of how health care is paid for is useful for developing an understanding of the general organization of health care in America.

Payment approaches for health care have been undergoing tremendous changes since the early 1980s. These changes have escalated during the 1990s. The basic approach for reimbursing hospital care has been completely restructured by many payers for care, and payment approaches for physicians and long-term care providers also are being restructured. As emphasized here, financing approaches vary from provider to provider and from payer to payer, and financing approaches will continue to evolve over time. Thus, this chapter attempts to explain not only the current structure of financing approaches but also the principles behind the financing system.

In explaining how the American health care financing system operates, this chapter focuses on

- What health care resources buy.
- Where resources come from.
- How health care providers are paid.
- Why health care expenditures have been increasing.

As displayed in Table 3.1, $988 billion, or 13.6% of the gross domestic product (GDP), was spent for health purposes in 1995. These expenditures represent

TABLE 3.1 Aggregate and Per Capita National Health Expenditures, by Source of Funds and Percentage of Gross National Product, Selected Calendar Years, 1929–1995

Calendar year	Total GNP[a]	Total health expenditures			Private health expenditures			Public health expenditures		
		Amount[a]	Per capita	Percentage of GNP	Amount[a]	Per capita	Percentage of total	Amount[a]	Per capita	Percentage of GNP
1929	$103.3	$3.6	$29	3.5	$3.2	$25	86.4	$0.5	$4	13.6
1935	72.2	2.9	23	4.0	2.4	18	80.8	0.6	4	19.2
1940	99.7	4.0	30	4.0	3.2	24	79.7	0.8	6	20.3
1960	503.7	26.9	146	5.3	20.3	110	75.3	6.6	36	24.7
1970	982.4	74.7	359	7.6	47.5	228	63.5	27.3	131	36.5
1980	2,631.7	248.0	1,049	9.4	142.2	601	57.3	105.8	448	42.7
1990	5,542.9	675.0	2,601	12.2	390.0	1,502	57.8	285.1	1,098	42.2
1991	5,917	761.7	2,901	12.9	441.4	1681	58	320.3	1,220	42.0
1992	6,244[b]	834.2	3,145	13.4[c]	478.8	1,805	57.4	355.4	1,340	42.6
1993	6,553[b]	892.1	3,330	13.6[c]	505.5	1,887	56.7	386.5	1,443	43.3
1995	7,254[b]	988.5	3,621	13.6[c]	532.1	1,949	53.8	456.4	1,673	46.2

[a]In billions of dollars.
[b]Gross Domestic Product.
[c]Percentage of Gross Domestic Product.

Sources: Adapted from Katherine Lewit et al., "National Health Expenditures, 1995," *Health Care Financing Review*, 18, Fall 1996; R. M. Gibson et al., "National Health Expenditures, 1983," *Health Care Financing Review*, 6, Winter 1984; R. M. Gibson, "National Health Expenditures, 1978," *Health Care Financing Review*, 1, Fall 1992 (pp. 14 and 19).

$3,621 per year for each person. Thus, the health care sector represents a major element of the American economy. As a component of the economy, health care has been growing at a fast rate over the past 30 years, though growth has slowed substantially during the past couple of years. As a point of comparison, health expenditures totaled only $43 billion in 1965, or 5.8% of the GDP. From 1965 onward, outlays for health rose, on the average, 11.7% each year. Although the rate of increase in costs between 1990 and 1991 was 11.4%, which was much lower than the peak inflation rate of 15.3%, growth in health care expenditures continues to exceed by a wide margin the overall inflation rates prevalent in the American economy. Since 1991, however, health care expenditures have risen 6.7% per year—still above inflation but lower than measured in previous years. An important element of the study of health care finance, therefore, is an analysis to understand the dynamics of spending in the United States and to understand what is being achieved by the ever-increasing health care expenditure levels.

What the Money Buys

National health care expenditures, as measured by the federal Health Care Financing Administration (HCFA), are grouped into two categories: (1) research and medical facilities construction and (2) payments for health services and supplies (see Table 3.2). Personal health care expenses constitute the bulk of the latter—$879 billion in 1995. Five types of personal health care expenditures account for over 75% of the 1995 total: 35.4% went to hospitals, 20.4% to physicians, 7.9% for nursing home care, 8.4% for drugs and drug sundries, and 4.6% for dentists' services. The other categories of expenditures are "other professional services," such as podiatry and private speech therapy, 5.3%; "other health services," 2.5%; administrative expenses, 5.4%; government public health activities, 3.2%; and construction, 3.1%. The costs of medical education are not included in these HCFA figures except insofar as they are inseparable from hospital expenditures and biomedical research.

Where the Money Comes from

Ultimately, the people pay all health care costs. Thus, when we say health care monies come from different sources, we really mean that dollars take different routes on their way from consumers to providers: through government, private insurance companies, and independent plans, in addition to out-of-pocket payments. In 1995 close to 21% of personal health care expenditures were directly out-of-pocket ($182.6 billion). At the same time, the government share was nearly 45% (about $392.1 billion), with the federal government bearing nearly three

TABLE 3.2   Aggregate and Per Capita Amount and Percentage Distribution of National Health Expenditures, Selected Calendar Years 1960–1995

Type of expenditure	Aggregate amount ($Billions)			
	1960	1980	1990	1995
Total	27.1	250.1	697.5	988.5
Health services and supplies	25.4	238.9	672.9	957.8
Personal health care	23.9	219.4	614.7	878.8
Hospital care	9.3	102.4	256.4	350.1
Physicians' services	5.3	41.9	146.3	201.6
Dentists' services	2.0	14.4	31.6	45.8
Other professional services	0.6	8.7	34.7	52.6
Home health care	0.0	1.3	13.1	28.6
Drugs and drug sundries	4.2	21.6	59.9	83.4
Eyeglasses and appliances	0.8	4.6	10.5	13.8
Nursing home care	1.0	20.0	50.9	77.9
Other health services	0.7	4.6	11.2	25.0
Expenses for repayment and administration	1.2	12.2	38.6	47.7
Government public health activities	0.4	7.2	19.6	31.4
Research and medical facilities construction	1.7	11.3	24.5	30.7
Research	0.7	5.4	12.2	16.6
Construction	1.0	5.8	12.3	14.0

Type of expenditure	Per capita amount ($)			
	1960	1980	1990	1995
Total	142.56	1063.80	2,683	3,621
Health services and supplies	133.61	1016.16	2,589	3,508
Personal health care	125.72	933.22	2,364	3,219
Hospital care	48.92	435.56	986	1,282
Physicians' services	27.88	178.22	563	738
Dentists' services	10.52	61.25	122	168
Other professional services	3.16	37.01	133	193
Home health care	0.0	5.53	50	105
Drugs and drug sundries	22.09	91.88	230	306

Source: Health Care Financing Administration, Office of the Actuary, Data from the Office of National Health Statistics.

fourths of that. Finally, almost 32% was paid through insurance companies ($302.7 billion) (Levit et al., 1996).

Public Outlays

The 45% of personal health care expenditures transferred by the public sector in 1995 ($392.1 billion) compares with 40% in 1980, 22% in 1965, 22% in 1950, and 9% in 1929. The increase, especially since 1965, is largely a result of greater federal expenditures. Proportionately, state and local government outlays have remained rather constant over time, in the 10% to 13% range. The significant rise in federal spending is accounted for by the Medicare and Medicaid programs, Title XVIII and XIX, respectively, of the Social Security Act.

Medicare. Medicare was inaugurated on July 1, 1966. It provides a range of medical care benefits for persons aged 65 and over who are covered by the Social Security system. The 1972 amendments to the Social Security Act extended benefits to persons aged 65 and older who do not meet the criteria for the regular Social Security program but who are willing to pay a premium for coverage. In July 1973 benefits were further extended to the disabled and their dependents and those suffering from chronic kidney disease (Russell et al., 1974).

Part A of the program, financed by payroll taxes collected under the Social Security system, provides coverage for care rendered in a hospital, an extended-care facility, or the patient's home. Part B, a voluntary supplemental program that pays certain costs of physicians' services and other medical expenses, is supported in part by general tax revenues and in part by contributions paid by the elderly (Somers & Somers, 1961). Neither Part A nor Part B of Medicare, however, offers comprehensive coverage. Built into the program are deductibles (set amounts the patient must pay for each type of service before Medicare begins to pay) and coinsurance (a percentage of charges paid by the patient). Limitations on the amount of coverage exist as well. Hospital benefits cease after 90 days if the patient has exhausted his or her lifetime reserve pool of 60 additional days; extended-care facility benefits end after 100 days. Unlike most private insurance, the Medicare program does not include an annual limitation on out-of-pocket spending. As a result, the Medicare program pays a relatively small share of total spending on behalf of senior citizens. The high out-of-pocket spending facing Medicare beneficiaries has created a large demand for supplemental insurance coverage.

In 1988, Congress passed a bill to substantially expand Medicare coverage. This legislation, the Medicare Catastrophic Coverage Act of 1988, set limits on the maximum out-of-pocket costs that beneficiaries were responsible for in the case of hospital care, physician services, and pharmaceuticals.

The Medicare catastrophic program, however, was greeted unenthusiastically by many elderly. In the fall of 1989, under heavy pressure from the elderly, Congress repealed the Catastrophic Coverage Act. The program's unpopularity was caused by its financing approach, which passed along the costs of the program to the elderly in the form of new premiums and income-related surcharges to the elderly's federal income tax. The elderly particularly objected to the added income tax, in part because many of the wealthy elderly who were required to pay the maximum tax already had arranged for similar supplementary insurance coverage through private insurance companies.

Quality and cost of care delivered by public programs have been long-standing issues. Medicare amendments passed in 1972 established professional standards review organizations (PSROs) to monitor the quality and quantity of institutional services delivered to Medicare and Medicaid recipients. The 1982 Tax Equity and Fiscal Responsibility Act (TEFRA), discussed below, replaced the PSROs with a "utilization and quality control peer review organization" (PRO). Subsequent legislation (P.L. 98-21) required that hospitals covered under Medicare's new case payment system contract with a PRO by 1984. The new PROs differ substantially from the old PSROs: PROs are to be statewide organizations unless exceptional circumstances pertain; they may be for-profit as well as nonprofit operations; they require participation of only a small segment of area physicians; and they operate under contract with the Health Care Financing Administration, with performance judged against preestablished and quantifiable contract objectives.

As with quality and cost reviews, recent changes in Medicare provisions have radically changed the way Medicare pays for hospital care. The TEFRA legislation of 1982 was designed to provide incentives for cost containment. Most important, TEFRA established a case-based reimbursement system (DRGs, or diagnosis related groups) while also placing limits on the rates of increase in hospital revenues. TEFRA was followed in 1983 by Title VI of P.L. 98-21, which established a prospective payment system. Discussion of the principles of these 1983 amendments is provided later in this chapter.

In the Omnibus Budget Reconciliation Act of 1989 (OBRA 1989), Medicare changed the way physicians are paid. Previously, Medicare payment rates for a service were based on the amounts physicians charged. The new payment system is a national fee schedule that assigns relative values to services based on the time, skill, and intensity it takes to provide them. The relative values are then adjusted for geographic variations of payment. This system went into effect on January 1, 1992.

OBRA 1989 also limited the amount that physicians are allowed to charge patients above the amount that Medicare pays and implemented a system intended to help Congress limit growth in Medicare expenditures for physician payments. Further discussion of these changes is provided later in this chapter.

The Balanced Budget Act of 1997 included several key changes in the Medicare program. The act increased substantially the variety of health plans that may receive Medicare payments and enrollees. Medicare beneficiaries can now choose among several types of managed care. In addition, the act added several new services to the Medicare benefit package, including preventive screening for prostate cancer, mammography, and colorectal screening, among other preventive benefits. As part of Congress's larger effort to balance the budget by the year 2002, the act produced $116 billion in Medicare savings between federal fiscal years 1998 and 2002.

Medicaid. Unlike Medicare, Medicaid is a program run jointly by federal and state governments; the name is more or less a blanket label for 50 different state programs designed specifically to serve the poor. Beginning in January 1967, Medicaid provided federal funds to states on a cost-sharing basis (according to each state's per capita income) so that welfare recipients could be guaranteed medical services. Payment in full was to be afforded to the aged poor, the blind, the disabled, and families with dependent children if one parent was absent, unemployed, or unable to work. Four types of care were required to be covered: (1) inpatient and outpatient hospital care, (2) other laboratory and x-ray services, (3) physician services, and (4) nursing facility care for persons over age 21. Legislation enacted in subsequent years added coverage of home health services for those entitled to nursing facility services and early and periodic screening, as well as diagnostic and treatment services for persons under age 21.

The 1972 Social Security Act amendments added family planning to the list of "musts." States must also now cover the services of rural health clinics, community and migrant health centers, health centers for the homeless, and similar qualified centers, as well as nurse-midwives and nurse practitioners. Currently, the law specifies another 31 optional services that states may elect to cover, including prescription drugs, intermediate care facilities for the mentally retarded, optometrists' services, dental services, and eyeglasses. States may place certain limits on the extent to which services are covered. For example, they may limit the number of covered prescriptions or hospital days.

Eligibility for Medicaid is determined by the states within federal guidelines. By and large, Medicaid is available only to very low income persons. The program also has categorical restrictions; that is, only families with children, pregnant women, and those who are aged, blind, or disabled can qualify.

With few exceptions, recipients of cash assistance are automatically eligible for Medicaid. In addition, most states extend Medicaid to some "medically needy" groups that meet the nonfinancial criteria for Medicaid eligibility but exceed the income requirements. Individuals with great medical expenses may "spend down" to the medically needy standard. Aged or disabled persons receiving long-term care in institutions or in alternative community-based programs can, in some states, spend down to Medicaid eligibility and, in others, receive Medicaid if their income is below a federally specified level.

Historically, because of the linkage between Medicaid and welfare eligibility, state variation in eligibility criteria for cash assistance resulted in variable Medicaid coverage across states. However, legislation enacted since the mid-1980s has decoupled Medicaid eligibility to numerous groups—chiefly low-income pregnant women and children—producing greater uniformity in Medicaid eligibility.

Due to the expansions, state Medicaid programs must now cover all pregnant women and children up to age 6 with family income below 133% of the poverty level; children below 100% of poverty who are aged 12 or younger (all poor children under age 19 will be covered by 2002); for a transition period, poor families who lose cash assistance because of earnings from work; for a 12-month period, two-parent families in which the principal earner is unemployed; and disabled persons who lose eligibility for cash assistance due to earnings from work.

Medicaid also pays the Medicare premiums, deductibles, and coinsurance for certain low-income Medicare beneficiaries. Finally, states have the option to cover a variety of other groups. It should be noted that, even with the expansions, Medicaid covers only 40% of the poor.

Because of the gaps in insurance coverage for the poor and near poor that are not taken care of by the Medicaid programs, much recent debate and analysis has focused an how to pay for services to individuals not covered by Medicare, private insurance, or Medicaid. As of 1993, at least 25 states have established bad-debt and charity-care pools to pay for hospital services and, in some cases, physician services for individuals who have no source of payment for their medical care. These programs have developed, in part, to spread the burden of the costs of care to indigents across the hospital system. The pools are generally funded through some form of tax or surcharge on hospital revenues from third parties (Lewin & Lewin, 1988; Thorpe & Phelps, 1992).

Other Public Expenditures. In 1995 Medicare and Medicaid accounted for 80.8% of public outlays for personal health care services. The next-largest expenditure category, state and local government outlays, accounted for 10% of the $392.1 billion spent on public programs (Levit et al., 1996).

There are four remaining significant personal health care categories for which government monies are spent: (1) federal outlays for hospital and medical services for veterans ($15.6 billion in 1995, 1.8% of public personal health care expenditures); (2) provision of care by the Department of Defense for the armed forces and military dependents (in 1995, $13.5 billion; 1.5%); (3) worker's compensation medical benefits ($19.8 billion; 2.3%); and (4) other federal, state, and local outlays for personal health care ($10.6 billion, 1.2%), including support for maternal and child health programs, vocational rehabilitation, Public Health Service and other federal hospitals, the Indian Health Service, temporary disability insurance, and the Alcohol, Drug Abuse, and Mental Health Administration. In contrast, all government public health activities are recorded as costing only $31.4 billion in 1995. It must be noted, however, that federal prevention and control operations are included in this figure, excluded are funds expended by other than health departments at the state and local levels for air and water pollution control, sanitation, and sewage treatment (Letsch, Levit, & Waldo, 1988). The relatively low level of government funding for public health activities deserves special attention in view of the growing recognition of the relationship between the environment and health and the importance of preventive care and health promotion.

Worker's compensation is an insurance system operated by the states, each with its own law and program, that provides covered workers with some protection against the costs of medical care and loss of income resulting from work-related injury and, in some cases, sickness (Congressional Research Service, 1976; Price, 1979a, 1979b; U.S. National Commission on State Workmen's Compensation Laws, 1973). The first worker's compensation law was enacted in New York in 1910; by 1948 all states had enacted such laws. The theory underlying worker's compensation is that all accidents, irrespective of fault, must be regarded as risks of industry and that the employer and employee shall share the burden of loss.

Private Health Care Expenditures

The bulk of private health care expenditures comes from two sources: individuals receiving treatment and private insurers making payments on the behalf of patients. In 1995 private expenditures totaled $459.3 billion, 52.3 % of all personal health care expenditures. In 1965, prior to the advent of Medicare and Medicaid, private expenditures accounted for 76.9% of all personal health care expenditures; in 1935, 82.4%; in 1929, 88.4% (Gibson, 1979). This recent decline in the private share of total expenditures is due to the sharp drop in out-of-pocket payments associated with increased federal spending as well as the slower growth in private health insurance payments. In 1965, 53% of personal health care expenditures was paid directly by the patient; in 1995, it was 21%. Yet because of inflation and other factors, the per capita dollar amount paid directly in 1995 was over eight times what it was in 1970 (Levit et al., 1995).

Private insurers have paid between 20% and 32% of personal health care costs since 1965. Their share was $45.3 billion in 1978, 27% of the total; in 1995, it was $276.8 billion, or 31.5% of the total.

Before considering private health insurance in any depth, the manner in which the term *insurance* is used in the health care industry should be clarified. Insurance originally meant and still usually refers to the contribution by individuals to a fund for the purpose of providing protection against financial losses following relatively unlikely but damaging events. Thus, there is insurance against fire, theft, and death at an early age. All of those events occur within a group of people at a predictable rate but are rare occurrences for any one individual in the group.

When medical insurance began, it was in this tradition. From 1847, when the first commercial insurance plan designed to defray the costs of medical care was organized, to the 1930s, health insurance consisted essentially of cash payments by commercial carriers to offset income losses resulting from disability attributable to accidents. Sickness benefits (cash payments during sickness) began as an extra, a "frill," on accident insurance policies. As with accident insurance, emphasis was on the replacement of income lost, in this instance as a result of contracting certain specified and catastrophic communicable diseases, such as typhoid, scarlet fever, and smallpox (Health Insurance Institute, 1975). With the organization of Blue Cross and Blue Shield, a new policy developed: reimbursing health care costs in general.

Health care utilization is not a rare occurrence. On average, each person in the United States visits a physician five times a year. One of every six Americans is admitted to a hospital at least once a year. Other than coverage for catastrophic illness, a fairly rare event, health insurance has become a mechanism for offsetting expected rather than unexpected costs. The experience of the many is pooled in an effort to reduce outlays for any one individual to a manageable prepayment size. Perhaps the term *assurance* more appropriately describes the health care payment system that has evolved. In Britain, assurance is used to denote coverage for contingencies that must eventually happen (e.g., life assurance), whereas insurance is reserved for coverage of those contingencies, like fire and theft, that may never occur.

Structure of the Private Insurance Industry. The organization of private insurance in the United States is undergoing dramatic changes. The most notable change, described below, is the growth in managed care and the rapid consolidation of health plans. Before 1980 virtually all private insurance was provided by either the national system of Blue Cross and Blue Shield plans or by commercial insurance companies, which offered health care insurance as one of many types of insurance products available to employers. These insurance companies charged employers or individuals annual premiums and generally paid health care providers on what is termed a fee-for-service basis. A set amount, often prescribed by the insurance plan or negotiated between the insurer and the provider, was paid by the insurance company to a provider each time a beneficiary used a covered service.

Starting in the early 1980s, however, a range of new insurance approaches and a range of new relationships between insurers and providers have emerged. Health maintenance organizations (HMOs), which deliver services on a capitated basis rather than a fee-for-service basis, have been expanding rapidly. Between 1990 and 1995, the number of Americans enrolled in HMOs increased by 27 million persons, to 63.3 million (Interstudy, 1997). Preferred provider organizations (PPOs), which either limit beneficiaries to a set list of physicians and other providers or provide economic incentives to use physicians who have offered discounts to the insurer, are also expanding rapidly; they accounted for 25% of all private insurance in 1992 (see Table 3.3). Point of service plans, which generally require members to go to providers within their networks for certain services but which give them the option to go to nonnetwork providers for other services, generally at a much higher cost, accounted for 16%.

The most dramatic change in the private insurance market during the 1990s has been the dramatic growth in managed care. As of 1996, nearly 75% of all workers were enrolled in some form of managed care. This represents a dramatic change: only 55% of workers were enrolled in managed care plans just 2 years earlier.

A second major change in the structure of the insurance industry is the growth of self-insured or self-funded health plans. Self-insurance refers to the assumption of claim risk by an employer, union, or other group, whereas self-funding refers to the payment of insurance claims from an established bank or trust account (Arnett & Trapnell, 1984). Self-insurance offers potential advantages to employers: they are exempt from most premium taxes and are able to retain interest on reserves (Arnett & Trapnell, 1984). Moreover, they have generally been exempt from state laws mandating minimum benefits under the Employee Retirement

TABLE 3.3 Enrollment in Managed and Unmanaged Group Health Plans, 1996

Plan type	Percentage of enrollment
Conventional FFS	26
HMO	33
PPO	25
POS	16

Source: KPMG Peat Marwick, *Health Benefits*, 1996, Table 9.

Income Security Act of 1974 (ERISA); however, a U.S. Supreme Court decision ruled that a Massachusetts mandated-benefit law is not preempted by ERISA because it applies to insurance contracts purchased for plans subject to ERISA. Such decisions could provide the states additional leverage to pursue health care reform that includes the uninsured and those with traditional insurance as well as the self-insured plans.

The growth in self-insurance has been significant. In 1996, 66% of firms with 200 or more workers were at least partially self-insured for their employees' health care costs, up from 46% in 1986 (Gabel, Ginsburg, & Hunt, 1997). One common operational mode of self-insured plans is the administrative services only (ASO) plan. Under an ASO plan, the insurance carrier handles the claims and benefits paperwork for the self-insured group. Insurance claims are normally paid from an employer bank account.

The prevalence of self-insurance differs by plan type. In 1995, 63% of FFS enrollees, 60% of PPO enrollees, and 53% of POS enrollees were in self-insured plans. In contrast, only 85% of HMO enrollees were in plans underwritten by an insurer (Jensen, Morrisey, Gaffney, & Liston, 1997).

Blue Cross and Blue Shield. The establishment of payment mechanisms to defray the costs of illness can be traced to the Great Depression. Previously hospitals had sought to assure reimbursement for their services through public education campaigns directed at encouraging their users, middle-income Americans, to put money aside for unpredictable medical expenses (Law, 1974). When hard times proved the inadequacy of the savings approach, attention turned to the development of a stable income mechanism. A model was at hand in the independent prepayment plan pioneered in 1929 at Baylor University Hospital in Texas to assure certain area schoolteachers of some hospital coverage. Under the plan, 1,250 teachers prepaid 50 cents a month to provide themselves with up to 21 days of semiprivate hospitalization annually.

In the early 1930s nonprofit prepayment programs offering care at a number of hospitals were organized in several cities. The American Hospital Association (AHA) vigorously supported the growth and development of these plans, soon to be named Blue Cross, and the special insurance legislation that was required for their establishment in each state (Law, 1974). The AHA set standards for plans and then offered its seal of approval to plans meeting the standards. A provider-insurer partnership was firmly established; indeed, not until 1972 did national Blue Cross formally separate from the AHA.

Whereas Blue Cross developed as a hospital insurance system, Blue Shield developed independently, beginning in 1939 as an insurer for physician services. These two insurers tend to be financially and organizationally distinct, but they have many similarities and most often work together to provide hospital and physician coverage. Blue Cross and Blue Shield both are organized for the most part under special state enabling acts. In most states a department or commissioner of insurance supervises the "Blues," issuing or approving their certificates of incorporation, reviewing their annual income and expenditure reports, and monitoring the rates subscribers pay into the program and the rates the programs pay to the providers (Law, 1974).

In line with their nonprofit status, both programs, at least initially, were committed to "community rating." Under such a policy a set of benefits is offered at a single rate to all individuals and groups within a community, regardless of age, sex, health status, or occupation. In essence, the rate represents an averaging out of high- and low-cost individuals and groups so that the community as a whole can be served with adequate benefits at reasonable cost (Somers & Somers, 1961). When commercial for-profit insurance companies entered the field, however, they did so with a policy of "experience rating," charging different individuals and population subgroups different premiums, based on their use of services. Low-risk groups could secure benefits at lower premiums. As a result, the Blues began to offer a multiplicity of policies with differing rate and benefits structures, and they generally have adopted experience rating. Had they not, their health insurance portfolios would have been heavily composed of adverse risks (Krizay & Wilson, 1974). Over the past several years, however, interest by purchasers to control spending have virtually eliminated community rating in the large group markets. Both commercial insurers and Blue Cross plans now largely sell experience-rated insurance products (both indemnity and managed care).

Commercial Insurance. Commercial insurance companies (Aetna, Metropolitan Life, etc.) entered the general health insurance market cautiously. They had realized losses on income-replacement policies during the Depression and were leery of the Blues' initial emphasis on comprehensive benefits. However, a Supreme Court decision recognizing fringe benefits as a legitimate part of the collective bargaining process, following as it did the freezing of industrial wages during World War II, proved too much of a temptation.

In the main, Blue Cross offered hospitalization insurance; Blue Shield covered in-hospital physician services and a limited amount of office-based care. The commercials offer both. As in the case of the Blues, commercial insurance is primarily provided to groups through employee fringe-benefit packages negotiated through collective bargaining. Individual coverage can be purchased, but it is usually quite expensive or has limited coverage. The commercials also sell major medical and cash payment policies The former, directed primarily at catastrophic illness, pay all or part of the treatment costs beyond those covered by basic plans. They are sold on both a group and an individual basis. Cash payment policies pay the insured a flat sum of money per day of hospitalization and are usually sold directly to individuals, often through mass advertising campaigns. Although the daily cash payment sum is usually small, it can help defray costs left uncovered by other insurance.

Like the Blues, the commercials are subject to supervision by state insurance commissioners, although such supervision does not include rate regulation. One general requirement is that commercials establish premium rates high enough to cover claims made under the insurance they provide. Solvency of the insurer is the principal aim of insurance commission surveillance in this instance (Krizay & Wilson, 1974).

During the 1990s, however, the distinction between many of the commercial and Blue Cross plans has blurred. To enhance their competitive pricing position vis-à-vis their commercial counterparts, several Blue Cross plans have converted to for-profit status or plan to. This shift has been accompanied by the establishment of companion foundations designed to continue the provision of "community-benefits/functions" performed previously. In addition, the range of products offered through commercial and Blue Cross/Blue Shield plans has become virtually identical. Both of these trends were precipitated by the increasing demands placed on the industry to deliver cost containment.

HMOs. The form of health insurance that is reshaping the way many Americans relate to the health sector is the HMO. HMOs integrate the delivery of health care and insurance for health care. Although there are many different types of HMOs, the essential idea is that an annual payment is made by or for beneficiaries and then a group of providers delivers all covered services for this "capitated" payment. The HMO concept fundamentally changes the traditional approach of paying physicians and other providers on a fee-for-service, "piece-work" basis. An HMO is paid a capitated amount to "maintain" (and when necessary, to restore) the health of an enrollee. Both commercial insurers and Blue Cross plans have actively entered the managed care market place.

Table 3.4 displays the growth in HMO members between 1976 and 1996, when 63.3 million Americans received care through HMOs. The 1995 membership is over 10 times that of 1976. The number of HMOs has grown from 174 in 1976 to 636 in 1996.

There are four distinct types of HMOs, which vary in how the fiscal agent relates to the providers of care group (Group Health Association of America, 1986). The traditional type of HMO is a "staff" model in which the fiscal agent employs salaried physicians who generally spend all their time delivering services to the HMO's enrollees. A "group" model is a slight variant of this in that the physicians as a single group contract with the fiscal agent to deliver services. In a "network" type of HMO the fiscal agent has contracts with multiple physician groups to provide services to enrollees; often the physician groups deliver services

TABLE 3.4   Number of HMO Members (in Millions), 1976–1987

Year	As of June	As of December
1976	6.0	na
1977	6.3	na
1978	7.6	na
1979	8.2	na
1980	9.1	na
1981	10.2	na
1982	10.8	na
1983	12.5	na
1984	15.1	na
1985	18.9	na
1986	23.7	25.7
1987	28.6	29.3
1988	na	32.7
1989	na	34.7
1990	na	36.5
1991	na	38.6
1992	na	41.4
1996	na	63.3

na, data not available.
Sources: Adapted from Gruber, R., Shadle, M., & Polich, C. L., "From Movement to Industry: The Growth of HMOs," *Health Affairs, 7*(3), p. 198, 1988. Group Health Association of America's *National Directory of HMOs Database, Health Affairs*, Summer 1988. *Interstudy*, Competitive Edge, HMO Directory 7.1, Excelsior, MN, 1997.

to non-HMO patients also. The fourth HMO type is the "independent practice association" (IPA) model, in which the fiscal agent contracts with a range of physicians, who work in independent practices or multispecialty group practices to provide services to HMO enrollees. Again, IPA physicians generally provide services to both HMO enrollees and patients with other forms of insurance.

HMOs vary in how they relate to hospitals. Some HMOs own their own hospitals, and others have varying forms of fiscal arrangements with community hospitals. The fiscal arrangements can include some version of a capitation payment or some form of discounted per diem or per case reimbursement mechanism.

The reason for increased enrollment in HMOs in recent years is principally the expectation and claim that HMOs reduce health care costs while providing coverage that has fewer copayment features and uncovered services. Many studies have found that HMOs, particularly group and staff models, reduce hospital use and total costs (Arnould, Debruck, & Pollard, 1984; Congressional Budget Office, 1995; Luft, 1978, 1981; Manning, 1984; Roemer & Shonick, 1973; Wolinsky, 1980). Physicians working in HMOs generally have a strong incentive to use resources efficiently because of the capitated payment approach. Most important, HMO providers have strong incentives to avoid hospitalizations. Studies consistently indicate that even after adjusting for demographic differences, HMO patients are hospitalized 15% to 40% less often than fee-for-service patients (Luft, 1981).

PPOs. In addition to HMOs, the other growing form of insurance coverage is that which uses PPOs. As with HMOs, there are many different types of PPOs. However, the general concept involves beneficiaries using physicians who have agreed to give price discounts to the insurer. The beneficiary usually is provided some incentive to use a preferred provider, in the form of either lower insurance premiums or waiver of cost-sharing requirements.

As indicated in Table 3.3, PPOs accounted for 25% of the private insurance market in 1995. PPOs have been growing, especially in areas where there is significant competition for patients among physicians and other health care providers. In competitive markets, insurers are best able to persuade providers to offer price discounts in return for a chance to increase patient volume. PPOs are often established not by insurers but by groups of physicians interested in maintaining patients in the face of competition from HMOs.

Managed care plans deliver cost savings through negotiated price discounts and reductions in hospital days. The demands by purchasers to sustain these savings have generated changes in the supply side of the health care marketplace. In addition to the growth in managed care, one of the most important trends over the past 5 years has been the substantial consolidation in the industry. Much of the consolidation has been driven by the economics of bargaining power; size and volume deliver higher discounts and more leverage on providers. When including Blue Cross plans collectively, the largest nine managed care plans currently control over 80% of the market (see Table 3.5). These trends are likely to continue as even some of the largest providers (i.e., Prudential) are examining further consolidations.

Extent of Private Health Insurance Coverage in the United States.

Private health insurance coverage for Americans is extensive but far from complete. As of 1996, all but 41.7 million, some 15.6% of the population, had some form of health insurance. These latest figures indicate that, despite the recent strong growth in the economy, the percentage uninsured continues to rise. For instance, during 1993, the start of the recovery, 15.2 % of Americans were uninsured (tabulations from March 1994 and March 1997 *Current Population*

TABLE 3.5 Managed Care Enrollment of the Ten Largest Plans, 1995

Plan	Enrollment (millions)	Cumulative Enrollment (%)
Blue Cross	8.5	15.7
United Healthcare	6.7	28.1
Kaiser Permanente	6.7	40.6
Aetna/U.S. Healthcare	5.7	51.1
Prudential	4.7	59.8
Cigna	3.9	67.0
PacifiCare/FHP[a]	3.6	73.7
Humana	2.1	77.6
Health Systems[b]	1.8	80.9
All other plans	10.3	100.0
Total all plans	54.0	100.0

[a]Data reflect PacifiCare's buyout of FHP; prior to acquisition, each plan enrolled approximately 1.8 million subscribers.
[b]Health Systems is involved in merger discussion with Foundation Health Plan.
Source: K. E. Thorpe, "The Health System in Transition: Care, Costs and Coverage," *Journal of Health Politics, Policy and Law, 22*(2), 344, April 1997.

Survey). The rising share of Americans without insurance, even as the economy has improved, is a cause for ongoing policy concern.

Although large numbers of individuals have some health insurance, the breadth of their coverage is uneven. An examination of the proportion of total consumer expenditures met by private insurance for various types of care indicates variations in coverage (see Table 3.6). As noted earlier, in 1995 expenditures made through private health insurance amounted to about 32.5 % of the total. Table 3.5 translates that percentage for 1995 and prior years into the proportions of expenditures met for the several categories of health care covered by such insurance. It is clear that many individuals have some coverage for drugs, physicians' office visits, and dental care, although the coverage often does not go very far.

One type of service that has very poor insurance coverage is long-term care that is custodial in nature. In discussing Medicare, it was noted that coverage for long-term care that involves rehabilitation has recently been expanded. However, very few long-term care services are for rehabilitation; most are custodial, involving chronic care of the frail elderly. Medicare pays less than 7% of all nursing care costs, and private insurance pays less than 1%.

The current system of financing long-term care relies on out-of-pocket expenditures by the elderly who can afford such expenditures. In most states, after an elderly person becomes impoverished by the costs of services, the state Medicaid program will cover services.

Although private insurance has played a very small role in insuring long-term care services, in recent years a market for private insurance has been emerging, and the number of policies has been expanding. In addition, numerous proposals have been made for developing an integrated public-private insurance system for long-term care services that would combine private insurance and some public resources now devoted to Medicaid long-term care services (Knickman, 1988; Health Security Act, 1993).

How the Money Is Paid Out

Paying Physicians

As indicated in Table 3.2, physician services account for approximately 20% of all health care expenditures. However, the method used to pay physicians influences not only this 20% of the health care bill but also the large share of health care costs that are controlled largely by physicians' decisions. It is important to emphasize the role of physicians in deciding when a patient uses hospital resources and in prescribing drugs and medical tests.

As already mentioned, methods used by insurers to reimburse physicians are undergoing substantial change. The growth of HMOs and PPOs is changing the ability of physicians to set prices freely. Increased regulation of fees by Medicare also is affecting the way physicians are reimbursed.

Fee for Service. The dominant approach to paying physicians continues to be some variation of a fee-for-service approach, though this is rapidly giving ground to various capitation arrangements. A traditional fee-for-service approach is a simple system in which a physician sets a price for each type of service delivered, and then the patient or the insurer pays this price.

For individuals who have no insurance for physician services, traditional fee-for-service generally is used. Even when an individual has private insurance, fee-for-service rates are generally charged, with the patient paying any share of the rate the insurer judges to be above a stated payment scale. Insurers use a wide range of methods for establishing payment scales for covered services.

The Medicare program's system for paying physicians is based on the fee-for-service approach. Prior to 1992, the system was based in part on a comparison of each doctor's fee schedule for a given type of service with those of other physicians in a community. Medicare never paid an individual physician an

TABLE 3.6 Percentage of Consumer Health Expenditures Met by Private Health Insurance, 1950–1991, Selected Years

Year	Total	Hospital care	Physicians' services	Prescribed drugs (out of hospital)	Dental Care
1950	12.2%	37.1%	12.0%	a	a
1960	27.8	64.7	30.0	a	a
1965	30.5	70.1	34.0	2.4%	1.6%
1966	30.4	71.0	34.0	2.7	2.0
1967	32.8	76.7	36.7	3.5	2.5
1968	34.5	78.8	40.5	3.6	3.1
1969	35.5	77.7	41.1	4.0	3.9
1970	37.2	77.7	43.7	3.9	5.3
1971	39.1	80.9	43.7	4.9	6.3
1972	39.0	76.5	45.8	5.0	7.2
1973	39.0	75.4	46.0	5.6	8.1
1974	41.4	77.3	49.8	6.2	11.0
1975	45.0	82.6	51.3	6.7	15.8
1976	47.0	84.6	53.1	7.9	19.6
1977	45.5	79.3	52.9	7.9	20.2
1981	54.5	82.9	58.9	13.4	34.9
1982	56.2	83.2	60.4	14.6	34.4
1983	56.5	83.5	60.6	14.8	34.9
1984	56.0	80.0	62.6	14.6	35.7
1985	55.5	79.4	62.2	14.8	36.5
1986	55.8	79.4	62.9	15.1	37.4
1987	56.2	79.5	62.9	15.6	37.6
1988	59.4	87.1	70.1	15.6	43.2
1989	61.0	88.6	70.5	15.2	43.7
1990	61.9	90.1	71.6	15.9	44.0
1991	62.9	91.1	72.2	16.9	44.7
1995	62.5	91.6	73.2	na	50.2

a, coverage insignificant.
Sources: Adapted from M. S. Carroll & R. H. Arnett II, "Private Health Insurance Plans in 1977: Coverage, Enrollment and Financial Experience," *Health Care Financing Reviews, 1,* Fall 1979, p. 14; R. M. Gibson, K. R. Levitt, H. Lazenby, & D. Waldo, "National Health Expenditures, 1983," *Health Care Financing Review, 6,* Winter 1984, Table 3; S. Letsch et al., "National Health Expenditures, 1987, *Health Care Financing Review, 10,* Winter 1988, Table 1, and *Health Care Financing Review,* Fall 1991, Table 10; and Levit et al., 1996, Table 16.

amount that exceeded the 75th percentile of charges by all physicians in a community (this was termed the "prevailing" fee). However, the Medicare program also used a cost of living index, termed the Medicare Economic Index, to constrain the growth in the maximum amount it would pay in a community for each type of physician service (Congressional Budget Office, 1986).

In OBRA 1989, Medicare substantially changed its system for paying physicians. Under the new payment system, each physician service is assigned a "relative value" based on the time, skill, and intensity it takes to provide it. The relative values are then adjusted for geographic variations and multiplied by a national conversion factor to determine the dollar amount of payment. This fee schedule, called the resource-based relative-value scale (RBRVS) went into effect on January 1, 1992.

This approach was intended to lead to a relative increase in payment for cognitive services (i.e., physicals and diagnostic visits) and relative decreases for services that involve procedures. This rebalancing would occur because the previous system led to higher rates for procedures than makes sense based on objective measures involving time, training, or relative expertise. Preliminary evidence suggests, however, that the RBRVS system has led to less change in relative payment rates than originally anticipated.

Preferred Provider Approaches. An alternative to traditional fee-for-service payment approaches is the use of negotiated discounts by physicians or groups of physicians. PPOs used this discounting approach to set reimbursement rates for patients covered by a participating insurer. In many ways, however, the discounting approaches inherent to PPOs are not distinct from fee-for-service approaches but rather a variation on the fee-for-service idea. Physicians continue to be paid on a service-by-service basis but at a somewhat lower rate than is charged for non-PPO patients.

Capitation and Salary. The alternative forms of provider reimbursement are capitation and salary. The latter approach is self-explanatory; its use as a payment mechanism for health professionals is widespread. Certainly, from the employer's point of view, a salary system has the merit of administrative simplicity. When the employer is the government, there is the added benefit of flexibility: the movement of providers into areas of medical scarcity and unpopular jobs is more easily accomplished under a salary system than under other payment mechanisms. From the provider's point of view, he or she has an income protected from sudden fluctuation in supply and demand, has no bill collection problems, and usually receives extensive fringe benefits (Roemer, 1962).

Various types of capitation approaches are used by individual practice associations to compensate physicians. Some pay individual physicians using discounted fee-for-service plans, but most put physicians at some financial risk for the costs of their patient's care. Often a physician receives a capitated annual payment for each patient who uses that physician as a primary provider. The capitated payment is meant to cover certain forms of primary care and, depending on the arrangement, some share of specialty care ancillary services and hospital care. The physician thus has strong incentives to manage resources efficiently.

Another form of capitation is to have a group of IPA physicians receive some percentage of a fee-for-service rate, with the remaining percentage held in escrow to assure that aggregate health care costs across the group do not exceed targets. The escrow amounts are distributed to the physicians at the end of the year if utilization targets are met.

Paying Hospitals

There are two major approaches to hospital reimbursement: retrospective and prospective, although there are numerous modes of payment within these two categories.

Retrospective Payment. Retrospective rates for payment to hospitals by third-party payers and individuals are set after services are provided. There are two major modes of retrospective payment: charges and cost. Most commercial insurers and some Blue Cross plans reimburse hospitals on the basis of submitted charges (charges are simply prices set by hospitals). Most hospitals set charges for basic and intensive-care room and board, as well as for each service provided. These prices may or may not reflect the true economic costs of the particular service. Often the variation above cost is a function of patient mix. Charges will exceed actual costs to the extent that a hospital serves a large number of nonpaying patients and to the extent that "cost-based" insurers actually pay amounts that are less than actual costs.

The more sophisticated retrospective payment mode is based on cost. The determination of cost never involves individual patients; rather, it is a matter of negotiation between hospitals and third-party payers such as Blue Cross and Medicaid. Cost reimbursement is used when insured patients receive their benefits as service rather than as dollar indemnities. Almost all group health insurance policies in the United States now provide service benefits rather than dollar indemnities. To determine reimbursable costs, third-party payers sum-total hospital costs, decide which costs are "allowable," then, using a formula, reimburse hospitals on a per-patient-day basis.

Prospective Payment. The most significant change in hospital payment methodologies in the past 10 years has been the recent expansion in prospective payment services. Of special importance were the changes in the method used by Medicare to pay hospitals. In the Tax Equity and Fiscal Responsibility Act (TEFRA) of 1982, Congress established a cost-per-case basis for hospital payment. TEFRA also placed a ceiling on the rate of increase in hospital revenues that would be supported by the Medicare program.

The 1983 amendments to the Social Security Act further defined the case payment system. These amendments created a revolutionary method of paying hospitals for inpatient care to Medicare patients, one that is based on DRGs. Under this system, hospitals are paid a preestablished amount per case treated, with payment rates varying by type of case. The DRGs measure hospital output by originally classifying patients into 23 major diagnostic categories (MDCs), based on major body systems. The MDCs are divided further into 47 diagnostic groups based on the patient's diagnosis or the surgical procedure used and on age, sex, and other clinical information. One additional group is also used for cases in which diagnosis and surgical procedure do not match (Grimaldi & Micheletti, 1982).

Not all hospitals are included in Medicare's case payment system. Certain specialty hospitals. such as children's long-term care, rehabilitation, and psychiatric hospitals are exempt. So are certain states, such as Maryland, that have approved alternative payment systems. Moreover, certain hospital costs, such as direct medical education and capital-related costs, continue to be reimbursed on a cost basis and are excluded from costs used to calculate case payment rates. There is continuing debate, however, about how to include these in the case payment system.

Payment that an individual hospital receives for treating Medicare patients in a given DRG depends on the DRG's "cost" weight multiplied by a "standardized" average cost for all Medicare patients. The standardization process includes adjustments for differences in wages and teaching intensity. Also, different rates are set for urban and rural hospitals. Payment amounts to hospitals are also adjusted each year by an update factor consisting of a measure of the price of goods and services purchased by hospitals. In addition, a discretionary adjustment factor (DAF) accounts for changes in new technology and productivity.

Two aspects of this payment system depart significantly from previous methods used to pay for Medicare patients. First, the DRG concept holds that the "best" measure of hospital output is the diagnosis treated rather than individual services provided or length of stay. That is, the basis of payment is the case treated rather than ancillary or routine inputs to hospital care.

Second, unlike retrospective payment methodologies, DRG payments are determined prospectively and are fixed. Although a portion of the initial rates for fiscal year 1984 were determined by historical costs, subsequent rates of increase in the payments are controlled before payment is made. Hence, Medicare now has the ability to control the rate of increase for Medicare patients.

The use of DRGs as a basis for hospital payment transcends Medicare and is spreading rapidly to other payers. At least 21 states, such as Pennsylvania, Utah, Ohio, Michigan, and Washington, have adopted case-based systems to pay for hospital care received by Medicaid patients. Thirty-two states, including Arizona, Oklahoma, and Kansas, employ a DRG system to pay for Blue Cross patients. As of 1993, Maryland was the only state that uses a DRG system for all third-party payers.

Use of classification schemes as the basis for hospital payment assumes that the classifications are clinically meaningful and "reasonably" homogeneous with respect to resource consumption. There is, however, evidence that some of the DRG categories do not satisfy either requirement (Prospective Payment Assessment Commission, 1985). Perhaps the most common criticism of the DRG categories is that they include patients with dissimilar resource needs because they often do not account adequately for differences in patient complexity or severity of illness (Horn et al., 1984). Variation in severity within each DRG category is cause for concern if patient complexity can be assessed before admission to the hospital; this can create an incentive to divert more complex patients to other hospitals. Long-run consequences may include shedding unprofitable DRG "products" and expanding the volume of "profitable" services to ensure hospital financing viability. Changes in hospital service mix may not be entirely undesirable, however, if increased patient volume allows hospitals to eliminate facility duplication and exploit economies of scale. On the other hand, narrowing the scope of services may adversely affect access to care in some cases.

Research concerning the impacts of the new Medicare DRG payment system indicates that the approach is significantly changing hospital utilization patterns. Medicare hospital admissions decreased 15.9% during the first 3 years of the new reimbursement system, and average length of stay decreased 17% (Guterman, Eggers, Riley, Greene, & Terrell, 1987). Although it is difficult to determine exactly how much of these dramatic reductions in utilization are attributable to DRGs, research studies do document that utilization rates fell much more quickly in states where the DRG system was implemented, compared to the states that received waivers to delay or avoid implementation.

The reduction in hospital use has not been without side effects, however. In particular, evidence consistently indicates sharp increases in posthospital use of services, including home health care and nursing home care, as well as increased readmissions (Guterman et al., 1987). The tighter regulation of Medicare payment rates also may be responsible for part of the rapid growth in cost of private insurance as hospitals shift some of their costs from Medicare to private insurance. That is, higher rates may be charged for individuals with private insurance to compensate for any operating losses associated with care delivered to Medicare patients.

Whereas inpatient care under Medicare relies on prospective case payment, outpatient care remains largely a cost-based system. A major problem in moving outpatient hospital spending into a per-visit or per-episode world is the ongoing problem of defining a clinically relevant case-mix system. However, as part of the 1997 Balanced Budget Act, Congress has directed the Department of Health and Human Services to accelerate the development of prospective payment systems for hospital outpatient care as well as certain post-acute-care benefits (i.e., skilled nursing facilities, home health care).

The Rising Costs of Health Care

National spending for health care grew an average of 12.4% per year from 1970 to 1991. Since 1991, however, the growth in national spending decreased to 6.7% per year. Yet despite this lower rate of growth, the rate of increase in health care costs has consistently far exceeded the rate of inflation in the general economy. Thus, health care expenses each year account for an increasing share of the nation's GNP.

Several factors have contributed to the rise in medical costs: general inflation in the economy, population growth, the development of new medical technology, and an increased "intensity" of services provided to all patients. Rapid development of medical technology and intensity of medical care services have been encouraged by growth in the extent of health insurance coverage and previous retrospective, cost-based payment systems that rewarded higher reported costs with higher payments (Feldstein, 1971). As insurance coverage increases, the out-of-pocket cost to the patient is reduced, leading to increases in demand for higher quality medical care and hence to rising prices. The growth in the comprehensiveness of third-party insurance coverage is stimulated in part through the federal government's tax law (Phelps, 1984). Under current tax law, employer payments to employees for health insurance are not considered taxable income. Because these tax subsidies reduce the price of health insurance, they provide incentives to purchase more health insurance.

Despite the theoretical connection between the extent of health insurance and costs, until the early 1980s there was little persuasive empirical evidence that increased health insurance coverage led to greater use of health care services. Some even argued that more comprehensive insurance, especially for ambulatory care, would reduce total spending by encouraging preventive health care and more "appropriate" hospital use (Roemer et al., 1975).

Data from the Rand Corporation's widely cited Health Insurance Experiment (Newhouse, Hopkins, Carr, & Gartside, 1981) provide considerable insight into the connection between insurance coverage and utilization. The experiment ran from 1974 through January 1982 and enrolled 7,716 individuals between the ages of 14 and 61 who belonged to 2,756 families. Families were assigned randomly to one of four mayor types of experimental plans:

1. A "free-care" plan, in which all care was received without charge (i.e., there were no coinsurance or deductible requirements).
2. An individual deductible plan, which imposed a 95% coinsurance rate on outpatient care, up to a maximum out-of-pocket expenditure of $450 per family, with all care beyond that amount (either inpatient or outpatient) free at time of service.
3. A series of intermediate coinsurance plans with cost-sharing requirements of either 25% or 50%.
4. "Income-related catastrophic" plans that included a 95% coinsurance requirement with income-related maximum dollar spending caps.

The results of the experiment were quite robust. Health care spending was almost 50% lower in plans with 95% cost sharing, compared to those in the free-care plans. Perhaps of more interest was the finding that any cost sharing, even for ambulatory care services, reduced costs, compared to the free-care plans.

Another important finding from the experiment was that, in general, the reduced utilization of health care due to cost sharing did not affect most measures of health status. However, two exceptions to those findings were slight increases in blood pressure for individuals with high blood pressure at the start of the study and for individuals who had low incomes (Brook et al., 1983).

The system of third-party reimbursement also has been implicated as a primary factor spurring the recent growth in new medical technology. Although in certain instances new technology has increased the length and quality of life, it is often very costly. As one observer of the system has noted, "with some important exceptions, the norm for hospital care in the United States approximates the maxim 'if you think it will help, do it' " (Aaron & Schwartz, 1984, p. 7). Because most patients are insulated from the true social costs of medical care through health insurance, our present system encourages the uses of services that may yield only slight, if any, positive diagnostic information, often regardless of cost. The HCFA, for example, found that the increased per-admission intensity of care accounted for over 20% of the growth in expenditures for community hospital inpatient care over the past 10 years (Freeland & Schendler, 1983).

Although the spread of new technology undoubtedly offers unprecedented medical benefits, some innovations are of marginal value. Further, facilities and services unavailable in the late 1970s or found only in medical centers are now offered in a substantial number of community hospitals. The increase in diagnostic imaging by computerized axial tomography (CAT) has been impressive, more than doubling since 1980 (Office of Technology Assessment, 1981). Similarly, rapid diffusion of magnetic resonance imaging (MRI) has occurred. The medical benefits of CAT scanning are well known; for instance, it has reduced the need for exploratory surgery. Yet growth in new technology has expanded the potential pool of recipients as well as symptoms diagnosed. Thus, although it is true that new technology provides unprecedented medical benefits, the downside is that new technology increases expenditures.

The battle over medical efficacy, new technology, and health care expenditures has escalated with the advent of Medicare's DRG payment system. Under the DRG system, hospitals may become more reluctant to purchase new technologies that add significantly to their operating costs because reimbursement rates will not automatically increase with an expenditure for technology. Moreover, the rate of technological diffusion in the industry will be sensitive to the method ultimately chosen by the HCFA to reimburse hospitals for capital expenditures. Yet, to date, the tremendous growth in new medical technology shows no perceptible signs of abating. Each year new, more expensive technologies with the potential for saving and improving the quality of life appear. Many consider cost increases resulting from advances in and greater use of medical technology as the necessary price of improvements in health care, if not health. Opponents suggest that a substantial portion of the utilization of technology is generally unnecessary. They link a proportion of the increase in ancillary service to physician fear of exposure to malpractice claims. Indeed, small increases in diagnostic accuracy often require substantial increases in the health care bill. This concern has increased interest in redirecting resources into programs—especially public health intervention—with more favorable cost-benefit implications.

Some observe that any appreciable reduction in spending can be accomplished only by denying medical benefits (Aaron & Schwartz, 1984). Others note that increased cost sharing may reduce spending and utilization, often without deleterious effects on health status (Brook et al., 1983). Thus, the debate continues surrounding the health implications of recent attempts, such as the expansion of the DRG system, to reduce the rate of growth of health care costs. A central feature of the debate is the role assumed by the "march of science." According to various estimates, innovation in medical technology has accounted for approximately half of the yearly rise in health care spending (Newhouse, 1993; Schwartz, 1987). Advances in medical technology continue at a rapid pace, with several promising new innovations currently in the pipeline (Schwartz, 1994). These include continued innovations in drug therapies, the treatment of autoimmune diseases, advances in molecular cell biology, and the study of genetics and its implications for the incidence of disease. Each of these promising innovations will yield substantial improvements in the quality and length of life. However, they are likely to be accompanied by a high price tag. Thus, the debate continues concerning the ability of public and private payees to "appropriately" balance their desires to control the growth in spending while encouraging the diffusion of new and promising technologies.

Conclusions

Money funds the health care delivery system, but the routes dollars take from consumers to providers can be labyrinthine. Some dollars go directly, some via the government, and some through insurance companies. Most health care providers are paid by salary, but some are paid on a piecework basis. Hospitals are paid for services provided in numerous ways. Some insurers base payments on what the hospital charges, whereas others pay on the basis of allowable average costs. Still others, notably Medicare and some Medicaid and Blue Cross plans, pay hospitals on a "case" basis, with the payment rate set in advance.

In the United States in the 1960s and 1970s a health insurance system that emphasized coverage for hospital care, with physician service in hospitals generally being more lucrative than in the office setting, tilted the system in the direction of utilization of the most expensive component of the system. Technological change, a significant factor in rising health care costs, was often poorly planned and evaluated, with decisions frequently made on the basis of universal access rather than cost-effectiveness.

The 1980s and 1990s, however, witnessed a virtual revolution in the financing and structure of medical care delivery. Fundamental changes in the methods used to pay health care providers, growing involvement by employers and employees in direct negotiation with providers, and a projected aggregate surplus of physicians have led to the changes in the structure of the delivery system. Notable has been the move from retrospective to prospective modes of payment. Although prospective per-case payment systems are generally restricted to inpatient hospital care, considerable research and development efforts—aimed at designing prospective case payment systems for long-term care, home health care, and outpatient care—are currently under way. In some quarters, across-the-board capitation payments may prove feasible.

The 1980s also saw the beginning of dramatic changes in the organization of medical practice. The growth in prepaid group practice, ambulatory surgery, and the "unbundling" of hospital services are indicative of the magnitude of recent changes in the delivery system. New alignments between providers, employers, and employees—in the form of HMOs, PPOs, and self-insurance ventures—also reflect the recent entrance of the consumer into direct financial negotiation with health care providers. Efforts by providers to unbundle services designed in part to increase revenues have been supplemented by the rise in capitation and integrated delivery systems. The impressive rise in efforts by purchasers to control costs, accompanied by the new dominance of managed care, truly represents a major change in the organization and delivery of services in the 1990s.

These changes have accelerated during the 1990s. Managed care is now the dominant force by which consumers receive their care. Indeed, 75% of working Americans, 40% of Medicaid beneficiaries, and nearly 15% of the Medicare population is enrolled in managed care. The shift to managed care has been credited by many as the primary factor accounting for the substantial reduction in the growth of health care costs, though the precise role that managed care has played in these savings remains an issue. Implications of this major change in the delivery system on the quality of care and access to come will, however, have to be carefully monitored.

What remains unresolved, however, is the future for the 41.7 million Americans who lack health insurance. Although Congress recently passed an important new insurance program designed to provide insurance to low-income children (as part of the 1997 Balanced Budget Act), left unresolved is how the remaining uninsured will access the system as the desire to control spending intensifies. The unresolved issues concerning financing care for the uninsured, combined with the financial pressures placed on providers as cost-containment efforts mount, arguably represent the major policy financing issues facing the system.

Mini-Case Study

The private sector has dramatically increased its desire and ability to extract cost savings from providers largely through the use of managed care. These savings were generated, however, during a time when hospitals were making substantial profits from Medicare. The Balanced Budget Act of 1997 has reduced substantially the rate of growth in Medicare payments to providers. What impact do you expect this legislation will have on

- the ability of the private sector to sustain its cost-containment efforts?
- pressures for even more productivity from the health care industry?
- consolidations among health plans and providers?
- access to care for the uninsured (i.e., the amount of charity care and bad debt provided by hospitals and other providers)?

Discussion Questions

1. One of the more significant changes in the structure of insurance over the past two decades is the economic actors who are at risk for higher health care spending. How has risk shifted throughout the system over the past two decades, and to what extent do these changes influence the yearly growth in health care spending?

2. What processes would be effective or desirable to balance society's desire to promote the introduction and diffusion of new lifesaving or quality-enhancing technologies yet at the same time assuring ourselves that health care costs will not continue to rise even faster?

3. In addition to health care, several other sectors of the economy are rising faster than the overall rate of economic growth. For instance, like health care, the computer and information industry continues to account for a rising share of GDP. Yet despite the rising share of GDP assumed by the information and computer industry, there is not a substantial concern or body of literature examining options for "computer cost containment." Why the concern in the health care industry?

References

Aaron, H., & Schwartz, W., *The Painful Prescription: Rationing Hospital Care*. Washington, DC: The Brookings Institution, 1984.

Arnett, R., II, & Trapnell, G., "Private Health Insurance: New Measures of a Complex and Changing Industry," *Health Care Financing Review, 6*(2), Winter 1984.

Arnould, R., Debrock, L. W., & Pollard, J. W., "Do HMOs Produce Services More Efficiently?" *Inquiry, 21*(3), Fall 1984.

Brook, R. et al., "Does Free Care Improve Adults' Health? Results from a Randomized Controlled Trial," *New England Journal of Medicine, 319*, 1426, 1983.

Carroll, M. S., & Arnett, R. H., II, "Private Health Insurance Plans in 1977: Coverage, Enrollment and Financial Experience," *Health Care Financing Review, 1*(3), Fall 1979.

Christensen, S., & Kasten, R., "Covering Catastrophic Expenses under Medicare," *Health Affairs, 3*(5), 79, 1988.

Congressional Budget Office, *Physician Reimbursement under Medicare: Options for Change*. Washington, DC: U.S. Government Printing Office, 1986.

Congressional Budget Office, *The Effects of Managed Care and Managed Competition*. Washington, DC: U.S. Government Printing Office, 1995.

Congressional Research Service, *Workmen's Compensation: Role of the Federal Government*. (IB75054). Washington, DC: Library of Congress, 1976.

Davis, K., & Rowland, D., "Uninsured and Underserved: Inequities in Health Care in the United States," *Milbank Memorial Fund Quarterly: Health and Society, 61*, 149, 1983.

de Lissovoy, G., Rice, T., Ermann, D., & Gabel, 1., "Preferred Provider Organizations: Today's Models and Tomorrow's Prospect," *Inquiry, 23*, 7, 1986.

Feldstein, M. S., *The Rising Cost of Hospital Care*. Washington, DC: Information Resources Press, 1971.

Freeland, M. S., & Schendler, C. E., "National Health Expenditure Growth in the 1980's: An Aging Population, New Technologies, and Increasing Competition," *Health Care Financing Review, 4*(3), 1983.

Gabel, J. R., Ginsburg, P. B., & Hunt, K. A., "Small Employers and Their Health Benefits, 1988–1996: An Awkward Adolescence," *Health Affairs, 16*(5), 103–110, 1997.

Gabel, J., DiCarlo, S., Fink, S., & de Lissovoy, G., "Employer-Sponsored Health Insurance in America: Preliminary Results from the 1988 Survey." *Research Bulletin*. Washington, DC: Health Insurance Association of America, January 1989.

Gibson, R. M., "National Health Expenditures, 1978," *Health Care Financing Review, 1*(1), 1979.

Gibson, R. M., Levitt, K., Lazenby, H., & Waldo, D., "National Health Expenditures, 1983," *Social Security Bulletin, 6*(2), 1984.

Grimaldi, P., & Micheletti, J., *Diagnosis Related Groups: A Practitioner's Guide.* Chicago: Pluribus Press, 1982.

Group Health Association of America, *HMO Industry Profile: Trends, 1985–1986* (Vol. 4). Washington, DC: Author, 1986.

Gruber, L. R., Shadle, M., & Polich, C. L., "From Movement to Industry: The Growth of HMOs," *Health Affairs, 7*(3), 197, 1988.

Guterman, S., Eggers, P. W., Riley, G., Greene, T. F., & Terrell, S. A., "The First 3 Years of Medicare Prospective Payment: An Overview," *Health Care Financing Review, 9*(1), 67, 1987.

Health Insurance Association of America, *Sourcebook of Health Insurance Data, 1984 Update.* New York: Author, 1985.

Health Insurance Institute, *Source Book of Health Insurance Data, 1974–75.* New York: Health Insurance Institute, 1975.

Health Security Act. White House Domestic Policy Council, Washington, DC, 1993.

Hellinger, F., "Recent Evidence on Case-Based Systems for Setting Hospital Rates," *Inquiry, 22*(1), 1985.

Horn, S., et al., "The Severity of Illness Index as a Severity Adjustment to Diagnosis-Related Groups," *Health Care Financing Review, 5*(Suppl.), 1984.

Hsiao, W., & Stason, W., "Toward Developing a Relative Value Scale for Medical and Surgical Services," *Health Care Financing Review, 1*, 23, 1979.

InterStudy, Competitive Edge, *HMO Directory 7.1*, Excelsior, Minnesota, 1997.

Jensen, G., Morrisey, M., Gaffney, S., & Liston, D., "The New Dominance of Managed Care: Insurance Trends in the 1990s," *Health Affairs, 16*(1), January/February, 1997.

Knickman, J., "Private Long-Term Care Insurance: Alleviating Market Problems with Public-Private Partnership," *Health Economics and Health Service Research, 9*, 13S, 1988.

Krizay, J., & Wilson, A., *The Patient as Consumer.* Lexington, MA: D. C. Health, 1974.

Laudicina, S., "State Health Risk Pools: Insuring the Uninsurable," *Health Affairs, 7*(4), 7, 1988.

Law, S. A., *Blue Cross. What Went Wrong?* New Haven, CT: Yale University Press, 1974.

Letsch, S., Levit, K., & Waldo, D., "National Health Expenditures, 1987," *Health Care Financing Review, 10*, 109, 1988.

Levit, K., Lazenby, H., Braden, B., Cowan, C., McDonnell, P., Sivarajan, L., Stiller, J., Wan, D., Donham, C., Long, A., & Stewart, M., "National Health Expenditures, 1995," *Health Care Financing Review, 18*(1), 1996.

Lewin, L., & Lewin, M., "Financing Charity Care in an Era of Competition," *Health Affairs, 6*(1), 47, 1988.

Luft, H., "How Do Health Maintenance Organizations Achieve Their Savings?" *New England Journal of Medicine, 298*, 1366, 1978.

Luft, H., *Health Maintenance Organization: Dimensions of Performance.* New York: Wiley, 1981.

Manning, W., "A Controlled Trial of the Effects of a Prepaid Group Practice on Use of Services," *New England Journal of Medicine, 310*(23), 1984.

McCarthy, C. M., "Incentive Reimbursement as an Impetus to Cost Containment," *Inquiry,* *12,* 320, 1975.

Muse, D. N., & Sawyer, D., *The Medicare and Medicaid Data Book, 1981* (HCFA Pub. No. 03128). Washington, DC: U.S. Department of Health and Human Services, 1982.

Newhouse, J. P., "An Iconoclastic View of Health Care Cost Containment," *Health Affairs*(Suppl.), 152–171, 1993.

Newhouse, J. P., Manning, W., Morris, C., Orr, L., Duan, N., Keeler, E., Leibowitz, A., Marquis, K., Marquis, S., Phelps, C., & Brooks, R., "Some Interim Results from a Controlled Trial of Cost Sharing in Health Insurance," *New England Journal of Medicine, 305,* 1501, 1981.

Office of Technology Assessment, *Policy Implications of the CT Scanner: An Update.* Washington, DC: Author, 1981.

Phelps, C. E., "Taxing Health Insurance: How Much Is Enough?" *Contemporary Policy Issues, 3*(2), 1984.

Price, D. N., "Workers' Compensation Programs in the 1970s," *Social Security Bulletin, 42*(5), 3, 1979a.

Price, D. N., "Workers' Compensation Coverage, Payments and Costs, 1977," *Social Security Bulletin, 42*(10), 18, 1979b.

Prospective Payment Assessment Commission, *Report and Recommendation to the Secretary, U.S. Department of Health and Human Services.* Washington, DC: U.S. Government Printing Office, 1985.

Roemer, M. I., "On Paying the Doctor and the Implications of Different Methods," *Journal of Health and Human Behavior, 3*(4), Spring, 1962.

Roemer, M. I., Hopkins, C. E., Carr, L., & Gartside, F., "Copayments for Ambulatory Care: Penny-Wise and Pound-Foolish," *Medical Care, 13,* 457, 1975.

Roemer, M., & Shonick, V., "HMO Performance: The Recent Evidence," *Health and Society, 51,* 271, 1973.

Russell, et al., *Federal Loyalty Spending, 1969–74.* Washington, DC: National Planning Association, 1974.

Schwartz, W. B., "The Inevitable Failure of Current Cost-Containment Strategies: Why They Can Provide Only Temporary Relief," *Journal of the American Medical Association,* 220–224, 1987, Jan. 9.

Schwartz, W. B., "In the Pipeline: A Wave of Valuable Medical Technology," *Health Affairs, 13*(3), 70–80, 1994.

Somers, H., & Somers, A. R., *Doctors, Patients and Health Insurance.* Washington, DC: The Brookings Institution, 1961.

Swartz, K., *The Uninsured with a Special Focus on Workers.* Unpublished report, The Urban Institute, 1989.

Thorpe, K. E., "The Health Care System In Transition: Care, Cost and Coverage," *Journal of Health Politics, Policy and Law, 22*(2), April 1997.

Thorpe, K. E., & Phelps, C., "The Social Role of Not-for-Profit Organizations: Hospital Provision of Charity Care," *Economic Inquiry, 29,* 472–484, 1992.

U.S. National Commission on State Workmen's Compensation Laws, *Report.* Washington, DC: U.S. Government Printing Office, 1973.

Wilensky, G., "Filling the Gaps in Health Insurance," *Health Affairs, 7*(3), 133, 1988.

Wolinsky, F., "The Performance of Health Maintenance Organizations: An Analytic Review," *Milbank Memorial Fund Quarterly, 58*(4), 4, 1980.

4

The Health Care Workforce

Christine Kovner and Edward S. Salsberg

Learning Objectives

After completing this chapter, the reader will be able to:

1. Describe the types of health care workers in the United States and the types of facilities in which they work.
2. Describe the impact of the changing health care system on the health care workforce.
3. Discuss professional licensure as a mechanism for health care worker quality assurance.
4. Identify areas of overlap among several health professionals.
5. Recognize the difficulties in estimating the future demand for and supply of health care workers.

Topical Outline

The workforce
Counting health workers: Problems and pitfalls
Nursing
Medicine
Other health workers
Current issues

Key Words: Supply, demand, need, unlicensed assistive personnel, graduate medical education, nurse practitioner, full-time equivalent, certification, licensure.

The health care workforce is the backbone of the health care delivery system. Even with major technological advances, it is the health care worker who ultimately determines the availability, quality, and cost of health services. Any effort to improve health care services or control costs must consider the supply, distribution, use, and education of the health care workforce. Conversely, any change in financing, organization, or technology will affect health care personnel.

The rapidly changing health care system is having a dramatic impact on the health care workforce, including the numbers and types of workers that will be needed and where and how they will practice and work. The transformation of health care is disrupting historic roles for physicians, nurses, and other health care professionals. Increasing corporatization of health care, competition, the expansion of managed care, the development of integrated delivery systems, and new technologies—all have an impact on the workforce. Health care workers are reassessing their roles and their relationship to the delivery system and other workers, and health professions education programs are reassessing their curricula and approaches. Although the American health care system is still in the early stages of this transformation, many implications for the workforce have emerged.

Among the factors affecting the workforce are the following:

- As competition expands, health care facilities and organizations are far more concerned with costs, productivity, and outcomes than in the past, leading to a reassessment of how many workers are needed and how they are used.
- Hospitals, the largest source of employment in the health field, are under pressure to reduce costs. Many are reducing staff and redesigning their operations.
- Care is shifting from inpatient to ambulatory care settings.
- HMOs, other managed care arrangements, and other purchasers of service are constraining and limiting the roles of physicians reducing their autonomy.
- Many settings are substituting lower cost workers.
- All settings are concerned with customer relations and patient satisfaction, and most sites want workers who are flexible, computer-literate, and customer-oriented.

The Workforce

The health care workforce is large and diverse. It includes many of society's most educated, and highly paid professionals, such as physicians. It includes a wide range of caregivers, from nurses to therapists. It includes millions of skilled technicians who work in hospitals, laboratories, and other settings; and it includes millions of semi-skilled workers, such as aides, clerks, and housekeeping staff.

Large numbers of managers, administrators, analysts, lawyers, computer opera-tors, and insurance sales personnel also work in health care organizations.

Health services are labor-intensive. This is true whether the services are provided in hospitals, in nursing homes, or in physicians' offices. In 1994 nearly 12 million people were employed in health care settings and/or as health profes-sionals, approximately 10% of the nation's total workforce (Bureau of Labor Statistics, 1994).

Over the last fifty years, health care employment has consistently grown at a faster rate than the overall employment in the American economy. From 1974 through 1994, employment in health care settings more than doubled (Franklin, 1995; Kahl, 1986). Even in national recessions, health care employment has risen sharply.

The changes now under way in health care are expected to slow the growth in jobs significantly and may even lead to a short-term decrease. However, the aging of the population and efforts to address specific health problems, such as high rates of infant mortality, will contribute to the need for health personnel. The federal Bureau of Labor Statistics projects that employment in health care settings will to rise over 33% between 1996 and 2006 (Franklin, 1997), but others believe that the changing health care system will slow the growth in jobs and may even lead to a loss of jobs (Berliner & Kovner, 1994; Center for Health Workforce Studies, 1997; Pew Health Professions Commission, 1995).

Health care employment can be viewed in two ways: by where health personnel work or by occupation. Health care workers are employed in settings such as hospitals, nursing homes, ambulatory care facilities, and other health service delivery sites. Persons educated as health care professionals or who provide health-related services work in many settings in addition to health facilities. For example, physicians teach at medical schools; nurses work in school health offices; pharmacists work for the pharmaceutical firms; and nurse aides assist the frail and elderly in their homes. Figure 4.1 shows the distribution of the health workforce by practice setting, including those in health professions working outside of the health industry.

Although the vast majority of health personnel work in the health settings such as hospitals, nursing homes, and doctors' offices, nearly 16% of the total health care workforce are in settings that are not considered part of the health industry. Table 4.1 presents the distribution by type of occupation of those who work in health facilities and other settings.

Table 4.2 shows health sector employment growth by major type of health setting for the years 1983 through 1994 (Bureau of Labor Statistics, 1994). During this period, the total U.S. workforce (nonfarm) grew by 24%; the total health industry workforce grew by 42% (Bureau of Labor Statistics, 1994). Noteworthy is that the hospital workforce (public and private) grew by only 17%, reflecting

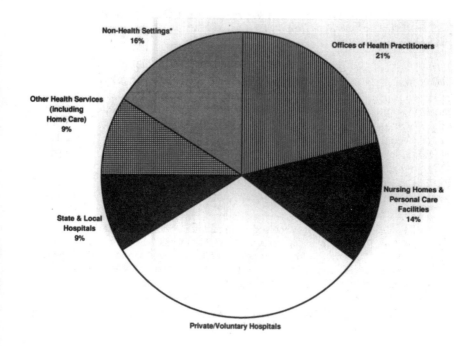

FIGURE 4.1   National health workforce: Distribution by practice setting, 1994.
Source: Bureau of Labor Statistics, Office of Employment Projections, National Industry Occupational Matrix, 1994.

*Employment in health care occupations outside the health care industry.

the early stages of the impact of the changing health care system, including the shift in care from more costly institutional settings to ambulatory care settings.

Counting Health Workers: Problems and Pitfalls

Counting and tracking health workers can be very confusing. Often figures on health care employment just report health "sector" employment, excluding health professionals in other settings. Yet, as noted above, close to 16% of health professionals work outside health settings.

Some data sources count the number of individuals in a setting or occupation regardless of how much they work. This is a body count, such as there are *x*

TABLE 4.1   The Health Care Workforce by Occupation and Type of Setting, 1994

Workforce	Health Settings	Other Settings	Total
Health Diagnosing[1]	507,957	86,408	594,365
Health Assessing[2]	1,993,512	511,129	2,504,641
Health Technicians[3]	1,552,929	617,181	2,170,110
Health Service[4]	1,689,722	375,349	2,065,071
Home Health[5]	287,247	296,946	584,193
Other Occupations[6]	4,050,633	N/A	4,050,633
Total	10,082,000	1,887,013	11,969,013

[1]Includes physicians, dentists, chiropractors, optometrists, and podiatrists.
[2]Includes RNs, PAs, pharmacists, dieticians, and therapists.
[3]Includes LPNs, lab and radiologic technicians, dental hygienists, and other technicians.
[4]Includes nurse aides, medical, dental and pharmacy assistants, OTAs and PTAs.
[5]Includes home health aides and personal and home care aides.
[6]Includes all health care occupations not elsewhere classified.

Source: Bureau of Labor Statistics, Office of Employment Projections, National Industry Occupational Matrix, 1994.

TABLE 4.2   The Health Industry Workforce by Setting* (in Thousands)

Workforce	1983	1994	% Change	Average annual % change
Offices of Physicians, Dentists, and Other Health Practitioners	1,503	2,546	69.4	4.9
Nursing Homes and Personal Care Facilities	1,106	1,649	49.1	3.7
Private/Voluntary Hospitals	3,037	3,774	24.3	2.0
State and Local Hospitals	1,115	1,081	−3.0	−0.3
Other Health Services (including home care)	341	1,032	202.6	10.6
Total of All Health Industries	7,102	10,082	42.0	3.2

*Excludes health workers outside of health industry.

Source: Bureau of Labor Statistics, Office of Employment Projections, National Industry Occupational Matrix, 1994.

number of nurses licensed in a state. Other data sets, to account for the fact that some people work only part-time, count full-time equivalents (FTEs). Two half-time workers represent two individuals but only one FTE. The American Hospital Association (AHA) reports FTEs, which allows analysts and hospitals to compare staffing across hospitals. The Department of Labor uses a third method of counting: they count the number of paychecks. This is similar to a body count except that a person working at two facilities would be counted twice. If hospitals substitute part-time workers for full-time workers, the Labor Department data might show an increase in employment, whereas the AHA data might show a decrease in FTEs.

Another problem is defining the organization or reporting unit. As integrated delivery systems develop, the distinction between hospitals and other settings, such as ambulatory and long-term care, is likely to blur, especially as some workers may move among sites. Also, if a facility contracts or outsources an activity (e.g., food service), then those workers may no longer be reported as health workers, even if they still work in the same location.

State licensing boards count all individuals with a license in those occupations that require a license. However, not all licensed individuals practice in their field. The number of licenses sets the upper limit on the number that can practice in that profession in a state. The percentage that is actually working or actively looking for work is generally referred to as the "labor force participation rate."

There is no single "right" way to count. This is not meant to discourage data analysis but to caution the reader to be aware of these differences and comparisons across data sources. For additional information on health workforce data issues, see *Data Systems to Support State Health Personnel Planning and Policymaking* (Wing & Salsberg, 1992).

Hospitals

As shown in Figure 4.1, hospitals are still the setting with the greatest number of health care workers; public and private hospitals combined employ 40% of all health care workers. But hospitals are undergoing major organizational changes and challenges as competition and managed care spread. After decades of growth, hospital employment has stabilized and some even predict that it will decline over the next decade (Pew Health Professions Commission, 1995). Some policy analysts see this as a positive sign—cost control is finally working. On the other hand, many groups, such as nurses and health worker labor leaders, have decried these cutbacks and workforce changes as undercutting the quality of care. This ersy is likely to continue for sometime as the health care system evolves. ils employ a wide range of workers. The single largest category is registered nursing, representing 24% of all hospital workers.

Long-Term Care Facilities

Over 1.5 million elderly and chronically ill Americans were residing in nursing homes in 1995 (U.S. Department of Health and Human Services, 1997). As the population ages, the number of nursing home residents is expected to increase. A total of 1.3 million FTEs were employed in nursing homes, 1 million (77%) of which provided nursing service, including registered nurses (RNs), licensed practical nurses (LPNs), and nurse aides. However, because of the high costs of maintaining a person in a nursing home and public distaste for nursing homes, public and private efforts are under way to develop less costly, more appealing alternatives. This includes the expansion of "life care communities" that provide limited support services and the expansion of home care. Although this will lead to a lower rate of nursing home use, it will also leave the more ill and needy in the nursing home, increasing patient acuity.

Many of the alternatives to nursing homes for supportive living for the elderly will not be considered health care facilities. Although some health workers, such as RNs, will be employed in these settings, the focus will be on housing and living arrangements rather than on health services. The nursing home workforce consists primarily of nurses (RNs and LPNs) and support staff.

Home Health Care

All of the forces for change are expected to lead to an increase in the use of home care services. As patients are moved quickly out of inpatient settings and as managed care organizations and payers seek to avoid costly, institutional settings, more patients will be treated in their homes. New and improved technology for monitoring patients will also facilitate the expansion of care in the home. As sicker patients with more complex needs are cared for at home, additional nurses and therapists (physical, occupational, and respiratory) will be employed in home care in the future.

The development of improved telecommunications technology, combined with pressures to constrain costs, may significantly change the way that home care services are delivered. The core of home care has been the visit by the nurse to the home. It is now possible for the nurse (or even a doctor) to "visit" the patient through a two-way visual and audio hookup. Even the patient's vital signs can be monitored remotely. The attraction for home care agencies is that this system drastically reduces travel time and significantly increases the number of patients that can be "seen" each day. With discussions under way regarding "capitating" home care (i.e., a set fee for a specific diagnosis or episode of illness), home care organizations will have a strong incentive to limit their costs. This may lead to a moderation in the future growth of home care employment.

Nevertheless, the Department of Labor expects the home care workforce to grow in the coming years. They project a growth of 550,000 home health workers and personal care aide positions, an increase of 79% between 1990 and 2006 (Silvestri, 1997). Although this growth is significant for home care, the absolute numbers are relatively modest compared to the numbers employed in hospitals.

Ambulatory Care Services

The changing health care system is shifting more care to nonhospital settings. This includes physician's offices, community health centers, ambulatory surgical centers, urgent care clinics, and offices of other practitioners (such as dentists and therapists). These sites have a variety of health workers, including physicians, other doctors, registered nurses, nurse practitioners, therapists, physician assistants, medical assistants, and technicians as well as a host of clerical and administrative support staff.

Employment in ambulatory settings is expected to grow significantly over the next few years. However, because it is relatively small compared to hospitals, the overall impact on health sector employment may be limited. In addition, marketplace pressures of competition will also have an impact on ambulatory care sites and constrain job growth. For example, in part to improve market position and to restrain costs, many solo practitioners are merging to form group practices, small groups are merging into larger groups, and some groups are affiliating or even being purchased by hospitals and for-profit chains. In addition, many purchasers/payers of care are trying to limit expenditures, including payment for physician services. These factors may moderate the growth of total jobs in ambulatory care settings.

An area where there has been significant growth in employment is in support services for health maintenance organizations (HMOs) and other managed care organizations. This includes nurses, physicians, and clerical staff for utilization review, quality monitoring, case management, customer relations, and other functions.

Nursing

This section presents an overview of the nursing profession. After a brief history of nursing, the section looks at how nursing is defined in law and by professional nurses. The various educational programs for nurses are described, as well as the levels of practice. Finally, current issues in nursing are analyzed within the context of the health care system. *Nurse* is a generic term that is applied to a variety of practitioners, from nurses' aides and assistants to nurse researchers with PhDs. The focus of this section will be the professional registered nurse and the licensed practical nurse.

Although English, Florence Nightingale (1820–1910) had a profound influence on American nursing. She advocated formal training for nurses and an administrative order for the hospital, with the matron (head nurse) as head (Rosenberg, 1987). After her success in decreasing the death rate of soldiers serving in the Crimean War, Nightingale opened a training school at St. Thomas's Hospital in England. The first training program in the United States was begun in 1872 at the New England Hospital for Women and Children in Boston. Training schools increased from 15 in 1880 to 1,105 by 1909, all under the direction of hospitals; nursing students provided much of the care in these institutions. Married women and those over 30 were excluded, along with divorced women (Kelly, 1987). Nurses were treated as subservient to both physicians and hospital administrators. According to Rosenberg (1987), until the 1920s the nurses' status was somewhat above that of a domestic servant. However, Wilkerson (1985) suggests that the public health nurse was "disciplined and well bred" (p. 1155), an "associate or co-worker of the physician" (p. 1157). In the early 1920s, soul searching and reform were beginning. Prior to World War I, Presbyterian Hospital, in conjunction with Teachers College, Columbia University, developed a 5-year combined college-diploma program.

A classic definition of nursing is that of Virginia Henderson (1966), who states: "The unique function of the nurse is to assist the individual (sick or well), in the performance of those activities contributing to health or its recovery (or peaceful death) that he would perform unaided if he had the necessary strength, will, or knowledge. And to do this in such a way as to help him gain independence as rapidly as possible" (p. 15).

There are many conceptual models and theories currently used and studied in nursing. Fawcett (1989) proposes that nursing is concerned with four concepts: patient, nurse, environment, and health. These four concepts are viewed differently in various models. Orem (1980) proposes that nursing is helping the patient with self-care. When the patient is unable to provide self-care, this role is assumed by the nurse. She states five methods to help others:

- Acting for or doing for another;
- Guiding another;
- Supporting another (physically or psychologically);
- Providing an environment that promotes personal development in relation to becoming; able to meet present or future demands for action; and
- Teaching another (p. 61).

Rogers, another popular nursing theorist, describes the person as an energy field, having no real boundaries. She proposes that the energy field of each person is in constant interaction with the environment, which is itself an energy field that is everything outside the human field. Wellness and illness are not differentiated within this model; rather, they are value judgments of society. Rogers differentiates nursing from other professions in that nursing's central concern is unitary human beings and their environments. Rogers indicates that the goal of nursing is promotion of health (Fawcett, 1989).

These two examples of nursing theory indicate what is either nursing's greatest strength or its greatest weakness—the diversity of opinion on what it is. It is a strength that nurses are open to new ideas and are not stagnant in a traditional view of nursing. Such an attitude will aid nurses in adapting to changes in the health care delivery system and creatively responding to clients' needs. But a problem with diversity is the lack of a cohesive voice for nursing.

Legal Definition

The American Nurses Association (ANA, 1995) suggests that authority for nursing is based on a social contract between society and the profession. The regulation of health professionals is a state responsibility. As such, each state has its own legal definition of the practice of nursing. Each state board of nursing defines and interprets the authority and scope of practice of registered nurses, although it is usually defined as the diagnosis and treatment of human responses. By 1923, legislation was enacted in all states for voluntary registration (Bullough, 1975). The first mandatory licensing law went into effect in New York State in 1947. It required that, with certain exceptions, only licensed professional nurses could legally use the title registered nurse.

For example, in New York State a registered professional nurse is described as "diagnosing and treating human responses to actual or potential health problems through such services as casefinding, health teaching, health counseling, and provision of care supportive to or restorative of life and well-being, and executing medical regimens prescribed by a licensed or otherwise legally authorized physician or dentist. A nursing regimen shall be consistent with and shall not vary from any existing medical regimen" (NY Education Law Article 139, Section 6902, 1989).

All states require that prospective registered nurses attend an approved nursing program and take a national licensing exam, the National Council Exam for Registered Nurses (NCLEX-RN) developed by the National Council of State Boards of Nursing. In 1996, of the 96,910 first-time candidates educated in the United States and its territories taking the exam, almost 87.7% passed (National Council of State Boards of Nursing, personal communication, March 3, 1997).

In some states, nurses (or certain categories of nurses) may prescribe pharmacologic agents or deliver a baby; in other states they may not. In addition, some states require continuing education for license renewal.

Licensed Practical Nurse. Licensed practical nurses (LPNs) and licensed vocational nurses (LVNs) work under the supervision of registered nurses or physicians and perform caregiving tasks such as medication administration and wound dressing change. LPN and LVNs must pass a national examination and are licensed in each state. In 1996 a total of 49,091 took the exam and 90.4% passed (National Council of State Boards of Nursing, personal communication, March 3, 1997).

Like other states, New York differentiates professional nursing from practical nursing, defining the later as "performing tasks and responsibilities . . . under the direction of a registered, professional nurse or licensed or otherwise legally authorized physician or dentist" (NY Education Law Article 139 Section 6902, 1989).

Other Nursing Personnel. Other nursing personnel include nurse aides, assistants, orderlies, technicians, and unlicensed assistive personnel (UAP). These personnel also work under the supervision of registered nurses and perform such simple tasks as temperature taking and comfort measures such as bathing and linen change. These occupations are not licensed by the states, although federal regulations require that nurse aides who work in long-term care facilities that are reimbursed by Medicare and Medicaid must complete a specified educational program and pass a written and practical test.

Education of Nurses

One of the most confusing aspects of nursing is the variety of programs for educating nurses. Unlike medicine, which has consistent educational requirements, nursing offers the student a number of options.

Although the American Nurses Association recommends that states require a baccalaureate degree to practice nursing, students can attend a 2-year college program, a 3-year hospital-based (diploma) program, a 4-year college program, a 2-year master's degree program, or a nursing doctoral (ND) program. North Dakota requires a baccalaureate degree, while all other state boards of nursing accept any of these programs as appropriate preparation for the registered nurse licensing exam. The practical nurse can attend programs in high schools, hospitals, junior colleges, or vocational schools.

Registered Professional Nursing. In January 1996 there were 1,516 basic educational programs for registered nurses in the United States, at the following educational levels: associate degree (876); baccalaureate degree (521); diploma (119) (National League for Nursing, 1996a). In addition, there were programs at the graduate level to prepare students for professional licensure. Total enrollments in professional nursing programs (as shown in Figure 4.2) were 261,219 in 1995, a 2.7% decrease from 1994. Graduations from professional nursing programs rose 2.3% (to 97,052) over the same period. Minorities comprised about 17.6% of enrollments (National League for Nursing, 1996a). Accreditation standards do not specify individual course requirements. Consequently, curricula vary widely from school to school, and transfer of nursing course credits is extremely difficult.

The first associate degree program began in 1952 (Anastas, 1984). The typical associate degree program requires basic liberal arts courses such as English and sociology. In addition, science courses, such as anatomy and physiology, are required. Nursing courses usually include fundamentals of nursing (clinical skills), maternal and child health, and care of acutely ill hospitalized adult patients. Experience is gained by practicing skills in the campus laboratory and in care of patients in institutional settings such as hospitals. The nurses enrolled in

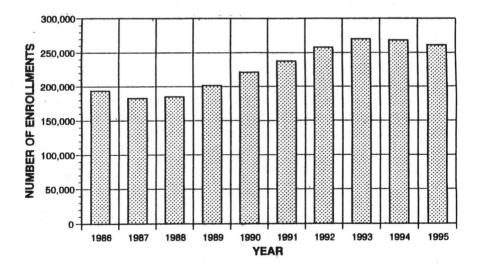

FIGURE 4.2   RN enrollments.
Source: National League for Nursing, 1996a.

associate degree programs are educated to be direct providers of care at the patient bedside. The programs are 2 academic years to 2 calendar years in length.

The typical diploma program is similar to the associate degree program, though usually under the auspices of a hospital. Often students are required to take liberal arts courses at a local college, and they receive college credit that can later be transferred to other colleges. The practical-experience sessions are usually longer than in the associate degree program, and the entire course takes about 3 years, with an emphasis on acute care (hospital-based) nursing. Diploma graduates who attend college often are not able to transfer the credits earned in the diploma program because until recently most of these were not degree-granting institutions.

The curriculum of the baccalaureate program is similar to that of liberal arts programs in other fields. Because the program is at least eight semesters long, the student takes more courses than in either the associate or the diploma program. Students take liberal arts courses such as English, math, and psychology and are required to take science courses such as microbiology, anatomy, and physiology. In addition, approximately half of the credits are usually in nursing courses. The organization of these courses varies from school to school. Some schools organize curricula developmentally and have courses devoted to care of infants, children, adults, and older people. Others base the curriculum on the relative health of populations and offer courses on prevention, episodic care, continuous care, and critical care. In addition, students learn to read and interpret research. Baccalaureate-prepared nurses are ready to work in community settings and leadership positions as well as in acute care settings. They are generalists who can provide care to individuals, groups, and families. Graduates are also prepared for advanced education in nursing.

Another opportunity for education in nursing is the external degree program, such as that offered by the Board of Regents of New York State. In 1971 an associate degree program was begun, followed by a baccalaureate degree program in 1976. Students obtain either degree by completing equivalency testing in liberal arts, sciences, and nursing. Students also must complete a practical exam. The program's philosophy centers on a person's knowledge and skills, rather than on how the information and skills were acquired. California's state education system has a similar program. Graduates of these programs are eligible for state licensure (Anastas, 1984).

Licensed Practical Nursing. Licensed practical nurses are educated in one of approximately 1,107 state-approved programs in the United States. More than half of these programs are in trade, technical, or vocational schools; the remainder are in colleges, community colleges, high schools, and hospitals. The programs typically are 1 year in duration and include classroom and clinical education. Although in 1996, 49,091 persons took the national licensing examination (National Council of State Boards of Nursing, personal communication), many of those who took the examination were actually students in professional nursing programs who took the examination to become LPNs prior to taking the RN examination. The typical LPN program includes basic courses in physical and social sciences and simple nursing procedures.

As shown in Figure 4.3, the National League for Nursing (1996b) reports that enrollments in 1995 were 56,028, down 5.7% from 1994. Graduates in 1995 numbered 44,234, a decrease of 1.9% from 1994, and the first decrease since 1988.

Other Nursing Personnel. Educational requirements for other nursing personnel, such as nurse aides, varies by employment setting. Some are educated in the setting in which they work, some in programs in high schools, and others in not-for-profit or for-profit vocational schools. Training takes from a few hours to 6 months or more.

Graduate Nursing Education

Nursing degree programs at the master's and doctoral level concentrate on nursing courses, with the assumption that the nurse baccalaureate graduate has had the

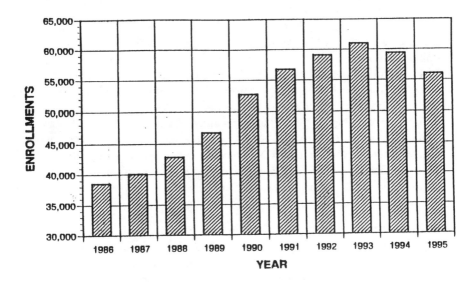

FIGURE 4.3 LPN enrollments.
Source: National League for Nursing, 1996b.

basic liberal arts and science courses. Historically, specialists in nursing were educated in specialized hospitals or became specialists based on clinical practice with a particular type of patient. In the 1950s colleges and universities began offering academic programs for specialty education. By the 1960s postgraduate education for clinical practice specialization was concentrated in universities.

Registered nurses with baccalaureate degrees can earn master's degrees in advanced clinical practice, teaching, and nursing administration/management. Within these three broad areas students usually focus on a nursing content area such as adult health, maternal-child health, psychiatric-mental health, or community health. Specific programs include everything from nursing informatics (computers) to home health care management to geriatrics to pediatric nursing. Most students choose to focus on advanced clinical practice. People with a baccalaureate in another field can earn a master's degree to prepare them for professional practice.

Within the generic category of advanced practice nurses, those with a clinical practice focus include clinical nurse specialists (CNSs), nurse practitioners (NPs), nurse midwives, and nurse anesthetists. Clinical nurse specialists have advanced degrees with expert skills in a particular area, such as mental health, cancer, or women's health. Nurse practitioners are educated to perform an expanded nursing role, usually in primary care. Nurse midwives are educated to provide pre-, intra-, and postpostpartum care and to provide family planning services and routine gynecological care, as well as caring for newborns. Nurse anesthetists are educated to administer anesthetics.

By 1995 there were 306 programs offering a master's degree in nursing, an increase of 30 over 1994. As shown in Figure 4.4, in 1995 there were 35,707 students enrolled in master's degree programs. This was an increase over the 34,157 enrolled in 1994. Only 29.6% were full-time, however, reflecting a rise of 11.9% from 1994 but a decrease from 68% full-time in 1972. The number of graduates per year continued to increase slightly to 9,261. About 13.2% were from minority groups, a percentage remaining essentially unchanged from 1994 (National League for Nursing, 1996c). In addition to clinical practice, master's degree programs also prepare RNs in management and teaching. By 1995 NP programs had 52.3% of enrollment in master's degree programs. Adult health continues to be the most popular specialty.

Doctoral Programs. Nurses can also earn doctoral degrees in nursing. There are three types of degrees offered. The ND (doctor of nursing) is similar to the MD; that is, it is the first professional degree, building on the earlier liberal arts or scientific education and preparing the student to take the state licensing exam to practice as a registered nurse. The DSN and DNSc are professional doctorates that prepare the nurse for advanced clinical practice. The PhD is a

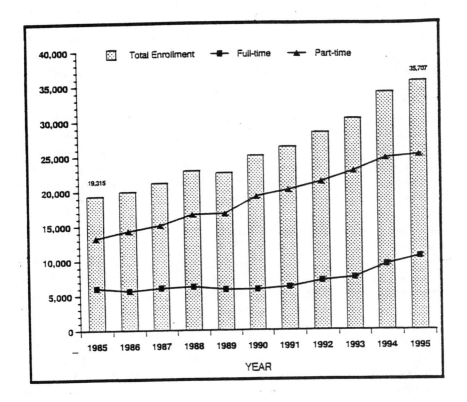

FIGURE 4.4   Master's enrollment.
Source: National League for Nursing, 1996c.

research degree, with requirements similar to the PhD in other fields: extensive preparation in a narrow field and a dissertation. In 1995 there were 64 doctoral programs in nursing in the United States, having grown from 5 programs in 1967. In 1995 a record 3,230 RNs were enrolled in these programs, and 425 graduated (National League for Nursing, 1996c).

Nurse Supply and Distribution

Historically, the major focus of nurses has been the care of the sick in institutions, particularly hospitals. Although most nurses still work in hospitals, the focus of nursing is moving away from that of dependent worker with a focus on illness to that of an independent practitioner with a focus on health. Porter-O'Grady (1986) proposes that the role of the nurse will shift from one in which responsibility for the care and safety of the patient is defined by the institution to one that focuses on health, with responsibility determined by the client. He suggests that functions will move from direct care dominated by the physician to team interaction focused on prevention. For many nurses this transition has already occurred.

Nurses have many options for the nature of their work, the hours they work, and the settings in which they work. Most people think of a nurse as a person in white, caring for a patient in the hospital; and although the majority of nurses have such jobs, many nurses work in other settings. Nurses work on a fee-for-service basis for clients who have mood disturbances, they deliver babies, and they work for government agencies developing policies for health care in certain geographic or political areas. Nurses teach schoolchildren about health, provide family planning services, administer intravenous nutritional therapy to people at home, and serve as patient advocates.

Nurses act as care integrators as well as caregivers (McClure & Nelson, 1982). As care integrators, nurses manage communication and coordination of activities of other care providers. Hospital nurses are the one type of health care provider who is with the patient 24 hours a day. Nurses provide direct care, which may include personal care such as bathing and help with toileting. Nurses administer medications and treatments, from intravenous fluids to dressing changes. Nurses teach the patient about his or her illness and about treatments that may be needed, and nurses assist patients to assume lifestyle changes that will improve their health. Nurses organize patient care across hospital departments, including radiology and laboratory. Nurses are usually the first persons to recognize an emergency and mobilize others to respond.

Another type of nurse manages a home care agency that provides nursing care to patients in their homes. She or he hires staff, assumes the financial responsibility for the agency, and serves as its manager. The nursing care must be coordinated so that the patient is getting the right care at the right time. In addition, nurses supervise the care provided by home health aides. They are responsible for the quality of care provided and for assuring that all government and accreditation regulations are met.

The nurse providing direct patient care in such an agency performs many of the same functions as those of the hospital nurse. There is, however, a greater focus on the patient (and family) assuming responsibility for the care. The nurse teaches the family along with providing the care. Nurses at home provide intravenous therapy, change dressings, administer medications, supervise respirators, and help families cope with the death of a loved one.

Nurse researchers review journals, collect and analyze data, and write reports. They usually have a doctorate. Areas of research interest to nurses include nursing practice, such as decision making and validating the efficacy of nursing practice; nursing education, such as learning strategies and methods to assess competence; and the administration, organization, and delivery of nursing services, such as cost-effectiveness of nursing services and delivery models (Welch, 1988).

Public health nurses usually work for a government agency and typically see clients in a clinic setting, trace contacts of communicable disease patients, and provide community education. They may work in a school or in an immunization clinic. They may design community education programs to prevent adolescent pregnancies or to decrease the spread of AIDS. Their focus is truly prevention and education to promote the health of a community.

Geographic Distribution and Educational Preparation. About 2.6 million people had licenses to practice as registered nurses (RNs) in the United States in 1996 (Division of Nursing, 1997). About 2.1 million (83%) were employed in nursing; 59% were working full-time. There was wide variation in the number of RNs in relation to the population. California, the state with the lowest ratio, had 566 RNs per 100,000; Massachusetts, the state with the highest ratio, had 1,128 RNs per 100,000 (Division of Nursing, personal communication, June 1997). Registered nurses are getting older, with a mean age of 44.3 in 1996. In part, this aging results from the high average age at graduation of associate-degree nurses. As shown in Figure 4.5, about 10% were minorities (defined as non-Whites). Although the percentage of male nurses is 5.4%, it has been increasing (Division of Nursing, 1997). The percentage of minority RNs is inconsistent with their representation in the general population and has been a concern of nursing and government for many years.

The 2.1 million employed RNs were prepared in a variety of educational programs, with 58.4% having less than a baccalaureate degree. The number of graduates from associate degree programs exceeded that from baccalaureate programs. Although fewer nurses are now prepared at the diploma level, about 35% of employed RNs had a diploma as their highest level of education. Only 193,159 (9.1%) had master's degrees and only .6% (14,300) were doctorally prepared (Division of Nursing, 1997).

Employment Settings. Although the percentage decreased from 1992, most RNs continued to work in general areas of hospitals caring for medical or surgical patients, as shown in Figure 4.6. About 1.3 million (60%) worked in hospitals, whereas only 170,856 (8.1%) worked in nursing homes. About 8% of RNs worked in ambulatory care settings. Staff nurses typically work in direct patient care, where they provide nursing care to individuals who may be acutely ill, as in a hospital; chronically ill or recovering from illness, as in a home

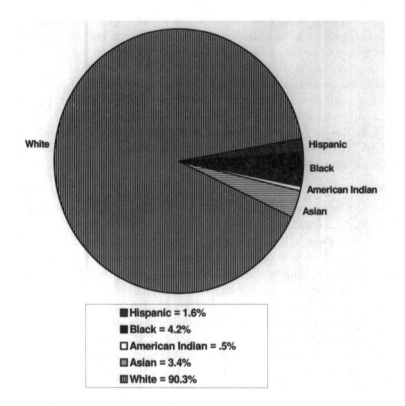

FIGURE 4.5   Registered nurses: Percentage of ethnic backgrounds—1996.
Source: Division of Nursing HRSA, 1997.

setting; or well but requiring preventive care, as in a health department or health maintenance organization (HMO) (Division of Nursing, 1997).

The average salary for full-time nurses was $42,071 per year in 1996, an increase of 11% over 1992. Salaries varied by geographic area, by setting, and by position. Nurses with more education had higher average salaries than those with less education, with staff nurses averaging $38,567 per year.

Advanced Practice Nursing. The Division of Nursing (1997) estimated that there were about 161,711 (6.3%) RNs academically prepared for advanced nursing practice in 1996, with 53,799 prepared as clinical nurse specialists. In addition, there were about 63,191 nurse practitioners, 30,386 nurse anesthetists, and 6,534 nurse midwives. All but nurse midwives increased in number over

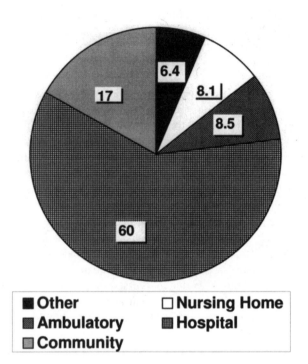

FIGURE 4.6 Registered nurses: Percentage in various employment settings—1996.
Source: Division of Nursing, HRSA, 1997.

1992. As discussed earlier, advanced practice nurses practice in a variety of settings. Legal limitations on such practice vary considerably from state to state. Numerous studies support the position that nurse practitioners provide health care equal in quality to that provided by physicians (Brown & Grimes, 1994), and it costs substantially less to educate a nurse practitioner than a physician.

Safriet (1992) points out that many more RNs are educated as nurse practitioners (NPs) than are those who practice as nurse practitioners. She attributes this difference to the regulatory constraints imposed by states. Examples include regulations or statutes limiting the care that practitioners can provide and restrictive reimbursement policies. In many cases NPs are reimbursed at a lower rate than that received by physicians who provide the same care with the same outcomes.

Safriet (1992) describes practice as prevention, diagnosis, prescription, and treatment and says that states have used a variety of approaches to expand the scope of practice for NPs, including revision of Nurse and Medical Practice Acts.

In addition to roles and title variations in different jurisdictions, restrictions on practice may vary. They fall into two general areas: the relationship between the NP and the physician (e.g., formal practice relationships, written practice protocols, and physician supervision) and restrictions on site of practice (e.g., to rural areas, to clinics only).

State regulations on nurses prescribing pharmaceuticals are inconsistent. In Oregon, NPs can prescribe pharmaceuticals, with no conditions of physician oversight (Safriet, 1992). In some states (Oregon, Washington, Alaska, and Montana) advanced practice nurses can prescribe without physician collaboration or authorizations, and in other states the nurse must have a practice arrangement with a physician. Some states limit prescriptive authority to central sites, to formularies, or to specific drugs (Carson, 1993).

Reimbursement continues to be a restriction on practice. Medicaid mandates direct Medicaid reimbursement of pediatric and family nurse practitioners (PNPs and FNPs) and midwives. Of 47 states responding to a federal study, 41 allow FNPs and PNPs to bill directly (Physician Payment Review Commission, 1993). In 1988 midwifery care became a covered Medicare service (e.g., for dialysis patients). Gynecologic care is excluded. Nurse practitioner care is covered if the NP works in collaboration with a physician and meets practice site restrictions (Safriet, 1992). Since January, 1997, Medicare has reimbursed advanced practice nurses.

The issues for the 21st century will likely focus on scope of practice, prescriptive authority, and reimbursement. If the United States moves to a system where financial barriers to health care are removed, the use of advanced practice nurses, especially NPs and nurse midwives will likely expand. It remains to be seen what physician reaction will be.

Organized Nursing

The ANA is the national professional organization for nurses. Founded in 1897, its members are not nurses but state or territorial nurses associations. The so-called tri-level system is composed of individual nurses who may join local and/ or district nurses associations. These in turn are usually organized by city or county into state associations. Delegates from the state associations meet annually at a national convention to set policy for the ANA.

The ANA also offers voluntary certification exams in a variety of nursing specialty areas, such as community health nursing, mental health nursing, and nursing administration. It serves as a lobbying association for nursing; its headquarters are in Washington, DC.

The National League for Nursing, founded in 1893 and unrelated to the ANA, serves as an accreditation body for the schools of nursing. Its subsidiary Community Health Accreditation Program (CHAP) accredits home health agencies. Membership is open to agencies, nurses, and nonnurses, although most members are in the nursing profession.

The American Association of Colleges of Nursing (AACN) is the organization of baccalaureate and higher degree programs. AACN has begun accrediting nursing programs, an activity that until 1996 was the responsibility of the National League for Nursing.

Sigma Theta Tau International is the honor society for nursing. An international organization located in St. Louis, its primary purpose is to foster scholarship in nursing. Membership is by election and restricted to those nurses who meet its academic and community service criteria.

In addition to the general organizations described above, nurses belong to numerous specialty groups. The groups tend to have as a focus the specialty area or site of practice for nurses. The first such organization was the American Association of Nurse Anesthetists (Kelly, 1987). Examples of other organizations include the American College of Nurse Midwives, the National Nurses Society of Addictions, the National Black Nurses Association, and the Society for Nursing History.

The National Institute for Nursing Research (NINR) is part of the National Institutes of Health (NIH). Prior to its establishment, funding for nursing research was under the auspices of the Division of Nursing in the Health Resources and Services Administration. The purpose of the NINR is to conduct and fund nursing research. Funding for fiscal year 1997 was $59.7 million. The primary focus is support of extramural research. Organized nursing viewed authorization of the institute as a milestone in the acceptance of nursing as a research-based profession.

Medicine

American medicine is undergoing a major transformation. Changes in the health care system are challenging physicians and transforming their traditional role in health care from the dominant, controlling force to one of many players. The world of fee-for-service, solo practice medicine is rapidly being replaced with managed care, capitation, and integrated delivery systems. The use of nurse practitioners, physician assistants, and other health care professionals is forcing greater collaboration and cooperation. Physicians still command responsibility for determining what type of care is provided, admitting patients into health facilities, ordering tests, prescribing medicine, and referrals to therapists, but they must now share the responsibility with other professionals and managed care organizations.

Undergraduate Medical Education

There are two types of medical education: allopathic (MD) and osteopathic (DO). Allopathic medicine is "a system of medicine based on the theory that successful therapy depends on creating a condition antagonistic to or incompatible with the condition to be treated" (Slee & Slee, 1986). Osteopathic medicine "emphasizes a theory that the body can make its own remedies, given normal structural relationships, environmental conditions, and nutrition. It differs from allopathy primarily in its greater attention to body mechanics and manipulative methods in diagnosis and therapy" (Slee & Slee, 1986). Once educated and trained, allopathic and osteopathic physicians are licensed by each state and have the same scope of practice.

There are 125 allopathic medical schools in the United States. The majority are part of academic medical centers that include tertiary hospitals and medical complexes. These medical schools graduated 16,029 physicians in 1996 (Barzansky, Jonas, & Etzel, 1996). In addition, there are 17 osteopathic schools, which graduated 1,843 physicians in 1995 (American Association of Colleges of Osteopathic Medicine, 1996). Of the 125 allopathic schools, 74 (59%) are publicly sponsored medical schools. The remainder are privately operated not-for-profit schools.

Medical school, the first formal step in the professional education of physicians, usually requires 4 years following baccalaureate education. The first 2 years are usually didactic (instruction taught in the classroom), and the second 2 years are primarily clinical experience. Numerous questions have been raised regarding the adequacy and appropriateness of the traditional medical education model and curriculum. Medical schools have been criticized for not encouraging primary care, for overemphasizing high-tech tertiary care, for emphasizing organ systems rather than the whole patient, for not educating more underrepresented minorities, and for not preparing physicians to work in the managed care environment.

As a result of these criticisms, there has been a major reassessment of medical school curricula, and many schools have modified or are considering modifying the traditional curriculum. Medical schools are becoming actively involved in primary care service delivery and many are developing affiliations with managed care organizations (Barzansky et al., 1996). In other cases, schools are beginning clinical training earlier in the education process.

Enrollment. Despite high tuition and a lengthy education, medicine is a highly sought profession, and applicants far exceed available slots. In 1995–96 there were 46,591 applicants to allopathic medical schools for 17,024 positions (Barzansky et al., 1996).

Allopathic medical school enrollment has been relatively stable since 1980 with graduations ranging between 15,300 and 16,300. However, as indicated in Table 4.3, female graduates have increased significantly, rising from 16.2% of graduates in 1975–76 to 40.9% in 1995–96. In that same year, 43% of new medical students were female (Association of American Medical Colleges, 1997).

TABLE 4.3 Allopathic Medical School Enrollment and Demographics

Academic year	Number of applicants	Applicant/ acceptance ratio	First-year enrollment	Graduates	Percentage of women graduates	Percentage of under- repre- sented minority graduates
1975–76	42,303	2.8	15,295	13,634	16.2	6.8
1985–86	32,893	1.9	16,963	16,117	30.8	7.4
1995–96	45,591	2.7	17,058	15,907	40.9	9.0

Source: American Association of Medical Colleges, 1997 Data Book, Tables B1, B6, and B8.

This has implications for the health care system, as female physicians have specialty and practice patterns different from those of male physicians.

The Association of American Medical Colleges (AAMC) defines underrepresented minorities as African American, Native American, Latino/Hispanic students/residents from Puerto Rico, and Mexicans and Chicanos. They exclude other Latino/Hispanics and Asians. The failure of American medical schools to enroll underrepresented minorities consistent with their representation in the general population has been of concern for many years. In 1975–76, 6.2% of allopathic medical school graduates were underrepresented minorities. In 1985–86 they were 10.4% of graduates; in 1995–96, 13.4% of medical graduates. Although this is encouraging, in 1990, 22% of Americans were African American, Native American, and Latino/Hispanic. This percentage has grown and is expected to continue to increase in future years. This underrepresentation is important not only in terms of social equity but also because of the potential impact on the outcomes of care (AAMC, 1997).

Financing. Because medical schools are part of educational/service enterprises, it is extremely difficult to determine what it actually costs to educate a physician. In 1994–95, allopathic medical schools reported revenues of $29.3 billion; the major sources of funding were faculty practice plans (33%), hospital and medical school programs (13.5%), and federal research and contracts (19%) (AAMC, 1997). This includes patient care services, research, and other related health professions education. By this method of accounting, student tuition accounted for only 4% of medical school revenues. Nearly 18% of revenues from public medical schools came from state and local government. One estimate of the cost of instruction for medical students for 1990–91 was $68,000 per year (Ginzberg, Ostow, & Dutka, 1993).

Tuition in private medical schools went up nearly $10,000 per year in the past decade, rising from an average of $15,023 in 1986–87 to $24,925 in 1996–97. Over the same period, tuition in public medical schools doubled, increasing from $4,574 in 1986–87 for in-state students to $9,107 in 1996–97 (AAMC, 1997). Scholarship funding did not keep pace with this rise in tuition. The mean debt of graduating medical students increased from $33,499 in 1986 to $75,103 in 1996 (AAMC, 1997).

Although physicians can anticipate higher than average incomes once they begin practice, the very lengthy period for education and training, with its relatively low salaries, combined with most loans coming due in the second year of residency training, may discourage medical students from choosing primary care. One recent survey found that higher debt had a significant impact on career decisions by medical students (Ginzberg et al., 1993).

Graduate Medical Education

Medicine is the only profession in which graduation from professional school is not sufficient for entry into active practice. To be licensed as a physician, to practice independently, and to be recognized by the profession as fully prepared, a physician must complete at least some supervised practical clinical experience through graduate medical education (GME), known as residency training. Until the early part of the 20th century, most physicians went directly from medical school to clinical practice. In response to the 1910 Flexner Report, a period of 1 or 2 years of internship was established to provide physicians with practical experience (Flexner, 1910/1960). Following this internship, most physicians practiced as generalists, providing a full range of services to their patients. As medicine became more complex and the number of physicians grew, there has been greater specialization and more advanced training. After specialty training, a physician may choose to "subspecialize." For example, after training for 3 years in internal medicine, a physician can choose 2 years additional training and subspecialize in such fields as cardiology and gastroenterology. Figure 4.7 shows the number of years beyond medical school needed for major specialty credentialing.

Graduate medical education has become a major financial and political issue in numerous states. It is a central determinant of the number and types of physicians available in a state. It is also a major source of funding for teaching hospitals, and in many states it has a major impact on Medicaid costs. The expansion of managed care, growing competition in health care, and other devel-

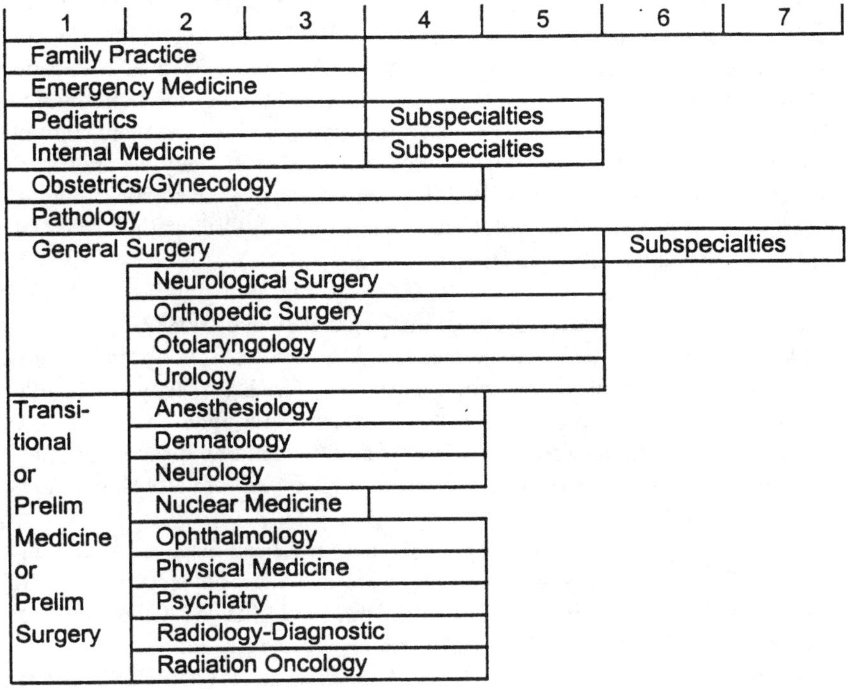

1	2	3	4	5	6	7
Family Practice						
Emergency Medicine						
Pediatrics			Subspecialties			
Internal Medicine			Subspecialties			
Obstetrics/Gynecology						
Pathology						
General Surgery					Subspecialties	
	Neurological Surgery					
	Orthopedic Surgery					
	Otolaryngology					
	Urology					
Transi-	Anesthesiology					
tional	Dermatology					
or	Neurology					
Prelim	Nuclear Medicine					
Medicine	Ophthalmology					
or	Physical Medicine					
Prelim	Psychiatry					
Surgery	Radiology-Diagnostic					
	Radiation Oncology					

FIGURE 4.7   Required number of years in residencies by specialty.
Source: NRMP Directory: Updated from AMA, 1996–1997 Graduate Medical Education Directory.

opments have brought a series of GME issues to the foreground nationally, in state capitals, and at teaching hospitals. The federal government and many states are considering legislation related to financing GME nationally.

Historically, the vast majority of residency training has taken place in large teaching hospitals. These hospitals offer residents an opportunity to see a wide range of patient conditions, and in many cases these hospitals are where medical schools and their faculty are located. Although the primary purpose of GME is the education of the resident, residents are also extensively involved in research, patient care, and teaching medical students. The concentration of training in large teaching hospitals has been criticized as resulting in the overuse of high-cost technology and inpatient services (Council on Graduate Medical Education, 1992; Physician Payment Review Commission, 1993). As services shift to ambulatory settings, there is a growing effort to provide more training outside hospitals to better prepare physicians for future practice and to encourage primary care.

The Growth of Residency Programs and Specialties. In 1995 there were 7,657 allopathic residency programs accredited by the Accreditation Council for Graduate Medical Education (ACGME) ("Graduate Medical Education," 1996). The ACGME is a private national body that oversees the accreditation of allopathic residency programs. In each specialty, a residency review committee (RRC) establishes standards and assesses individual residency program performance against those standards. In 1996 there were 594 osteopathic internship and residency programs accredited by the American Osteopathic Association (American Osteopathic Association, 1996).

In 1995 there were more than 98,000 physicians in training in ACGME-accredited allopathic residency programs. This included 21,372 new first-year residents, of whom 16,072 were graduates of U.S. medical schools; the remaining 5,300 were graduates of foreign medical schools ("Graduate Medical Education," 1996). Thus, there were 33% more first-year residents than graduates of U.S. medical schools. There were 6,078 interns and residents in osteopathic training programs (American Osteopathic Association, 1996). All of these were graduates of U.S. schools.

Throughout the 1980s and early 1990s there has been a sharp increase in the total number of residents and specialty areas in which physicians could train. The number of residents increased by 42% from 1982 to 1995 ("Graduate Medical Education," 1993, 1996). During this same period, the number of first-year residents rose only about 13%, from 18,972 in 1982 to 21,372 in 1995. The rapid growth in the total number of residents reflects the sharp increase in the number of residents going on to subspecialty training.

The number of subspecialty residents grew at a substantially higher rate than that of primary care residents. Although there was some subspecialty training in 1982, there were no accredited programs. The growth in residency positions and subspecialties may have been appropriate when there was a perceived shortage of physicians. Furthermore, specialization may lead to improved quality. However, there is a growing concern that there will be a significant oversupply of specialists in the United States (Pew Health Professions Commission, 1995). It is generally recognized that the key determinant is the number and mix of physicians in residency training (Wennberg, Goodman, Nease, & Keller, 1993).

Women are far more likely to go into those specialties generally considered primary care. Although women made up 34% of all residents in 1995, they constituted 42% of the residents in family practice, 61% in pediatrics, and 58% in obstetrics. On the other hand, they represented only 18% in surgery and 7% in orthopedic surgery ("Graduate Medical Education," 1996).

International Medical Graduates. Foreign medical school graduates, referred to as international medical school graduates (IMGs), are eligible to apply for residency training if they pass specific examinations testing medical knowledge and English proficiency and meet other conditions. Because of the concern with shortages in the 1950s and 1960s, immigration requirements for physicians were reduced. As noted above, in 1995 the number of new, allopathic residents was nearly one third above the number of U.S. allopathic medical graduates. This gap was filled primarily by foreign medical school graduates. Numerous groups have recommended that the total number of residency slots in the United States be sharply reduced ("Consensus Statement," 1997; Council on Graduate Medical Education, 1992; 1997; Institute of Medicine, 1996; Physician Payment Review Commission, 1993).

Forty-seven percent of IMGs in training in the United States are on exchange visas that allow them to learn American medicine but require that they return to their native country ("Graduate Medical Education," 1996). However, many of these physicians have obtained waivers and have been permitted to stay in the United States (Institute of Medicine, 1996).

Financing Graduate Medical Education. Historically, generous federal, state and private insurance reimbursement rates for hospitals, a robust hospital sector, and federal investment in research supported the training of physicians as part of the basic function of academic medical centers and hundreds of other hospitals. These hospitals are facing major challenges; the new marketplace has little tolerance for expenses that are not directly related to patient care.

Embedded in complex hospital reimbursement formulas used by Medicare and most Medicaid programs are costs for GME. In federal fiscal year 1995, Medicare provided an estimated $6.6 billion (Institute of Medicine, 1997) and Medicaid an estimated $2 billion (Salsberg, 1997), and Mullan, Rivo, and Politzer estimated that private payers paid $5 billion. The total reimbursement in 1993 was estimated to be equal to $184,000 for each resident for each year of training (Mullan, Rivo, & Politzer, 1993). Residents and teaching hospitals are involved in a number of activities, such as research and care for the poor. Despite numerous attempts, there is no consensus on the actual cost or the reasonable cost of training a physician (Salsberg, 1997).

The evolution of the health care system, particularly increased competition, is leading to fundamental changes in the financing of GME. It is no longer possible to support the higher costs of teaching hospitals through generous and hidden reimbursement policies. As managed care enrollment increases (especially for Medicaid and Medicare recipients) and competition expands, there is growing pressure to revise the financing of GME.

Physician Supply and Distribution

In 1995 there were approximately 582,000 allopathic physicians involved in patient care in the United States (American Medical Association, 1996-97b). As

**TABLE 4.4   Distribution of Allopathic Physicians by Activity
in 1995**

Activity	Number	Percentage
Patient Care	582131	80.8
Office-Based Practice	427275	59.3
Hospital-Based Practice	154856	21.5
Residents/Fellows	96352	13.4
Full-Time Staff	58504	8.1
Other Professional Activity	43312	6.0
Medical Teaching	9469	1.3
Administration	16345	2.3
Research	14340	2.0
Other	3158	0.4
Not Classified	20579	2.9
Inactive	72326	10.0
Address Unknown	1977	0.3
Total	720325	100.0

Source: AMA, 1996/97 Physician Characteristics and Distribution in the U.S., Table A-1.

seen in Table 4.4, the majority of these physicians are in office-based practice, which includes solo and group practice as well as other ambulatory care settings, such as HMOs.

The number of allopathic patient care physicians nearly doubled between 1975 and 1995 (American Medical Association, 1996-97b). The physician-to-population ratio increased from 135 patient care physicians per 100,000 people in 1975 to 216 in 1995, or about 60%.

Geographic Distribution. The supply of physicians is not evenly distributed across the United States. The majority of physicians are concentrated in urban areas. In 1992 there were nearly 2,200 urban and rural areas that were classified by the federal government as health professional shortage areas (HPSAs). In total, these areas needed about 4,500 additional physicians to adequately serve their populations (Rivo & Satcher, 1993). The lower physician-to-population ratio in most rural areas reflects, in part, the need for a minimum population base required to support a physician practice and to maintain skill levels for certain specialties.

Doubling the total U.S. physician supply over time has led to some dispersal of physicians to rural areas, but the vast majority of new physicians locate in urban areas. From 1980 to 1995, the supply of allopathic physicians grew by

TABLE 4.5   Allopathic Patient Care Physicians; Total, Total to Population Ratio, Female and IMGs

	Total patient care physicians	Physician to population ratio*	Female physicians Number	Percentage	International medical graduates (IMG) Number	Percentage
1975	311,937	135	24,345	7.8	61,416	19.7
1980	376,512	159	39,969	10.6	72,935	19.4
1985	448,820	180	64,424	14.4	95,362	21.2
1990	503,870	198	86,376	17.1	106,515	21.1
1995	582,131	216	126,583	21.7	136,812	23.5

*The ratio of nonfederal allopathic physicians to civilians.

Source: AMA, 1996/97 Physician Characteristics and Distribution in the U.S., Tables A-1, A-9, and A-13.

231,000 in metropolitan statistical areas, an increase of 60%. During the same period, the number of physicians in nonmetropolitan areas went up 22,600, an increase of 39 % (American Medical Association, 1996-97b). Despite the growth in total physician supply, serious access problems remain in rural areas (National Rural Health Association, 1992).

Gender, Ethnicity, and Nationality. One of the most striking recent changes in the physician supply in the United States has been the steady growth in the number of female physicians. The percentage of female patient care physicians grew from 7.8 % in 1975 to 21.7% in 1995, as seen in Table 4.5 (American Medical Association, 1996-97b). This trend will continue as the number of women in medical school continues to increase. However, because most physicians practice for 30 to 40 years and only a small percentage leave or enter practice each year, it takes many years to significantly modify the composition of the physician workforce (Kindig & Libby, 1996). The growth in the number of IMGs has been steady, although far less dramatic than for women. This growth is likely to continue for several years, given the current number of IMGs in training.

Specialty Distribution. Table 4.6 presents the number of allopathic physicians in selected specialties from 1975 to 1995. Although in 1995 there were more than 130,000 physicians in the four specialties generally considered primary care (internal medicine, family practice, pediatrics, and general practice), non-

TABLE 4.6   Allopathic Physicians by Specialty 1975, 1985, and 1995

Specialty	1975	1985	1995	Percentage of change (85–95)	Average annual percentage of change (85–95)
Total Physicians	393,742	552,716	720,325	30.3	1.3
Anesthesiology	12,861	22,021	32,853	49.2	2.0
Cardiology	6,933	13,224	18,998	43.7	1.8
Dermatology	4,661	6,582	8,563	30.1	1.3
Emergency Medicine	0	11,283	19,112	69.4	2.7
Family Practice	12,183	40,021	59,345	48.3	2.0
Gastroenterology	2,381	5,917	9,551	61.4	2.4
General Practice	42,374	27,030	16,867	–37.6	–2.3
General Surgery	31,562	38,169	37,569	–1.6	–0.1
Internal Medicine	54,331	88,862	115,168	29.6	1.3
Neurology	4,131	7,776	11,397	46.6	1.9
Obstetrics/ Gynecology	21,731	30,867	37,652	22.0	1.0
Ophthalmology	11,129	14,881	17,464	17.4	0.8
Orthopedic Surgery	11,379	17,166	22,037	28.4	1.3
Otolaryngology	5,745	7,267	9,086	25.0	1.1
Pathology	11,720	15,456	17,824	15.3	0.7
Pediatrics	22,192	36,026	50,620	40.5	1.7
Psychiatry	23,922	32,255	38,098	18.1	0.8
Radiology (Diag. & Ther.)	15,071	21,644	27,846	28.7	1.3
Urology	6,667	8,836	9,886	11.6	0.6

Source: AMA, 1996/97 Physician Characteristics and Distribution in the U.S., Table A-2.

P care

primary-care physicians comprised two thirds of all practicing physicians. This distribution is significantly different from most other countries, such as Canada, Great Britain, and Germany, where more than 50% of physicians are in primary care specialties (Physician Payment Review Commission, 1993).

As indicated in Table 4.6, the rapid increase in physicians between 1975 and 1995 has not been evenly spread among specialties, with non-primary-care specialties growing far more rapidly than primary care. However, there are a

TABLE 4.7   Comparison of Metropolitan* to Nonmetropolitan Physicians

Specialty	Mean patient visits/week		Mean fee for office visit		Mean net income	
	Metropolitan	Nonmetro	Metropolitan	Nonmetro	Metropolitan	Nonmetro
All Physicians	98.4	135.4	$66.20	$41.47	$150,000	$146,000
General/ Family Practice	116.3	163.4	$53.26	$38.84	$108,000	$112,000
Internal Medicine	93.4	137.4	$71.04	$50.52	$142,000	$150,000
Surgery	91.8	133.0	$66.74	$38.43	$200,000	$250,000

*Metropolitan includes locations with populations of 1,000,000 or more.

Source: AMA, Socioeconomic Characteristics of Medical Practice 1996, Tables 15, 27, and 50.

number of strong indications that the number of U.S. medical school graduates interested in primary care is increasing (Association of American Medical Colleges, 1997; Physician Payment Review Commission, 1997).

Physician Practice Patterns. Practice patterns vary between urban and rural settings. As indicated in Table 4.7, physicians in nonmetropolitan areas provide more visits per week. Fees are also lower in nonmetropolitan areas; although overall average income is less in rural areas, this appears to reflect the different mix of specialties. When analyzed by specialty, rural physicians had a higher net average income in many specialties, reflecting longer hours and more visits per week.

Physician Income

Physicians are among the highest paid professionals in the United States, and their income through the 1980s grew faster than that of any other profession (Pope & Schneider, 1992). Figure 4.8 indicates the median net income after expenses but before taxes for some of the major specialties. Of particular interest is the much lower level of net income for primary care physicians.

Market forces may have affected the income of physicians. In 1994 average physician income declined almost 4% from the prior year (Simon & Born, 1996). This was the first time since the AMA collected these data that income had declined. A recent study by Simon and Born (1996) attributes at least part of this decline to the expansion of managed care. However, they found that specialists' incomes declined similarly in markets with and without extensive managed care penetration. One possible explanation may be the general increase in competitiveness in the marketplace simultaneous with the sharp increase in the number of specialists.

Organized Medicine

The American Medical Association (AMA) represents the interests of some physicians by lobbying at the national and state level, by collecting and analyzing data, and by producing and distributing reports on subjects of importance to physicians. Recently, the association has become concerned with the anticipated surplus of physicians and the impact of the expansion of managed care on the physician workforce.

The National Medical Association is the professional society for Black physicians. With membership of about 14,500, it has councils in areas such as maternal and child health, and medical education and sections on the major medical specialties (Daniels & Schwartz, 1994).

Specialty societies, such as the American Academy of Pediatrics and the American Society of Obstetricians and Gynecologists, represent the professional interests of specific specialties. According to Jones (1993), there are 12,200 medical organizations, boards, and groups in the United States.

The American Association of Medical Colleges (AAMC) represents American medical schools and teaching hospitals. The AAMC has been very active promoting medical school and GME reform and efforts to increase underrepresented minorities in medicine.

The new health care system is likely to create a serious challenge to organized medicine. Physicians may grow increasingly disillusioned and frustrated: their incomes are being squeezed by managed care, there is increased competition, practices are being bought and sold by for-profit companies or aggressive not-for-profits, and managed care organizations and health care networks have significant control over where and how physicians practice. Although organized medicine remains influential on a political level, physicians may look to other organizations to represent them in their everyday struggle with the health system. For example, as more physicians become employees of larger organizations, unionization is

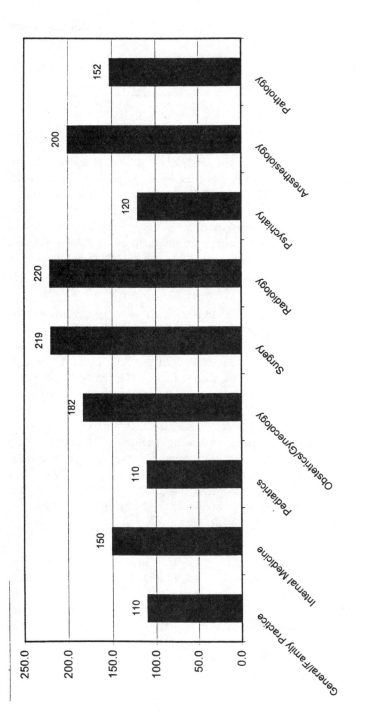

FIGURE 4.8 Median physician net income (in thousands of dollars) after expenses before taxes, by specialty, 1994.

Source: AMA, 1996 Socioeconomic Characteristics of Medical Practice, Figure 17.

likely to grow. It is unclear how far this will spread and what its impact will be on organized medicine.

Physician Assistants

Physician assistants (PAs) work under the direct supervision of physicians. Regulation of PAs varies from state to state, but supervision does not mean on-site supervision. In most states the amount of delegation to a PA is a decision between the physician and the PA.

Both demand and supply of PAs have been increasing rapidly. PAs can expand access to primary care and improve physician productivity, both of which are promoted by the expansion of managed care; PAs can substitute for physicians in hospitals; and in some areas, PAs may replace residents in training.

Physician Assistant Education. Physician assistants are a relatively new profession. The first PA educational program was established by Duke University Medical Center in 1965, in part to allow an opportunity for medics who had gained clinical experience in the Vietnam War to practice in the health care system. In 1971, with the passage of the Comprehensive Health Manpower Act, federal financial support became available and contributed to the rapid expansion of programs. In 1996 a total of 2,532 PAs graduated from 71 accredited PA programs (American Academy of Physician Assistants, 1997b). Physician assistant programs are located in a number of academic settings and offer a variety of credentials; most programs are 24 months long. The average cost to educate a PA student in 1993 was estimated to be $7,045 per year (Oliver, 1993). More than half the 1992 entering PA students already had a bachelor's degree or higher. Most students entered with extensive experience in the health field (American Academy of Physician Assistants, 1997a).

Practicing Physician Assistants. In 1997, there were about 34, 683 PAs practicing in the United States, and they work in a wide variety of specialties. The largest number of PAs (11,035) work in family practice (40%); the second largest concentration (4,361 or 16% of PAs) is in surgery. As the effectiveness and efficacy of PAs is demonstrated in more and more specialty areas, PAs may be drawn away from primary care specialties. The ratio of PAs to population varies widely between states, from 391 per million population in Alaska to 15.9 per million in Mississippi. PAs work in a wide array of practice settings, providing over 129 million patient visits in 1996 (American Academy of Physician Assistants, 1997a). In 1996, the average of total annual income for full-time clinically practicing PAs was $64,584 (American Academy of Physician Assistants, 1997b).

Other Health Workers

Other "Doctors"

In addition to physicians, there are a variety of other health professionals educated in graduate programs beyond the baccalaureate who use the title "doctor." These doctors tend to specialize in specific areas of the body. Each specialty has its own body of knowledge, professional association, and educational requirements.

Dentists. In 1997 there were approximately 155,000 practicing doctors of dental science (DDS). About 79% of these dentists were generalists, and 91% were in private practice. Only about 32% of dentists were in practice with other dentists. Although the 1995–96 first-year dental class had 35% minorities and 35% women, only 8% of practicing dentists were women. Dentistry has far fewer graduate training opportunities than medicine, and there are more dental school graduates who would like advanced training than there are opportunities (American Dental Association, 1997).

Podiatrists. Podiatrists diagnose, treat, and prevent abnormal foot conditions. Educated at one of the seven podiatric medicine schools in the United States, they perform surgery and prescribe and administer pharmaceuticals. Licensed by individual states, they deliver a wide range of medical and surgical services. There were about 11,000 practitioners in 1997 (American Podiatric Medical Association, 1997; U.S. Department of Health and Human Services, 1992).

Chiropractors. Chiropractors treat problems of the body's structural and neurological systems. Chiropractors are educated in 4-year programs, which follow at least 2 years of undergraduate education. There are 17 chiropractic schools; 14 were accredited by the Council on Chiropractic Education (CCE) (U.S. Department of Health and Human Services, 1992). Their graduates are eligible for licensure in all 50 states. In 1994, there were approximately 50,000 licensed chiropractors (Cooper & Stofler, 1996).

Optometrists. Optometrists are licensed to diagnose and provide selective eye treatment. In some states they are licensed to prescribe a limited range of pharmaceuticals. There were about 26,000 practicing optometrists in the United States in 1997 (American Optometric Association, 1997). Educated at one of the 16 schools of optometry, students have 4 years of professional training following undergraduate school. Optometrists, while having far less formal education than ophthalmologists (physicians with residency training in ophthalmology), provide many of the same services as these physicians, usually at a lower cost. As state government considers increasing the scope of practice of optometrists and as managed care expands, there has been conflict about the overlapping roles of optometrists and ophthalmologists.

Allied Health Personnel

The Committee on Allied Health Education and Accreditation of the American Medical Association, which oversees nearly 3,000 educational programs, defines allied health as "a large cluster of health care related professions and personnel whose functions include assisting, facilitating, or complementing the work of physicians and other specialists in the health care system, and who choose to be identified as allied health personnel" (U.S. Department of Health and Human Services, 1992, p. 177). This general definition allows for occupations to be added and subtracted as the health care system evolves.

Allied health occupations are among the fastest growing in health care. The number of allied health professionals is difficult to estimate and depends on the definition of allied health (U.S. Department of Health and Human Services, 1995). The U.S. Department of Health and Human Services, Bureau of Health Professions, estimates that there were approximately 1.8 million allied health personnel in the United States in 1990 (U.S. Department of Health and Human Services, 1992). Unlike medicine, women dominate most of the allied health professions, representing between 75% and 95% of most of the occupations. For some allied health professions (physical therapists) all states require licensure, while others (occupational therapy) are required to be licensed in only some states. The following briefly describes some of the major occupations usually included under the allied health rubric.

Clinical Laboratory Personnel. Clinical laboratory workers perform a wide array of tests on body fluids, tissues, and cells to assist in the detection, diagnosis, and treatment of diseases and illnesses.

Diagnostic Imaging Personnel. Originally referred to as x-ray technicians and then radiologic technologists and technicians, this field is now more appropriately referred to as diagnostic imaging, as it continues to expand to include nuclear medicine technologists, radiation therapists, sonographers or ultrasound technologists, and magnetic resonance technologists.

Dietetic Personnel. Dietitians are trained in nutrition and are responsible for providing nutritional care to individuals and for overseeing nutrition and food services in a variety of settings, ranging from hospitals to schools.

Emergency Medical Personnel. Emergency medical technicians (EMTs) are responsible for providing a wide range of services on an emergency basis for trauma and other emergency situations and in the transport of emergency patients.

Medical Record Personnel. Overseeing medical information to assure that it meets the medical, administrative, and legal requirements is the responsibility of medical record administrators, medical record technicians, and medical record coders.

Occupational Therapy Personnel. Occupational therapists are registered by the American Occupational Therapy Association (AOTA) if they graduate from an accredited educational program and pass the AOTA certification examination.

Physical Therapy Personnel. Physical therapists (PTs) evaluate and treat patients to improve functional mobility, reduce pain, maintain cardiopulmonary function, and limit disability. Physical therapists treat movement dysfunction resulting from accidents, trauma, stroke, fractures, multiple sclerosis, cerebral palsy, arthritis, and heart and respiratory illness. Physical therapy assistants (PTAs) work under the direction of PTs and help carry out the treatment plans developed by PTs.

Respiratory Therapy Personnel. Respiratory therapy personnel evaluate, treat, and care for patients with breathing disorders. They work under the direction of qualified physicians and provide such services as emergency care for stroke, heart failure, and shock and treat patients with emphysema and asthma.

Speech-Language Pathology and Audiology. Speech-language pathologists and audiologists identify, assess and provide treatment for individuals with speech, language, or hearing problems.

In addition to physicians, nurses, and allied health personnel, there are a variety of other health care practitioners. Space does not permit a thorough discussion of each of these workers, but several examples will be given.

Pharmacists. Pharmacists have traditionally prepared pharmaceutical prescriptions; however, their role has expanded to include providing information to patients about pharmaceuticals and drug interactions. All states require pharmacists to be licensed. Pharmacists are educated in 5-year bachelor of science programs or 6-year PharmD programs. In 1995 there were 75 colleges of pharmacy, with only 25 offering just the BS degree. Pharmacists can specialize by obtaining advanced degrees in pharmacy and through residency programs. Pharmacy technicians assist pharmacists with activities not requiring the judgment of a pharmacist.

Public Health Personnel. Public health includes a variety of health workers. Whereas most health practitioners work with individual patients, public health workers are concerned with the health of entire communities and population groups. Many work in state and local health departments. The U.S. Department of Health and Human Services (1992) estimates that in 1989 there were approximately 500,000 professionals working in public health. Of these a substantial proportion were educated in a specific clinical discipline, such as nursing, medicine, or other professions discussed in this chapter. Some public health professionals are graduates of the nation's 24 accredited schools of public health (U.S. Department of Health and Human Services, 1992). In 1989 these schools had an enrollment of 10,000 students. Their graduates are prepared in such areas as epidemiology, nutrition, health education, environmental health, health administration, and health policy. Other schools also prepare students in these areas.

Alternative Healers. Alternative healers include naturopaths and practitioners of acupuncture and oriental medicine. Several states have now begun to license these alternative healers.

Current Issues

The rapid changes in health care in America present both a crisis and an opportunity for health workers. Competition, managed care, for-profit health care, integrated delivery systems, new technologies, and improved telecommunications are among the major factors influencing health care.

The Patient/Consumer as Part of the Health Care Team

One of the changes likely to have an impact on health workers is the changing role of patients, now also referred to as consumers, clients, and customers.

Consumers are becoming more involved in their health and in the health care they obtain. They have access to more information than ever before from their health care providers, on television, in print, and via the Internet. For example, the Agency for Health Care Policy and Research developed clinical practice guidelines on topics such as smoking cessation and cancer pain. Each of these clinical practice guidelines had a "patient's guide" that reviewed the types of treatment available and how to work with health providers to obtain care. Another example: pharmacologic agents that were once available only by prescription are now available over the counter at pharmacies.

In the competitive market, many managed care organizations and hospitals are trying harder to involve and please patients. Many health care organizations now ask consumers how satisfied they are with their care, in part to appeal to what consumers want from health care. Many hospitals have been "reengineered" to be more "patient focused."

The Role of Professionalism in Assuring Quality of Care

Historically, the nation has relied heavily on licensure, accreditation, and certification of health professionals to assure health care of high quality. But as the health care system has become more competitive and consumers demand improved outcomes, the health care system's efforts to improve quality have expanded significantly. They are reviewed in depth in chapter 14. This section briefly reviews the role of professionalism and individual accreditation in assuring quality. As managed care expands, it is likely that there will be numerous skirmishes among professionals, government, and managed care organizations as to who should determine who is qualified to perform what activities and who should monitor the quality of care. Freidson (1973) stated that the autonomy of medicine is a characteristic of a profession:

> First, the claim is that there is such an unusual degree of skill and knowledge involved in professional work that non-professionals are not equipped to evaluate or regulate it. Second, it is claimed that professionals are responsible—that they may be trusted to work conscientiously without supervision. Third, the claim is that the profession itself may be trusted to undertake the proper regulatory action on those rare occasions when an individual does not perform his work competently or ethically. (p. 137)

Health professional licensure is the government's primary method of assuring qualified professionals. Most health professionals are licensed by states. Licensure requires graduation from an approved school and passage of an examination. In addition to formal licensure, government also exerts considerable control over the practice of medicine through requirements for and monitoring of performance under Medicaid and Medicare. Government also has an impact on practitioners through its regulation of health facilities, such as hospitals, that provide care.

Another way to promote quality is through certification and accreditation. Beyond licensure, physicians can be certified for specialty practice in medicine and nurses can be certified for specialty practice in nursing. Each medical specialty establishes standards for physicians seeking to be board-certified. This includes, at a minimum, satisfactory completion of an accredited residency program and passage of an exam. It may also include several years of practice and completion of a minimum number of specific procedures. In a few specialties, such as family practice, a physician must periodically pass an exam or demonstrate continuing competency. Board certification provides professional recognition within a specialty and sets minimum qualifications for practice as a board-certified physician. This is an important example of the self-regulation of the medical profession by physicians.

Another approach to promoting high quality of care is through the regulation of health facilities, including requiring that they monitor the professionals who practice in their facility. For example, the Joint Commission on Accreditation of Health Care Organizations (JCAHO) requires that hospitals and other facilities monitor physicians who practice in their facilities. The JCAHO requires hospitals to set criteria for staff privileges. For example, the hospital's medical by-laws may state that only board-eligible or board-certified surgeons may conduct surgery. They may further state that only physicians with certain training or experience, as evaluated by the hospital's medical board, may perform certain complex procedures. In this way, although all physicians in the same state may have the same license, physicians are restricted by health facilities in the types of care they can provide. Unlike licensure, which is usually for life, health facilities are expected to monitor performance on an ongoing basis. Nevertheless, as indicated in chapter 14, the public's concern with quality is likely to go well beyond relying on the profession to regulate itself.

Growing Competition Among Professionals

Although the future health care system is expected to make extensive use of health care teams—multiple caregivers working together—there is also likely to be greater competition between and among professions. Attractive professional careers, good incomes, professional autonomy, and/or an opportunity to help others have helped to fuel an increasing supply of health professionals. When combined with pressures from purchasers and insurers to constrain costs, this growing supply is likely to lead to conflicts, which probably will be greatest where different professions or subgroups provide similar or overlapping services. Among the potential conflicts are nurse practitioners and physicians; primary care physicians and specialists; nurses and unlicensed assistive personnel; psychiatrists, psychologists, and social workers; and ophthalmologists and optometrists.

In a competitive marketplace, price often becomes the determining factor in the competition between providers (this assumes that they can provide similar products of similar quality). Thus, if there is a surplus of providers, which is likely in many communities, there may be growing competition based on price. Overtly, the competition will not be about price or turf but about qualifications, with each group claiming it is better qualified than the other to provide a specific service.

Advanced practice nurses, including nurse practitioners, are likely to increasingly compete with physicians. The conflict is expected to be especially strong between those physicians and nurses who provide primary care because of the overlap in the care they provide. Nurse practitioner education is substantially less expensive than physician education—which requires 7 to 10 years, including GME. After education to become a registered nurse, the average cost (including overhead) per graduate of primary care nurse practitioner programs was about $34,096 (Lewin-VHI, Inc., 1994). This compares to more than the $68,000 cost per year for medical school (Ginzberg et al., 1993) and $184,000 per year in third-party reimbursement for graduate medical education (Mullan et al., 1993).

As the supply of specialty physicians outpaces the demand, more and more specialists will attempt to provide primary care. Many primary care physicians argue that specialists do not have the skills or orientation to provide primary care. At the same time, many specialists argue that, having gone through a generalist education before subspecializing, they are qualified to provide primary care. For example, a gastroenterologist completes an internal medicine residency program before subspecializing. Some primary care physicians may also provide services that the specialist believes only the specialist should provide. For example, many primary care physicians believe they are able to provide care for all but the most psychotic and complex patient, whereas many psychiatrists argue that patients with depression are often misdiagnosed yet treated by primary care physicians.

In addition to competition among professionals, there will be increased competition between professionals and assistive personnel because of the overlap in the care they provide. Examples of the occupations with overlap include physical therapy assistants and physical therapists and unlicensed assistive personnel and registered nurses. Although most people would agree that it is clear that for some activities, such as making a patient bed, unlicensed assistive personnel can provide the same quality of care as registered nurses; for other activities, such as starting an intravenous line, the quality comparison is less clear and research evidence sparse. There is some concern that the increased use of unlicensed assistive personnel may compromise the quality of care patients receive. This is likely to be an area in which professionals disagree with health care managers.

The Supply and Demand for Physicians

Some of the more hotly debated health workforce policy issues in the 1990s have concerned issues of physician workforce planning. At the core of the debate is how to encourage the production of a physician workforce that can best meet the health needs of the nation. The debate has been fueled by lack of agreement as to whether the current and projected supply is adequate to meet the nation's needs as well as whether the marketplace, without specific government interventions, will produce the appropriate role number, mix, and distribution of physicians (Cooper, 1995; Ginzberg, 1996; Mullan, 1996; Reinhardt, 1996; Rivo & Kindig, 1996).

The National Council on Graduate Medical Education has been in the forefront of efforts to encourage a physician supply and distribution better able to meet the medical needs of the nation. Their findings are summarized in the box that follows (Cooper, 1995; Ginzberg, 1996; Mullan, 1996; Reinhart, 1996; Rivo, 1996).

The increase in the supply of physicians is expected to continue for the next several decades. Simultaneous with the steady growth in supply has been the expansion of managed care. It is well documented that HMOs use fewer physician resources than the fee-for-service system: several studies have found HMO staffing to range from 120 to 138 per 100,000 (Politzer et al., 1996). The COGME (1996) estimated that there is generally a need for between 145 and 185 physicians per 100,000 population. There are signs, such as the drop in physician incomes (Simon & Born, 1996), that the surplus is beginning to be felt by practicing physicians.

There are some benefits of a surplus. It may drive prices down; it may make it easier to get physicians to underserved areas; and it may make physicians more sensitive to patients. On the other hand, physicians could generate their own demand by ordering tests and revisits. In a surplus, physicians may not have sufficient volume to maintain their skills; society and individual physicians will have wasted a large investment; and there is little public benefit for the investment (Wennberg et al., 1993).

Another reason for concern has been the high level of public financing for GME. Medicare and Medicaid provided an estimated $8.6 billion in 1995 (Institute of Medicine, 1997). With a growing expectation of a physician surplus, it is hard to justify massive public support. Congress has considered legislation to decrease this financing, but efforts have been blocked by concerns with the impact on teaching hospitals and care for the poor in inner cities that are served by residents (Iglehart, 1996).

Findings of the Council on Graduate Medical Education

The Council on Graduate Medical Education (COGME) was authorized by Congress in 1986 to advise the federal government and the Congress on issues related to the supply, distribution, and use of physicians. The council issued its third report with specific findings and recommendations for physician workforce reform (COGME, 1992). The following is a brief summary of the council's findings and recommendations. These issues and concerns continue to be of significance.

1. The nation has too few generalists and too many specialists.
2. Problems of access to medical care persist in rural and inner-city areas despite large increases in the number of physicians.
3. The racial/ethnic composition of the nation's physicians does not reflect the general population and contributes to access problems for underrepresented minorities.
4. Shortages exist in the specialties of general surgery, adult and child psychiatry, and preventive medicine and among generalist physicians with geriatrics training.
5. Within the framework of the present health care system, current physician-to-population ratio in the nation is adequate. Further increases in this ratio will do little to enhance the health of the public or to address the nation's problems of access to care. Continued increases in this ratio will hinder efforts to contain costs.
6. The nation's medical education system can be more responsive to public needs for more generalists, underrepresented minority physicians, and physicians for medically underserved rural and inner-city areas.
7. The absence of a national physician workforce plan, combined with financial and other disincentives are barriers to improved access to care (COGME, 1992).

The Role of Government and the Market. The Clinton administration proposal for national health care reform included an extensive role for government in determining how many doctors should be trained in each specialty. This proposal had little support. Others have argued that the market should decide, not government (Foreman, 1996). There are some indications that the market can work. For example, after reports that new anesthesiologists could not find jobs, the number of U.S. medical school graduates selecting anesthesiology dropped significantly (Association of American Medical Colleges, 1997). However, there are other factors that deter an effective market for the production of physicians: hospitals decide how many residents to train—often based on their service and financial needs, not community needs; Medicare hospital reimbursement, a government program, includes generous support for residents; a large supply of IMGs is available and anxious to enter American medicine regardless of the market (the percentage of IMGs training in anesthesiology went up as U.S. medical graduates selected other specialties); and there is no systematic information available to medical students on demand by specialty.

The Medical School Versus GME Cutback Debate. The Pew Health Professions Commission (1995) recommended that U.S. medical schools reduce graduates by 20% in anticipation of the surplus and increased managed care. This brought a strong objection from the medical school community, which expressed concern that reducing U.S. medical school graduates in the absence of constraints on IMGs would just substitute IMGs for U.S. graduates. This would not reduce the growing supply of doctors but would cut U.S. admissions when applicants were at an all-time high. Although this debate is not resolved, some U.S. medical schools have begun to reduce admissions.

An Emerging Consensus. The shortcomings of relying totally on government or totally on the market is leading to proposals that have a role for both. Numerous groups have made proposals to reform GME that involve revising federal GME payment policies, the establishment of a GME trust fund, reducing the number of IMGs and supporting a transition for alternatives to residents as caregivers ("Consensus Statement," 1997; Council on Graduate Medical Education, 1997; Institute of Medicine, 1996; Physician Payment Review Commission, 1997).

In early 1997 the federal government approved a Medicare demonstration in New York that provides financial incentives for downsizing (Health Care Financing Administration, 1997). Several states are providing financial incentives to achieve public policy goals, including additional primary care physicians (Salsberg, 1997). In addition, several studies have been undertaken to better estimate the demand in specific specialties (Meyer et al., 1996; Politzer et al., 1996).

Nurse Supply and Demand

Cyclical shortages and surpluses of registered nurses (RNs) have occurred during the 20th century. This reflects, in part, the difference in the wages between nurses and nonnurses and within nursing and the lag in response of the educational system to changes in demand. In response to severe shortages in the late 1980s, salaries for RNs rose significantly; these higher salaries led to an increase in the numbers of RNs being educated. In the 1990s, as RN salaries rose, including relative to LPNs and unlicensed assistive personnel, employers increasingly sought ways to substitute lower cost personnel for RNs.

The Role of the Government and the Market. In addition to changes in salaries, in the early 1990s other approaches were implemented in part through government subsidy to balance supply and demand. These include recruiting more people into nursing (such as through scholarships and marketing), improving retention (such as through raising starting salaries and increasing salary progression), and decreasing the demand.

Health organizations have reorganized to decrease the demand for nurses. Approaches included case management, work redesign, and the use of technology, among others. Case management had as its goal the prudent use of health resources, often leading to decreased length of stay. Redesign interventions varied from partnerships between nurses and unlicensed assistive personnel to rethinking the components of care required by patients during an episode of illness. An example of technology was the use of computerized information systems to improve communication and decrease paperwork. Many hospitals have expanded the use of unlicensed assistive personnel to reduce the number of nurses needed.

The Ideal Workforce

Since the turn of the 20th century, educators, clinicians, and government have debated about the best way to assure that the United States has an appropriate health care workforce. The criteria that characterize an appropriate health workforce are (1) enough health care workers; (2) adequate distribution of those workers among the geographic regions, including urban and rural areas; (3) broad-banded workers; (4) efficient workers; and (5) informed consumers.

The ideal workforce would have an adequate supply of health care workers. As discussed in "Counting Health Workers" (p. 67), assessing the current supply of health care workers is difficult. Establishing the number and type of health care workers we need is a major challenge that balances the interests of the existing health professions, the payers, and the government. Having the right health care workers at an accessible place at the time a person, family, or community needs the provider is equally difficult. Ideally, the least expensive health care worker who has the requisite skills would provide the care.

Health care workers have traditionally had well-defined legally prescribed roles. Although there is obvious overlap among many health professions, each profession continues to define its area of expertise. From a community's point of view, health care workers who are "broad banded" (competent in a number of areas) would improve access to care. For example, if an RN could perform physical therapy, then small rural hospitals might not have to hire both RNs and physical therapists. If the food service worker could also perform housekeeping functions, then hospitals would not have to hire housekeepers but could have one worker perform both activities.

The efficiency of the health care work force is an obvious need in an era that is increasingly cost-conscious. Not only must health care workers provide effective care, but that care must be provided efficiently.

Finally, the informed and well-educated consumer will know when a health problem requires a health care worker and which worker can provide the needed care most efficiently.

Americans, through their government representatives, have developed the current system. This system uses professional licensure and regulation of providers—both the clinicians and organizations in which clinicians work—in addition to voluntary certification and accreditation. Another approach to this method is "competency-based." Rather than a health worker being licensed as a general provider, such as a physician, if providers are competent to provide care, they provide it. Thus, a nurse may become competent at prescribing pharamocologic agents, through a formal education program, through individual study, and/or from clinical practice. The nurse would then be able to prescribe. Criticism of this approach is primarily focused on the concept that health care cannot be divided into a number of tasks.

Although health care employment has grown consistently for the past several decades, pressure to control costs and the changing health care system may lead to fewer health workers in the future. Most health workers work in hospitals; as hospitals close beds and facilities, the health workers who worked in those hospitals will not be needed. Although many of them will find employment in other settings, some will not (Berliner & Kovner, 1994; Center for Health Workforce Studies, 1997).

Conclusions

The rapid changes in the health care delivery system will undoubtedly lead to changes in the roles of health professionals and their relationships. Managed care will require greater collaboration among health professionals. It will also mean greater supervision and management of health professionals by nonhealth professionals. Some health professionals may resist this inevitable oversight as an intrusion on their professionalism. New relationships and even a new definition of professionalism may need to be developed.

The provision of health care in the early 21st century will require the cooperation and coordination of the many health workers currently providing health care and those who will be educated in these health careers in the future and will likely include health care workers educated in new careers. There are large areas of overlap in the care provided by health professionals. Physicians, nurses, and physical therapists all work with patients in performing range-of-motion exercises. Physicians, nurses, and pharmacists all teach patients about medications and their side effects. Nurses and respiratory therapists teach and supervise patients in deep breathing following surgery. It is not surprising that patients in hospitals complain because they cannot tell who is who—everyone is wearing a white uniform or lab coat or, more recently, many health care workers are wearing street clothes.

Most health care professionals today are educated in their own professional schools, in health facilities, and in divisions of colleges and universities. Few health professionals currently take any courses together, nor do many even share the same faculty. In many cases, students in a variety of professions receive their clinical training in the same institutions. However, there is rarely any shared clinical teaching or learning. To provide effective care in the future, health care professionals should share much of their initial academic health experiences. If most health professionals take pathophysiology, why shouldn't they take it together? Others suggest that there should be a core curriculum for health professionals, with specialization into physical therapy, respiratory therapy, or imaging occurring at the upper division in the undergraduate curriculum.

It seems clear that as health care moves from the hospital to the community, even more coordination of patient care and cooperation among health providers will be required. It is also likely that any one of a variety of health professionals will be the primary caregiver or coordinator, and that will vary depending on the health problems of the clients.

Discussion Questions

1. How should graduate medical education be funded?
2. How should health professional education be funded?
3. Discuss the pros and cons of professional licensure.
4. How should the need for health workers be determined?
5. What should the role of employers be in assuring the quality of professional services?
6. Discuss the pros and cons of competition between specialists and generalists; and competition among professionals.
7. What should the government's role be in the supply and demand for health professionals?
8. Discuss the characteristics of the ideal health work force.

References

American Academy of Physician Assistants, Division of Research and Data Services, *Information Update*. Alexandria, VA: Author, 1997a.

American Academy of Physician Assistants, Division of Research and Data Services, *Physician Assistants: Statistics and Trends, 1991—1996.* Alexandria, VA: Author, 1997b.

American Association of Colleges of Osteopathic Medicine (AACOM), *1992 Annual Statistical Report.* Rockville, MD: Author, 1992.

American Association of Colleges of Osteopathic Medicine (AACOM), *1996 Annual Statistical Report.* Rockville, MD: Author, 1996.

American Dental Association, "Dental Education and Career Information Fact Sheet" (Internet), www.ada.org/prac/careers/fs-dent.html (June 12, 1997).

American Hospital Association, *Hospital Statistics: Emerging Trends in Hospitals the AHA Profile of United States Hospitals.* Chicago: Author, 1996–97.

American Medical Association, *Graduate Medical Education Directory.* Chicago: Author, 1996–97a.

American Medical Association, *Physician Characteristics and Distribution in the U.S.* Chicago: Department of Physician Data Services, 1996–97b.

American Nurses Association, *Nursing's Social Policy Statement.* Washington, DC: Author, 1995.

American Optometric Association, 1997, http://www.aoanet.org

American Podiatric Medical Association, 1997, http//www.apma.org

American Osteopathic Association, *Opportunities: 1996–97 Directory of Osteopathic Postdoctoral Education Programs,* (Vol. 5). Chicago: Department of Education, 1996.

Anastas, L., *Your Career in Nursing.* New York: National League for Nursing, 1984.

Association of American Medical Colleges, *AAMC Data Book Statistical Information Related to Medical Education.* Washington, DC: Author, 1997.

Association of American Medical Colleges (AAMC), "U.S. Medical School Graduates' Rising Interest in Primary Care Indicates Trend," [Internet], http://aamcinfo.aamc.org/about/progemph/nrmp/release.htm (June 19, 1997).

Barzansky, B., Jonas, H., & Etzel, S., "Educational Programs in US Medical Schools, 1995–1996," *Journal of the American Medical Association, 276,* 714–719, 1996.

Berliner, H. S., & Kovner, C. T., *The Supply and Demand for Health Workers in New York City: 1995–97.* New York: New York State Department of Health, 1994.

Brown, S. L., & Grimes, D., "A Meta-Analysis of Nurse Practitioners and Nurse Midwives in Primary Care." *Nursing Research 44*(6), 332–339, 1995.

Bullough, N., "Barriers to the Nurse Practitioner Movement: Problem of Women in a Women's Field," *International Journal of Health Sciences,* 5, 225, 1975.

Bureau of Labor Statistics, "Occupational Outlook Handbook" (Internet), available: http://www.bls.gov/oco/ocos079.htm (June 16, 1997).

Carson, W., "Gains and Challenges in Prescriptive Authority," *American Nurse, 25*(6), 19, 20, 1993.

Center for Health Workforce Studies and New Century Concepts, *The Changing Health Care System in New York City: Implications for the Health Workforce.* New York: Planning and Placement Fund of 1199/ League Employment, Training, and Job Security Fund, 1997.

"Consensus Statement on Physician Workforce," Association of American Colleges, (Internet), available: http://www.aamc.org/meded/edres/workforce/consen.htm (1997).

Cooper, R. A., "Perspectives on the Physician Workforce to the Year 2020," *Journal of the American Medical Association, 274,* 1534–1543, 1995.

Cooper, R. A., & Stoflet, S. J., "Trends in the Education and Practice of Alternative Medicine Clinicians," *Health Affairs, 15,* 226–238, 1996.

Council on Graduate Medical Education, *Patient Care Physician Supply and Requirements: Testing COGME Recommendations* (DHHD Publication No. HRSA-P-DM95-3). Rockville, MD: Bureau of Health Professions, Health Resources and Services Administration, 1996.

Council on Graduate Medical Education. *1997 Recommendations to the Congress and the Secretary of Health and Human Services on Graduate Medical Education Payment Reform.* Rockville, MD: U.S. Department of Health and Human Services. 1997.

Council on Graduate Medical Education, *Third Report: Improving Access to Health Care Through Physician Workforce Reform: Directions for the 21st Century.* Rockville, MD: U.S. Department of Health and Human Services, Human Resources Services and Administration, 1992.

Daniels, P., & Schwartz, C. A. (Eds.), *Encyclopedia of Associations* (28th ed., Vol. 1, pt. 2). Washington, DC: Gale Research, 1994.

Division of Nursing, Bureau of Health Professions HRSA, *Advance Notes from the National Sample Survey of Registered Nurses.* Rockville, MD: Author, 1997.

Fawcett, L., *Analysis and Evaluation of Conceptual Models of Nursing* (2nd ed.). Philadelphia: F. A. Davis, 1989.

Flexner, A., *Medical Education in the United States and Canada.* Washington, DC: Science and Health Publications, 1960. (Original work published 1910)

Foreman, S., "Managing the Physician Workforce: Hands Off, the Market Is Working," *Health Affairs, 15*(2), 243–249, 1996.

Franklin, J. C., "Industry Output and Employment Projections to 2005," *Monthly Labor Review, 118*(11), 45–60, 1995.

Franklin, J. C., "Industry Output and Employment Projections to 2006." *Monthly Labor Review, 120*(11), 39–57, 1997.

Freidson, E., *Profession of Medicine.* New York: Dodd, Mead & Company, 1973.

Ginzberg, E., "The Future Supply of Physicians," *Academic Medicine, 71,* 1147–1153, 1996.

Ginzberg, E., Ostow, M., & Dutka, A., *The Economics of Medical Education.* New York: Josiah Macy Jr. Foundation, 1993.

"Graduate Medical Education," *Journal of American Medical Association, 270,* 1116–1122, Appendix II, 1993.

"Graduate Medical Education," *Journal of the American Medical Association, 276,* 739, Appendix II, Table 1, 1996.

Health Care Financing Administration, U.S. Department of Health and Human Services, "New York Teaching Hospitals Participating in Graduate Medical Education Demonstration," *HHS News,* February 1997.

Henderson, V., *The Nature of Nursing.* New York: Macmillan, 1966.

Iglehart, J. K., "Health Policy Report: The Struggle to Reform Medicare," *New England Journal of Medicine, 334,* 1071–1075, 1996.

Institute of Medicine, *The Nation's Physician Workforce: Options for Balancing Supply and Requirements.* Washington DC: National Academy Press, 1996.

Institute of Medicine, *On Implementing a National Graduate Medical Education Trust Fund.* Washington, DC: National Academy Press, 1997.

Jones, S. R., "Organized Medicine in the United States," *Annals of Surgery, 217,* 423–429, 1993.

Kahl, A., & Clark, D., "Employment in Health Services: Long Term Trends and Projections," *Monthly Labor Review,* 30–55, August 1986.

Kelly, L. Y., *The Nursing Experience.* New York: Macmillan, 1987.

Kindig, D. A., & Libby, D. L., "Domestic Production vs. International Immigration. Options for the US Physician Workforce," *Journal of American Medical Association, 276,*978–982, 1996.

Lewin-VHI, Inc., *Federal support for the training of Nurse Practitioners and Nurse-Midwives* (Contract No. 240-93-0043). Washington, DC: Health Resources and Services Administration, Bureau of Health Professions, Division of Nursing, 1994.

McClure, M. L., & Nelson, M. J., "Trends in Hospital Nursing," in L. H. Aiken (Ed.), *Nursing in the 1980s: Crisis, Opportunities, Challenges* (pp. 59–73). Philadelphia: Lippincott, 1982.

Meyer, G. S., Jacoby, I., Krakauer, H., Powell, W., Aurand, J., & McCardle, P., "Gastroenterology Workforce Modeling,"*Journal of the American Medical Association, 276,* 689–694, 1996.

Moses, E., *The Registered Nurse Population. Finding from the National Sample Survey of Registered Nurses, March 1992.* U.S. Department of Health and Human Services, Public Health Service, Health Resources and Services Administration, 1992.

Mullan, F., "Powerful Hands: Making the Most of Graduate Medical Education," *Health Affairs, 15*(2), 250–254, 1996.

Mullan, F., Rivo, M., & Politzer, R. M., "Doctors, Dollars, and Determination: Making Physician Work-force Policy," *Health Affairs, 12* (Suppl.), 138–151, 1993.

National League for Nursing, *Nursing Data Source 1996* vol. 1 (Publication No. 19-6932). New York: Author, 1996a.

National League for Nursing, *Nursing Data Source 1996* vol. 2 (Publication No. 19-6959). New York: Author, 1996b.

National League for Nursing, *Nursing Data Source 1996* vol. 3 (Publication No. 19-6940). New York: Author, 1996c.

National Rural Health Association, *Study of Models to Meet Rural Health Care Needs through Mobilization of Health Profession Education and Services Resources.* Rockville, MD: U.S. Department of Health and Human Services, Health Resources and Services Administration, 1992.

Oliver, D. R., *Ninth Annual Report on Physician Educational Programs in the United States, 1992–1993.* Iowa City, IA: Association of Physician Assistant Programs, 1993.

Orem, D. E., *Nursing: Concepts of Practice.* New York: McGraw-Hill, 1980.

Pew Health Professions Commission, *Critical Challenges: Revitalizing the Health Professions for the Twenty-first Century.* San Francisco: University of California, San Francisco, Center for Health Professions, 1995.

Physician Payment Review Commission (PPRC), *Annual Report to Congress 1993.* Washington, DC: Author, 1993.

Physician Payment Review Commission (PPRC), *Annual Report to Congress 1997.* Washington, DC: Author, 1997.

Politzer, R., Gamliel, S., Cultice, J., Bazell, C., Rivo, M., & Mullan, F., "Matching Physician Supply and Requirements: Testing Policy Recommendations," *Inquiry*, *33*, 181–194, 1996.

Pope, G., & Schneider, J., "Trends in Physician Income," *Health Affairs*, 181–193, Spring 1992.

Porter-O'Grady, T., *Creative Nursing Administration: Participative Management into the 21st Century*. Rockville, MD: Aspen, 1986.

Reinhardt, U. E., "The Economic and Moral Case for Letting the Market Determine the Health Workforce," in *The U.S. Health Workforce Power, Politics and Policy*. Washington, DC: Association of Academic Health Centers, 1996.

Rivo, M. L., & Kindig, D., "A Report, on the Physician Work Force in the United States," *New England Journal of Medicine*, *334*, 892–896, 1996.

Rivo, M. L., & Satcher, D., "Improving Access to Health Care Through Physician Workforce Reform: Directions for the 21st Century," *Journal of American Medical Association*, *270*, 1074–1078, 1993.

Rosenberg, C., *The Care of Strangers*. New York: Basic Books, 1987.

Safriet, B., "Health Care Dollars and Regulatory Sense: Role of Advanced Practice Nursing," *Yale Journal on Regulation*, *9*(2), 149–220, 1992.

Salsberg, E., *State Strategies for Financing Graduate Medical Education*. New York: United Hospital Fund, 1997.

Silvestri, G. T., "Occupational Employment to 2006," *Monthly Labor Review*, *120*(11), 58–83, 1997.

Simon, C. J., & Born, P. H., "Trends: Physician Earnings in a Changing Managed Care Environment," *Health Affairs*, *15*, 124–133, 1996.

Slee, V. M., & Slee, D. A., *Health Care Terms* (2nd ed.). St. Paul, MN: Tringa Press, 1986.

U.S. Department of Health and Human Services, "Americans Less Likely to Use Nursing Home Care Today," *HHS News* [Internet], available: http://www.cdc.gov/nchswww/releases/97news/97news/nurshome.htm (June 12, 1997).

U.S. Department of Health and Human Services, *Health Personnel in the United States: Eighth Report to Congress: 1991* (DHAS Publication No. HRSPOD 92-1). Washington, DC: Resources and Services Administration, 1992.

Welch, C., "Conference Report: Directions for Nursing Research in New York State," *Journal of the New York State Nurses Association*, *19*(3), 16, 1988.

Wennberg, J., Goodman, D. C., Nease, R. F., & Keller, R. B., "Finding Equilibrium in U.S. Physician Supply," *Health Affairs*, 89–103, Summer 1993.

Wilkerson, K. B., "Public Health in Nursing: In Sickness or in Health," *American Journal of Public Health*, *75*, 1155–1157, 1985.

Wing, P., & Salsberg, E. S., *Data Systems to Support State Health Personnel Planning and Policymaking: A Resource Guide for State Agencies*. Albany, NY: New York State Department of Health, 1992.

5

Comparative Analysis of Health Systems: An International Perspective

Victor G. Rodwin

Learning Objectives

1. Analyze conceptual and methodological issues in the study of health systems.
2. Identify common problems of health policy in diverse health systems.
3. Understand key features of health systems in France, Canada, and Britain.
4. Describe the U.S. health system in comparative perspective.
5. Think about the uses of comparative analysis in learning from abroad.

Topical Outline

Issues in the study of comparative health systems
    Conceptual issues
    Methodological issues
    Learning from abroad
Common problems of health policy in three countries
    France
    Canada
    Britain
The U.S. health system: A comparative perspective
    American values and popular opinion

The structure of health care financing and organization
Policy responses to health sector problems
The uses of comparative analysis in learning from abroad

Key Words: **Health systems, inputs and outputs, outcomes, inefficiency in the allocation of resources, determinants of health policies, national health insurance (NHI), national health service (NHS), socialized health service, direct vs. indirect third-party payment, policy learning.**

Comparative analysis of health systems in industrially advanced nations has produced a large and growing literature that provides profiles and improves our understanding of health care systems abroad.[1] This chapter begins with an overview of general issues in the comparative study of health systems. Next it assesses some common problems of health policy in three countries: France, Canada, and Britain. Finally, it analyzes the U.S. health system from a comparative perspective and examines the uses of comparative analysis, for Americans, in learning from abroad.

Issues in the Study of Comparative Health Systems

Three stages may be distinguished in the evolution of comparative health systems research (Dumbaugh & Neuhauser, 1979), all of which are apparent in contemporary studies of health systems abroad. The first stage dominated until the mid-1960's and continues today in the form of "travelogues" written by physicians returning from overseas tours (Corson, 1948). During the second stage, researchers described health systems from a variety of perspectives—often with hopes of promoting health care reform.[2] During the third stage there has been an attempt to make the comparative study of health systems into a kind of social science. The research has focused largely on explaining variation across health systems on

---

[1]Suggested readings on comparative health systems and policy appear at the end of this chapter.
[2]For examples of some classic books, see Douglas-Wilson and McLachlan (1974); Fry (1970); Raffel (1985); Roemer 1(1977, 1981, and 1991); Saltman (1988); Sidel and Sidel (1977). In addition, there are some excellent single country case studies: Andreopoulos (1975) on Canada; Forsyth (1966), Lindsey (1962), Edwards (1995) on Britain; Hyde (1974) and Siegrist (1947) on the former Soviet Union; Weinerman and Weinerman (1969) on Eastern Europe.

the basis of received theories within such disciplines as anthropology, sociology, political science, and economics.[3]

The social science approach to comparative health systems has the inherent defect of its virtues. To achieve a rigorous study design, it has classified descriptive data on health systems, formulated hypotheses, and tested them against available evidence. Among economists, for example, the focus has been largely on cross-sectional comparisons of health services utilization and expenditures, thus narrowing the scope of research questions and eroding the ideals shared by Stage 2 scholars, who were more motivated by the pragmatic concerns of improving the delivery of medical care.

Social scientists tend to display more interest in the theoretical concerns of their disciplines than in social change. Nevertheless, some excellent studies have been produced, and this has raised some conceptual and methodological issues that remain at the center of health services research.

Conceptual Issues

The concept of a "health system" is clearly central. And yet there is no fully satisfactory definition of this concept, for it is difficult to agree both on the boundaries of the system and on a definition of health. Blum (1981) provides a visual model of health, suggesting that health care services are merely one input into health among three others—heredity, behavior, and environment (Figure 5.1). Weinerman (1971) defines the health system as "all of the activities of a society which are designed to protect or restore health, whether directed to the individual, the community, or the environment." Anderson (1972) has outlined more concretely the "boundaries of a relatively easily defined system with entry and exit points, hierarchies of personnel, types of patients"—in short, what he calls "the officially and professionally recognized 'helping' services regarding disease, disability and death" (p. 22).

Viewing the concept of health system at a macrosociological level, Field (1973) proposes the following formal definition: "that societal mechanism that transforms generalized resources . . . into specialized outputs in the form of health

---

[3]For a good example of how anthropologists approach the comparative study of health systems, see Leslie (1976). For a sociological perspective, see Anderson (1989), Elling (1980), Field (1989) or Light and Schuller (1986). For an organization theory perspective, see Saltman and Van Otter (1992). For a political science approach, see Altenstetter (1978), Immergut (1992) and Leichter (1979, 1991). For an economic approach, see Hu (1976), Hurst (1992), McLachlan and Maynard (1982), and Schweitzer (1978). Also, for examples of single-country studies, see Eckstein (1959) and Klein (1995) on England, Wilsford (1991) on France, Stone (1980) on Germany, and Field (1967) on the former Soviet Union.

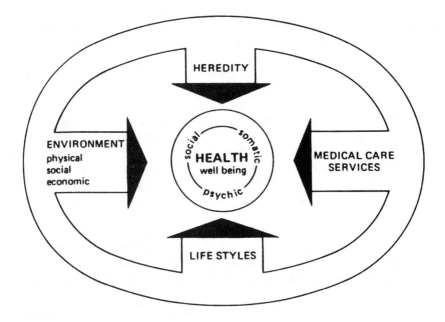

FIGURE 5.1   Inputs to health.
Adapted from H. Blum, *Planning for Health* (2nd ed.), New York: Human Sciences Press, 1981, p.3.

services." He adds that "the 'health system' of any society is that social mechanism that has arisen or been devised to deal with the incapacitating aspects of illness, trauma, and (to some degree) premature mortality . . . the five D's: death, disease, disability, discomfort, and dissatisfaction" (pp. 768, 772).

Another approach to the concept of health system is to define it implicitly by postulating a causal model of it. Thus, drawing on Weinerman's definition and on Elling and Kerr's (1975) proposed framework for studying health systems, De Miguel (1975) outlines four subsystem levels that influence health status: individual, institutional, societal, and environmental. Such an approach allows one to analyze a health system by investigating the effects of a hierarchy of independent variables on the dependent variable, health status. It also raises questions about the most effective levels at which to effect system change.

Methodological Issues

The fundamental methodological issue in comparative health systems research involves devising a study design and selecting alternative systems that allow the analyst to hold some variables constant while manipulating experimental ones. In the area of health policy, for example, how does one evaluate the success of cost-containment efforts in health systems characterized by diverse patterns of financing and provider reimbursement? Quasi-experimental research designs would suggest matching two health systems on all but a few policy-related factors. But "matching," let alone a real experiment, is rarely feasible in policy research.

One response to this difficulty has been to match health systems on at least some criteria (e.g., levels of health resources) and then to call for "in-depth studies of contrasting cases" (Elling & Kerr, 1975). Another response has been to use the language of natural experiment and view "most similar systems" as laboratories in which to assess the effects of alternative policy options at home (Marmor, Bridges, & Hoffman, 1978). A third response is to adopt a "modular approach" that examines systematically diverse components of health systems (Ellencweig, 1992).

Another methodological concern in the social science approach to comparative health systems research is whether the descriptive studies and data collected during stages 1 and 2 are actually comparable. If they are not, this casts great doubt on the utility of making international comparisons. If they are, qualifications must usually be made.

The most difficult methodological issues arise in evaluating health systems, for this involves specifying the relationship between the elements of a health system (inputs and outputs) and their impact on health status (outcomes). But how does one distinguish the effect of health services on health from the effects of improvements in social services, income security, education, and transportation, not to mention the social and physical environments? This question raises the problem of devising indicators of health status, It also explains why, in his comparative study of the United States, Sweden, and England, Odin Anderson (1972) found it impossible to attribute differences in the usual health indices of morbidity and mortality to patterns of medical care organization in these countries. To evaluate health systems, it is necessary to agree on consistent definitions of health system inputs and outputs and to devise health status indicators to measure outcomes.

Learning from Abroad

Although there is a large literature on the comparative analysis of health systems, there are rarely attempts to draw lessons from comparative experience. Comparative studies of health policy are sparse. Most often, they describe an experience in a range of policy areas; only rarely do they interpret, let alone evaluate, this experience. Exceptions to this general rule are of interest because they have contributed at least three ideas that have implications for learning from abroad.

First is the idea of evolutionary progress in health systems. Medical sociologists such as Field (1973) and Mechanic (1976) argue that health systems in Western industrialized nations are evolving in similar directions. Drawing on Field's typology, consisting of five systems—the private health system, the pluralistic one, the national health insurance (NHI) system, the national health service (NHS), and the socialized health service—such views would suggest that the direction of change in modern societies is from the system of Type 1 to that of Type 5 (Table 5.1). Unlike Field and Mechanic, who are not convinced that such change necessarily implies "progress," Milton Roemer (1977) describes similar trends as a march toward a health ideal.

The second idea, the notion of public policy learning, is methodological in nature. It is highlighted in Glaser's studies of health policy in Western Europe and Canada. *Paying the Doctor* (1970) analyzes systems of physician remuneration. *Health Insurance Bargaining* (1978) explains how alternative administrative arrangements affect the process of bargaining between the medical profession and the state. *Paying the Hospital* (1987) describes systems of hospital reimbursement and assesses the implications for the United States. *Health Insurance in Practice* (1991) reviews a wide range of issues related to the financing and organization of national health insurance in cross-national perspective. Each of these studies starts with the presumption that the United States has many problems and that the policies and experience of Western Europe and Canada can shed light on and provide a useful range of solutions for the United States.

The third idea focuses on understanding either determinants of health policies or at least their effects. Leichter (1979), for example, analyzes the determinants of health policies in Britain, Germany, Japan, and the Soviet Union. Similarly, Altenstetter (1974) and Stone (1980) show how different structures and processes explain the differences in policy between the United States and West Germany; and Hollingsworth (1986) attempts to relate differences in structure and performance by comparing the United States and Britain. This approach views "most similar systems" as laboratories in which to assess the effects of alternative policy options at home (Teune, 1978). It is exemplified by Evans (1984) and Marmor and his colleagues (1978), who used this approach in their studies of Canada.

The idea of evolutionary progress in the development of health systems suggests that the United States can learn about future policy issues by studying nations whose systems are more advanced. Similarly, the idea that policy learning brings foreign solutions to bear on American problems is a variation on this theme. Finally, the idea of using comparative analysis to understand the determinants and effects of policies abroad can assist us in evaluating alternative policy options at home.

There is, however, an important caveat to these views. The ideas summarized above, indeed most of the literature in comparative health policy, often minimize

TABLE 5.1 The Evolution of Health Systems

Health System	Type 1: Private	Type 2: Pluralistic	Type 3: National health insurance	Type 4: National health service	Type 5: Socialized health service
General definition	Health care as item of personal consumption	Health care as predominantly a consumer good or service	Health care as an insured, guaranteed consumer good or service	Health care as a state-supported consumer good or service	Health care as a state-provided public service
Position of the physician	Solo entrepreneur	Solo entrepreneur and member of variety of groups, organizations	Solo entrepreneur and member of medical organizations	Solo entrepreneur and member of medical organizations	State employee and member of medical organizations
Role of professional associations	Powerful	Very strong	Strong	Fairly strong	Weak or nonexistent
Ownership of facilities	Private	Private and public	Private and public	Mostly public	Entirely public
Economic transfers	Direct	Direct and indirect	Mostly indirect	Indirect	Entirely indirect
Prototypes	U.S., Western Europe, Russia in the 19th century	U.S. in 20th century	Sweden, France, Canada, Japan in 20th century	Great Britain in 20th century	Soviet Union in 20th century

Sources: V. G. Rodwin, *The Health Planning Predicament: France, Quebec, England, and the United States.* Berkeley: University of California Press, 1984, p. 245. Adapted from M. G. Field, *Comparative Health Systems: Differentiation and Convergence,* Final Report under Grant No. HS-00272, Rockville, MD: National Center for Health Services Research, 1978.

or overlook the substantial problems of health systems abroad. An alternative, problem-oriented approach might be to reverse this emphasis. For example, another way to think about learning from abroad is to begin with the recognition that most countries, irrespective of their particular health system, face serious common problems with regard to the efficient and equitable allocation of scarce health care resources. The Organization for Economic Cooperation and Development (OECD) and the World Bank have published important comparative studies that reflect this approach (see suggested readings).

Economists, for example, emphasize the problem of inefficiency in the allocation of health care resources. They point out that cost containment should not be confused with allocative efficiency in the use of health care resources, and they study the possibilities of obtaining more value for the money spent on health care. This applies not only with regard to improving health status but also with respect to altering input mixes in the provision of health services taking advantage of cost-effective treatment settings (e.g., ambulatory surgery) and personnel (e.g., nurse practitioners).

Public health and medical care analysts criticize the lack of continuity of care between, for example, the primary, secondary, and tertiary levels of health care. Although health planners have called for redistributing resources away from hospitals to community-based ambulatory care services and public health programs, the allocation of resources within health regions has been notoriously biased in favor of more costly technology-based medical care at the apex of the regional hierarchy (Fox, 1986; Rodwin, 1984). The consequence of this allocational pattern has been to weaken institutional capability for delivering primary care services and has exacerbated the separation between primary, secondary, and tertiary levels of care, thus making it difficult for providers to assure that the right patient receives the right kind of care, in the right place, and for the right reason.

Consumers have noted the inflexibility of bureaucratic decision-making procedures and the absence of opportunities for exercising for what Hirschman (1970) calls "voice" in most health care organizations. Indeed, the problem of control and how it should be shared among consumers, providers, managers, and payers is at the center of most criticisms leveled against the current structure of health systems in Western industrialized nations. In all of these systems, decisions about what medical services to provide, how and where they should be provided, by whom, and how often are separated from the responsibility for financing medical care.

Common Problems of Health Policy in Three Countries

Drawing on the problem-oriented approach presented above, this section assesses common problems with regard to the efficient and equitable allocation of scarce health care resources in four nations: France, Canada, Britain, and the United States (Table 5.2). The three other countries are far smaller than the United States in terms of population size. They have slightly less gross domestic product (GDP) per capita and spend less on health care as a percentage of GDP. But all three countries represent important models of health care financing and organization. France is a prototype model of a traditional European national health insurance (NHI) system; Canada is an example of a newer NHI system operating in a federal institutional structure that resembles more closely the United States; Britain is the model par excellence of a national health service (NHS).

Outside the system of health care financing in the United States (see chapter 3), there are two principal methods of health care financing: compulsory payroll taxes and general revenue taxation. France is an example of an employment-based NHI system financed by payroll taxes on employers and employees. Canada and Britain both rely on general revenue taxation. Whereas Canada uses national and provincial general tax revenues to finance a federal decentralized NHI system, Britain relies overwhelmingly on central government funds to finance an NHS. Despite these differences in health care financing and the differences in health care spending noted above, there are also some notable points of convergence between the United States and at least two of the selected countries with regard to certain health system characteristics as well as health outcome characteristics (Table 5.2).

France

The French health system combines NHI with solo-based fee-for-service private practice in the ambulatory care sector and a mixed hospital care sector of which two thirds of all acute beds are in the public sector and one third are in the private sector (Rodwin, 1981). Physicians in the ambulatory sector and in private hospitals (known as *cliniques*) are reimbursed on the basis of a negotiated fee schedule. Roughly 30% of all physicians selected the option to extra-bill beyond the negotiated fees that represent payment in full for the remaining 70% of physicians (Rodwin & Sandier, 1993). Physicians based in public hospitals are reimbursed on a part-time or full-time salaried basis. *Cliniques* are reimbursed on the basis of a negotiated per diem fee. Public hospitals used to be reimbursed on a retrospective, cost-based, per diem fee, but they have received prospectively set "global" budgets since 1984.

There are several problems in this system. From a public health point of view, there is inadequate communication between full-time salaried physicians in public hospitals and solo-based private practice physicians working in the community. Although general practitioners in the fee-for-service sector (roughly one-half of

TABLE 5.2. Country, Health System, and Health Characteristics: France, Canada, United Kingdom, and United States

Country Characteristics	Year	France	Canada	U.K	U.S.
Total population in thousands	1996	58,333	29,680	58,144	277,800
Percent of population over age 65	1996	15.4%	12.1%	15.8%	12.2%
GDP $ per capita[a]	1996	$20,525	$21,823	$18,852	$26,148

Health System Characteristics	Year	France	Canada	U.K	U.S.
Health expenditure as a percent of GDP	1996	9.6%	9.2%	6.9%	14.2%
Per capita health expenditures[a]	1994	$1,811	$1,950	$1,153	$3,408
Doctors' consultations per capita	1993	6.3	6.8	5.8	6.0
Acute care bed-days per 1000 population	1995	1,300	1,300	800	800

Health Outcome Characteristics	Year	France	Canada	U.K	U.S.
Health system perceived as "bad"[b]	1994	10.0%	12.0%	17.0%	28.0%
Infant mortality per 1000 live births	1995	5.0	6.0	6.0	8.0
Life expectancy (females) at age 65	1994	20.6	20.0	18.4	19.0
Life expectancy at birth (males)	1995	73.9	75.3	74.3	72.5
Self-evaluation as "less than good," population 16 and over[c]	1991	27.30%	46.30%	36.00%	N/A
Adverse effects from medicines, per million population[d]	1993	17.6	0.6	1.1	0.6

[a]In purchasing power parities.
[b]Percentage of population that perceives health systems as "bad" based on surveys reported by Blendon et al. (1990).
[c]Percentage of population that evaluates their own health status as "less than good" based on national surveys.
[d]Number of deaths caused by adverse effects from medicines as reported by *WHO World Statistics Manual* and complemented by national sources.

Source: OECD HealthData, 1997.

French physicians) have informal referral networks to specialists and public hospitals, there are no formal institutional relationships that assure continuity of medical care, disease prevention and health promotion services, posthospital follow-up care, and more generally systematic linkages and referral patterns between primary-, secondary-, and tertiary-level services.

From the point of view of economic efficiency criteria, there are additional problems in the French health care system. On the demand side, two factors encourage consumers to increase their use of medical care services: the uncertainty about the results of treatment and the availability of insurance coverage. To reduce the risk of misdiagnosis or improper therapy, physicians are always tempted to order more diagnostic tests. Since NHI covers most of the cost, there is no incentive—neither for the physician nor for the patient—to balance marginal changes in risk with marginal increases in costs. This results in excessive (and often inappropriate) use of services.

On the supply side, fee-for-service reimbursement of physicians provides incentives for them to increase their volume of services so as to raise their income. Likewise, per diem reimbursement of *cliniques* provides incentives to increase patient lengths of stay. The imposition of global budgets eliminated this problem, but the budgets represent a blunt policy tool—one that tends to support the existing allocation of resources within the hospital sector and possibly to jeopardize the quality of hospital care. It is relatively easy for a hospital to receive an annual budget to maintain its ongoing activities but extremely difficult to receive additional compensation for higher service levels, institutional innovation, or improvements in the quality of care. Even with prospective budgets, hospitals naturally seek to maximize the level of their annual allocations and to resist budget cutbacks.

In summary, under French NHI, providers have no financial incentives to achieve savings while holding quality constant or even improving it. Nor are there incentives—in public hospitals, for example—to increase service activity in exchange for more income. Consumers have few incentives, other than minimal copayments, to be economical in their use of medical care. And there are no incentives to move the French system away from hospital-centered services toward new organizational forms that encourage teamwork between general practitioners, specialists, and hospitals and greater responsiveness to emerging market demands (Rodwin, 1997).

Canada

Under Canadian NHI, although coverage for drugs is far less than in France, there are no copayments. This means that patients are not required to pay a proportion of their medical bills; there is "first-dollar" coverage for a comprehensive "package" of hospital and medical services. Physicians in ambulatory care are paid predominantly on a fee-for-service basis, according to fee schedules negotiated between physicians' associations and provincial governments. All physicians must accept these fees as payment in full. In contrast to France, physicians in hospitals are most often paid on a fee-for-service basis, as in the United States.

There are few private, for-profit hospitals in Canada, such as French *cliniques* and American proprietary or "investor-owned" institutions. Most acute-care hospitals in Canada are legally private, nonprofit institutions. But their operating expenditures are financed through the NHI system, and most of their capital expenditures are financed by the provincial governments. In the United States, Canada's health system is often depicted as a model for NHI (Himmelstein, Woolhandler, and the Writing Committee of the Working Group on Program Design, 1989). Its financing, through a complex shared federal and provincial tax revenue formula, is more progressive than the European NHI systems financed on the basis of payroll taxes. Canada's levels of health status are high by international standards. And in comparison to the United States, it has achieved notable success in controlling the growth of health care costs. What, then, are the problems in this system?

From the point of view of health care providers, there is, above all, a crisis of underfinancing. Physicians complain about low fee levels. Hospital administrators complain about draconian control of their budgets. And other health care professionals note that the combination of a physician "surplus" and excessive reliance on physicians prevents an expansion of their roles.

Although Evans (1992) contends that Canadian cost-control policies cannot be shown to have jeopardized the quality of care, providers and administrators alike claim that there has been deterioration since the imposition of restrictive prospective budgets. Leaving aside the issue of quality, the same issues discussed in the context of France are present in Canada with respect to economic efficiency. Neither the hospital, the physician, nor the patient has an incentive to be economical in the use of health care resources. On the demand side, because patients benefit from what is perceived as "free" tax-financed first-dollar coverage, they have no incentive to choose cost-effective forms of care. For example, in the case of a demand for urgent care, there is no incentive for a patient to use community health centers rather than rush directly to the emergency room.

On the supply side, physicians lack incentives to make efficient use of hospitals, which are essentially a free good at their disposal. There are no incentives for altering input mixes to affect practice style. Nor are there incentives for providers to evaluate service levels and the kinds of therapy performed in relation to improving health status. It could be argued that these problems are common to all health systems, but they are especially acute in a system characterized by a concentrated political interests—health care providers, on the one hand, and a "single payer," on the other—that tend to support the status quo. On the one hand, providers organized in strong associations have strong monopoly power, which they use to defend their legitimate interests; on the other, the monopoly power of sole-source financing (NHI) keeps provider interests in check at the cost of not intervening in the organizational practice of medicine.

Stoddard (1984) has characterized the problems of the Canadian health system as "financing without organization." In his view, Canadian provinces "adopted a 'pay the bills' philosophy, in which decisions about service provision—which services, in what amounts, produced how, by whom and where—were viewed as the legitimate domain of physicians and hospital administrators" (p. 3). The reason for this policy is that provincial governments were concerned about maintaining a good relationship with providers. This concern has not avoided tough negotiations and periodic confrontations. But there have been only limited efforts to devise new forms of medical care practice, for example, health maintenance organizations (HMOs) or new institutions to handle long-term care for the elderly. The side effect of Canadian NHI has been to support the separation of hospital and ambulatory care and to reinforce traditional organizational structures.

As in France there are, in essence, two strategies for managing the Canadian health system and making adjustments. The first involves greater regulation on the supply side: even stronger controls on hospital spending, more rationing of medical technology, and more hospital mergers and eventually closures. The second involves increased reliance on market forces on the demand side: various forms of user charges such as copayments and deductibles now advocated as a form of privatization. Neither strategy is likely to succeed on its own. The former will control health care expenditures in the short run, but it fails to affect practice styles. Its effectiveness runs the risk of exacerbating confrontations between providers and the state and jeopardizing health care needs. The latter deals with only part of the problem—the demand side—and neglects the issue of supply-side inefficiency. It provides no mechanism by which consumer decisions can generate signals to providers to adopt efficient practice styles. Moreover, it is likely to raise the level of total (public and private) expenditures.

Between these two strategies, there is increasing recognition among Canadian policymakers that the health sector requires significant reorganization. In Ontario, in 1996, the Health Services Restructuring Commission was formed; in Quebec the federation of GPs formed a task force on the reorganization of primary care. Both of these efforts have reinforced the trend toward "integrated health systems" and the use of gatekeepers in primary care.

Britain

There are many models of an NHS in Europe, ranging from decentralized systems in Sweden, Norway, Finland, and Denmark to more centralized systems in Spain,

Greece, Portugal, and Italy. Because the British NHS is one of the oldest and most thoroughly studied models, it stands as an exemplar. It is financed almost entirely through general revenue taxation and is accountable directly to the Department of Health and Social Security (DHSS) and Parliament. Access to health services is free of charge to all British subjects and to all legal residents. But despite the universal entitlement, health expenditures in the U.K. represent only 6.9% of the gross domestic product (GDP)—less than one half that in the United States (Table 5.3).

Although the NHS is cherished by most Britons, there are, nevertheless, some serious problems concerning both the equity and efficiency of resource allocation in the health sector. With regard to equity (defined as "equal care for those at equal risk") in 1976, the Resource Allocation Working Party (RAWP) developed a formula for the allocation of NHS funds between regions (DHSS, 1976). The formula represents one of the most far-reaching attempts to allocate health care funds because it incorporated regional differences in health status based on standardized mortality ratios. Slow progress was made in redistributing the aggregate NHS budget along the lines of RAWP, but substantial inequities still remain, from the point of view of both spatial distribution and social class (Townsend & Davidson, 1982).

With regard to efficiency, the problems are even more severe because NHS resources are extremely scarce by OECD standards. Because there is less slack, the marginal costs of inefficiency are higher than in Western Europe or the United States. And because the NHS faces the same demands as other systems to make available technology and to care for an increasingly aged population, British policymakers recognize that they must pursue innovations that improve efficiency. But there have been numerous obstacles in the way: opposition by professional bodies, difficulties in firing and redeploying health care personnel, and the institutional separation between hospitals, general practitioners, and community health programs.

The tripartite structure of the NHS has, since its establishment in 1948, been a source of inefficiency:

1. Regional Health Authorities (RHAs) have been responsible (until the mid-1990s) for allocating budgets to districts and hospitals. Hospital-based physicians, known as "consultants," are paid on a salaried basis, from these budgets, with distinguished clinicians receiving "merit awards"; and all consultants have the right to see a limited number of private, fee-paying patients in so-called pay beds within their service units.

2. Outside the RHA budget (until the mid-1990s) were the Family Practitioner Committees (FPCs) responsible for remunerating general practitioners (GPs), ophthalmologists, dentists, and pharmacists. The GPs are reimbursed on a capitation basis, with additional remuneration coming from special "practice

TABLE 5.3   Total Expenditures on Health Care as a Percentage of GDP: 1995–1996

Country	% Total Expenditure on Health in GDP
Australia	8.4
Austria	7.9
Belgium	7.9
Canada	9.2
Czech Republic	7.9
Denmark	6.4
Finland	7.5
France	9.6
Germany	10.5
Greece	5.9
Iceland	7.9
Ireland	4.9
Italy	7.6
Japan	7.2
Mexico	4.5
Netherlands	8.6
New Zealand	7.2
Norway	7.9
Portugal	8.2
Spain	7.6
Sweden	7.2
Switzerland	9.8
Turkey[a]	5.2
United Kingdom	6.9
United States	14.2

[a]1994.
Source: OECD Health Data File, 1997. Paris: OECD.

allowances" and fee-for-service payment for specific services (e.g., night visits and immunizations).

3.   Separate from both the RHAs and the FPCs have been the local authorities (LAs), which are responsible for the provision of social services, public health services, and certain community nursing services.

This institutional framework has created perverse incentives—for example, to shift borderline patients from GPs to hospital consultants, to the community, and back to the hospital. Until the reforms introduced by the Thatcher government in 1991, GPs had no incentive to minimize costs and could even impose costs on RHAs by referring patients to hospital consultants or for diagnostic services. NHS managers could shift costs from the NHS to social security by sending elderly hospitalized patients to private nursing homes. And consultants could shift costs back onto the patient by keeping long waiting lists, thereby increasing demand for their private services. As in France and Canada, neither the patient nor the physician in Britain bears the cost of the decisions they make; it is the taxpayer who pays the bill.

Four strategies—all of them inadequate—have attempted to deal with this problem. The first came promptly with the arrival of the first Thatcher government in 1991. After cautious attempts to denationalize the NHS by promoting a shift toward NHI and privatization, the conservative government backed off when they realized that such an approach would not merely provoke strong political opposition but also would increase public expenditure and therefore conflict with their budgetary objectives (McLachlan & Maynard, 1982). Instead, the strategy was narrowed in favor of encouraging competition and market incentives in limited areas. To begin with, the government allowed a slight increase in pay beds within NHS hospitals. In addition, it introduced tax incentives to encourage the purchase of private health insurance and the growth of charitable contributions. Also, the government encouraged local authorities to raise money through the sale of surplus property and to contract out to the private sector such services as laundry, cleaning, and catering.

The second response was the Griffiths Report (1983), which resulted in yet another reorganization in the long history of administrative reform within the NHS. Roy Griffiths, the former director of a large English department store chain, introduced the concept of a general manager at the department (DHSS), regional, district, and unit levels. This manager was presumably responsible for the efficient use of the budget at each level of the NHS. In summary, the report observed, in a sentence that has since become well known, "if Florence Nightingale were carrying her lamp through the corridors of the NHS today, she would almost certainly be searching for the people in charge" (Griffiths, 1983, p. 12). The problem, however, is that, following the Griffiths Report, the tripartite structure of the system remained largely unchanged; and the general managers had very little information about least-cost strategies (across the tripartite structure) for generating improvements in health status.

The third response to the problem of improving efficiency was to reduce the drug bill (Maynard, 1986). In April 1985, the government limited the list of reimbursable drugs and reduced the pharmaceutical industry's rate of return. These measures helped contain the costs of the formerly open-ended drug budget within the NHS, but there is no evidence that they had any impact on the efficiency of health care expenditures.

Finally, the fourth and most significant reform for improving efficiency was announced in a government White Paper, *Working for Patients* (1989) passed in 1990 (The National Health Service and Community Care Act) and implemented on April 1, 1991. The White Paper proposed a range of significant changes, all of which attempt to create "internal markets" within the public sector, by giving providers incentives to treat more patients and having "money follow patients." On the demand side, the government proposed that, instead of operating as monopoly suppliers of services, district health authorities be required to purchase services for the patients they serve. On the supply side, the government proposed that NHS hospitals be given the option to convert from purely "public" status to that of independent, self-governing "trusts." Also, the government proposed that GPs be given the option to serve as "fundholders" for their enrolled patients and thereby serve as purchasers on their behalf for basic specialty and hospital services.

In July 1990, RHAs were streamlined and FPCs were transformed into newly named Family Health Service Authorities (FHSAs) with stronger management over primary care. In 1996 the districts were merged with the FHSAs into roughly 80 health authorities (HAs) and placed under a new National Health Service Executive (NHSE) with eight regional offices. The HAs are supposed to function as integrated purchasing coalitions, thereby strengthening the role of internal markets in the allocation of health resources. There have been some preliminary evaluations of these reforms, but they are still too recent to permit one to conclude very much about the effects of internal markets on efficiency of resource allocation, continuity of care, and responsiveness to patient demands.[4]

The U.S. Health System: A Comparative Perspective

How does the U.S. health care system measure up in comparison to the health sector in France, Canada, and Great Britain? To answer this question, we will review the ways in which the U.S. health system differs from and resembles that of other Western industrialized nations. Let us examine this issue from the perspectives of three characteristics that typically distinguish the United States from Western Europe and Canada: (1) values and popular opinion, (2) the structure of health care financing and organization, and (3) policy responses to health sector problems.

---

[4]For recent discussion of the British reforms, see S. Glouberman (1996), I. Holliday (1995), R. Klein (1995), Robinson and Le Grand (1994), C. Smee, "Self-Governing Trusts and GP Fundholders: the British Experience," in Saltman and Von Otter (1995) and A. Wall (1996).

American Values and Popular Opinion

The prevailing image of American values and popular opinion is that of 19th-century liberalism, which has colored American perceptions of equity, the proper role of government, and citizenship. These perceptions represent a range of American values and popular opinions that distinguish the United States from Western Europe and Canada.

American attitudes about equity with regard to health care were formed in the 19th century as the country became populated by immigrant populations in urban centers. During this period the concept of "truly needy" emerged (Rosner, 1982). Many Americans developed a sense of responsibility to come to their aid, but there were also harsher attitudes inspired by social Darwinist notions that distinguished between the "truly needy" and the "undeserving" or "unworthy" poor. Whereas in Western Europe broadly based socialist parties viewed poverty as an outcome of the economic system, in the United States there was an inclination to regard poverty as an individual problem. Hence, the greater attention to *equality of opportunity* in the United States as compared with *equality of results* in the more left-leaning European social democracies.

As far as the proper role of government is concerned, in contrast to Western Europe and Canada, the United States has a history of antigovernment attitudes. The suspicion about excessive governmental authority and the attachment to individual liberties is a pervasive American value.

American perceptions of citizenship also present a striking contrast to Western European perceptions. In the United States individualistic values, on the one hand, and social and ethnic heterogeneity, on the other, have resulted in more "fractionalized understandings of citizenship" (Klass, 1985). In Western Europe and Canada, the understandings of citizenship are grounded in notions of solidarity and universal entitlements. The difference is that Western Europe and Canada have largely succeeded in covering all of their citizens under some form of national health insurance (NHI); the United States has not.

There is a general aversion among Americans to universal entitlements. As Reinhardt (1985) has observed, when Americans face a trade-off between establishing tax-financed entitlements and leaving the uninsured on their own, they prefer to do the latter. It would be misleading, however, to draw any conclusions about how generous Americans are or how much social welfare they provide based only on the image of liberalism outlined above. In contrast to Western Europe and Canada, Americans prefer to promote redistribution policies through local assistance and indirect subsidies to the voluntary sector via tax exemptions.

Clearly, in comparison to Western Europe and Canada, there are important differences in the United States with regard to values and popular opinion. But how much of a difference do these differences make?

The Structure of Health Care Financing and Organization

The prevailing image of the American health care system is one of a privately financed, privately organized system with multiple payers. These characteristics derive, in large part, from the absence of a publicly mandated NHI program. In comparison with Western European nations, Japan, and Canada, the United States is last with respect to the public share of total health care expenditures (Table 5.4). Although the United States has the highest per capita health care expenditures—public and private combined (Table 5.5)—and spends the highest percent-

TABLE 5.4 Sources of Finance and Health Care Expenditures: The Mix Between Public and Private in 1995–1996 as a Percentage of Total Expenditure on Health

Country	Public	Private
Australia	66.5	33.5
Austria	74.9	25.1
Belgium	87.7	12.3
Canada	71.4	28.6
Denmark	79.4	20.6
Finland	74.5	25.5
France	80.7	19.3
Germany	78.3	21.7
Greece	82.9	17.1
Iceland	83.5	16.5
Ireland	80.8	19.2
Italy	69.9	30.1
Japan	78.4	21.6
Mexico	59.4	40.6
Netherlands	77	23
New Zealand	75.9	24.1
Norway	82.5	17.5
Portugal	59.8	40.2
Spain	76.3	23.7
Sweden	80.2	19.8
Switzerland	71.9	28.1
Turkey[a]	50	50
United Kingdom	84.3	15.7
United States	47	53

[a]1994.
Source: OECD Health Data File, 1997.

TABLE 5.5   Per Capita Health Care Expenditures, 1995–1996 in $US Purchasing Power Parities (PPP)

Country	$US (PPP)
Australia	$1,776
Austria	$1,681
Belgium	$1,693
Canada	$2,002
Czech Republic	$749
Denmark	$1,430
Finland	$1,389
France	$1,978
Germany	$2,222
Greece	$748
Iceland	$1,839
Ireland	$923
Italy	$1,520
Japan	$1,581
Mexico	$384
Netherlands	$1,756
New Zealand	$1,251
Norway	$1,937
Portugal	$1,077
Spain	$1,131
Sweden	$1,405
Switzerland	$2,412
Turkey[a]	$272
United Kingdom	$1,304
United States	$3,708

[a]1994.
Source: OECD Health Data File, 1997.

age of its GDP on health care (Table 5.3), it retains the lowest share of public expenditure as a percentage of total health expenditures (Table 5.4).

The organization of health care in the United States is noted for being on the private end of the public-private spectrum. In comparison with Western Europe, the United States has one of the smallest public hospital sectors. In the organization of ambulatory care, American private fee-for-service practice corresponds to the norm, at least in comparison to NHI systems. However, the absence of an NHI program in the United States has resulted in a system of multiple payers and has encouraged a more pluralistic pattern of medical care organization and more innovative forms of medical practice—for example, multispecialty group practices, HMOs, ambulatory surgery centers, and preferred provider organizations (PPOs).

The United States is also different, in comparison to Canada and Western Europe, with regard to the ways in which health resources are used. For example, the United States (along with Spain and the United Kingdom) is among those OECD countries with the lowest number of acute care hospital beds per thousand population (Table 5.6). These data should not necessarily lead one to the conclusion that the United States is less prone to institutionalize patients than Western Europe and Canada. They probably reflect the size of the American private

TABLE 5.6 Acute Care Hospital Beds and Use of Inpatient Care, 1994–1995

Country	No. of beds per 1000 population	Bed days per 1000 population
Australia	4.3	1000
Austria	6.6	1800
Belgium	4.8	1300
Canada[a]	3.6	1400
Czech Republic	7.3	2000
Denmark	4	1200
Finland	4	1100
France	4.6	1300
Germany	6.9	2000
Greece[b]	3.9	—
Iceland	3.7	1100
Ireland	3.4	1000
Italy	5.3	1400
Netherlands	3.9	1000
Norway	3.4	1000
Portugal	3.4	800
Spain	3.2	900
Sweden	3.1	800
Switzerland[a]	6.1	1700
Turkey	2	400
United Kingdom	2	800
United States	3.3	800

[a]1993.
[b]1992.

Source: OECD Health Data File, 1997.

nursing home industry, which has no equivalent in Western Europe or Canada, where a large portion of long-term care for the elderly is provided in hospitals.

These are ways in which the American health care system is different from that of Western Europe and Canada. But there are also some noteworthy points of similarity. For example, most health systems in industrially advanced nations are centered around the hospital. They allocate roughly one half of total health care expenditures to the hospital sector. The United States corresponds to the norm in this regard (Table 5.7).

There is also a high degree of similarity among the United States, Canada, and Western Europe in the broad structure of health care financing and provider reimbursement (Figure 5.2). From the point of view of both consumers and providers, the essential feature of modern health care systems is the central role of third-party payment, by either government or health insurers. On the financing end, all health systems are supported primarily either by general revenue taxes or by payroll deductions in the from of compulsory taxes or voluntary health insurance premiums. On the payment end, the magnitude of third-party payment dwarfs the out-of-pocket payment by consumers.

For the consumer, what matters with regard to health care financing is not the relative public and private mix but rather the relative portion of *direct versus indirect* third-party payment. To emphasize that the largest portion of health care financing in the United States is private is misleading; for the more critical factor is that public and private health insurance are both forms of third-party payment.

TABLE 5.7   Components of Health Care Expenditure, 1994–1996

Country	Inpatient	Ambulatory	Pharmaceutical	Other
Australia	43.8	27.8	11	17.4
Austria	20.6	23.4	14.1	41.9
Belgium	37.4	37.7	18.9	6
Canada	45.6	23.3	14.3	16.8
Denmark	59.4	18.9	11.2	10.5
France	44.6	27	16.9	11.5
Germany	35	30.1	12.7	22.2
Iceland	54.3	23.8	16.3	5.6
Italy	47.9	30.2	18.6	3.3
Japan	31.1	42.3	21.2	5.4
Netherlands	52.5	28.1	10.7	8.7
Switzerland	51.7	37.4	7.6	3.3
United States	43.3	33.2	8.9	14.6

Source: OECD Health Data File, 1997.

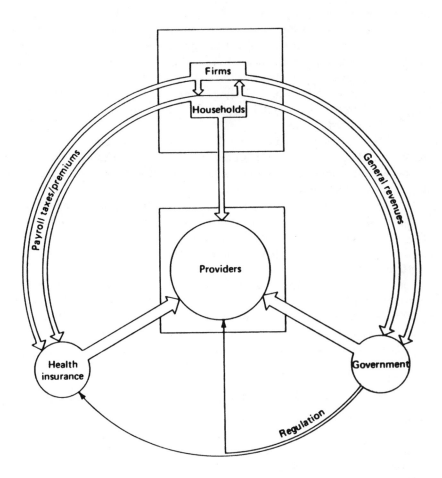

FIGURE 5.2   Health care financing and provider reimbursement.

This amount grew to 73.1% of national health expenditures in 1990, leaving consumers with direct out-of-pocket contributions equal to 23.3% of total health expenditures (Levit, 1991). The OECD does not routinely compare consumers' out-of-pocket payments to total expenditures. However, available data on this important indicator suggest that, once again, the United States is different (Figure 5.3). It has the highest share of direct out-of-pocket payments by consumers. Even under French NHI, consumers contribute roughly 14% of total health

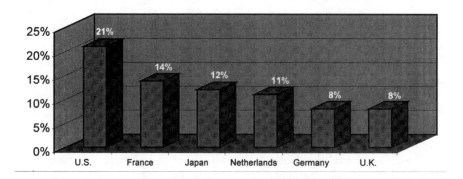

FIGURE 5.3   Share of patient out-of-pocket payments as a percentage of personal health care expenditures (1988–1996).

Sources: U.S.: Year 1994. Levit, K., Lazenby, H., & Sivarajan, L., "National Health Expenditures, 1994" *HCFA Review, 17*(3), 1996, Table 12.
France: Year 1996. *Comptes nationauz de la santé, 1996.* Ministry of Health.
Japan: Year 1990. Kousei Tokei Kyokai, *Kousei no Sninyou, 38*(9), 1991, p. 237, cited by Ikegami, "The Economics of Health Care in Japan," in *Science, 258,* 1992.
Netherlands: Year 1988. OECD, *The Reform of Health Care: A Comparative Analysis of Seven OECD Countries.* Paris: OECD, 1992, p. 89.
Germany: Year 1995. Busse, R., & Howorth, C., "Cost-containment in Germany, 1977–1997," unpublished paper, Department of Epidemiology and Social Medicine, Medizinische Hochschule Hannover, Hannover, Germany.
U.K.: Year 1989. OECD, *The Reform of Health Care; A Comparative Analysis of Seven OECD Countries.* Paris: OECD, 1992, p. 116.

expenditures in the form of out-of-pocket payments. The difference is not as large as the image of a private financing system would suggest.

The image of a private organizational structure in American health care is well founded. But that view, too, is incomplete. In spite of its *relatively* small size, there is an important role for the public sector in the United States—both in ambulatory services for the noninstitutionalized patient and in the provision of hospital services.

With regard to ambulatory care, there is a maze of special federal programs and a network of local government services largely for the poor. The services are provided in either county or municipal hospital emergency rooms, in local health departments, or in neighborhood health centers. As for hospitals, more than 30% of all acute-care institutions are owned and operated by governments. This includes the federal Veterans Administration hospitals and marine and military hospitals, as well as state, county, and municipal hospitals. Although Medicare and Medicaid were intended to bring the poor into "mainstream medicine," (i.e., into the private sector), local county governments continue to finance care for the "medically indigent" uninsured, either through private vendors or directly in public hospitals. These hospitals are a major source of care not only for Medicaid beneficiaries but also for more than half of the poverty population who do not meet Medicaid eligibility levels and consequently often do not have access to private physicians or voluntary hospitals.

To sum up, there are distinctive characteristics of health care financing and organization in the United States, but there are also striking points of similarity when compared with Western Europe and Canada. The distinctive characteristics include the absence of an NHI program, preferences for institutional flexibility, and innovative forms of medical care organization. The points of similarity—the coexistence of both public and private provision and third-party payment—are structural features of the American health system as well as those of most other OECD health systems.

Policy Responses to Health Sector Problems

Over a decade ago Abel-Smith (1985) referred to the United States as the "odd man out" when he noted the divergence between Western European and American policy responses to the problem of containing health care costs. He suggested that Western Europe relies on regulation, whereas the United States seeks to promote competition and greater reliance on market forces. Abel-Smith pointed to three examples of American policy responses to health sector problems: (1) the growth of deductibles, copayments, and other cost-sharing mechanisms; (2) the trend toward making those who benefit from insurance actually pay the whole cost—this implies, for example, reducing tax deductions and thus providing incentives for employers and employees to shop more prudently for insurance coverage; and (3) the growth of competitive bidding as a mechanism of forcing competition between alternative providers.

There were important insights behind this interpretation of the American policy response to health sector problems. But in retrospect, there are some errors. To begin with, the growth of cost-sharing was not limited to the United States. Many European countries followed similar revenue-enhancing strategies. In fact, although the share of out-of-pocket payments by consumers, as a percentage of total health expenditures, is larger in the United States than in Western Europe (Figure 5.3), the share in the United States has declined over the past decade (Levit et al., 1996). Second, the trend toward making those who benefit from insurance actually pay the whole cost was largely rhetorical because employer health insurance premiums remain tax deductible and tax-deductible employee spending accounts have been expanded in the 1990s. Third, despite the rhetoric and actual force of competition in the U.S. health systems, there has probably been more regulation in the eastern states with all-payer systems (e.g., New York, New Jersey, and Maryland) than in all of Western Europe. Even in well-known "pockets of competition" (e.g., California, Arizona, and Minnesota) regulation is essential, if only to enforce the rules of the competitive game. The prospective payment system (PPS) or Medicare provides a good illustration. Although one of its effects was to intensify competition between hospitals, the use of diagnosis-related groups (DRGs) for hospital reimbursement was actually a highly regulatory strategy of centralized price controls, one that falls well within Western Europe policy traditions.

In regulating physician activities, American policy has not backed off. Rather, since the creation of physician review organizations (PROs) under PPS, the regulation of physician behavior in the United States is surely stronger than any emerging European equivalent, including the French and Canadian systems of medical profiles, which are among the most developed outside the United States (Rodwin, 1989a).

Three characteristics distinguish American policy responses from those of Western Europe and Canada:

1.   The United States has long been concerned about the dangers of monopoly power and has pursued (until the recent wave of consolidation within the health sector) a strong antitrust policy. A notable case in point were the Federal Trade Commission's measures to curb the monopoly powers of physicians and hospitals and to eliminate restraints on trade in health care by allowing advertising.[5] In the United States, structural interests are not formally sanctioned and accepted as institutionalized counterparts for purposes of negotiating with the government. Instead, the more typical response of American health policy is to advocate proposals to fragment powerful groups that are presumed, as a consequence, to compete with one another.

2.   Following directly from the first characteristic of the American policy response is the absence in the United States of institutional structures for negotiating between major groups of health care providers and the government or an NHI board of directors, or both. In contrast to the adversarial American approach, which attempts to fragment both the medical profession and the hospital associations—a strategy of "divide and conquer"—the Western European and Canadian

---

[5]This change of policy was prompted by the 1977 U.S. Supreme Court decision in *Bates v. State Bar of Arizona*, 433 U.S. 350 (1977) allowing health care professionals to engage in advertising.

response consolidates the organization of provider groups and confronts them with countervailing organizations.

This important difference acts as a severe constraint, in the United States, on the possibilities of negotiating a national fee schedule for physicians or a uniform hospital payment system for all payers and hospitals (Rodwin, 1990). The constraint, however, has made it possible for individual payers (e.g., Medicare, Medicaid, and private health plans) to strike harder bargains with smaller groups and to foster competition and new organizational arrangements for medical care.

3.   In contrast to Western European and Canadian strategies of comprehensive health care reform and strong centralized regulation, American strategies (with the exception of PPS for Medicare) are characterized by far greater decentralization and by more persistent social experimentation. Although major policy initiatives have usually come from the federal level and a range of government programs at the county and municipal levels, when compared to unitary European states (e.g., France and Britain), American federalism provides a striking contrast. But even in comparison to other federal states, such as Canada and Germany, the United States is still characterized by more decentralization and experimentation in the policy-making process.

These three characteristics of American policy responses to health sector problems highlight the ways in which the United States is different from Western Europe and Canada. But if one compares the evolution of American health policy over the past four decades with that of Western Europe and Canada, there are also points of similarity.

For example, Brown (1988) identifies four American policy responses to health sector problems: (1) the subsidy strategy—government grants on the supply side; (2) the financing strategy—third-party financing on the demand side; (3) the reorganization strategy—government inducements to promote new organizations for delivering medical care; and (4) the regulatory strategy—government attempts to influence the "use, price and quality of services, and the size, location, and equipment of facilities." Three of the four categories—subsidy, financing, and regulatory—are equally good descriptors of the Western Europe and Canadian policy response to their health sector problems.

In the 1950s and 1960s, during the expansion phase of health care systems, there was extraordinary convergence among Western industrialized nations around both the subsidy and financing strategies (De Kervasdoué, Kimberly, & Rodwin, 1984). In the mid-1970s and 1980s, during the containment phase, there was also convergence around the regulatory and reorganization strategies. Although one can point to examples of the reorganization strategy in all countries, Canada (particularly Quebec) and Western Europe have focused more on administrative reorganizations in the public sector, whereas the United States has encouraged reorganization in the private sector at the level of the delivery system. This is perhaps the most notable aspect of the American health policy response to health sector problems.

The Uses of Comparative Analysis in Learning from Abroad

Given the ways in which the health sector in the United States resembles that of Western Europe and Canada and the ways in which it is exceptional, what inferences can one draw about the uses of comparative analysis for purposes of learning from abroad? If the United States is truly exceptional in the health sector, then one can argue that there is little to learn from Western Europe and Canada. Countries often rely on this "assumption of uniqueness" to reject ideas from abroad (Stone, 1981). To the extent that the United States is unexceptional, however, a case can be made for drawing lessons from comparative experience.

For example, there is a widely shared belief among American policymakers that a national program providing for universal entitlement to health care in the United States would result in runaway costs. In response to this presumption, nations that entitle all of their residents to a high level of medical care while spending less on administration and on medical care than does the United States, are often held up as models. The Canadian health system is the most celebrated example. French NHI, a prototype of Western European continental health systems, is another case in point. Britain's NHS, although typically considered a "painful prescription" for the United States (Aaron & Schwartz, 1984), nevertheless assures first-dollar coverage for basic health services to its entire population and, as we have seen, spends less than half as much money, per capita, as the United States (Table 5.5).

All of these countries have produced some of the leading physicians and hospitals in the world. Judging by various measures of health status, they are in the same league as, or better than, the United States (Table 5.8). But in the United States over 15% of the population remains uninsured for health care services while spending, as a percentage GDP, surpasses that of all industrially advanced nations (Table 5.3).

Should we adopt the Western European or Canadian models of health care financing and organization? Or should we maintain our present system and recognize that it is a manifestation of American exceptionalism, that is, of the ways in which the United States is fundamentally different from Western Europe and Canada? Both of these responses are probably inappropriate. The second response—that comparative analysis is not useful—insulates us from the experience of other nations. It smacks of ethnocentrism, makes us conservative, and thereby supports the status quo in the United States. The first response—that we should adopt the West European or Canadian model—relies too heavily on the experience of those nations. It is misleading because, as we have seen, there

TABLE 5.8   Health Care Expenditures and Health Status: 1994–1995

| Country | Total Expenditure on Health as a % of GDP | Life Expectancy | | | | Infant Mortality Per 1,000 Live Births |
| | | At Birth | | At Age 65 | | |
		Females	Males	Females	Males	
Canada	9.2	81.3	75.3	20.1	16.2	6
France	9.6	81.9	73.9	20.6	16.1	5
Germany	10.5	79.5	73	18.3	14.6	5.3
Italy	7.6	80.8	74.4	19.6	15.7	6.2
Japan	7.2	82.8	76.4	20.9	16.5	4.3
Spain	7.6	81.2	73.2	19.8	15.8	5.5
United Kingdom	6.9	79.7	74.3	18.4	14.7	6
United States	14.2	79.2	72.5	19	15.5	8

Source: OECD Health Data File, 1997.

are serious limitations in the Western European and Canadian health systems. Moreover, many of the present institutional arrangements of health care delivery in the United States are superior to those abroad.

The proliferation of medical technology combined with an aging demographic structure are trends common to all modern health care systems and have contributed to rising health care costs. Policymakers have responded largely by implementing systems with increasing control over expenditures on doctors' services as well as hospital budgets. Virtually no one in Canada or Western Europe views the American system as a model to emulate. Even under the government of Prime Minister Thatcher there was no significant challenge to the principle of an NHS in Britain (Klein, 1985; *Working for Patients*, 1989). Nor is there any question about eliminating NHI in such countries as France, Canada, Germany, Belgium, or the Netherlands.

Despite these attitudes, one striking aspect about how some common problems are currently being dealt with abroad is the extent to which a number of fashionable American themes have drifted north to Canada and across the Atlantic to Western Europe. In the context of the problems we identified earlier—inefficiency in the allocation of health care resources, lack of continuity between levels of care, and the absence of consumer "voice" in most health care organizations—the concept of a managed-care organization (MCO), in combination with elements of market competition, has a certain appeal. Since an MCO is by definition both an insurer and a provider of health services, it establishes a link between the financing and provision of health services. Because its managers have a budget to care for an enrolled population, they have powerful incentives to provide needed services in a cost-effective manner while simultaneously maintaining quality to minimize the risk of disenrollment.

The idea of introducing MCOs or similar kinds of health care organizations into national systems that provide universal entitlement to health care resembles, in many ways, the American experience of encouraging Medicare beneficiaries to enroll in federally qualified HMOs or competing medical plans (CMPs). The idea usually involves two reforms. It spurs policymakers to combine regulatory controls with competition on the supply side, and it encourages them to design market incentives for both providers and consumers of health care.

To the extent that the insertion of MCOs into NHI or NHS systems represents an American "solution" to *foreign* problems, it may provide a way in which Canada and Western Europe could learn from the United States (Rodwin, 1989b). It may also, paradoxically, have more practical implications for the United States than simply transposing a European NHI system into the American context. For example, the insertion of MCOs into NHI or NHS systems might provide insights on how to implement health care reform in the United States.

Just how policy learning occurs as a result of studying health care systems abroad is not thoroughly understood (Rodwin & Brecher, 1992). But there is no doubt that more policy research in the field of comparative health systems could potentially be helpful in learning from abroad.

Mini-Case Study

You have just been hired by Health Care Associates (HCA), a large U.S. consulting firm specializing in health care management and policy analysis. HCA's clients range from government agencies to large health care providers, insurers, and purveyors of information-based administrative technologies. The firm has grown rapidly over the past decade and thrives on its stellar reputation for quality work and advice that has helped many clients achieve their goals.

Because many of HCA's private clients are entering the global marketplace, the CEO calls you one day and asks you to prepare a memorandum on the market opportunities for techniques of managed care in health care systems abroad. What would you advise her to do? Include in your answer a discussion of the possibilities in national health insurance systems (e.g., France and Canada), as well as national health services systems (e.g., Britain). Also, based on your understanding of the financing and organization of their respective health care systems, provide some advice on potential clients for introducing elements of managed care within each system.

Discussion Questions

1. What are the strengths and weaknesses of the social science approach to comparative health systems?
2. How can the analysis of health systems abroad be used to promote policy learning?
3. What are three common problems in health policy development found in different countries?
4. How does the French NHI system differ from the Canadian NHI system in its financing?
5. Compare the organization and financing of the British and U.S. health systems.
6. Is there evidence of policy convergence in the evolution of the French, Canadian, and British health systems?
7. Are policy responses to health sector problems different in the United States than in France, Canada, and Britain? If so, how? If not, why not?

Acknowledgment

I wish to thank Xabier Boullon-Agrelo for his painstaking assistance in updating the OECD data and designing the tables in this chapter.

References

Aaron, H., & Schwartz, W., *The Painful Prescription: Rationing Hospital Care*. Washington, DC: Brookings Institution, 1984.

Abel-Smith, B., "Who Is the Odd Man Out? The Experiences of Western Europe in Containing the Costs of Health Care," *Milbank Memorial Fund Quarterly: Health and Society, 63*(1), 1–17, 1985.

Altenstetter, C., *Health Policy-Making and Administration in West Germany and the United States*. Beverly Hills, CA: Sage Publications, 1974.

Altenstetter, C., *Changing National-Subnational Relations in Health: Opportunities and Constraints* (DHEW Pub. No. 6, NIH 78-182). Washington, DC: U.S. Government Printing Office, 1978.

Anderson, O., *Health Care: Can There Be Equity? The United States, Sweden, and England*. New York: John Wiley & Sons, 1972.

Anderson, O., *The Health Services Continuum in Democratic States*. Ann Arbor, MI: Health Administration Press, 1989.

Andreopoulos, S., (Ed.), *National Health Insurance: Can We Learn from Canada?* New York: John Wiley & Sons, 1975.

Blendon, R., Leitman, R., Morrison, K. & Donelan, K., "Satisfaction with Health Systems in Ten Nations," *Health Affairs, 2*(9), 1990.

Blum, H., *Planning for Health*. New York: Human Sciences Press, 1981.

Brown, L., *Health Policy in the United States: Issues and Options*. New York: Ford Foundation, 1988.

Corson, J., *Loiterings in Europe*. New York: Harper, 1948.

De Kervasdoué, J., Kimberly, J., & Rodwin, V. (Eds.), *The End of an Illusion: The Future of Health Policy in Western Industrialized Nations*. Berkeley: University of California Press, 1984.

De Miguel, S., "A Framework for the Study of National Health Systems," *Inquiry, 12,* 10, 1975.

DHHS, *Sharing Resources for Health in England: Report of the Resource Allocation Working Party*. London: Her Majesty's Stationery Office, 1976.

Douglas-Wilson, I., & McLachlan, G. (Eds.), *Health Services Prospects: An International Survey*. London: Nuffield Provincial Hospitals Trust, 1974.

Dumbaugh, K., & Neuhauser, D., "International Comparisons of Health Services: Where Are We?" *Social Science and Medicine, 221,* 13B, 1979.

Eckstein, H., *The English National Health Services: Its Origins, Structure, and Achievements*. Cambridge, MA: Harvard University Press, 1959.

Edwards, B., *The National Health Service: A Manager's Tale*. London: Nuffield Provincial Hospitals Trust, l995.

Ellencweig, A., *Analyzing Health Systems: A Modular Approach*. New York: Oxford University Press, 1992.

Elling, R., *Cross-National Study of Health Systems: Concepts, Methods and Data Sources*. New Brunswick, NJ: Transaction Books, 1980.

Elling, R., & Kerr, H., "Selection of Contrasting National Health Systems for In-Depth Study," *Inquiry* (Suppl. 12), 2, 1975.

Evans, R., *Strained Mercy: The Economics of Canadian Health Care*. Toronto: Butterworths, 1984.

Evans, R., "Canada: The Real Issues," *Journal of Health Policy, Politics and Law, (17)*(4), 1992.

Field, M., *Soviet Socialized Medicine*. New York: Free Press, 1967.

Field, M., "The Concept of 'Health System' at the Macrosociological Level," *Social Science and Medicine, 7,* 763–785, 1973.

Field, N., *Success and Crisis in National Health Systems: A Comparative Approach*. New York: Routledge, 1989.

Forsyth, G., *Doctors and State Medicine: A Study of the British Health Service*. London: Pitman Medical, 1966.

Fox, D., *Health Policies, Health Politics*. Princeton, NJ: Princeton University Press, 1986.

Fry, J., *Medicine in Three Societies: Comparison of Medical Care in the USSR, USA and UK*. New York: Elsevier, 1970.

Glaser, W., *Paying the Doctor: Systems of Remuneration and Their Effects*. Baltimore: Johns Hopkins University Press, 1970.

Glaser, W., *Health Insurance Bargaining: Foreign Lessons for Americans*. New York: Gardner Press, 1978.

Glaser, W., *Paying the Hospital*. San Francisco: Jossey Bass, 1987.

Glaser, W., *Health Insurance in Practice: International Variations in Financing, Benefits, and Problems*. San Francisco: Jossey-Bass, 1991.

Glouberman, S., *Beyond Restructuring*. London: King's Fund, 1996.

Griffiths, R., *NHS Management Inquiry*. London: DHSS, 1983.

Himmelstein, D., Woolhandler, S. (and the Writing Committee of the Working Group on Program Design), "A National Health Program for the United States: A Physician's Proposal," *New England Journal of Medicine, 320*(2), 1989.

Hirschman, A., *Exit, Voice and Loyalty*. Cambridge, MA: Harvard University Press, 1970.

Holliday, I., *The NHS Transformed*. Manchester, UK: Baseline Books, 1992.

Hollingsworth, J., *A Political Economy of Medicine: Great Britain and the United States*. Baltimore: Johns Hopkins University Press, 1986.

Hu, T., *International Health Costs and Expenditures* (DHEW Pub. no. 78-184).Washington, DC: U.S. Government Printing Office, 1976.

Hurst, J., *The Reform of Health Care: A Comparative Analysis of Seven OECD Countries*. Paris: OECD, 1992.

Hyde, C., *The Soviet Health Service: A Historical and Comparative Study*. London: Lawrence and Wusharat, 1974.

Immergut, E., *Health Politics: Interests and Institutions in Western Europe*. New York: Cambridge University Press, 1992.

Klass, O., "Explaining America and the Welfare State: An Alternative Theory," *Health Affairs, 41*(Spring), 1985.

Klein, R., *The New Politics of the NHS* (3rd ed.). London: Longman, 1995.

Klein, R., "Why Britain's Conservatives Support a Socialist Health Care System," *Health Affairs, 41*, Spring 1985.

Leichter, H. M., *A Comparative Approach to Policy Analysis: Health Care Policy in Four Nations*. Cambridge: Cambridge University Press, 1979.

Leichter, H., *Free to Be Foolish: Politics and Health Promotion in the United States and Great Britain*. Princeton, NJ: Princeton University Press, 1991.

Leslie, C., Ed., "Theoretical Foundations for the Comparative Study of Medical Systems," *Social Science and Medicine, 12* (Special Issue), 1978.

Levit, K., Lazenby, H., & Sivarajan, L., "National Health Expenditures, 1994," *Health Care Financing Review, 3*(17), 52, 1996.

Light, D., & Schuler, A., *Political Values and Health Care: The German Experience*. Cambridge, MA: MIT Press, 1986.

Lindsey, A., *Socialized Medicine in England and Wales*. Chapel Hill: University of North Carolina Press, 1962.

Marmor, T., Bridges, A., & Hoffman, W., "Comparative Politics and Health Policies: Notes on Benefits, Costs, Limits." In D. Ashford (Ed.) , *Comparing Public Policies*. Beverly Hills, CA: Sage Publications, 1978.

Maynard, A., *Annual Report on the National Health Service*. New York: Center for Health Economics, 1986.

McLachlan, G., & Maynard, A. (Eds.), *The Public/Private Mix for Health: The Relevance and Effects of Change*. London: Nuffield Provincial Hospitals Trust, 1982.

Mechanic, D., "The Comparative Study of Health Care Delivery Systems," in *The Growth of Bureaucratic Medicine: An Inquiry into the Dynamics of Patient Behavior*. New York: John Wiley, 1976.

Raffel, N. (Ed.), *Comparative Health Systems*. University Park: Pennsylvania State University Press, 1985.

Reinhardt, U., "Hard Choices in Health Care: A Matter of Ethics," in L. Etheredge et al. (Eds.), *Health Care: How to Improve It and Pay for It*. Washington, DC: Center for National Policy, 1985.

Robinson, R., & Le Grand, J., *Evaluating the NHS Reforms*. London: King's Fund Institute, 1994.

Rodwin, V., "The Marriage of National Health Insurance and *la Médecine Libérale* in France: A Costly Union," *Milbank Memorial Fund Quarterly: Health and Society, 59,* 16, 1981.

Rodwin, V., *The Health Planning Predicament: France, Quebec, England and the United States*. Berkeley: University of California Press, 1984.

Rodwin, V., "Physician Payment Reform: Lessons from Abroad," *Health Affairs, 9*(1), 1989a.

Rodwin, V., "New Ideas for Health Policy in France, Canada, and Britain," in M. Field (Ed.), *Success and Crisis in National Health Systems: A Comparative Approach*. New York: Routledge, 1989b.

Rodwin, V., "The Rise of Managed Care in the United States: Lessons for French Health Policy," in C. Altenstetter & J. Bjorkman (Eds.), *Health Policy Reform, National Variations and Globalization*. New York: St. Martin's Press, 1997.

Rodwin, V., & Brecher, C., "Comparative Analysis and Mutual Learning," in Rodwin et al. (Eds.), *Public Hospital Systems in New York and Paris*. New York: New York University Press, 1992.

Rodwin, V., & Sandier, S., "Health Care under French National Health Insurance: A Public-Private Mix, Low Prices and High Volumes," *Health Affairs*, Fall, 110–131, 1993.

Roemer, M., *Comparative and National Policies on Health Care*. New York: Marcel Dekker, 1977.

Roemer, M., *National Health Systems of the World* (Vols. 1 and 2). New York: Oxford, 1991.

Roemer, M., & Roemer, R., *Health Care Systems and Comparative Manpower Policies*. New York: Marcel Dekker, 1981.

Rosner, D., "Health Care for the 'Truly Needy': Nineteenth-Century Origins of the Concept," *Milbank Memorial Fund Quarterly: Health and Society, 60* (Summer), 355, 1982.

Saltman, R. (Ed.), *The International Handbook of Health Care Systems*. New York: Greenwood Press, 1988.

Saltman, R., & Von Otter, C., *Planned Markets and Public Competition: Strategic Reform in Northern European Health Systems*. Philadelphia, Open University Press, 1992.

Saltman, R., & Von Otter, C., *Implementing Planned Markets in Health Care*. Bristol, PA: Open Society Press, 1995.

Schweitzer, S., *Policies for the Containment of Health Care Costs and Expenditures* (DHEW Publication No. 78-184). Washington, DC: U.S. Government Printing Office, 1978.

Sidel, V., & Sidel, R., *A Healthy State: An International Perspective on the Crisis in the United States Medical Care*. New York: Pantheon, 1977.

Siegrist, H., *Medicine and Health in the Soviet Union*. New York: Citadel Press, 1947.

Stoddard, D., *Rationalizing the Health Care System*. Paper presented at the Ontario Council Conference, Toronto, May 14–15, 1984.

Stone, D., *The Limits of Professional Power*. Chicago: University of Chicago Press, 1980.

Stone, D., "Drawing Lessons from Comparative Health Research," in R. A. Straetz, M. Lieberman, & A. Sardell (Eds.) , *Critical Issues in Health Policy* (pp. 135–148). Lexington, MA: D.C. Heath and Co., 1981.

Teune, H., "The Logic of Comparative Policy Analysis," in D. Ashford (Ed.), *Comparing Public Policies*. Beverly Hills, CA: Sage Publications, 1978.

Townsend, P., & Davidson, N. (Eds.), *Inequalities in Health: The Black Report*. London: Penguin, 1982.

Wall, A. (Ed.), *Health Care Systems in Liberal Democracies*. London, Routledge, 1996.

Weinerman, R., "Research on Comparative Health Systems," *Medical Care, 11*(9), 3, 1971.

Weinerman, R., & Weinerman, J., *Social Medicine in Eastern Europe: Organization of Health Services and the Education of Medical Personnel in Czechoslovakia, Hungary, and Poland*. Cambridge, MA: Harvard University Press, 1969.

Wilsford, D., *Doctors and the State: The Politics of Health Care in France and the United States*. Durham, NC: Duke University Press, 1991.

Working for Patients. London: Her Majesty's Stationery Office, 1989.

Suggested Readings on Comparative Health Systems and Policy

Altenstetter, C., & J. Björkman, eds., *Health Policy Reform, National Variations and Globalization*. New York: St. Martin's Press, 1997.

Anderson, O., *The Health Services Continuum in Democratic States*. Ann Arbor, MI: Health Administration Press, 1989.

Ellencweig, A., *Analyzing Health Systems: A Modular Approach*. New York: Oxford University Press, 1992.

Field, M., ed., *Success and Crisis in National Health Systems*. New York: Routledge, 1989.

Graig, L., *Health of Nations: An International Perspective on U.S. Health Care Reform*. Washington, DC: Congressional Quarterly Press, 1993.

Health Affairs, "Pursuit of Health Systems Reform" (Special Issue), *10* , Fall, 1991.

Hurst, J., *The Reform of Health Care: A Comparative Analysis of Seven OECD Countries*. Paris: OECD, 1992.

Investing in Health: World Bank Development Report. Washington, DC: World Bank, 1993.

Jérôme-Forget, M., J. White, & J. Weiner, eds., *Health Care Reform through Internal Markets: Experience and Proposals*. Washington, DC: Brookings Institute for Research on Public Policy, 1995.

Journal of Health Policy, Politics and Law, "Comparative Health Policy" Special Issue, *17*, Winter, 1992.

Lassey, M., Lassey, W., & Jinks, M., *Health Care Systems Around the World*. Upper Saddle River, NJ: Prentice Hall, 1997.

Merrill, J., *The Road to Health Care Reform*. New York: Plenum, 1994.

OECD, *Health Care Systems in Transition: The Search for Efficiency*. Paris: Author, 1990.

OECD Health Systems: Facts and Trends (1960–1991). Paris: OECD, 1993.

OECD Health Systems: The Socioeconomic Environment (Statistical References). Paris: OECD, 1993.

OECD, *Health: Quality and Choice.* Paris: Author, 1994.

OECD, *New Directions in Health Policy.* Paris: Author, 1995.

OECD, *Health Care Reform: The Will to Change.* Paris: Author, 1996.

OECD, *Internal Markets in the Making: Health Systems in Canada, Iceland and the United Kingdom.* Paris: Author, 1995.

Payer, L., *Medicine and Culture: Varieties of Treatment in the United States, England, West Germany and France.* New York: Henry Holt, Owl Book Edition, 1996.

Raffel, M. W., ed., *Comparative Health Systems.* University Park, PA: Pennsylvania State University Press, 1985.

Raffel, M., ed., *Health Care Reform in Industrial Countries.* University Park, PA: Pennsylvania State University Press, 1997.

Saltman, R., ed., *The International Handbook of Health Systems.* New York: Greenwood Press, 1988.

Saltman, R., & C. Von Otter, *Implementing Planned Markets in Health Care.* Bristol, PA: Open University Press, 1995.

White, J., *Competing Solutions: American Health Care Proposals and International Experience.* Washington, DC: Brookings, Institution, 1995.

II

Settings

Part II, "Settings," is divided into five chapters: on hospitals, ambulatory care, long-term care, mental health, and health maintenance organizations (HMOs) and managed care. Settings are places where health care is provided. Integrated health care systems provide or arrange for care of patients that crosses all these elements—acute care, primary care, chronic care, mental health care, and managed care—in a vertically connected fashion. The settings are not exclusive categories—for example, mental health care is provided in hospitals, in ambulatory care and long-term care settings, and in health maintenance organizations. (We have chosen to give mental health its own chapter because it is financed differently from physical and chronic care and because organizations and workers that provide only mental health care face certain different issues and concerns, such as legal questions regarding involuntary hospitalization.)

In chapter 6, A. R. Kovner explains how hospitals fit into the health care delivery system, describes their historical development in the United States, and presents current hospital statistics and characteristics. Some important types of hospitals—teaching, systems, public, and rural hospitals—are described. Next, the economic impact of hospitals is discussed. Hospital organizational structure is reviewed, as in the governance structure and processes of hospitals under different kinds of sponsorship—public, nonprofit, and for-profit. Forces compelling and constraining change in hospitals are detailed. Current issues are presented, including overcapacity, preferential ownership, physicians' relationship to hospitals, and ways to make hospitals more accountable for performance.

In chapter 7, Mezey introduces different concepts of ambulatory care and presents ambulatory care statistics. Next, he reviews the organization of ambulatory care services. He categorizes ambulatory care as primary, emergency, specialty, alternative, and self-care, each of which he discusses. He concludes with a discussion of current issues, including who will and should be future primary care providers and the impact of financing of delivery models, concluding with a discussion of the benefits of primarily providing care to populations or panels of patients for better social results.

In chapter 8, Richardson, Raphael, and Barton examine the long-term-care sector, which includes health, social, and housing services for those with chronic illness. They begin by describing the types of health and social services that are part of long-term care. Next they present the characteristics and health needs of people with chronic illness, and the demographic changes that will affect the future demand for long-term care. Long-term care is costly and, unlike acute care, most expenses are paid for by insurance. The authors review the characteristics and performances of the main institutional providers of long-term care: nursing homes, home health and hospice services, and other services in the community supporting the chronically ill. Finally, they conclude with examining some of the major reforms affecting the future demand and cost of long-term care, such as Medicare reform, managed care, private insurance, and integration of long-term and acute care.

In chapter 9, Sharfstein, Stoline, and Koran present definitions and an overview of mental illness. Included are the forms and prevalence of mental disorders and treatments and services for the mentally ill. Next, the historical development of the American mental health care system is traced. The authors discuss mental health personnel, trends in delivery, and settings for mental health services. This is followed by a discussion of insurance coverage for mental disorders. Some of the most important legal issues include commitment procedures, the right to treatment, the right to refuse treatment, and the insanity defense in criminal proceedings. Patient–therapist relationships and utilization review procedures have also been subjected to judicial and legislative scrutiny. The authors conclude with a discussion of current issues such as access to care, priorities for care, and the emphasis on cost control in recent years at the expense of patient care.

In the final chapter in Part II, a new chapter for the sixth edition, A. R. Kovner discusses recent developments in HMOs and managed care. He begins with a consideration of what purchasers of health care want and why this has resulted in the impressive growth of HMOs and managed care. This is followed by a historical description of managed care, a look at the organizational structure of HMOs, and a discussion of their important statistics and service characteristics. Prototype HMOs, such as Kaiser-Permanente and Humana are highlighted. Kovner next reviews how a typical HMO premium dollar is spent. There is a discussion of forces compelling and constraining change in managed care, such as pressure from regulators, large purchasers, competitors, providers, and advocates. The chapter concludes with a review of current issues, raising the following questions: Does provision of medical care by HMOs cost any less than that provided by traditional and other providers? To what extent do HMOs and managed care plans encourage too little care for members? Do health plans and insurers add sufficient value to justify spending 33%–40% of the premium on nonservice costs? And to what extent should HMOs and managed care share in the financing of medical education, research, and the cost of serving the uninsured?

6

Hospitals

Anthony R. Kovner

Learning Objectives

1. Explain why hospitals have developed as they have in the United States.
2. Differentiate among some important types of hospitals.
3. Describe the economic impact of hospitals.
4. Analyze the organizational structure of hospitals and the ways in which physicians are affiliated with them.
5. Describe the role of hospitals in health delivery systems.
6. Analyze the forces propelling and constraining change in hospitals.

Topical Outline

How hospitals fit into the health care delivery system
Historical development of hospitals
Hospital statistics and characteristics
Some important types of hospitals
    Teaching hospitals
    Hospital systems
    Public hospitals
    Rural hospitals
Economic impact of hospitals
    Importance to communities
    Jobs
    Cost
Hospital organizational structure
    Functional vs. divisional structure
    Models of medical service organization

Hospital mergers and affiliations
Accountability of hospitals
Forces compelling and constraining change in hospitals
Current issues
  Overcapacity
  Ownership
  How physicians should relate to hospitals
  Accountability for performance

Key Words: **Hospital, voluntary hospital, community hospital, teaching hospital, hospital case-mix, medical services organization, dual authority structure, hospital systems.**

To many Americans, hospitals are "a white labyrinth" (see Smith & Kaluzny, 1986)—large, complex, and subtle institutions. Until we are sick, we often know little about what goes on inside our local hospital, other than that very ill patients are being treated by doctors, expensive bills go out, and hospital care is complex and labor intensive. Hospitals are complicated places that carry out many different functions while caring for the sick. Even those who work in them often know little about departments or occupations other than their own. Yet hospitals, like other more familiar local organizations, open, grow, merge, and even close. A key theme of this chapter is the transformation of many hospitals away from being the center of health care in many communities to being an important part of a larger health care system that spans several communities.

This chapter covers the following topics concerning hospitals: historical development, statistics and characteristics, some important types, economic significance, organizational structure, ownership and accountability, forces compelling and constraining change, and current issues of overcapacity, type of ownership, the organizational relationship of the medical staff to the institution, and accountability for performance.

Historical Development

The development of American community hospitals (average length of stay of 30 days or less for patients and nonfederal in their ownership) can be divided into the following periods:

Early hospitals, built before 1870

First period of rapid growth, 1870–1910

Period of consolidation, 1910–1945

Second period of rapid growth, 1945–1980

Current period of consolidation, 1980 to the present

The first American hospitals were primarily religious and charitable, tending to provide care for the sick rather than medical cure (Freymann, 1974, pp. 28–29; Rosenberg, 1974; Starr, 1982). Private voluntary hospitals, founded and operated by community leaders in the United States, go back to the 18th century (Freymann, pp. 22–24). These hospitals could do little to cure their patients (the well-to-do were largely cared for by physicians in their homes). By 1873, there were an estimated 178 hospitals in the United States (Stevens, p. 52).

From 1870 to 1910, as biomedical science and technology developed more effective means of intervention, hospitals evolved into local workshops for physicians treating all classes of patients. Safer hospital care was achieved through advances in general hospital hygiene, including the development of trained nurses and techniques for asepsis and surgical anesthesia. Between 1870 and 1910 the number of hospitals grew spectacularly, increasing 20-fold to more than 4,300 in 1909 (Stevens, p. 52). Medical care had become too complex for physicians to carry their entire armamentarium in their black bags; the hospital's special equipment and consultation with other medical specialists had become essential parts of medical practice.

According to Starr (pp. 169–170) the period from 1750 to 1850 saw the formation of voluntary and public hospitals. From 1850 to 1890 local communities developed religious or ethnic institutions and specialized hospitals for certain diseases or categories of patients such as children and women. During the period 1890–1920 many physicians started their own for-profit hospitals. Fewer new hospitals were built during the period from 1910 to 1945 than before or after.

The types of patients in hospitals changed with each medical discovery. In 1923 the discovery of insulin drastically altered the nature of treatment for diabetes. Liver extract reduced the incidence of pernicious anemia in 1929. Sulfonamides began to affect treatment of pneumonia and some other infectious diseases in 1935, a trend that accelerated with the introduction of antibiotics beginning in 1943, as well as the continuing development of immunization techniques. The development of rehabilitation services began to bring more disabled patients to hospitals. In the 1950s hospital treatment became more important for chronic disease. As infectious diseases generally have been conquered (with the notable exception of AIDS), hospitals increasingly focused on the pathology of trauma and degenerative and neoplastic disease.

The years from 1945 to 1980 were a second major growth period, during which there was a tremendous increase in hospital services, costs, and technology and a more modest expansion in the number of hospitals. Many small rural hospitals were built during this period, financed by federal monies under federal legislation known as the Hill-Burton Act. A major factor influencing the increased breadth and intensity of hospital care was the rapid growth of insurance to pay for hospital care. The Blue Cross system originally was developed during the Great Depression to help assure payment to hospitals. Hospital insurance developed rapidly during World War II as a result of collective bargaining agreements. In that period the federal government limited the allowable amounts of wage increases but not of noncash benefits. In 1965 the Medicare and Medicaid programs were created, the former providing hospital and medical insurance for the elderly and the latter providing it for the poor. Over the 40-year period from 1935, the availability of a source of payment for hospital care (especially within the context of generally less widespread coverage for other types of care) was a major factor in the increase in hospital utilization, in terms both of admissions and average length of stay, that occurred during that period.

Since 1980 hospital discharge rates and average length of stay have decreased. Age-adjusted hospital discharge rates went from 159 per 1,000 in 1980 to 109 discharges per 1,000 population in 1993 (National Center for Health Statistics, 1996). Between 1984 and 1994, the number of hospitals decreased from 5,759 to 5,229 and the average daily census from 702,000 to 568,000 (AHA 1996–97). Because the average daily census decreased more rapidly than the number of beds, hospital occupancy has been decreasing as well, from 75.6% in 1980 to 62.9% in 1994 (AHA 1996–97). There are also fewer independent hospitals. According to the AHA's Annual Survey of Hospitals, 21% of community hospitals participated in health networks in 1994, up from 11% in 1993 (AHA 1995–96).

Hospital care is big business. In 1994 hospital expenditures amounted to $338.5 billion, representing 36% of the nation's health expenditures and 4.9% of the nation's gross national product or $1,264 per American spent on hospital care (National Center for Health Statistics 1996). Hospital profits were 5% of costs in 1994 (Thorpe, 1997).

Hospital Statistics and Characteristics

There are two major agencies that count and classify hospitals in the United States: the American Hospital Association (AHA) and the National Center for Health Statistics (NCHS) of the U.S. Department of Health and Human Services. (Another valuable resource is *The Sourcebook*, annually published by HCIA and Deloitte & Touche.) The AHA annually publishes the *AHA Guide to the Health Care Field* (AHA, 1995–96a), its journal *Hospitals*, and a companion publication, *Hospital Stat* (AHA, 1996–97). Together these publications list each AHA-registered hospital, giving its basic characteristics as well as much summary data. The NCHS publishes the results of its "Hospital Discharge Survey" periodically in *Monthly Vital Statistics Report* and *Health and Vital Statistics.* The "Hospital Discharge Survey" gathers and analyzes data from a sample of hospitals on demographic characteristics of patients, descriptors of hospitals, morbidity diagnoses, and surgical operations. Since 1976, a congressionally mandated annual report to the president, titled *Health: United States,* has appeared. It includes some data on hospitals, as well as health and financial data.

Hospital Statistics

Table 6.1 provides summary statistics on community hospitals. Community hospitals include general short-term hospitals under not-for-profit (voluntary), public (governmental), and investor-owned (proprietary) auspices. As of 1995, 69.8% of the beds and 60% of the hospitals are under nonprofit auspice; 18.0% of the beds and 25.9% of the hospitals are under governmental auspice; and 12.1% of the beds and 14.4% of the hospitals are under for-profit auspice (AHA, 1996–97). Other hospitals include federal hospitals and long-term mental and other hospitals.

From 1985 to 1995, as shown in Table 6.1, the number of community hospitals has decreased, by 9.4%, whereas their average size has decreased from 175 to 168 beds. During the 10 years the number of beds decreased by 12.8%, the number of admissions by 7.8%, and their average daily census by 15.6%. On the other hand, the number of surgical operations increased by 15.1% and the

TABLE 6.1 Selected Measures in Community Hospitals, 1995 and 1985

Measure	1995	1985
Hospitals	5,194	5,732
Beds (000s)	873	1,001
Average size (beds)	168	175
Admissions (000s)	30,945	33,449
Average daily census (000s)	548	649
Average length of stay, days	6.5	7.1
Inpatient days (000s)	199,876	236,619
Surgical operations (000s)	23,163	20,113
Births (000s)	3,765	3,521
Outpatient visits (000s)	414,345	218,716

Source: Adapted from the American Hospital Association, *Hospital Statistics*, 1996–97 (AHA 1996–97).

number of outpatient visits by 89.4%. Obviously, hospitals these days are focusing more attention on ambulatory than on inpatient care.

A different set of statistics is available from the *Sourcebook*, drawn primarily from Medicare cost reports and providing a 5-year financial and operational report card on 3,972 hospitals with 25 or more beds in service.

What Table 6.2 shows is that, despite provision of less inpatient care, hospitals remain profitable. According to *Hospital Stat*, the nation's hospitals' aggregate profit margin was 6.7% in 1996 (AHA, 1997–8). Hospitals have been able to accomplish this largely by reducing average length of stay and full-time-equivalent (FTE) staff per discharge rather than through reducing excess capacity by closing facilities or combining programs and services (Pallarito).

Hospital Characteristics

Hospitals differ from one another with respect to size, mission, ownership, complexity, competitive environment, population served, endowment and financial situation, physical facilities, costs per day for care, or patient diagnostic category.

Many hundreds of hospitals have fewer than 50 beds each. Many of these hospitals are in areas with sparse populations, the nearest hospital being an hour's drive away or more for many residents of the community. On the other hand, as of 1994, 273 hospitals had more than 500 beds (AHA, 1996–97); some have more than 1,000 beds. These are naturally found in densely populated cities, for some people the nearest hospital being literally across the street.

TABLE 6.2   Hospital Vital Signs

Vital signs	Median values, 1995
Occupancy rate, acute care	45.16%
Percentage of outpatient revenues	37.34%
Operating revenues per adjusted discharge	$4,797
Total profit margin	5.33%
FTEs per adjusted average daily census	5.23
FTEs per 100 adjusted discharges	6.10
Salaries and benefits per FTE	$38,411
Percentage of salary and benefits expense	50.90%

An example of the small hospital, according to the 1995–96 AHA hospital guide, Union County General Hospital in Clayton, New Mexico, had 28 beds and provided the following services: a birthing room; breast cancer screening; case management; community health reporting, health status assessment, and service planning; a diagnostic radioisotope facility; an emergency department; transportation; a health fair; home health services; a hospice; outpatient surgery; and ultrasound. At the other end of the spectrum, New York University Medical Center in New York City had 879 beds and was listed as providing all of the services that Union County General provided. In addition, NYU Medical Center provided alcoholism services; angioplasty; cardiac catheterization laboratory and intensive care unit; community outreach; crisis prevention; computerized axial tomography (CT) scanner; dental services; extracorporeal shock wave lithotripter; fitness center; geriatric services; health information center and health screenings; HIV-AIDS services; hospital-based outpatient care; magnetic resonance imaging (MRI); Meals-on-Wheels; medical-surgical, neonatal, and pediatric intensive care units; nutrition programs; obstetrics unit; occupational health services; oncology services; open heart and outpatient surgery; patient education center and patient representative services; physical rehabilitation inpatient unit and outpatient services; positron emission tomography scanner; primary care department; psychiatric care, including an inpatient unit, child adolescent services, consultation-liaison services, education, emergency, geriatric and outpatient services, and a partial hospitalization program; radiation therapy; reproductive health services; single photon emission computerized tomography; social work; sports medicine; support groups; teen outreach services; transplant services; trauma center; urgent care center; volunteer services; and a women's health center (AHA, 1995–96).

Hospitals are similar to one another in that they provide inpatient care by nurses and physicians, the latter having a good deal of autonomy in deciding whom to admit and what services patients will receive. Hospitals must be financially solvent to survive as organizations. Many of them also seek to grow. Hospitals provide services every day and at every hour of the day. Some hospital services are difficult to quantify and measure; for example, how can one measure the amount of health education service a patient receives? But all hospitals are organized so that standby capacity or arrangements are available to meet medical emergencies and to deal with critical and life-threatening situations. Hospitals are characterized by hierarchy and rules. There is increasing standardization of patient care, for example with regard to what drugs are available for certain diagnoses. There is general agreement about the principal objectives of hospitals: curing and caring.

Some Important Types of Hospitals

The American Hospital Association classifies hospitals in several ways. Those in which the average length of stay is 30 days or less are called short-term hospitals. In long-term hospitals the average length of stay is more than 30 days. There are specialty hospitals—for example, orthopedic or cancer—and general hospitals. There are teaching and nonteaching hospitals, hospitals that are independent or are part of multihospital systems, public and private hospitals, and nonprofit and for-profit (also called investor-owned) hospitals. The following important types of short-term hospitals will be discussed: teaching, those in multihospital systems, public, and rural. These categories are not mutually exclusive. For example, Bellevue Hospital in New York City is a public, teaching hospital that is part of a multihospital system.

Teaching Hospitals

In 1994 there were 274 short-term, general nonfederal hospitals belonging to the Council of Teaching Hospitals and Health Systems (COTH) of the Association of American Medical Colleges. These COTH hospitals represent 6% of all hospitals. Relative to other hospitals, COTH hospitals are larger and more generally in large urban areas. They offer more specialized services and provide more service for which they are paid from any source termed "uncompensated care" than are non-COTH hospitals. Although COTH hospitals represent only 6% of the nation's hospitals, in 1994, 22% of the nation's total outpatient visits were to COTH hospitals, as were 18% of total surgical operations. COTH hospitals employed 25% of the total full-time equivalent employees (FTEs) for all hospitals in 1994 (Association of American Colleges, personal communication, 1996).

Because of their commitment to the triad of teaching hospital missions—education, research, and patient care—COTH members also offer a large percentage of tertiary or highly complex services. For example, in 1994, 94% of COTH members reported having a cardiac catheterization function (vs. 31% for non-COTH members); 82% reported having megavoltage radiation services (only 36% for non-COTH hospitals); and 63% reported the capability to perform organ transplants (only 5% of non-COTH hospitals reported the capability to perform them).

In 1994, COTH members claimed 45% of the total deductions against charges for charity care (out of all short-term nonfederal hospitals); this was approximately $5.6 billion and 27% of the deductions for bad debt (approximately $3.8 billion) (Association of American Colleges, personal communication, 1996).

Multihospital Systems

Hospitals are part of a multihospital system when they are either leased under contract management by another hospital or are legally incorporated by or under the direction of a board that determines the control of two or more hospitals (Ermann & Gabel, 1984). Increasingly, hospitals are becoming parts of larger health systems that are more than systems of hospitals. Such health systems commonly provide diversified services, including surgery, ambulatory care, rehabilitation, home health services, skilled nursing, psychiatric care, and alcohol/drug dependency facilities and services.

The investor-owned corporation Columbia/HCA is the largest health system in the United States. As of 1995, it had over $20 billion in sales annually and owned 348 hospitals in 38 states as well as hundreds of outpatient diagnostic and surgery centers, nursing homes, home care units, blood centers, and psychiatric facilities. With 285,000 employees, Columbia/HCA is the ninth largest nongovernment employer in the United States. The company has been criticized for "making fat profits on hospitals at the expense of the poor and the sick" (Ginsburg, 1996), but they are certainly not alone in making money out of health care where each of the over $1 trillion of expense is a dollar of income for somebody. Let us not forget that Columbia/HCA's $20 billion in sales is about a 2% share of the health care market. In the automobile industry, General Motors has 33% of the market ("U.S. Vehicle Sales," 1996).

In 1994 more than 650 hospitals were involved in mergers or acquisitions with other hospitals (HCIA Inc.). There has also been increased merger activity among hospital alliances (whose participating members are in a federated entity composed of independent hospitals or hospital systems organized for joint ventures or to achieve joint action, such as lower purchasing costs). The year 1994 witnessed the merger of American Healthcare Systems and Premier Health Alliance, two of the larger alliances, with more than 1,400 hospitals and 25% of all U.S. hospital beds (HCIA Inc.).

Rural Hospitals

A rural area is territory falling outside a metropolitan statistical area (MSA), which is defined as territory containing a city with a population of at least 50,000 or an urban area with a population of at least 50,000 and a total metropolitan population of at least 100,000 (AHA, 1992). In 1995, 2,236 of the nation's hospitals (43%) were rural. Most of these had fewer than 100 beds (AHA, 1996–97). A rural hospital is often the first or second largest local employer and provides an essential element in the infrastructure needed for local economic development (Berry & Beaulieu, 1994).

Sixty rural hospitals closed in 1995 (AHA, 1996–97). Key problems of rural hospitals include threat of closure, thereby depriving local residents of access to care; the questionable financial viability of hospitals with fewer than 50 beds; difficulties in assuring quality of care in such hospitals when operated as independent units; and difficulties in attracting and retaining skilled professionals to work in isolated rural localities. Rural American counties face different kinds of problems depending on economic structure. Although they are often thought to consist only of farm areas, rural counties can be classified as economically dependent on farming; manufacturing; mining; oil and energy; large federal, state, or local government installations; federal lands; and retirement settlement communities; or they may be characterized by persistent poverty (AHA, 1992).

In 1994 a considerable number of rural hospitals joined together to serve sparsely populated regions. This promotes the sharing of expensive medical equipment among smaller hospitals that have little available capital and allows leverage in contract negotiations with managed care providers. Belonging to a system also gives rural hospitals a better chance of attracting and retaining physicians.

Public Hospitals

Public hospitals are owned by agencies of federal, state, and local governments. Federal hospitals typically have been designed for special beneficiaries: American Indians, merchant seamen, military personnel, and veterans. State hospitals typically have provided long-term psychiatric and chronic care, in the past especially for patients with tuberculosis. There are also state university or teaching hospitals that provide short-term general acute care.

There are two main types of local, short-term, general public hospitals by ownership. They may be owned by a city or county government department or by a freestanding governmental entity, such as an authority, a district, or a public benefit corporation. Increasingly, like those in the private sector, public hospitals are seeking alternative structures, including forming nonprofit corporations or entering into public-private mergers or partnerships. The first type has characteristics similar to the smaller nonprofit hospital, is located in small towns or cities of moderate size, is used by private attending physicians, and serves paying and indigent patients.

The second type is located in major urban areas. Physician staff is mostly salaried and works either for the hospital directly or for medical school clinical practice plans. The larger public hospitals typically rely heavily on medical residents in training to provide physician services. The deficits of some, though not all, public hospitals and systems are paid for from local taxes or federal Medicare and Medicaid "disproportionate share" hospital payments.

Hospital Organizational Structure

The basic departments of the short-term general hospital are medical and dental, nursing, other diagnostic and therapeutic support (such as pharmacy and social service), financial and information, human resources, and "hotel" services such as security and housekeeping. Most community hospitals provide services both to inpatients, who are admitted and assigned a bed (usually two patients to a room), and to outpatients who come to an emergency department, an ambulatory care department, or to a diagnostic or therapeutic service for a procedure not requiring admission as an inpatient.

Medical and Dental Staff

Physicians and dentists relate to community hospitals in different ways. Attending physicians on the hospital staff who are not salaried often conduct much of their business in private offices that they own or rent. These physicians may admit patients to more than one hospital and may compete with each other and any particular hospital for patients or customers. Other physicians may be full-time, either salaried or paid by the hospital in proportion to the amount of work they do. These physicians often see patients or perform related activities in offices that are provided to them by the hospital. Some hospitals employ physicians to provide primary care in competition with other physicians who are attendings or local nonhospital affiliated practitioners. Other hospitals contract with physician groups to provide emergency care or subspecialist services on hospital premises or in satellite centers. Some physicians are attendings who maintain their own practices distinct from the hospital but who also receive a part-time salary from the hospital for administrative work, such as being the chief of a service (e.g., obstetrics-gynecology).

When physicians admit patients to the hospital, they are free to order whatever tests or treatments they deem necessary within guidelines set out by the medical staff and approved by the hospital board of directors. The chief executive officer is responsible, usually through a chief medical officer, for assuring compliance with these guidelines. Traditionally, the physician has managed the care: determined the amount of services used and the consequent costs of patient care. This has been changing recently as others "manage" care and more physicians increasingly accept, given limited resources, the implications that follow from all patients (and plan members) not benefitting when physicians are allowed to order whatever they wish for particular patients.

Although the attending (nonsalaried) physician is technically a guest in the hospital (or indirectly acts as a subcontractor), the hospital is responsible for the care its staff renders patients on a physician's orders. Until several years ago, hospitals could not be held liable for the wrongful conduct of a physician, but this principle has been significantly changed by a series of judicial decisions, beginning in the 1970s (Southwick, 1978). Changing legal doctrines regarding negligence and the corporate liability of hospitals have established that hospitals are legally responsible and, to the extent that hospital negligence is involved, financially responsible for the care and the arrangements for care provided by their entire clinician and administrative staff.

Traditionally, physicians have been mostly organized along the lines of medical specialties (of which there are more than 20). But not all hospitals provide all specialty services, and in smaller hospitals, for organizational purposes, several specialties, such as surgical subspecialties, are combined. The larger the hospital and the more specialized the medical services, the greater the number of separate medical departments. There is no universal logic to the way in which the medical departments are categorized. Some are differentiated from the others based on the type of skill involved, some by the age or sex or the primary patient group, and others by the organ or organ system that primarily falls under their purview. They don't always agree as to which specialty can best treat certain patients with certain diagnoses. Departments found in most hospitals include the following:

- *Internal Medicine*: general diagnosis and therapy of adults for problems involving one or more internal organs or the skin, in which the principal tools do not involve a physical alteration of the patient's body by the physician.
- *Surgery*: diagnosis and therapy in which the principal tools involve a physical alteration of a part of the patient's body by the physician.
- *Pediatrics*: general diagnosis and therapy for children, primarily but not entirely with nonsurgical techniques.
- *Obstetrics/gynecology*: diagnosis and therapy relating to women's health and to the sexual and reproductive system of women, using both surgical and nonsurgical techniques.
- *Psychiatry/neurology*: diagnosis and therapy for people of all ages with mental, emotional, and nervous system problems, using primarily nonsurgical techniques.
- *Radiology/diagnostic imaging*: diagnosis and therapy, primarily through the use of x-ray and other internal imaging techniques.
- *Pathology*: diagnosis, both before and after treatment.
- *Anesthesiology*: principally concerned with preparing patients so that they may be surgically operated upon with no pain or discomfort during the procedure.

Other general medical departments include family and emergency medicine. More subspecialized medical departments tend to be organized around organs and organ systems, for example, ophthalmology (eye); otolaryngology (ear, nose, and throat); urology (male sexual/reproductive system and the renal system for both sexes); orthopedics (bones and joints), and so on.

There are 24 medical specializations for which professional certification may be attained by passing a medical specialty board examination. Specialties other than the ones previously mentioned include allergy and immunology, dermatology, neurosurgery, nuclear medicine, physical medicine and rehabilitation, plastic surgery, preventive medicine, proctology, and thoracic surgery. There are clinicians other than physicians who may be granted hospital medical staff privileges; these include dentists, clinical (PhD) psychologists, and podiatrists.

Physicians and dentists practicing in hospitals have their own medical and dental staff organization, with bylaws, rules, and regulations that must be approved by the hospital's governing board. The medical staff bylaws specify procedures for election of medical staff officers, who are given authority under the bylaws to enforce rules and regulations. These operate through a committee structure. The officers delineate privileges, such as what operations surgeons are being credentialed to perform, and recommend disciplinary action when necessary. The officers enforce the bylaws and must oversee the committee structure and submit reports of medical staff activities to the governing board.

There are numerous medical staff committees in hospitals, some of which include nonphysicians, particularly nurses, as members. The executive committee of the medical staff commonly coordinates all activity, sets general policies, and accepts and acts on recommendations from other committees. The joint conference committee, if there is one, is made up of board and medical staff members and deliberates on matters involving medical and nonmedical considerations, such as affiliations with other hospitals. The credentials committee reviews applications by physicians to join the medical staff and considers the qualifications of education, experience, and interests before making recommendations to the executive committee. It then makes recommendations regarding appointment to the hospital's governing board. In some hospitals the joint conference committee is also involved in the process.

The infections control committee is responsible for preventing infections in the hospital through routine preventive surveillance, tracking down of outbreaks of infection, and education of hospital personnel. The pharmacy and therapeutics committee reviews pharmacologic agents for inclusion in the list of drugs approved for hospital use. The tissue committee is responsible for ensuring quality control of surgery, principally by examining and evaluating bodily tissues removed during operations.

The medical records (health information) committee is responsible for certifying complete and clinically accurate documentation of the care given to patients. This committee also acts as a judge of clinical care, based on the written record. The utilization review committee evaluates the appropriateness of admissions and length of stay in the hospital and may review use of services and facilities for patients.

The tissue, quality assurance/improvement, and utilization review/management committees provide for review of the physician's professional work by other physicians. Due to the changing legal, regulatory, and competitive environment and the increasing size and complexity of many hospitals, physicians and the medical staff are being subjected to closer scrutiny. Traditionally, in the hospital the medical chain of authority has existed side by side with an administrative chain. Increasingly, these chains are being unified, usually under the direction of physicians whose jobs are primarily managerial. The day-to-day work of medical committees, such as quality improvement and utilization management, is increasingly carried out by paid nonphysicians, who are, of course, under physician direction. There are increasing numbers of salaried physicians in hospitals other than physicians in training. In some hospitals, intensivist physicians are responsible for medical care of patients with specific diseases, such as heart attacks, and provide care formerly provided by those attending physicians whose practice has increasingly shifted away from the hospital to HMOs and the ambulatory care office.

Models of Medical Services Organization

Shortell (1985) has conceptualized four different models of organization for physicians working in hospitals: traditional (departmental), divisional, independent-corporate, and parallel. Under the traditional model, each department includes relevant medical specialists but does not contain support services required by the physicians to provide care. These services are typically organized as functional departments such as nursing, housekeeping, and dietary. Figure 6.1 shows a traditional hospital organizational chart, in which support services are organized separately from medical services. The medical staff's relationship to the hospital is indirect, as shown by the dotted line. Physicians are not a part of the hospital chain of command, as are nurses and assistant administrators. In hospitals this is referred to as a *dual authority structure* (H. L. Smith, 1995). Under this model, most physicians see themselves as independent practitioners, not hospital employees, who must practice according to medical staff bylaws, rules, and regulations that they set themselves, although they must be approved by the hospital's board of trustees.

Shortell's second model of medical services organization, the divisional model, is characterized by the placement of functional support services within medical divisions, such as surgery, medicine, or women's health. Each division includes many of the support services such as nursing and clerical (and sometimes dietary, medical records, and even routine lab and x-ray). Each medical division leader is responsible for management of the division, including financial management, of both medical and support services. The Johns Hopkins Hospital in Baltimore, Maryland, is organized along these lines (Heyssel, Gaintner, Kues, Jones, & Lipstein, 1984).

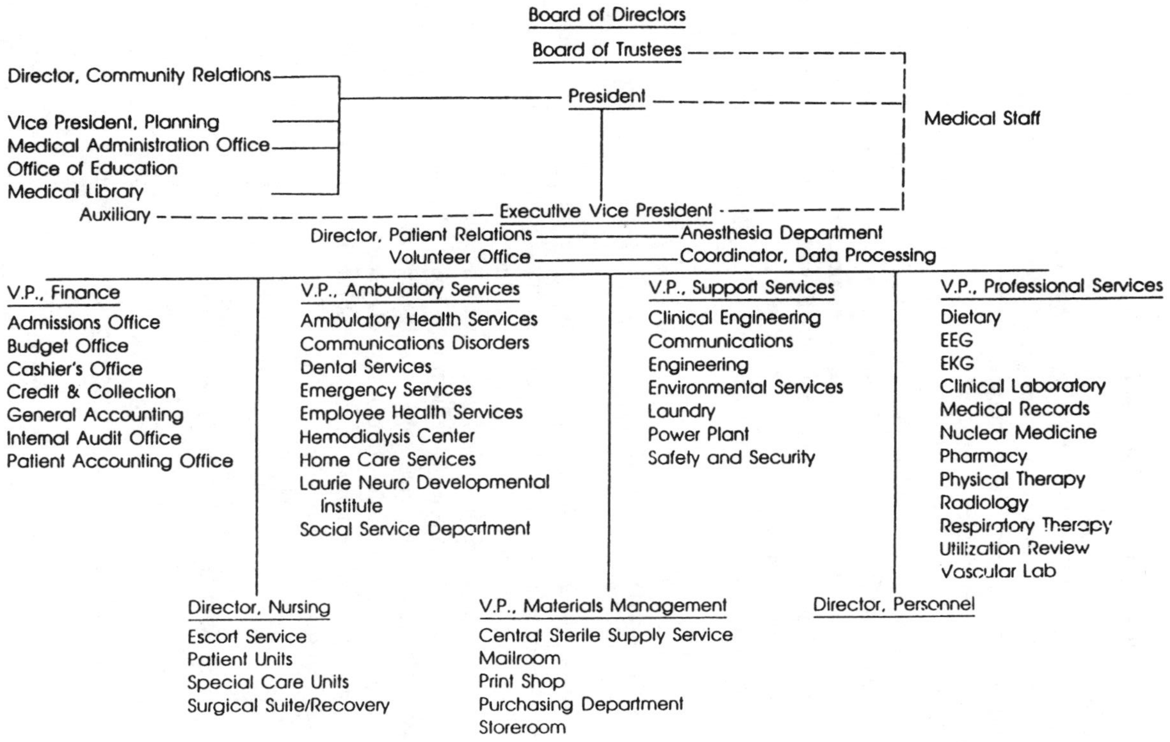

Board of Directors

Board of Trustees

President

Medical Staff

Executive Vice President

Director, Community Relations

Vice President, Planning
Medical Administration Office
Office of Education
Medical Library
Auxiliary

Director, Patient Relations
Volunteer Office
Anesthesia Department
Coordinator, Data Processing

V.P., Finance
Admissions Office
Budget Office
Cashier's Office
Credit & Collection
General Accounting
Internal Audit Office
Patient Accounting Office

V.P., Ambulatory Services
Ambulatory Health Services
Communications Disorders
Dental Services
Emergency Services
Employee Health Services
Hemodialysis Center
Home Care Services
Laurie Neuro Developmental
   Institute
Social Service Department

V.P., Support Services
Clinical Engineering
Communications
Engineering
Environmental Services
Laundry
Power Plant
Safety and Security

V.P., Professional Services
Dietary
EEG
EKG
Clinical Laboratory
Medical Records
Nuclear Medicine
Pharmacy
Physical Therapy
Radiology
Respiratory Therapy
Utilization Review
Vascular Lab

Director, Nursing
Escort Service
Patient Units
Special Care Units
Surgical Suite/Recovery

V.P., Materials Management
Central Sterile Supply Service
Mailroom
Print Shop
Purchasing Department
Storeroom

Director, Personnel

FIGURE 6.1 Traditional (departmental) organizational structure for hospital medical services.

171

Under Shortell's third model, the independent-corporate form, the medical staff becomes a separate legal entity that negotiates with the hospital to provide service. An independent group of physicians provides medical services to the hospital, under contract. A version of this model of organization is found in the Permanente medical groups. They contract with the various Kaiser health plans to form the Kaiser-Permanente medical care program, one of the nation's largest HMOs.

Shortell's fourth model involves the creation of a separate organization to conduct certain activities that are not handled well by the regular medical staff organization. Certain physicians are selected to participate in a parallel organization for some percentage of their time, typically to work on a more separate and focused agenda such as organization of a PHO (physician–hospital organization) for managed care contracting (see chapter 11) or a task force for strategic planning.

Other Patient Care Services

For a discussion of nursing services, see chapter 4 of this text. Other hospital diagnostic and therapeutic services that may or may not be part of a medical department include laboratory, usually under the direction of the department of pathology; electrocardiography, usually a part of internal medicine; electroencephalography, part of neurology; radiography, part of radiology; pharmacy; clinical psychology; social service; inhalation therapy (often part of anesthesiology or pulmonary medicine); nutrition; physical, occupational, and speech therapy, which are often in the department of rehabilitation medicine; home care; and medical records, among others.

Hospital Support Structure

The nonclinical services that a hospital provides can be categorized into four subsystems: finance, facilities and equipment (plant), human resources, and management.

The financial subsystem includes the provision of capital, operating costs, cash budgeting, pricing and allocation, long-range financial planning, and collection policies. In addition, some hospitals have endowments to invest and grants to prepare and administer.

The facilities and equipment subsystem includes dietary services (the preparation of food for patients and usually for staff and for visitors), engineering and environmental services, clinical engineering, power plant, grounds, housekeeping, communications, and purchasing and stores, among others.

The human resources subsystem includes job analysis and description, job evaluation, wage and salary administration, recruitment, screening and selection, communication to employees, training and development, organizational development, and collective bargaining and labor contract administration.

The management subsystem includes planning and marketing, community patient and public relations, data processing and management information, legal services, and compliance with governmental regulatory and accrediting organizations, among others.

The organizational structure for a multihospital or integrated delivery system is more complex and comprises a central headquarters, sometimes an intermediate divisional organization, often organized on a geographical basis (e.g., eastern and western region), as well as hospitals and other care organizations and agencies, as shown in Figure 6.2.

New Developments in Hospital Organization

Over the past five years, there has been continued pressure on hospitals to contain costs, improve quality, and justify resources used relative to contribution to community health. This is in the face of a great deal of overcapacity, which is related to incentive payment that has rewarded shorter hospital stays and lowered hospital admissions. Hospitals have adapted to these pressures in many ways. In the 1990s these have included integrated delivery networks, mergers and acquisitions, continuous quality improvement, patient-focused care, and community health benefit.

Integrated Delivery Networks, Mergers, and Acquisitions

Many hospitals are responding to local pressures by rapidly merging, acquiring, and entering into affiliations and other risk-sharing reimbursement agreements with other acute and nonacute care providers, hospital-based health care systems, physicians and physician group practices, and managed care organizations (HCIA Inc.). Transactions increasing at a rapid pace include mergers of nonprofit organizations into either investor-owned or other nonprofit entities. In 1994 mergers among hospitals, physicians, groups, HMOs, and other health care providers totaled more than $20 billion. More than 650 hospitals were involved.

According to Shortell, Gillies, and Devers (1995), the goal of integrated delivery networks is "to organize the entire continuum of care—from health promotion and disease prevention to primary and secondary acute, tertiary care,

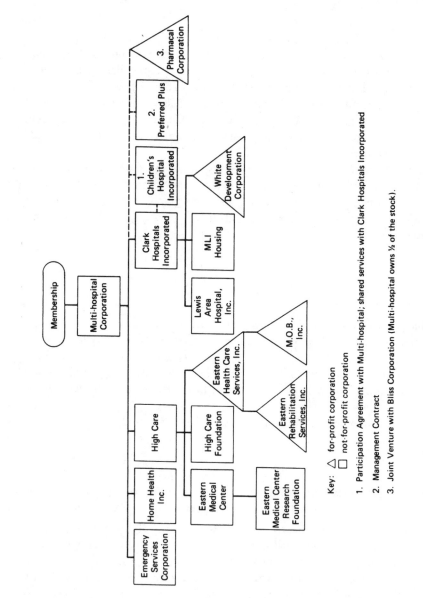

Key: △ for-profit corporation
      ☐ not-for-profit corporation

1. Participation Agreement with Multi-hospital; shared services with Clark Hospitals Incorporated

2. Management Contract

3. Joint Venture with Bliss Corporation (Multi-hospital owns ½ of the stock).

FIGURE 6.2 Multihospital system organizational chart.

174

long-term care and hospice care—so as to maximize its effectiveness across episodes of illness and pathways of wellness. A premium is placed on integration and holistic care, not fragmentation and specialist care" (pp. 39–40). Nevertheless, the study of 11 leading systems by Shortell et al. found that "their scores on physician-system integration and clinical integration are low, and progress is relatively slow" (pp. 39–40). The authors ask, "If this is true for some of the leading organizations, how much more so for the less advanced?" (Shortell, Gillies, Anderson, Erickson, & Mitchell, 1996).

It takes many years to truly integrate these new, often hospital-sponsored agglomerations of facilities and services into integrated systems for the delivery of health care. Barriers to doing so include failure to understand the new core business; inability to overcome the hospital paradigm, as it may not be consistent with system priorities; ambiguous roles and responsibilities throughout the system; inability to "manage" managed care; inability to execute the strategy; and a lack of alignment or match between various components, such as orientation toward the market versus managerial control of strategy (Shortell et al., 1996). Success is highly dependent on system investments in information technology, managerial leadership, and empowerment and shared system ownership with physicians.

Continuous Quality Improvement

Continuous quality improvement (CQI) is a concept that has been applied by many large American corporations. The basic approach is to measure variation in a work process, such as management of care for diabetes patients or of patient flow in an emergency department, in relation to a standard or benchmark and then to implement interventions to decrease process variation and to improve performance results.

The process of CQI begins with a definition of what good quality is for a particular process. Focus is on the consumer of the product or service, whether it is a physician who wishes a quick turnaround in x-ray reports or a patient or potential patient seeking a diagnosis or cure. Everyone involved in providing the product or service learns how quality is measured and participates in improving quality. Rather than focusing on poor quality outcomes and how to avoid them, the work team becomes involved in continuously improving standards for better performance and in finding ways to meet those standards.

The benefits of CQI can perhaps best be understood by comparing CQI with traditional ways of working in which managers are in charge, focus is on production and slogans, and emphasis is placed on getting the work done in the cheapest way, assuming given levels of quality, rather than on meeting or exceeding consumer or user expectations.

The steps of the CQI process are as follows: find a process to improve, organize a team that knows the process, clarify current knowledge of the process, understand the causes of variation in the process, select the process improvement and continue data collection, do the improvement data collection and analysis, check the results and lessons learned from the team effort, and act to hold the gain and to continue to improve the process.

Examples of hospital processes that can be improved are increasing the preadmission testing rate to reduce turnaround time in the operating room (in this way there are fewer delays for patients scheduled for surgery due to tests not being done or having to be redone), making maximum use of registered nurse skills and employing fewer agency nurses, improving the recruitment and retention of staff nurses, and lowering the hospital cesarean section rate (e.g., by focusing on education to avoid repeat C-sections).

According to Deming (1986), there are 14 points that must be followed to implement CQI successfully, as follows: create constancy of purpose for improvement of product and service; adopt the new philosophy; cease dependence on inspection to achieve quality; don't award business on the basis of price alone; improve constantly every process for planning, production, and service; institute on-the-job training; institute leadership; drive out fear; break down the barriers between staff areas; eliminate slogans, exhortations, and targets for the workforce; eliminate numerical quotas for the workforce and numerical goals for management; remove barriers that rob people of pride of workmanship; institute a vigorous program of education and self-improvement for everyone; and put everyone in the organization to work to accomplish the transformation.

The Patient-Focused Hospital

In "patient-focusing" the hospital attempts to contain hospital inpatient costs and improve quality by restructuring services so that more of them take place in the nursing units (patient floors), rather than in specialized units in dispersed hospital locations and by cross-training staff in the nursing units so that they can perform a variety of functions for a small group of patients, rather than one set of functions for a large number of patients. Thus, for example, x-ray and lab services can both be done in the nursing units by staff who are so trained. Or alternatively, the same staff can serve a few patients food, clean their rooms, and assist in their nursing care.

As services have been customarily organized in hospitals, to get a routine x-ray for an inpatient can require 40 separate steps and consume 140 minutes of personnel time. Up to 24 hours may elapse from the doctor's initial request to receipt of the report, and it can involve 15–20 employees. Moreover, most of the steps are not medical or clinical activities.

According to J. Smith (1990), hospital staff spend most of their time on nine activity categories: medical, technical, and clinical; hotel and patient services; medical documentation; institutional documentation; scheduling and coordination; patient transportation; staff transportation; management and supervision; and being "ready for action" (i.e., standing by in the emergency department whether or not patients are there requiring service). In a study at Lakeland Regional Medical Center, a 750-bed hospital in central Florida, Smith (1990) found that only one sixth of personnel-related costs were consumed by medical, technical, and clinical activity and that almost twice that amount of time was spent on writing things down. Scheduling and coordination took as much time as medical activity, and ready-for-action time consumed more.

J. Smith (1990) suggests that restructuring services can result in reducing the number of staff required for patient care activities at Lakeland from 2,200 to 1,200–1,300, and that this can actually improve quality of care and levels of service. Lakeland has been reorganized into five 125-bed operating units. The physical space allotted to each unit is sufficient to contain a mini-lab, diagnostic radiology rooms, linen and general supply, stock rooms, and so on. Medical documentation can be reduced by almost two thirds, scheduling and coordination service by more than two thirds, and ready-for-action time by two thirds.

Patient-focused care has been difficult for those hospitals attempting it to fully and rapidly implement for among the following reasons: high cost of conversion, extensive physical renovations required, resistance from functional departments, and other priorities for management, such as mergers and considering potential mergers.

Hospital Community Benefit Programs

Rising public concern about the high cost and inaccessibility of quality health services has focused on the hospital as one of the major causes of the problem, rather than as a catalyst for reform. Increasingly, the hospital and other segments of the health care industry are perceived as more interested in making money than in caring for patients.

The Hospital Community Benefit Standards Program (Kovner, 1994) was funded by the W. K. Kellogg Foundation to demonstrate that new credible standards could assist and encourage leading hospitals to manage highly effective community benefit programs and that community benefit programs based on these standards can help put hospitals in the forefront of efforts to reform the health care system.

The program adopted four standards (Kovner & Hattis, 1990): (1) there is evidence of the hospital's formal commitment to a community benefit program for a designated community; (2) the scope of the program includes hospital-sponsored projects for the designated community to improve health status and access to care and contain the growth of community health costs; (3) the hospital's program includes activities designed to stimulate other organizations and individuals to join in carrying out a broad health agenda in the designated community; and (4) the hospital fosters an internal environment that encourages hospital-wide involvement in the program.

Community benefit can be viewed as an extension of continuous quality improvement and of the patient-focused hospital beyond hospital walls and into the community. The focus is on problems of health status, access to care, and containment of community health care costs, about which the hospital, other health care providers, and local leaders can do something meaningful, based on national standards that can be adapted locally and will alter current resource distribution patterns.

Examples of such reallocations include providing more prenatal care, especially to at-risk mothers, thereby improving the health status of mother and child, while improving access to care and reducing health care costs, such as for care of low-weight babies resulting in part from the absence of prenatal care; closing duplicative facilities and services; and establishing special programs to reach groups lacking access to health care for economic, social, linguistic, and cultural reasons.

Again, it has been difficult for many hospitals to implement community benefit programs for reasons such as other time-consuming priorities, such as mergers and acquisitions; competitive cost pressures that militate against development of nonrevenue-producing programs; competition with other local providers; and a lack of skills and experience in working with community leaders and of data needed to develop the programs.

Current Issues

Some current issues affecting hospitals include the following: (1) what to do about hospital overcapacity, (2) who should own community hospitals, (3) how physicians should relate to hospitals, and (4) how hospitals should be accountable for performance.

Hospital Overcapacity

According to Shortell, Gillies, and Devers (1995), hospitals that will succeed in the years ahead will in many cases have to downsize acute inpatient bed capacity by up to 50%. Assuming four hospitals in a city require 600 beds but presently have 1,000 beds, this could mean four 150-bed hospitals, three 200-bed hospitals, two 300-bed hospitals, or one 600-bed hospital. Let's assume for the moment that the technical best solution—for reasons of economies of scale and consumer and provider choice and convenience—is two 300-bed hospitals. The issue is how to get from where we are to where we want to be.

The way we seem to be going about this is "letting the market take care of things," as has occurred in other industries, from banking to hotels to airlines. In fact, this is a recipe for how Columbia/HCA has entered a market and reduced its costs through consolidation, closings, and integrations of service. The political implications of letting the market take care of things, however, includes the loss of jobs by those working in the downsized or closed hospitals, many of whose employees cannot get comparable jobs, and the loss of convenience to doctors and patients when services are no longer available locally. Advocates for these interests then often call on government for legislative and other remedies.

Local Ownership

To what extent should hospitals be locally owned? According to Seay and Vladeck (1987), the benefit of not-for-profit ownership in health care is that these hospitals are more geographically bound and community-responsive, providing a continuing presence and service capability, thus giving patients and the community an institution that will exist tomorrow as well as today. For hospitals to do what is appropriate from the perspective of community need is not always profitable. The issue remains the same if a local hospital is sold to a large not-for-profit system whose interest is not primarily being in the community and staying in the community.

A related question is, of course, is the community willing to pay whatever extra it takes to keep a less efficient hospital locally based? And is there any government or public interest in keeping community hospitals locally owned? In some states, such as New York, this issue has been articulated in terms of keeping investor-owned hospitals out of the state so that profits cannot be taken out of the state and local nonprofits are less threatened by competitors. The same issue is raised with regard to public hospitals, which may no longer be as needed as they were previously because there is already too much inpatient capacity in the community; that is, although employees, patients, and advocates maintain that public hospitals serve their clients much better than do other hospitals, which mainly serve commercial and Medicare clienteles.

Physician–Hospital Relationships

Traditionally, in most hospitals physicians have related to the hospital as independent contractors. They have been part of the hospital medical staff but are mainly in business for themselves. In an era of managed care, hospitals find it increasingly difficult to survive and grow unless they are more closely tied to their physicians and unless most physicians on the medical staff are closely tied to the hospital as part of a network for delivering managed care. Hospitals are increasingly buying physician practices and employing physicians to create this unity of purpose.

Coming from a different direction, particularly in the western and southern United States, physicians and physician corporations are organizing to take a primary role in managing care. They contract directly with employers and third-party payers in order to retain any funds earned from successfully managing risk (utilization and related expenses will be less than that paid for under capitation; see chapter 10 of this text on Health Maintenance Organizations and Managed Care). Such physicians can choose to ally with hospitals or more commonly to contract with hospitals, paying them a discounted fee per diem. Such contracting forces the hospital to become a supplier, similar to a drug company or provider of durable medical equipment. For some hospitals this is a painful departure from their traditional valued role of providing leadership in the organization of health care services in a community, often providing as well services to the poor and teaching services for physicians and nurses.

Accountability for Performance

What does society expect from our hospitals? That they will do no harm; that, for the patients who should come to them, hospitals will provide effective, efficient, and humane diagnosis and treatment; that hospital costs will be closely related to benefits, that quality will be predictable, and that access when hospital services are required will be assured. One can go further and expect from hospitals a leadership role in assuring better health care for the community; that is, if we can find some consensus about what "better" care and "community" is.

Alternatively, Americans can expect that hospitals will meet the expectations of their owners: that hospitals generate a good return on investment for investors and do not lose any votes for politicians (if hospitals are publicly owned), and that hospitals, as nonprofits, meet community needs as defined by trustees serving as owners in trust for the community served.

However we define accountability, we can expect that there will be fewer freestanding hospitals, fewer hospitals, and fewer beds staffed five years from now than there are in 1998. Given the increasing development of protocols for care, clinical pathways, and hospital information systems and the increasing interest in quality on the part of purchasers of care, we can expect more accountability demanded of hospitals—expressed quantitatively such as in terms of bad outcomes avoided relative to a particular diagnosis, treatments provided or not provided, or length of waits to be seen by a clinician in the hospital emergency department.

Mini-Case Study

St. George Hospital has an inpatient capacity of 60% and lost $6 million last year on annual revenues of $200 million. St. George is located in a large eastern city and competes with four other hospitals, two of which are having merger discussions. Most of St. George's medical staff is in private practice, and many physicians admit to other hospitals as well. Managed care companies have 20% of the market in town; St. George has contracts with most of these companies.

You are Charlie Sweat, board chair. You've been approached by Glenn Morris, board chair of the Victory Hospital (which made $100,000 last year). He has asked you to persuade your board to merge with his hospital. Victory Hospital is 20% smaller than St. George and is not religiously sponsored. Morris is suggesting a full merger, with 50% of the board from each hospital.

What are some of the factors that St. George Hospital should consider before continuing discussions with Victory?

Discussion Questions

1. Why are hospitals organized the way they are, particularly as this concerns nonpaid trustees and hospital medical staffs?
2. What role should hospitals play in organized health care delivery systems?
3. What are the advantages and disadvantages of different models of physician affiliation with hospitals?
4. How should those operating hospitals themselves deal with the problem of overcapacity?
5. To what extent should hospitals be regulated and by whom?

References

American Hospital Association, *Environmental Assessment for Rural Hospitals*. Chicago: Author, 1992.

American Hospital Association, *AHA Guide: The AHA Guide to the Health Care Field*. Chicago: Author, 1995–96.

American Hospital Association, *Hospital Stat: Emerging Trends in Hospitals*. Chicago: Author, 1996–97.

American Hospital Association, *Hospital Stat: Emerging Trends in Hospitals*. Chicago: Author, 1997–98.

Berry, D. E., & Beaulieu, J. E., "Supply of Hospital and Long Term Care Services in Rural Areas," in J. E. Beaulieu & D. E. Berry (eds.), *Rural Health Services: A Management Perspective.* Ann Arbor, MI: Health Administration Press, 1994.

Deming, W. E., *Out of Crisis.* Cambridge, MA: MIT-CAES, 1986.

Ermann, D., & Gabel, J., "Multi-Hospital Systems: Issues and Empirical Findings," *Health Affairs, 3*(1), 50, 1984.

Freymann, J. G., *The American Health Care System: Its Genesis and Trajectory.* New York: Medcom Press, 1974.

Ginsburg, C., "The Patient as Profit Center: Hospital Inc. Comes to Town," *Nation,* November 18, 1996, pp. 18–22.

HCIA Inc. & Deloitte & Touche LLP, *The Comparative Performance of U.S. Hospitals: The Sourcebook,* Baltimore: Author, 1995.

Heyssel, R. M., Gaintner, R., Kues, I., Jones, A. A., & Lipstein S. H., "Decentralized Management in a Teaching Hospital: Ten Years Later at Johns Hopkins," *New England Journal of Medicine, 310,* 1477, 1984.

Kovner, A. R., & Hattis, P. A., "Benefitting Communities," *HMQ,* Fourth Quarter 1990, pp 6–10.

Kovner, A. R., "The Hospital Community Benefit Standards Program and Health Reform," *Hospital & Health Services Administration, 39*(2), 1994.

National Center For Health Statistics, *Health United States: 1995.* Hyattsville, MD: Public Health Service, 1996.

Pallarito, K., "Hospitals Withstanding Managed Care," *Modern Healthcare, 26,* p. 62, December 1996.

Rosenberg, C. E., *The Care of Strangers.* New York: Basic Books, 1987.

Seay, J. D., & Vladeck, B. C., *Mission Matters: A Report on the Future of Voluntary Health Institutions.* New York: United Hospital Fund of New York, 1987.

Shortell, S. M., "The Medical Staff of the Future: Replanting the Garden," *Frontiers of Health Services Management, 1*(3), 3, 1985.

Shortell, S. S., Gillies, R. R., Anderson, D. A., Erickson, K. M., & Mitchell, J. B., *Remaking Health Care in America: Building Organized Systems.* San Francisco: Jossey-Bass, 1996.

Shortell, S. S., Gillies, R. R., & Devers, K. J., "Reinventing the American Hospital," *Milbank Quarterly, 73*(2), 131–160, 1995.

Smith, D. B., & Kaluzny, A. D., *The White Labyrinth* (2nd ed.). Ann Arbor, MI: Health Administration Press, 1986.

Smith, H. L., "Two Lines of Authority Are One Too Many," *Modern Hospital,* March 1955, pp. 59–64.

Smith, J., "The Patient-Focused Hospital," *Hospital Management International,* 1990, pp. 185–187.

Southwick, A., *The Law of Hospital and Health Care Administration.* Ann Arbor, MI: Health Administration Press, 1978.

Starr, P., *The Social Transformation of American Medicine.* New York: Basic Books, 1982.

Stevens, R., *American Medicine and the Public Interest.* New Haven, CT: Yale University Press, 1971.

Thorpe, K. E., "The Health System in Transition: Care, Cost and Coverage," *Journal of Health Politics, Policy and Law, 22,* 355, April 1997.

"U.S. Vehicle Sales in September," *New York Times,* October 4, 1996.

7

Ambulatory Care

Andrew P. Mezey

Learning Objectives

1. Explain what is meant by ambulatory care.
2. Explain what is meant by primary care.
3. Describe where and how primary care is delivered.
4. Describe how the delivery of primary care is changing due to managed care.
5. Describe the role of emergency services in the spectrum of ambulatory care.

Topical Outline

Ambulatory care
   Ambulatory care statistics
   Organization of ambulatory care services
Primary care
   Primary care providers
   Sites of care
Emergency care
   Hospital emergency services
      General description and statistics
      Staffing
   Freestanding emergi-centers and urgi-centers
   Prehospital emergency care
Specialty ambulatory care
   Medical
   Surgical
   Imaging
Complementary and alternative care

Patient networks and support groups
Summary and current issues

Key Words: **Ambulatory care, primary care, primary care provider, emergency care, specialty ambulatory care, home health care, complementary and alternative care, patient networks and support groups.**

Ambulatory care is personal health care provided to individuals or a population of individuals who are not occupying a bed in a health care institution or at home. It encompasses all health services provided to individual patients, including community services, such as general information about the hazards of smoking or substance abuse, and some of the services delivered by public health departments, such as information about immunizations and sexually transmitted diseases. Primary care, emergency care, and ambulatory specialty care, including ambulatory surgery, are all subsets of ambulatory care. They are provided in a variety of settings—freestanding provider offices, hospital-based clinics, school-based clinics, public health clinics, and neighborhood and community health centers.

Current practice is to attempt to provide health care services in the least costly setting. This has led to decreased utilization of emergency services, increased utilization of nonemergent ambulatory facilities, and a corresponding decrease in hospital admissions and hospital days. The types and severity of those illnesses that physicians and other providers are able and willing to treat in ambulatory settings have also increased. Patients admitted to hospitals are therefore sicker and stay for shorter periods than they did formerly. At discharge they often require support services for variable lengths of time after they leave the hospital. Some of these services are provided in the home, others in ambulatory care settings. This has changed the principal locus of care for certain services, such as rehabilitation services (physical therapy, etc.), and invasive diagnostic and surgical procedures from the hospital to ambulatory facilities and to the home.

What has been the standard of practice but is now beginning to change is the single episodic encounter, usually between a physician and a patient, driven by the patient's perceived need for medical care. For example, an individual with a rash that has not responded to usual remedies sees a dermatologist to whom he has been referred by a friend, not by the patient's personal physician. No record of the encounter is communicated by the dermatologist to another physician. The rash recurs, and the patient seeks advice from another dermatologist, with the same result—improvement followed by recurrence. The third physician encounter may be with the personal physician, who may recognize the cause of the rash as related to a condition that the patient has but that was not communicated to the previous two dermatologists. Though the patient has had the luxury of ultimate choice, it may not have been in the patient's best interests to have exercised that choice.

The problem facing us in this rapidly changing health care delivery system is how to maintain an individual's ability to choose while containing costs, providing quality care, and maintaining satisfaction with the care received. In this latter regard, an aspect of these changes deals with the need to preserve the pleasure that both providers of care and patients derive from establishing long-term relationships. It is similar to the pleasure one gets from maintaining long-term friendships, friendships that are full of shared experiences that allow people to connect easily even after long absences. Long-term relationships between patients and their physicians are involuntarily ruptured when a patient changes jobs and the new employer has a health insurance contract that does not include the patient's physician. This has the effect of diminishing the effort both physicians and patients will make in building trusting relationships.

The need to reduce the costs of health care has had a number of other effects. Primary care providers have taken on patient responsibilities previously referred to specialists. This, in turn, has decreased the reliance on specialists and is one cause of the apparent oversupply of specialists found in some parts of the United States. Consumers have become concerned that controlling costs leads to a decrease in the quality of care. Abuses of the system in the name of controlling costs are difficult to document, but the health care marketplace is adjusting to the concerns of consumers, either through legislation or through market pressures (Bodenheimer, 1996).

This chapter looks at how ambulatory services are provided—who provides those services and where—with particular emphasis on the characteristics of the provision of primary care. The intent is to give the reader an understanding of how and where individuals receive the great bulk of their health care in the United States. The chapter will not discuss mental health, public health, or rehabilitative services.

Ambulatory Care Statistics

In 1994 the average person made 6.0 visits to a physician and spent 0.55 days in an acute-care hospital (549.4 short-stay hospital days per 1,000 population). Thus, 11 times more ambulatory care episodes than hospital days of care occurred (USDHHS, 1995, Tables 74, 83). This ratio is up from 4.7 in 1980, as the number of ambulatory visits increased from just under 5 per person and the number of hospital days declined sharply from 1,163 per 1,000 population in 1980

(USDHHS, 1982, Tables 35, 43). The unprecedented shifts away from inpatient care of the two last decades have had an enormous impact on the organization, staffing, and financing of ambulatory services in the United States. The number of Americans who reported a visit to a physician in the past year increased slightly, from 75% in 1980 to 79.2% in 1994. A full 90.5% of the population in 1994 had seen a physician in the past 2 years (USDHHS, 1986, Table 58; 1995, Table 77). Meanwhile, the average length of stay in nonfederal acute-care hospitals decreased from 7.3 days in 1980 to 6.0 in 1993 (USDHHS, 1982, Table 42; 1995, Table 85). Thus, in sum, most patient-physician contacts now take place on an ambulatory basis.

The rates of visits to physicians vary by age, gender, race, and socioeconomic status. About 94.8% of the very young (under 5 years) and 91.4% of the very old (75 years and over) have an annual visit with a physician; 74.2% of males and 84.1% of females report an annual physician visit; and 79.6% of Whites and 79.5% of Blacks saw a physician in 1994, compared with 75.4% and 74%, respectively, in 1980 (USDHHS, 1982, Table 36; 1995, Table 77). The eradication of the gap observed between the races also occurred for differences of physician use by the rich and the poor. In 1964, 58.6% of those with a family income of less than $14,000 reported seeing a physician; 73.6% of persons living in families earning *more* than $50,000 did so. By 1994 these rates had increased to 78.0% and 83.7%, respectively (USDHHS, 1995, Table 77). The enactment of Medicaid and Medicare accounts for much of the increased use of physicians by lower-income groups.

Somewhat paradoxically, the number of physician visits per person is actually higher among lower-income groups (those with less than $14,000 annual family income) than among those with annual family incomes above $50,000; the reported rates are 7.6% and 6.0%, respectively (USDHHS, 1995, Table 74). Thus, access, as measured by the percentage seeing a physician yearly, has improved for the poor but still lags; whereas utilization, as measured by the number of physician visits per person per year, is higher because there is more sickness among the poor (Wilensky & Berk, 1982). For the elderly poor, ambulatory visits actually decreased by 20% between 1982 and 1986, when the federal government reduced support for health services (R. W. Johnson Foundation, 1987).

In 1994 Whites reported 6.1 visits per year; Blacks, 5.7 (USDHHS, 1995, Table 74). Although a larger proportion of Blacks live in poverty (a condition associated with higher utilization rates), they experience more problems with access to physician services than do Whites, who constitute the majority of poor people. The percentage of visits occurring in hospital outpatient departments is slightly less than double for Blacks (20.3%), compared with Whites (12.5%) (USDHHS, 1995, Table 75). Similar differences in hospital outpatient use exist for socioeconomic class. The inverse holds true for visits to doctors' offices and use of telephone contact with physicians when analyzed by race or socioeconomic status.

Organization of Ambulatory Care Services

There are two major categories of ambulatory care. The dominant form is that care provided by private physicians in solo, partnership, or private group practice on a fee-for-service basis. The other, growing dramatically in the past decade, is ambulatory care in organized settings that have an identity independent from that of the individual physicians practicing in it. These categories are not strictly exclusive, as most physicians practicing in their own offices have contracts with one or more managed care organizations (see chapter 10, on managed care). Other forms of ambulatory health care delivery in this latter category are hospital-based ambulatory services, including clinics, walk-in, and emergency services; hospital-sponsored group practices and health promotion centers; freestanding "surgi-centers" and "urgi"- or "emergi-centers"; health department clinics; neighborhood and community health centers (NHCs and CHCs); organized home care; community mental health centers; school and workplace health services; and prison health services.

Different ambulatory care settings provide services for diverse groups in the population. Results in utilization and quality of services provided also differ by demographic group. Almost 20 years ago Dutton (1979) analyzed the impact of the major forms of ambulatory care on patients in Washington, DC, in terms that still apply today:

> Sources used primarily by the poor—hospital outpatient departments, emergency rooms, and public clinics—contained important structural and financial barriers, and had the lowest rates of patient-initiated use. The prepaid system, in contrast, maximized patient's access to both preventive care and symptomatic care, and did not seem to inhibit physician-controlled follow-up care. The results suggest some perverse effects of fee-for-service payment: patients, especially poor patients, appeared to be deterred from seeking preventive and symptomatic care, while physicians were encouraged to expand follow-up services. Moreover, services in fee-for-service systems were distributed less equitably relative to both income and medical need than in the prepaid system. (p. 221)

Primary Care

Primary care, as defined by the Institute of Medicine (Institute of Medicine, 1996) is "the provision of integrated, accessible care services by clinicians who are accountable for addressing a large majority of the personal health care needs, developing a sustained partnership with patients, and practicing in the context of family and community" (p. 1). Embedded within this definition is the concept that a primary care clinician should be able to address an individual's health needs over a long period of time, that the health needs will vary over time, and that the individual may sometimes need others to care for those health needs (e.g., physician subspecialists, physical therapists, social workers). It is also implicit in this definition that the primary care provider must act as a coordinator for those health needs. It is obvious that primary care, when defined in this way, is much broader than the provision of the primary health care needs of patients in an ambulatory setting.

This definition of primary care is also much broader than that of "first contact" care. First-contact care occurs when an individual, faced with a new symptom or sign, whether real or perceived, asks some other individual for advice. That person can be a friend or family member who has medical expertise beyond that of the general population—nurses, pharmacists, physical and occupational therapists, respiratory therapists, and the like. It can also be advice sought from someone who has had personal or family experience with an illness that seems to be related to the symptoms or signs at hand. These types of interchange are common everyday occurrences. The situation may be as mundane as when the parent of a first child seeks help for what to do about the infant's fever, cold, or diarrhea from a neighbor with several children. It can be as complex as seeking advice from a friend about the possibility of serious heart disease or cancer, when that friend's family member has had a recent experience with cancer or heart disease.

On the other hand, it is possible that, with more and more of the population becoming computer-literate, greater use of information about health and disease will become commonplace. The Internet is an amazing source of up-to-date information easily available to anyone with access to it. The National Institutes of Health maintain a section called "Consumer Health Information" (http://www.nih-gov/health/consumer/conicd.html). It not only lists publications on a variety of subjects but also provides information about how to manage common complaints associated with disease treatments. For the patient with cancer desiring information about diet and nutrition there is an extensive guide that is easy to read for most individuals. It contains headings dealing with such questions as "What kinds of food do I need?" and "Can good nutrition treat cancer?" It discusses how to manage eating problems that may occur during the treatment of cancer, such as loss of appetite, vomiting, dry mouth, and a changed sense of taste or smell.

Combined with official government information are a growing number of publications, accessible in print and on the Internet, that can lead the individual to sites on the Internet with information on a variety of health-related subjects (Your Personal Net Doctor, 1996). Subjects include "The Home Hypochondriac," with headings asking "Am I an Addict?" "Do you have diabetes and not know it?" and "Are you at high risk for stroke?" It lists areas to go to for a self-administered health questionnaire, for depression screening, for parenting advice, and for information on sleep apnea. There are sections on how to live a healthy life, how to find information on specific diseases, and how to find out about alternatives to traditional medical treatments. Hospitals have also entered the consumer information field, offering advice on wellness as well as on illness and providing information on how to access care at their own institutions. Although clearly a marketing attempt, the information is useful and readily available. It is likely that patients will use these sources of information on health care prior to calling their primary care provider. Rather than speaking with family members or friends, they may find it more appealing and less threatening to utilize "chat rooms" on the Internet to "speak" with others on a variety of subjects dealing with everyday issues, such as otitis media in children, parenting problems, work-related stress, and depression, as well as such major life-threatening problems as cancer.

With increasing numbers of Americans receiving their health insurance through managed care organizations (MCOs), other responsibilities of primary care providers have emerged. In a fee-for-service model, the primary care provider is responsible only for those patients who happen to come into his or her office. The provider's practice is viewed as being made up of individual patients, not as a discrete population. In managed care settings, especially when the provider is paid through a capitation system rather than by a modified fee-for-service system, the provider can be held responsible for providing appropriate health services to the entire population of patients assigned to him or her. The MCO can perform an audit of the provider's practice to see if standards of care have been met. Thus, the provider is held responsible for all the patients in his or her panel, even if they have never shown up for a visit. For example, if the standard of care set by the MCO for a pediatric practice requires 90% of children to have received all their immunizations by 2 years of age, the denominator used is the total number of children 2 years of age and older in the provider's panel of patients, not just those that have actually been seen in the office. Standards of care, benchmarks against which the adequacy of care provided by the primary care practitioner is judged, exist for preventive services such as blood pressure screening, breast cancer screening (mammogram, self-breast-exam education), diabetes screening, and colorectal cancer screening, as well as for the appropriateness of illness management. Although quality assurance measures have been required in hospital settings for a long time, it is only since 1991, with the advent of standards for accreditation of MCOs by the National Committee on Quality Assurance (NCQA), the accrediting body for MCOs, that standards of care in ambulatory settings have begun to be monitored.

The definition of primary care has also expanded to include the integration of needed services across disciplines and across settings. To a large extent this is being driven by a capitated financing system that must deliver services in the least costly manner while preserving quality of care. This is especially true for full-risk contracts. As more of the market moves toward this form of financing, the role played by the primary care provider will be larger. In the fully mature integrated health care system, the primary care provider will likely be a primary care team. This team, composed of nurses, social workers, physicians, nurse practitioners, physician assistants, pharmacists, and others, will manage the care of a panel of patients in the least costly way and in the least costly setting. These settings, sometimes called an integrated delivery system (IDS), include the whole spectrum of care currently utilized: ambulatory primary and specialty care, hospital inpatient and outpatient settings, home care, nursing home care, skilled nursing care facilities, and freestanding outpatient rehabilitation facilities. To do this, either an organization will own all the various parts of the health care delivery system or partnerships will have to be created among the various players. IDS models currently exist in both urban and rural settings, and development of the approach to care provision will likely continue and expand (*Primary Care*, 1996).

Primary Care Providers

The providers of primary care fall into four major disciplines: physicians, nurse practitioners (NPs), midwives, and physician assistants (PAs). Although they take very different pathways to become primary care providers, at the completion of their training they are very similar in their capabilities in ambulatory primary care settings. It is estimated that NPs and PAs can perform typically 75% of services that physicians provide in adult practices and 90% in pediatric practices (Scheffler, 1996).

This is also a period when training programs for nurse practitioners, midwives, and physician assistants are increasing in number and size. At the same time there is a nationwide effort, at both federal and state levels, to increase the number of physicians being trained in primary care. It will be interesting to see how much of primary care services will be provided by which profession in the coming years.

Sites for the Provision of Primary Care Services

Primary care in the United States is provided in a number of settings, with private physician offices continuing to be the dominant site even in this era of increasing penetration of MCOs. This is unlikely to change because independent practice associations (IPAs) continue their dominance in an expanding managed care market. On the other hand, as many states have applied for and received waivers from the Health Care Financing Administration (HCFA) to introduce mandatory Medicaid managed care, it is likely that neighborhood- and community-based organizations and hospital-based primary care clinics will expand their primary care capabilities. In the past these hospital-based primary care sites were actually located in the hospital or on the hospital grounds. More recently, hospitals have aggressively sought to maintain their inpatient base by moving their ambulatory facilities away from the hospital. At the same time, especially in the case of some public hospitals that have expanded into rural areas and inner cities, expansion of clinics into the community improves access to health care for underserved populations. These organizations have been the traditional providers of care to patients with Medicaid-financed insurance and wish to continue to be. They will have to expand services to cover evening, night, and weekend hours for their patients, they will have to develop the information systems and the efficiency seen in the private for-profit and not-for-profit sectors, and they will have to develop partnerships with other providers of care so that they can offer a system of integrated care across a variety of settings.

Academic medical centers (AMCs), those teaching hospitals closely aligned with medical schools, have been particularly aggressive in expanding their primary care operations in order to maintain their missions of patient care, education of residents and medical students, and clinical research. Montefiore Medical Center in the Bronx, New York, is one of the more aggressive in this regard, establishing 25 offsite primary care offices in the past 5 years, planning to establish 15 more, employing 250 primary care physicians, and expecting to hire 250 more in the next 5 years. Montefiore is also seeking full-risk capitation from MCOs so that it can manage all the care for its patients (S. F. Foreman, personal communication, February 20, 1997).

Emergency Care

The United States has developed a complex system of emergency care for its citizens, beginning with the national 911 emergency response system, continuing with hospital-based emergency services and specialized emergency services such as Level I trauma centers with their 24-hour, 7-day availability of a complete array of medical and surgical specialists, diagnostic imaging, and operating rooms and complemented by well-staffed and well-equipped intensive care units.

Hospital Emergency Services

General Description and Statistics. Most U.S. hospitals provide emergency services, and over 93% of community hospitals have emergency departments (AHA, 1992–93, Table 12A). These units serve several functions, from caring for the acutely ill or injured patient to providing walk-in services to less acutely ill patients. Many physicians on the hospital staff also use the emergency room as a setting to assess a patient with a problem that either may lead to inpatient admission or require equipment or diagnostic imaging facilities not available in the physician's office. Increasingly, extended care facilities such as nursing homes and chronic disease hospitals may use the emergency services of an acute care facility for evaluation of a patient with a sudden change in medical status. Emergency services function as a major source of unscheduled admissions to the hospital, averaging about 40% nationwide (AHA, 1993–94), and higher than that in many inner-city institutions (Schroeder, 1993). Throughout the 1980s and early 1990s emergency department (ED) visits increased; however, there was a decline in 1994 for the first time since 1983 (AHA, 1994). In 1993 over 75% of all admissions and 90% of pediatric admissions at Jacobi Medical Center, a hospital caring for a large number of the medically indigent and Medicaid-insured and a member hospital of the New York City Health and Hospitals Corporation, were through the ED (Jacobi Medical Center, 1993).

Three decades ago Weinerman, Ratner, Robbins, and Lavenber (1966) defined three categories of patients presenting themselves to emergency units:

> *Nonurgent:* "Condition does not require the resources of an emergency service; referral for routine medical care may or may not be needed; disorder is nonacute or minor in severity."

> *Urgent:* "Condition requires medical attention within the period of a few hours; there is a possible danger to the patient if medically unattended; disorder is acute but not necessarily severe."

> *Emergent:* "Condition requires immediate medical attention; time delay is harmful to patient; disorder is acute and potentially threatening to life or function." (p. 1037)

These terms derive from a professional perspective and are based on medical diagnoses. Most patients cannot make these distinctions and err in both overinterpreting and underinterpreting the gravity of symptoms. Most patients presenting to an emergency service feel that they need immediate attention, regardless of what the professional staff may think. Others know that they do not have an urgent or emergent problem. They simply use the emergency service because it is all that is available to them. Young, Wagner, Kellerman, Ellis, and Bonley (1996) reported that 37% of total ED visits but 49% of ambulatory patients were assessed as nonurgent at triage. The General Accounting Office in 1993 reported that 43% of patients seen in hospital EDs were classified as "nonurgent" (U.S. GAO, 1993). However, a University of California study showed that the emergency staff was able to move only 20% of its patients to other settings (Shesser, 1995).

Some hospitals have developed walk-in units to relieve the emergency services of the burden of the nonurgent patients and to respond to the competition from freestanding walk-in services or urgi-centers. By organizing group practices in the outpatient clinics some hospitals have been able to provide "add-on" slots in the appointment schedule to accommodate the nonurgent patient demanding urgent attention. Financial incentives are forcing hospitals to make every effort to reduce the costly care of nonurgent patients in the emergency setting. These efforts include evening and weekend hours for walk-in units and after-hours telephone access for clinic patients. One study, however, found no difference in emergency service visits or hospitalizations between a group of patients randomized to telephone access to physicians, who in turn had access to computerized medical records, and control patients (Darnell et al., 1985).

Managed systems of care often require subscribers to get prior approval before authorizing emergency services, and unauthorized use may not be covered. As the roles of provider and insurer become commingled, it is easier to design and to enforce the use of more efficient and less expensive methods of providing nonurgent care. Some states that have been able to show marked declines in emergency department use by the introduction of Medicaid managed care programs (American College of Healthcare Executives, 1993). This trend is likely to increase as more states apply for and receive mandated Medicaid managed care waivers from the Health Care Financing Administration.

Staffing. Dramatic changes in the staffing of emergency departments have occurred in the past two decades. Teaching hospitals once relied almost exclusively on junior house officers to staff their emergency services, with backup supervision by more senior house officers or staff members. Nonteaching hospitals either had physicians with staff privileges cover the emergency services in rotation or relied on "moonlighters" from residency programs of nearby teaching hospitals. Many teaching hospitals have developed residency programs in emergency medicine, run by full-time, board-certified emergency medicine specialists interested in academic careers. Many medical schools have established academic departments of emergency medicine in recognition that the field has developed its own particular body of knowledge and areas for research.

Community hospitals have also shifted to full-time emergency medicine specialists, frequently contracting with a physician group serving several hospitals in the area. The hospitals that contract for coverage from an emergency medicine group are willing to pay a premium in return for reliable staffing.

Freestanding Emergi-Centers and Urgi-Centers

First established in Delaware and Rhode Island in 1973, freestanding ambulatory care facilities providing emergency services and urgent care for nonurgent patients now operate throughout the United States. Some, such as the emergi-center, have the 24-hour, 7-day access that hospital emergency services provide. Others, so-called urgi-centers or Doc in the Box, provide less comprehensive emergency services and are commonly open 12 hours a day, 7 days a week. These centers do not serve truly emergent patients, and most do not receive ambulance cases.

Two groups of patients find these centers attractive: those seeking the convenience and access of emergency services without the delays and other forms of negative feedback associated with using hospital services for nonurgent problems and those whose insurance treats emergi-centers preferentially compared with physicians' offices (Chesteen, Warren, & Woodley, 1986). Both hospitals and private practitioners feel the competitive pressures from these new centers. Hospitals have responded by sponsoring or buying emergi-centers and urgi-centers, and physicians have formed them. Several thousand of these facilities now exist. Precise data, however, are not available. There is no clear definition for the spectrum of services provided by an emergi-center. It can range from a group practice that has simply expanded hours and eased access for walk-in patients to hospitals with satellite services that are geographically separate but organizationally and administratively far from freestanding.

As these centers have increased in number and become familiar to more patients, many have evolved to offer a combination of walk-in and appointment services. The appointment services initially provided follow-up for the presenting complaint. They have evolved into more comprehensive routine ambulatory services, especially among the urgi-centers. Many now market their services as having all of the advantages of the personal relationship with a primary care physician plus the convenience of expanded hours and short waiting times. In many geographic areas the chain-sponsored urgi-center is a convenient and economic method for a newly trained primary care physician to enter practice without the expense of acquiring an office and equipment. The flexible hours of employment are attractive to nurses and other health workers.

Prehospital Emergency Care. Emergency medical services extend beyond the hospital emergency department or the freestanding emergi-center to include other services provided to accident victims or individuals suffering acute, life-threatening illnesses such as acute myocardial infarction or stroke. The goals of these services are to preserve life and reduce disability by providing prompt treatment and transportation to comprehensive treatment facilities. The intended recipients of care are patients with emergent or urgent problems.

Large urban areas have developed sophisticated emergency medical services (EMS), run either as separate agencies of a city or county government or as part of another service, such as the police or fire department. Ambulances provided by such an EMS are staffed by emergency medical technicians (EMTs), individuals who have received specialized training in life support. There are two levels of EMTs: those with training in the basic aspects of life support (EMT-A) and those with advanced life support training (paramedics or EMT-P) (Kellerman, 1994). In rural and in many suburban settings the emergency response is through volunteer ambulance services; these are staffed mainly by EMT-As.

The emergency prehospital care for these problems requires a functioning EMS system. Its 15 core elements, though described almost 20 years ago (Hoffer, 1979) still pertain today: provision of labor force, training of personnel, communications, transportation, facilities, critical care units, use of public safety agencies, consumer participation, accessibility to care, transfer of patients, standard medical record keeping, consumer information and education, independent review and evaluation, disaster linkage, and mutual-aid agreements. A principal goal has been to provide for the whole nation a set of coordinated emergency care dispatch centers, using the uniform emergency telephone number, 911.

Specialty Ambulatory Care

In this section, specialty ambulatory care is defined as care given by physicians who are not generalists. Generalists are defined as individuals practicing family medicine, general pediatrics, general internal medicine, geriatric medicine, and general obstetrics and gynecology. Patients can be referred to specialists for conditions that their primary care providers feel they cannot or should not handle. Patients can also choose to bypass the generalist physician and go directly to a specialist. This route has become less common because of financial penalties associated with self-referral to specialists imposed by managed care health insurance plans. Despite this, the proportion of ambulatory care visits to other than generalist physicians does not appear to have changed since 1985 (USDHHS, 1995, Table 80). This may be explained by the observation that more services, both medical and surgical can and are being performed on an ambulatory basis.

Ambulatory Medical Specialty Care

Medical specialists can be defined as physicians who have had training beyond that required for certification in their primary specialty. They are often referred to as subspecialists. General internists must receive 3 years of training in an accredited internal medicine residency program prior to becoming eligible to sit for the examination for primary certification in internal medicine given by the American Board of Internal Medicine. Internists who wish to become further specialized (subspecialized) must take another 2 to 3 years of training in an accredited specialty residency (fellowship) program. They then become eligible to sit for a "subboard" examination in that specialty, also administered by the American Board of Internal Medicine. Thus, a physician qualified, for example, as a cardiologist will have passed examinations in both internal medicine and cardiology. Similar training requirements apply to the specialty areas within other disciplines, such as pediatrics, radiology, and obstetrics and gynecology.

Internists who have received subspecialty training often practice general internal medicine in addition to their area of specialization. This is true for internists in private practice, whether solo, small group, or large multispecialty group practice. This is generally not true for those internal medicine specialists who are part of the full-time staff at large academic medical centers, such as those associated with medical schools.

A level of tension exists currently between physicians in medical subspecialties wanting to practice as generalists and MCOs and between generalists and subspecialists. In the first case, MCOs believe that subspecialists practice a more costly form of medical care than do generalists and that this increase in cost carries over even when subspecialists perform generalist activities. In addition, MCOs believe that subspecialists tend not to perform the preventive and screening tasks required of a primary care provider (PCP) to the same degree that generalists do. Thus, MCOs would prefer not to select subspecialists as PCPs if at all possible and may deselect them when the opportunity arises.

In the second instance, generalists come into conflict with subspecialists over who should be treating patients for a variety of conditions. This is especially true for patients with chronic illness, a group whose medical expenses total $425 billion per year (Jeffrey, 1996). Ware, Bayliss, Rogers, Kosinski, and Tailor (1996) reported that chronically ill elderly and poor patients treated in HMOs had worse physical outcomes than patients treated in fee-for-service (FFS) systems. Yellin et al. (Yellin, Criswell, & Feigenbaum, 1996) reported no differences in utilization and outcomes among persons with rheumatoid arthritis treated in FFS or prepaid group practice settings. Because of this lack of clarity about cost of care and quality of care, some MCOs are contracting with subspecialists to provide care to their patients without first accessing a PCP. How this ultimately plays out will have significant impact on physician workforce needs.

Surgical Ambulatory Care

Surgical ambulatory care is defined as surgical procedures performed on patients not admitted to an inpatient bed (outpatients). From 1980 to 1993 the percentage of surgeries done on an outpatient basis rose from 16.4% to 54.9% of the total number of surgeries performed. Some hospitals report over 60% of total surgical procedures performed on outpatients (USDHHS, 1995, Table 90). This marked change can be attributed to improved technology, economic pressures, and the demands of both patients and third-party payers. These procedures take place not only in hospital-based settings but in freestanding ambulatory surgical centers. Patient satisfaction and outcomes appear to be good for all forms of ambulatory surgery.

Ambulatory Imaging Facilities

Ambulatory imaging facilities can be located in hospitals, be part of a large multispecialty group practice, or be freestanding. All offer similar services, such as standard radiographic studies (x rays), ultrasound, echocardiography, nuclear medicine studies (bone scans, thyroid scans), computed axial tomography (CT scans), and magnetic resonance imaging (MRI). Some of the more esoteric imaging techniques, such as positron emission tomography (PET) scans, and most imaging associated with invasive techniques, such as cardiac and cerebral angiography, are done in hospitals, the latter as inpatient studies.

In addition to the above, imaging procedures are done by specialist physicians in their own offices. There are many gastroenterologists, urologists, and cardiologists who perform diagnostic imaging in their private offices rather than use the local hospital's facilities. Pulmonary specialists may be set up to perform a whole array of diagnostic tests in their own offices, including radiographic studies.

All of this causes competition among the various providers, and although competition may keep costs down in usual markets, it does not necessarily appear to be true of the health marketplace. All these facilities require expensive equipment and rely on referrals from other physicians to succeed. Ethical, legal, and financial problems emerge, especially when some of the referring physicians have financial interests in the success of the freestanding imaging centers. On the other hand, this competitive market makes life convenient for patients because some of the centers are open for business 24 hours a day, 7 days per week.

Home Health Care

Home health care services are the fastest growing sector of Medicare by percentage of increase in expenditures per year. The primary reason for this increase has been economic pressure—the need to get patients out of the hospital quicker—but it has not caused a general outcry from the public as have "drive-through" mastectomies and 24-hour hospital stays after delivery. This is likely related to three factors: patients prefer to be cared for in their own homes; most patients, no matter how complex their medical problems, can be cared for as well in the home as in a rehabilitation or skilled nursing facility; and outcomes of home care are similar to other settings for similar conditions (Mezey, personal communication, March 28, 1997). In addition, in 1989, following a lawsuit, Medicare rules for home care services were clarified, making it easier for Medicare recipients to receive home health services, with expenditures increasing at an average annual rate of 40% between 1988 and 1991 and reaching $5.4 billion (Bishop & Skwara, 1993). Overall home health care expenditures in 1993 were estimated to be $23 billion, increasing at an annual rate of 19.1% between 1982 and 1992, and 12.9% between 1992 and 1993 (NIHCM, 1996).

Patients are eligible to receive home health services from a qualified Medicare provider if they are homebound, if they are under the care of a specified physician who will establish a home health plan, and if they need physical or occupational therapy, speech therapy, or intermittent skilled nursing care. Skilled nursing care is defined both as technical procedures, such as tube feedings or catheter care, and as skilled nursing observations. *Intermittent* is defined as up to 28 hours per week for nursing care and 35 hours per week for home health aide care. Many hospitals have formed their own home health care agencies, finding this a useful way to increase revenues while enabling them to discharge patients from the hospital earlier. In most communities, however, the bulk of home health services is still provided by not-for-profit agencies, such as the Visiting Nurse Service of New York.

Complementary and Alternative Medical Care

In 1992, Congress established the Office of Alternative Medicine (OAM) at the National Institutes of Health (NIH) with the stated purpose of evaluating complementary and alternative medical treatment modalities to determine their effectiveness and to integrate these treatments into mainstream medical practice. A number of OAM centers were established, including those at the Universities of Minnesota, Texas, and California (Davis) and Stanford and Columbia Universities. All of them have mission statements emphasizing the use of alternative/complementary medicine in dealing with various conditions such as HIV infection/AIDS, substance abuse, asthma and allergy, cancer, and cardiovascular and musculoskeletal diseases. Research into the use of such interventions as biofeedback, botanical remedies, and non-Western medicine treatments, among others, is ongoing. At present the OAM is developing an operational definition for complementary and alternative therapies to aid in their study and evaluation. Two definitions that may be useful are "an unrelated group of non-orthodox therapeutic practices, often with explanatory systems that do not follow conventional biomedical explanations" or "medical interventions not taught at United States medical schools or not available at United States hospitals" (*Alternative Medicine Homepage*, 1997).

There are numerous types of practitioners of alternative and complementary medicine. They call themselves by a variety of names: acupuncturists, homeopaths, naturopaths, aroma therapists, nutritional healers, herbalists, massage therapists, music therapists, and so on. They too are listed on the Internet. Although there are no reliable statistics regarding the total number of visits made to practitioners of alternative and complementary medicine or how many people self-administer these types of treatments, Eisenberg et al. (1993) showed that 34% of 1,539 adults surveyed reported using one or another form of alternative medicine. In two studies of HIV-infected gay or bisexual men, over half stated that they used complementary or alternative treatments (Anderson, 1993; O'Connor, Lazar, & Anderson, 1992).

Patient Networks and Support Groups

Patient networks and support groups exist for virtually every illness. They can be accessed in a variety of ways—through the Internet, through the social work department of the local hospital, through community organizations such as the YMCA, or through organizations established for specific diseases or needs (e.g., AIDS/HIV disease, diabetes mellitus, blindness, breastfeeding, cancer, colostomies, multiple sclerosis, and cardiovascular diseases). They are a useful adjunct to care, allowing patients to share experiences and concerns. As discussed in the section on primary care, "chat rooms" accessed on the Internet allow two or more individuals to "speak" to each other about issues of mutual concern. This method of patient networking and support will likely increase markedly, offering as it does a combination of the convenience of remaining at home, the flexibility of the hours of use, and perhaps the advantage of anonymity.

Summary and Current Issues

In this chapter we have attempted to give the reader a picture of the status of ambulatory care available to the average American. We have emphasized the provision of primary care because we believe that it is through a continuous, mutually trusting relationship between the individual and the provider of primary care that health and emotional needs will best be served. We have tried to show how that continuum starts when an individual, concerned about a specific problem, tries to deal with it. There are a number of options available: asking a knowledgeable relative or friend, using resources available in print or on the Internet, or discussion with a health care provider, either a practitioner of alternative medicine or a traditional practitioner, over the telephone, by e-mail, or in person.

The Primary Care Provider of the Future

The definitions of the providers of primary care will expand to include individuals other than those described in the section on primary care. There are, for example, infectious disease specialists—internists with specialty training in infectious diseases—who act as primary care practitioners for individuals with infection due to human immunodeficiency virus (HIV), including but not limited to AIDS. HIV disease was initially recognized as an acute infection but has become a chronic infection with the advent of new and improved therapies. These infectious disease specialists are being recognized as true primary care providers for a subset of patients with special needs.

The above is true of other diseases, such as many types of cancer and genetic diseases such as cystic fibrosis. The list will expand as medical knowledge and effective treatments for many disease entities expands. It is likely that, as the treatment of mental illness becomes more and more pharmacologic, its treatment will become an effort managed by primary care teams that will include psychiatrists, psychologists, social workers, and nurse practitioners or physician assistants, with internists or family practitioners acting as consultants rather than as primary care providers in this setting. The use of primary care provider teams will expand to cover a whole host of diseases now primarily cared for by single practitioners.

Current practice is for patients to access their primary care provider when deciding that they need more information than is available to them through other means. This trend was initially driven by health cost considerations; it has now gone beyond that to the recognition that everyone should have a medical "home," a place one can go to for the full spectrum of care, both for wellness and for sickness, for advice and education about remaining healthy, and for advice about returning to a prior level of health. This primary care medical home will, in the future, consist of teams of individuals with overlapping areas of expertise, offering a spectrum of services—from the management of minor acute illness and advice about diet, exercise, and vitamin supplements to the management of psychosocial issues such as domestic violence, alcoholism, and substance abuse and the coordination of care for serious life-threatening or chronic conditions. Individuals may be referred to health care providers outside their primary care teams, but the responsibility for the coordination and monitoring of their care will continue to rest within their medical homes.

Drivers of Change

This change in how primary care is delivered will be driven by changes in how health care is financed. Capitation, specifically full-risk capitation, will by and large replace fee-for-service payments. Health care practitioners and health care institutions—hospitals, nursing homes, home health care agencies, ambulatory surgical and imaging facilities—will become aligned financially and will integrate their systems. They will be dependent on each other to provide health care for a large population of individuals, offering three things: cost-effectiveness, high patient satisfaction, and medical outcomes that meet or exceed expected benchmarks. To do this, they will need real teamwork. Health care managers will have to be trained to function effectively in this new paradigm. This will be easier to do than to train physicians to act as members of a health care team because, historically, the culture of medical practice has rewarded individual, not team efforts.

These changes will occur, but they will occur slowly, driven by changes in the education of primary care physicians. The requirements for the accreditation of primary care residency programs are changing. Experience in the continuity of care of panels of patients in community-based settings, as opposed to hospital-based outpatient clinics, is now beginning to be developed. Primary care residency programs are required to develop a formal curriculum that documents training in many aspects of medicine that are currently not specifically covered in most programs. Aspects of medicine, such as biomedical ethics, epidemiology, medical legal issues, cost issues in health care, and the responsibility of health care providers for an entire population of individuals, as opposed to responsibility for the episodic care of individual patients, will become the educational standard for all primary care providers.

Benefits of Change

This latter philosophy of care, that of populations or panels of patients, was originally driven by cost concerns. Giving influenza vaccine to an entire population of elderly patients, for example, might save money by decreasing the seasonal number of admissions for pneumonia and other influenza-related complications. Strict adherence to yearly mammograms for women over the age of 40 or 50 might save money by allowing earlier detection of breast cancer and therefore less costly interventions. Early recognition of illness might also decrease the costs of care for prostate cancer, colorectal cancer, and adult-onset diabetes. Emphasis on wellness programs, such as decreasing the incidence of obesity; education on the importance of exercise for weight control; decreasing the risk for the development of, for example, osteoporosis and heart disease; and promotion of smoking cessation to decrease the incidence of lung and heart disease, will become standard features of the care offered by primary care providers, either directly or indirectly, to their populations of patients.

The data on whether or not these practices do save money for specific groups of people insured by a single HMO are not clear, but accrediting organizations like the NCQA are demanding that HMOs adhere to these recommendations. And HMOs, in turn, are demanding that practitioners listed on their panels adhere to these standards as well. In the early 1990s the majority of medical school deans responsible for the oversight of residency education were concerned about the impact that managed care was having on their training programs. That has changed. In the 1997 meeting in Santa Fe, New Mexico, of the Group on Residency Affairs (GRA) of the Association of American Medical Colleges (AAMC), the tone of the discussion changed. There was an emphasis on how to teach the "new medicine" to residents, not based on cost of care concerns but based on the best interests of patients.

Each year approximately 12,000 residents complete training in generalist specialties in the United States. It will be from this group of individuals, trained in a different paradigm of what constitutes primary care, that the changes in how ambulatory care is delivered will come. They will be joined by other providers of primary care—nurse practitioners, midwives, physician assistants, and social workers—and formed into primary care teams. They will have profound influences on all aspects of care because these primary care providers/teams have the greatest number of patient contacts. They will demand that their surgical and medical subspecialist colleagues pay attention to their concerns. This will be easier to do as the financial incentives among all providers of care become more clearly aligned.

In conclusion, the changes in the provision of ambulatory care services to individuals and to populations of individuals, with its emphasis on health education, an increased role for the primary care provider as a coordinator of care, an ever decreasing reliance on the provision of care of patients in hospital settings, and a greater reliance on cooperation among providers from different disciplines—doctors, nurse practitioners, physician assistants, midwives, social workers, mental health workers—holds great promise for improving the health of the people of the United States. It also has the potential to offer greater value—comprehensive care and improved quality of care at a reduced cost—for both the individual and for the entire population. The challenge will be to retain the ideal of the classical patient-provider relationship, that of a long and trusting association, in the face of the rapid movement away from the delivery of medical care as a cottage industry to a system dominated by the development of coordinated groups of providers practicing in integrated delivery systems.

Mini-Case Study

As a health care consultant you have been asked by Dr. Irving Freedom, a 48-year-old internist with subspecialty training in pulmonary disease, to give him

---

Mini-Case Study *(cont.)*

some advice. For the past 20 years, Dr. Freedom has been practicing general internal medicine as a solo practitioner in an affluent suburb of a large eastern U.S. city. He estimates that 75% of his time is spent as a primary care doctor for approximately 1,000 individuals. The remainder of his time is spent taking care of patients with complicated pulmonary problems, both inside and outside the local community hospital, generally as a consultant to other physicians.

Times are changing in the area. The penetration of managed care health insurance has increased from 10% of eligible patients 5 years ago to 40% today. You believe that it is likely to increase to 65%–70% within the next 2 to 3 years. Dr. Freedom has told you that he has not signed contracts with any of the managed care organizations operating in his area yet.

What should you advise him to do? Include in your answer a discussion of what he should do about his solo practitioner status and the likelihood of his being able to continue as a primary care doctor or as a pulmonary specialist or both. Include, as well, what you believe Dr. Freedom needs to learn in order to function effectively in this new environment.

Discussion Questions

1. What factors are driving the delivery of health care away from emergency care and inpatient hospital stays?
2. How has the role of the primary care practitioner expanded?
3. For what groups of patients do medical specialists function as primary care providers?
4. In the context of this chapter, what is meant by the integrated delivery of health care services?
5. What are three factors that have contributed to the increase in patients learning to provide more of their own health care?

References

Alternative Medicine Homepage, World Wide Web, http//:www.pitt.edu/~cbw/oam.html (1997).

American College of Healthcare Executives, *Managed Care in Medicaid: Lessons for Policy and Program Design*. Melrose Park, IL: Author, 1993.

American Hospital Association, *Hospital Statistics*. Chicago: Author, 1992–93.

American Hospital Association, *Hospital Statistics: Annual Survey of Hospitals*. Chicago: Author, 1993–94 .

American Hospital Association, *Hospital Statistics: Emerging Trends in Hospitals 94/5*. Chicago: Author, 1994.

Anderson, W. H., et al., "Patient Use and Assessment of Conventional and Alternative Therapies for HIV Infection and AIDS," *AIDS, 74,* 561–564, 1993.

Bishop, C., & Skwara, K. C., "Recent Growth of Medicare Home Health," *Health Affairs, 12,* 95–107, 1993.

Bodenheimer, T., "Sounding Board: The HMO Backlash—Righteous or Reactionary," *New England Journal of Medicine, 335,* 1601–1603, 1996.

Chesteen, S. A., Warren, S. E., & Woolley, F. R., "A Comparison of Family Practice Clinics and Free-standing Emergency Centers: Organization Characteristics, Process of Care, and Patient Satisfaction," *Journal of Family Practice, 23,* 377, 1986.

Darnell, J. C., Hiner, S. L, Neill, P. J., & Mamlin, J. J., "After-hours Telephone Access to Physicians with Access to Computerized Medical Records: Experience in an Inner-City General Medicine Clinic," *Medical Care, 23*(1), 20, 1985.

Dutton, D. B., "Patterns of Ambulatory Health Care in Five Different Delivery Systems," *Medical Care, 17,* 221, 1979.

Eisenberg, D. M., Kessler, R. C., Foster, C., Norlock, F. E., Calkins, D. R., & Delbanco, T. L., "Unconventional Medicine in the United States: Prevalence, Costs, and Patterns of Use," *New England Journal of Medicine, 328,* 248–252, 1993.

Institute of Medicine, *Primary Care: America's Health in a New Era.* Washington, DC: National Academy Press, 1996.

Jacobi Medical Center, *1993 Finance Department Statistical Report.* New York: Author, 1993.

Jeffrey, M. A., "Doctors Battle Over Who Treats Chronically Ill," *Wall Street Journal,* December 11, 1996.

Kellerman, A., "What Is Clinical Emergency Medicine," in *The Role of Emergency Medicine in the Future of American Medical Care.* New York: Josiah Macy, Jr. Foundation, 1995.

National Institute for Health Care Management, *Health Care System DataSource.* San Francisco, CA: Institute for Health Policy Studies, University of California, 1996.

O'Connor, B. B., Lazar, J. S., & Anderson, W. H., "Ethnographic Study of HIV Alternative Therapies," poster, VIII International Conference on AIDS, Amsterdam, June 1992.

Primary Care: America's Health in a New Era. Washington, DC: National Academy Press, 1996.

Robert Wood Johnson Foundation, *Special Report: Access to Health Care in the United States: Results of a 1986 Survey.* Princeton, NJ: Author, 1987.

Scheffler, R. M., "Life in the Kaleidoscope: The Impact of Managed Care on the U.S. Health Care Workforce and a New Model for the Delivery of Primary Care." In *Primary Care: America's Health in a New Era* (pp. 312–340). Washington, DC: National Academy Press, 1996.

Schroeder, S. A., "Training an Appropriate Mix of Physicians to Meet the Nation's Needs," *Academic Medicine, 68,* 1993.

Shesser, R., "What Is Clinical Emergency Medicine? Session I: Proceedings of the Conference." In *The Role of Emergency Medicine in the Future of American Medical Care,* Josiah Macy Jr. Foundation, 1995.

U.S. Department of Health and Human Services, *Health United States, 1982* (DHHS Publication No. 83-1232). Washington, DC: U.S. Government Printing Office, 1982.

U.S. Department of Health and Human Services, *Health United States, 1986* (DHHS Publication No. PHS 87-1232). Washington, DC: U.S. Government Printing Office, 1986.

U.S. Department of Health and Human Services, *Health United States, 1995* (DHHS Publication No. PHS 96-1232). Washington, DC: U.S. Government Printing Office, 1995.

U.S. General Accounting Office, "Emergency Departments: Unevenly Affected by Growth and Change in Patient Use," in Committee on Finance, U.S. Senate, *Report to the Chairman, Subcommittee on Health for Families and the Uninsured* (GAO/HRD-93-4). Washington, DC: Author, 1993.

Ware, J. E., Bayliss, M. E., Rogers, W. H., Kosinski, M. A., & Tailor, A. R., "Differences in 4-Year Health Outcomes for Elderly and Poor, Chronically Ill Patients Treated in HMO and Fee-for Service Systems," *Journal of the American Medical Association, 276*, 1039–1047, 1996.

Weinerman, E. R., Ratner, R. S., Robbins, A., & Lavenbar, M. A., "Yale Studies in Ambulatory Medical Care: 5. Determinants of Use of Hospital Emergency Services," *American Journal of Public Health, 56*, 1037, 1966.

Wilensky, G. R., & Berk, M. L., "The Health Care of the Poor and the Role of Medicaid," *Health Affairs, 1*(4), 50, 1982.

Yellin, E. H., Criswell, L. A., & Feigenbaum, P. G., "Health Care Utilization and Outcomes among Persons with Rheumatoid Arthritis in Fee-For-Service and Prepaid Group Settings," *Journal of the American Medical Association, 276*, 1048–1053, 1996.

Young, G. P., Wagner, M. B., Kellerman, A. C., Ellis, J., & Bonley, D., "Ambulatory Visits to Hospital Emergency Departments, Patterns and Reasons for Use," *Journal of the American Medical Association, 276*, 460–465, 1996.

Your Personal Net Doctor: Your Guide to Health and Medical Advice. New York: Wolf New Media, 1996.

8

Long-Term Care: Health, Social, and Housing Services for Those with Chronic Illness

Hila Richardson, Carol Raphael, and Lynne Barton

Learning Objectives

1. Define long-term care and the long-term care population.
2. Differentiate between long-term and acute care services.
3. Describe the different types of services that are part of the long-term care spectrum.
4. Describe the major policy issues in long-term care.
5. Analyze the political and economic forces influencing long-term care services in the future.

Topical Outline

The types of health and social services that are part of long-term care

The characteristics and health needs of people with chronic illness

The effect of demographic changes in the 21st century on the demand for long-term care

The increasing cost of long-term care to the Medicare and Medicaid programs

Nursing homes

    Number and characteristics of people using them

Financing
Quality issues
Home health and hospice services
   Ownership and capacity
   Personnel
   Financing
   Quality issues
Services in the community supporting the chronically ill
Types of residential settings with supportive services
   Availability
   Cost
The major reforms addressing the future demand and cost of long-term care
   Medicare reforms
   Managed care
   Private insurance
   Integrating long-term and acute care
Future direction

Key Words: **Long-term care, chronic health conditions, activities of daily living, formal and informal services, home care, Certified Home Health Agency, hospice services, adult day care, respite services, assisted living, board-and-care homes, continuing care retirement communities (CCRCs), Medigap insurance, Medicaid "spend-down," dual eligibility, integrated long-term and acute care services.**

Long-term care is one of the most important health issues facing the United States as it enters the 21st century. The steady growth in the number of elderly people, the growing numbers of people surviving previously fatal conditions and living longer with chronic diseases, and the aging of the baby boomer generation have created a burgeoning need for long-term care services. This growth is expected to worsen the drain on federal and state budgets that fund long-term care programs. As these trends converge, debate about the health policies to lessen their impact is limited by a political climate characterized by holding the line on public spending. There is deepening concern over whether there will be sufficient resources to meet the growing need for long-term care.

Long-term care encompasses a wide array of health, personal care, social support, and housing programs. Unfortunately, these programs often lack coordination, and they are underfunded, unevenly distributed, and plagued by quality problems. Services are provided to people of all ages in institutions, community-based settings, and private homes, but most people needing assistance with daily living receive help from families and friends outside the formal or established long-term care system. The formal services are paid for by a patchwork of federal, state, and personal resources. People who do not meet the eligibility criteria for federal and state-funded programs and do not have sufficient income to pay for the services incur great financial hardship and can even become impoverished during the course of obtaining the services they need. These problems in access, financing, and quality in long-term care services have existed for decades. Federal and state reforms have been undertaken but have been mostly limited to the economic issues of increasing cost-sharing by individuals and providers and implementing new payment mechanisms. Given these problems in long-term care, the influx of larger numbers of people needing services will only place further stress on a system that is already lagging in its ability to pay for and meet existing needs in a cost-efficient way.

This chapter will provide the background for understanding the importance of long-term care as a major health care issue. The discussion starts with a description of the current long-term care services—whom they serve and how they are financed—and concerns about their quality. This is followed by a review of the major reforms being proposed to address long-term care costs. The chapter ends with a discussion about what the future holds.

Definition of and Need for Long-Term Care

Long-term care is a range of health, personal care, social, and housing services provided to people of all ages with chronic health conditions that limit their ability to carry out normal daily activities without assistance. People needing long-term care have many different types of physical and mental disabilities, and their need for the mix and intensity of long-term care services can change over time. Long-term care is mainly rehabilitative and supportive rather than curative. It can be provided in either the home or in residential or institutional settings by health care workers other than physicians and, for the most part, requires little or no technology.

Much of the need for long-term care results from either chronic conditions or the aging process that leads to mental or physical impairment. Chronic conditions refer to both chronic illnesses (the presence of long-term disease) and impairments (an abnormality of bodily function or structure (Table 8.1). By definition, chronic conditions cannot be cured. But good chronic care includes prevention of secondary conditions such as urinary tract infections, bedsores, and depression. Although people use the acute care system during an exacerbation of a chronic condition and for treatment of secondary conditions, most chronic care needs are nonmedical and include such services as transportation, supportive housing, and shopping assistance.

TABLE 8.1 Examples of Conditions and Impairments Requiring Long-Term Care Services

Chronic illness
  Arthritis
  Cancer
  Heart disease
  Emphysema
  Alzheimer's disease
  Cystic fibrosis

Impairments
  Blindness
  Hearing loss
  Paralysis

Developmental disabilities
  Cerebral palsy
  Genetic or congenital defects
  Seizure disorders

Injuries
  Paralysis from head and spinal cord injuries
  Burns

Determination of the need for long-term care cannot be based solely on a diagnosis or type of impairment. For example, some people with arthritis function independently, whereas others need assistance with basic activities. Also, people's needs vary as they experience acute episodes followed by periods of stability in their condition. The need for long-term care does not depend on a diagnosis; it is determined by other means. For the elderly it is usually determined by measuring limitations in performing daily activities. Two measures are most commonly used: activities of daily living (ADLs) and instrumental activities of daily living (IADLs). The ADLs are a measure of a person's dependence on others for assistance with personal care functions (i.e., bathing, dressing, feeding oneself, toileting, and transferring from bed to chair). The IADLs measure a person's ability to perform household and social tasks such as preparing meals, shopping, housework, getting around the community, and managing money. Other functions, such as the ability to attend school or work also may be used. Not all people with ADL or IADL limitations need assistance from another person. Some can perform the tasks independently with aids such as canes, walkers, and adaptive devices for kitchens and bathrooms.

A person can need long-term care at any age. The most familiar example is an elderly person needing minimal help in performing basic activities at home: bathing, dressing, walking, shopping, meal preparation, transportation, house-cleaning, and other activities important for self-sufficiency. On the other end of the continuum, a young person paralyzed by an automobile accident may be completely dependent on nursing services in a nursing home for all basic activities, plus care for such needs as ventilator-assisted breathing and tube feedings. Long-term care can be continuous or intermittent, but it is assumed that most people will need it with increasing intensity for years, often for the remainder of their lives (Kane & Kane, 1987). The goal of all long-term care services is to enable people to regain or maintain the highest level of independent functioning possible.

Chronic conditions are the major cause of illness, disability, and death in the United States today, accounting for three of four deaths (Institute for Health and Aging, 1996). In 1995, one in six Americans—41 million people—had a chronic condition that limited activity to some degree and put him or her at risk of needing long-term care services. Of these, more than 12 million said they needed assistance to perform activities and were unable to attend school, work, or live independently. Eighty percent of them reported that they needed assistance to live at home or in community residential settings. The remaining 20 percent were residing in institutions. Of the total 12 million who needed assistance, 57% were over 65 years of age, but 5 million (40%) were working-age adults. Children and youth represented 3% (400,000) of those needing long-term care services (Figure 8.1).

As Figure 8.2 shows, the growing need for long-term care services is due to both the increase in the number of persons with limitations resulting from chronic conditions and the increase in the elderly population, which have the highest prevalence of chronic conditions by the year 2050. Projections for that year estimate that the number of people with chronic conditions will reach 42 million, representing nearly 17% of the population (Institute for Health and Aging, 1996). New types of technology and pharmaceuticals now ensure the survival of premature infants and victims of accidents who would otherwise die. Many of those who survive have permanent disabilities and can require long-term care services for a lifetime.

However, most of the increase in the demand for long-term services will result from the growth in the number of elderly people, because this population develops chronic conditions more often and with greater severity than younger age groups. As Figure 8.2 shows, the percentage of persons between 65 and 84 years of age is expected to double by the year 2020, growing from 7% (33.5 million) in 1995 to almost 15% (53 million). By 2050, persons over 65 years of age will represent 20% of the population (78 million). The percentage of the oldest elderly, those over 85 years, is projected to triple from just over 1% of the population in 1995

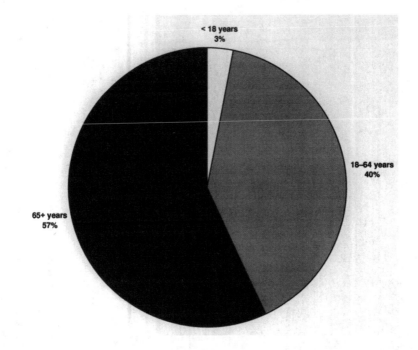

FIGURE 8.1 Long-term care need by age, 1995 (12 million persons).
Source: GAO, *Long-Term Care: Current Issues and Future Directions* (GAO/HEHS-95-109),
Figure 2, p. 7. Washington, DC: U.S. Government Printing Office, April 1995.

to over 3% in 2050 (U.S. Bureau of the Census, 1996). Based on current trends, by 2020 up to 14 million of those over 65 will need long-term care—double the 7 million who need long-term care today (Institute for Health and Aging, 1996).

The current and anticipated future cost of care for the elderly and others with chronic conditions has significant implications for national health care expenditures. A study of enrollees in a health maintenance organization (HMO) found that the population with at least one chronic condition had average costs at least twice those of the population with no chronic conditions. Enrollees with chronic conditions (38% of the population) accounted for 71% of the total costs (Fishman, Von Koff, Lozano, & Hecht, 1997). The direct costs for all services provided to persons with chronic disease was $425 billion in 1990—70% of the $612 billion in total national expenditures on personal health care. Of the amount

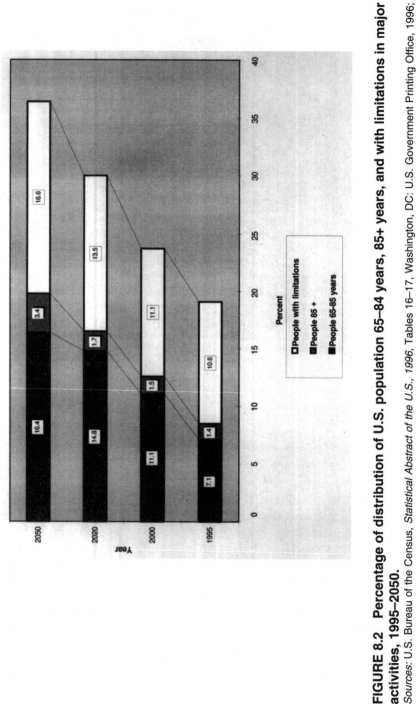

FIGURE 8.2 Percentage of distribution of U.S. population 65–84 years, 85+ years, and with limitations in major activities, 1995–2050.

Sources: U.S. Bureau of the Census, *Statistical Abstract of the U.S., 1996*, Tables 16–17, Washington, DC: U.S. Government Printing Office, 1996; Hoffman, C., & Rice, D.P., in *Chronic Care in America: A 21st Century Challenge* (p. 18). Princeton, NJ: Robert Wood Johnson Foundation, 1996.

spent, the largest share (40%) was for hospital care (Institute for Health and Aging, 1996).

Because long-term care is largely publicly financed, the growth in demand has strained public coffers. In 1995 spending for nursing homes and home health care alone was $106.5 billion with public programs, mainly Medicaid and Medicare, financing 57.4%. Out-of-pocket payments by patients and family accounted for the remaining 42.6%. The spending for Medicare and Medicaid was 12% of all personal health care expenditures in that year. Medicaid bears the greatest share of the public financing for long-term care because it provides coverage for more nursing home care than Medicare does. In 1995, Medicaid spending on long-term care services was 38% of the total $106.5 billion, with the federal government paying 21% and state and local governments paying 17% of $18 billion. Medicare expenditures for long-term care, although only 18% of total expenditures, more than doubled from 1990 to 1995 (Levit et al., 1996).

It is difficult to exactly predict the future need for and costs of long-term care. The influence of different lifestyles and better medical management and prevention of chronic conditions for the baby boomer generation could postpone or decrease the need for services. At the same time, the increase in life expectancy and the growth in the elderly population will cause the absolute numbers of people who need long-term care services to grow. On balance, there will be an increasing need for services. However, the magnitude may not be as great as the worst predictions indicate.

Long-Term Care Services: Delivery and Financing

Long-term care is provided in both institutional and community-based settings. In recent years the use of formal home and community-based services has grown while the number of people in nursing homes has declined (Moon, 1996). However, the long-term care market remains characterized by reliance on more costly institutional services and uneven availability of home and community-based care, with the exception of a few states that are innovators in this market. One distinguishing aspect of long-term care as compared to acute care is the substitution of informal, unpaid care for health care providers. Roughly 75% of those with long-term care needs living in the community receive only informal care provided and paid for by family members and to a lesser degree by friends (Congressional Budget Office, 1991). The services provided through established programs are funded almost equally by out-of-pocket income of individuals and public funding through Medicare, Medicaid, and federal block grants.

Nursing Homes

The most important providers of formal long-term care services are nursing homes. In 1995 there were 16,700 nursing homes with 1.8 million beds in which

1.5 million people received care. The number of nursing homes decreased 12.6% between 1985 and 1995, whereas the number of beds increased 9%. The decline in the total number of nursing homes in the United States is occurring while the number of nursing home beds is increasing. As a result, the number of beds per home has increased from 75 beds per home in 1974 to 106 beds per home in 1995 (Strahan, 1997).

For-profit organizations own just over 66% of nursing homes, not-for-profit groups own nearly 26%, and 8% are government-owned. Nursing homes are operated either independently or as members of a group of facilities operating under one general authority or ownership called a chain. In 1995, 45% of nursing homes were operated independently, whereas 54% were operating as part of a chain. A significant increase in the number of nursing homes operated by chains has occurred in the past two decades. In 1977, nursing homes with chain affiliations were 28% of total homes; in 1985 they were 41%; and by 1995, 54% of nursing homes were part of chains (Strahan, 1997).

The cost of nursing home care is largely paid by Medicaid (47%), with individuals and their families paying 37% (see Figure 8.3). Medicare paid only 9% of nursing home care in 1995; the remaining 7% was paid by other government sources (i.e., Veteran's Administration) and private insurers. In 1995, spending for nursing home care was $78 billion, which is on average $127 per day (Levitt et al., 1996). However, there is a wide variation in nursing home costs from state to state (Kane, 1996).

Most states use a case-mix system for the Medicaid payment to nursing homes. Nursing homes receive payment based on the intensity of care their residents need (Kane, 1996). The case mix is determined through assessment of the physical and mental functioning of the resident. With this approach, the nursing home gets paid more for sicker and more dependent residents, thus creating an incentive not to help residents improve their functioning. To minimize this possibility, states and the federal government monitor the quality of care in nursing homes and, as part of this function, require the homes to document the resident's progress or the reasons for lack of progress.

Although nursing home care is the service most closely associated with long-term care, only a small percentage of the elderly are living in nursing homes on any given day. In 1995, 4% of the persons over 65 years of age lived in a nursing home (Strahan, 1997). This proportion of the total elderly population in nursing homes is slightly lower than in 1985, when it was 5% (Strahan, 1997). The rate of nursing home admissions is declining along with the decline in occupancy rates, from 93% in 1985 to 87% in 1995. States have encouraged the growth in the home care industry and residential services at the same time that they have put tighter controls on the construction of nursing home beds. This has shifted the site of care for the elderly to their homes and communities.

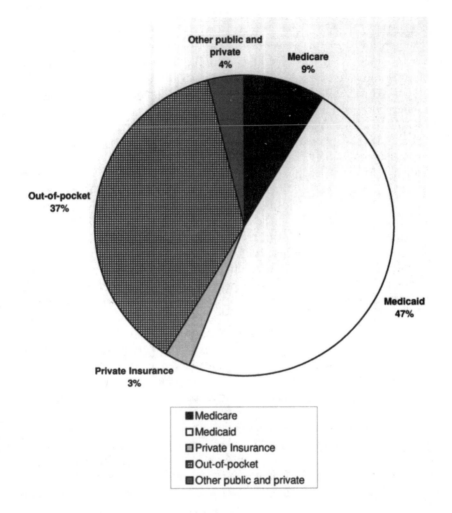

FIGURE 8.3 Distribution of nursing home expenditures by payer, 1995 (total expenditure: $77.9 billion).
Source: Health Care Financing Administration, *Health Care Financing Review, 18*(1), 211–212, 1996.

In 1995 those in nursing homes were typically the older elderly. The largest percentage of the people were 75–84 years and older (38%), followed by those aged 85 years and older (36%) and those 65–74 years (16%) (Strahan, 1997). The rate of nursing home use increases with age, with just over 1% of persons between 65 and 74 years in nursing homes, compared to 24% of those 85 years and older (U.S. Bureau of the Census, 1996). It has been projected that if past utilization patterns continue, over half of the women and almost one third of the men who turned 65 in 1990 can be expected to use a nursing home sometime before they die (Murtaugh, Kemper, & Spillman, 1990).

Elderly White people are most likely to use nursing homes, representing 88% of nursing home residents in 1995 (Strahan, 1997). More reliance on informal care within Black communities and discriminatory admission practices by nursing homes are two possible reasons given for the underrepresentation of Blacks and other races among nursing home residents.

Although 90% of nursing home residents are elderly, many very frail, the remaining 10% are under 65 years of age. These residents have physical and mental disabilities due to accidents or congenital abnormalities that prevent them from living in the community. The number, but not necessarily the proportion, of younger nursing home residents is expected to grow because (1) persons born with lifelong disabilities during the baby boom of the 1940s and 1950s have aging parents who are dying or becoming too old to care for them; (2) medical technology can now keep alive people who are severely disabled at birth or who experience traumatic injuries and require institutional long-term care for decades; (3) people with HIV illness and AIDS who cannot function in the community need nursing home care during medical crises or at the end of life. This younger institutionalized population often requires very different activities and support services from those needed by the typical frail elderly residents of nursing homes. Nursing homes have to adapt their recreation programs and institutional routines (such as times for getting up and going to bed) and provide more private space to meet the needs of younger residents (Blustein et al., 1992).

Nursing homes are feared by older people as places where they will be neglected, abused, and left to die alone. This image, although not applicable to most nursing homes, has been reinforced by continual scandals related to physical danger, filthy conditions, patient abuse, and negligence (Institute of Medicine, 1986; U.S. Senate Special Committee on Aging, 1986; Vladeck, 1980). Defining and measuring quality of care in nursing homes is particularly difficult because it must be measured over an extended period, with periodic and careful assessment of the medical, functional, social, and psychological needs of the resident.

The quality of care in a nursing home is closely related to quality of life; the resident's ability to make decisions about food, activities, clothing, and pursuing personal interests; having privacy; and being treated courteously and kindly by staff. These goals can be difficult and costly for even the best nursing homes to achieve. One of the critical elements of quality of life in nursing homes is the quality of the resident-staff relationship. Most of the care in nursing homes is provided by nurse's aides, who usually are low-paid, in many states receive relatively little training, and are often inadequately supervised. They are often required to care for a large number of frail, very old residents, many of whom have mental impairments as well as physical disabilities. Not surprisingly, the turnover rate for nurse's aides ranges from 70% to over 100% a year (Institute of Medicine, 1986).

To make recommendations on how to address these universal and persistent quality problems, the Institute of Medicine sponsored a 2-year study of state and federal nursing home regulations. The panel's report led to the nursing home reforms in the Omnibus Reconciliation Act of 1987. The provision included specific requirements for nurse aide training and nurse staffing; resident assessments that could lead to measuring outcomes and quality-of-life improvements, like reducing the use of physical restraints; and providing more protection of patient self-determination.

Home-Based Services

Home care encompasses a broad array of health care and social services provided to individuals and their families in their home or other residential settings. Generally, home care is classified as services related to either medical needs or personal care and social needs. The medically related services are often referred to as home health care and consist of home visits by health professionals (i.e., nurses, physical therapists, occupational therapists, and/or a paraprofessional "home health aide") to provide assistance with ADLs. For medically related home health care there must be a plan of care prescribed by a physician, and the care provided in the home must be supervised by a professional, usually a nurse. Medically related services include giving oral medications and injections, changing surgical dressings and other nursing treatments, teaching the patient and family, and assistance with ADLs.

Personal care and social services are usually referred to broadly as home care. These services include assistance with direct personal needs such as bathing, dressing, and grooming. These services are performed by a personal care aide or a home health aide. In addition, this classification of services includes help with IADLs such as shopping, cooking, and cleaning, which are performed by "homemakers," "housekeepers," or personal care aides.

The National Association for Home Care (NAHC, 1996), a trade association that represents home care and hospice agencies, has identified a total of 18,874 home care agencies in the United States in 1995. These agencies included 9,120 home health agencies certified by Medicare to provide medically related services, 1,857 hospices certified by Medicare, and 7,897 home health agencies, home care aide organizations, and hospices that do not participate in Medicare. When Medicare included home health services, primarily short-term skilled-nursing and restorative therapy, as one of its covered services, the Medicare-certified home health agency grew very rapidly and became the major type of home care agency. In 1967 there were 1,753 Medicare-certified home health agencies (CHHAs), in 1985 there were 5,983 CHHAs, and in 1995 the number had risen to the high of 9,120 (NAHC, 1996). To become certified by Medicare, an agency has to meet the conditions of participation that include required policies, record-keeping practices, training of workers, utilization review, and quality assurance.

As the numbers indicate, many home care agencies do not become Medicare-certified because they provide services only to private-pay clients, they do not provide all the services Medicare requires, or they do not want to meet all the conditions of participation. The noncertified agencies can be licensed by the state, if the state has licensure requirements, or the agency can operate on a nonlicensed basis. As an example of the complexity and fragmentation of the home care system, a comparative study of formal home care providers in California showed that at least seven types deliver home care and related services: licensed only, noncertified home health agencies, licensed and certified home health agencies, nurse registries, employment agencies, unlicensed temporary personnel agencies, other unlicensed agencies, and unlicensed individual providers. These providers varied in the kinds of services provided, sources of payment, payment arrangements, regulatory agencies and requirements, duration of care, supervision of care, and utilization of services (Harrington & Grant, 1990).

The growth in the number of CHHAs has been accompanied by changes in the mix of organizations that own or sponsor them. As Figure 8.4 shows, Visiting Nurse Associations (VNAs), usually not-for-profit agencies, and public agencies represented 90% of the 1,700 CHHAs in 1967. There were no for-profit or not-for-profit (PNP) agencies that year because originally Medicare legislation prohibited the certification of agencies with such ownership. However, the prohibition was lifted in 1980, and a dramatic growth in the number of for-profit CHHAs occurred. By 1985 for-profit CHHAs accounted for 32% of over 4,000 CHHAs. Also, the hospital-based CHHA experienced a rapid growth, going from 7.6% in 1967 to 21% in 1985. In 1995 the proprietary and PNP agencies represented over 50% of the more than 8,000 CHHAs; the hospital-based agencies, many of which also had proprietary and PNP ownership, represented slightly less than 30%. The VNAs and the public agencies stabilized at 6% and 13%, respectively, after experiencing a dramatic decrease between 1967 and 1985 (NAHC, 1996).

In addition to the array of formal direct providers of home care services, the home care sector now includes the home medical equipment and home infusion therapy industries. Advancements in technology have made it possible to provide in-home therapies that previously could be provided only in the hospital (e.g., intravenous therapy, respirators, and parenteral nutrition). This sector has experienced a high growth rate, with estimated expenditures for infusion therapies, as

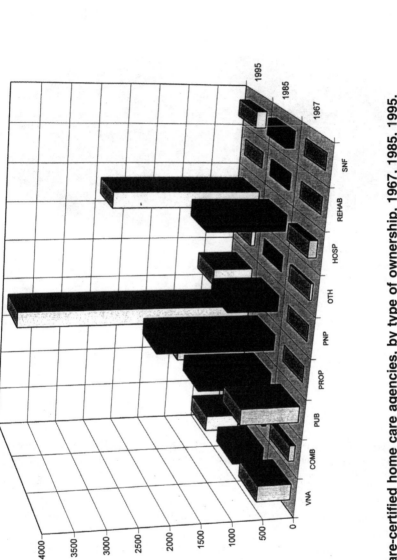

FIGURE 8.4 Medicare-certified home care agencies, by type of ownership, 1967, 1985, 1995.
VNA = Visiting Nurse Associations, COMB = combination agencies (government and voluntary), PUB = Public agencies, PROP = Proprietary agencies, PNP = Private not-for-profit agencies, OTH = Other freestanding agencies, HOSP = Hospital-based agencies, REHAB = Rehabilitation facility-based agencies, SNF = Skilled Nursing Facility-based agencies.

Source: National Association for Home Care, *Basic Statistics About Home Care,* 1996, p. 3.

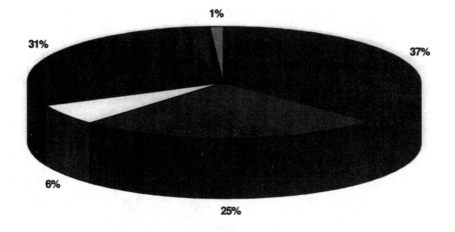

1%

31%   37%

6%

25%

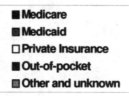

■ Medicare
■ Medicaid
☐ Private Insurance
■ Out-of-pocket
▨ Other and unknown

FIGURE 8.5   Sources of payment for home care, 1992.
Source: National Medical Expenditure Survey 1987 data and Lewin-VHI Inc., Fairfax, Virginia,
analysis for 1992.

an example, growing from $684 million in 1986 to almost $3 billion in 1992
(NAHC, 1993).

   An estimated total of $52 billion was spent on all types of home health services
in 1996 (NAHC, 1996). The mean annual expense per patient in that year was
$1,967, with annual expenditures increasing with age. For those 85 years and
older the average spent was $3,292 per person, whereas those 65 to 74 years of
age spent an average of $2,014. In 1992, the latest year for which a breakdown
by payer for all home health services is available (Figure 8.5), 31.4% was paid
out of pocket by individuals; Medicaid paid 24.7% and Medicare paid 37.8%,
for a total of public payments of 62.5%. Private insurance paid only 5.5% of
annual home health expenditures. The other programs that pay for some home

health services are the Older Americans Act, Title XX of the Social Services Block Grants, the Veterans Administration, and the Civilian Health and Medical Program Uniform Services (CHAMPUS).

In contrast to Medicare, Medicaid benefits for home health services can be extensive, depending on the state. They can include services by nurses, home health aides, social workers, housekeepers, and various therapists. Most states expanded their home health and community-based services under Section 2176 waivers (Home and Community Based Waiver Program) in the 1981 Omnibus Reconciliation Act.

Quality of home health services is particularly difficult to monitor because most of the time it cannot be observed. The patient contact occurs in the patient's home, often with only a home health aide or attendant and the patient present. Visits to the patient by a professional supervisor may occur only once every 2 weeks and then may not include an observation of the care being provided by the aide.

As in the nursing home industry, quality problems in home care often are related to the difficulty home health agencies have in attracting and retaining experienced and reliable staff and to the varying state requirements for training and supervision of unskilled home health workers. The wages of home health workers lag behind those of most unskilled positions available, such as hotel, laundry, and cleaning work (Kane & Kane, 1987). In 1996 national average hourly wages for home health aides ranged from a low of $6.45 to a high of $10.14 (Hoechst Marion Roussel, 1996).

As with nursing homes, improving the quality of home care staff can also increase the costs of providing care. As Medicare and Medicaid develop more stringent limitations on eligibility for home health services and ratchet down rates, agencies may be less likely to undertake efforts that will improve quality of care. The considerable physical and emotional strain of home health work, together with the geographic difficulty of supervision, makes quality assurance not only a challenging but also an expensive endeavor for management.

Hospice Services

Hospice services are mainly provided in the home to the terminally ill and their families. Hospice is based on a philosophy of care imported from England and Canada that holds that during the course of terminal illness the patient should be able to live life as fully and comfortably as possible but without artificial or mechanical efforts to prolong life. In the hospice approach the family is the unit of treatment. An interdisciplinary team provides medical, nursing, psychological, therapeutic, pharmacological, and spiritual support during the final stages of illness, at the time of death, and during bereavement. The main goals are to control pain, maintain independence, and minimize the stress and trauma of death.

Increased federal and private insurance has spurred a boom in hospice care. In 1983, Medicare added hospice benefits and the number of programs increased from 516 in 1983 to 1,857 in 1995 (NAHC, 1996). Medicare hospice expenditures have grown significantly, increasing 35.7% in 1 year alone. In 1994, Medicare spending for hospice services was $1.4 billion, and in 1995 it was $1.9 billion (Health Care Financing Administration, 1996a).

The funding for hospice under Medicare strongly reinforces the intent that, among other things, hospices be used as a way of avoiding hospital expenses. For example, at least 80% of hospice care must be provided in the home, not in an inpatient setting like a hospital or nursing home. Also, the patient must waive other types of acute care, the patient's doctor must certify that life expectancy is 6 months or less, and 5% of services have to be furnished by volunteers in the patient's home, with documentation of the cost savings from volunteers' services.

Hospice services have gained acceptance as an alternative to hospital care for the terminally ill. It is likely that the number of hospices will continue to grow because their philosophy toward caring for those at end of life has become a model for the nation.

Community-Based Services

Services based in the community are provided through voluntary, public, or proprietary organizations and include adult day care, hospice, respite, meals, transportation, and case management programs for the frail elderly, chronically ill children, and persons with developmental disabilities. These services are supported by a combination of funds from Medicare, Medicaid, Title III of the Older Americans Act, and other federal, state, and local social services programs. The extent of the services provided and the eligibility requirements vary by funding source and by state and locality.

As Table 8.2 summarizes, states use the social services block grant program to provide homemaker, home health aide, chore, adult day care, and adult foster care services. Under Title III of the Older Americans Act, established in 1965, available services include transportation, homemakers, and chore and home health aide services. Amendments to the Older Americans Act in 1987 authorized funds for nonmedical in-home services that included visiting and telephone reassurance, chore maintenance, and in-home respite and adult day care respite for families (General Accounting Office, 1988).

Adult Day Care Services

Adult day care is a program that offers a wide range of health and social services to elderly persons during the day and out of the home. Adult day care services are usually targeted to elderly in families where the caregivers work or to elderly persons living alone. Their goal is to delay or prevent institutionalization and provide respite for the caregiver. The services offered follow a medical or social model.

Data on adult day care programs are still limited, but a 1994 survey found that there were about 2,756 licensed adult day care centers in 27 states in 1994 (Graves & Bectel, 1996). Most adult day care programs offer social services, crafts, current events discussions, family counseling, reminiscence therapy, nursing assessment, physical exercise, ADL rehabilitation, psychiatric assessment, and medical care. States finance adult day services with Medicaid funds and Social Security block grants for those who qualify. Medicare does not cover adult day care. Most elderly people and their families pay for adult day care out of pocket.

Respite Services

Respite services provide a temporary respite, or break, for the caregivers of the frail elderly or disabled chronically ill. There is no uniform definition of respite care. Programs can be provided in or out of the person's home. In-home respite provides temporary homemaker, chore, or home health services while the main caregiver is away. Out-of-home care includes adult day care and temporary stays in nursing homes, hospitals, group homes, or foster care homes. The type and scope of services and eligibility for services vary considerably among states (Kane & Kane, 1987; Meltzer, 1982). States started using respite services for developmentally disabled and mentally retarded children in the 1960s. The concept was extended to the elderly to reduce the stress of informal caregivers and the costs of institutionalization.

Respite care may be paid for by Medicaid, a social services block grant, Older Americans Act funds, state general revenues, or privately. Medicaid rules require that respite care be provided only to elderly at risk of institutionalization. With the passage of the Medicare Catastrophic Coverage Act in 1988, Medicare coverage was temporarily extended to respite services. This benefit was lost when the act was repealed in 1989.

Long-Term Care Residential Services

New living environments that are more homelike and less institutional are the focus of much attention in the current long-term care market and are seen as playing a growing role in the continuum of long-term care services. Having

TABLE 8.2 Major Federal Programs Supporting Long-Term Care Services for the Elderly and Persons with Disabilities

Program	Services	Population
Medicare (Title XVIII of the Social Security Act)	100 days posthospital nursing home care, intermittent skilled home care, limited hospice care	All persons eligible for Social Security: persons 65+, permanently disabled, or with end-stage renal disease
Medicaid (Title XIX of the Social Security Act)	Nursing home care, facilities for persons with mental retardation and chronic care hospitals; home health, transportation, homemaking	Persons whose income meets the definition of "needy" or who "spend down" their assets to meet the definition, those who qualify for disability payments under supplemental security income (SSI) or Aid to Families with Dependent Children (AFDC)
Social services block grant (Title XX of the Social Security Act)	States have option to spend funds, can include home-delivered meals, transportation, respite, day care, protective services, housekeeping, legal services	Eligibility established by the state but largely for low-income persons
Older Americans Act	Allocations made to states for senior centers, congregate meals, home-delivered meals, transportation, housekeeping, chore services, telephone reassurance, information and referral, and other supportive services	Persons 60+ regardless of income, although usually low income; mentally impaired; and isolated elderly persons

(continued)

TABLE 8.2 *(cont.)*

Program	Services	Population
Rehabilitation Act	Vocational rehabilitation services, independent living services such as attendant and personal care, and centers for independent living	Disabled

Sources: Kane & Kane, 1987, pp. 72–75; General Accounting Office, *Long-Term Care: Current Issues and Future Directions* (GAO/HEHS-95-109), Washington, DC: Author, 1995, p. 10.

affordable and appropriate housing available for elderly and disabled people can reduce the level of need for institutional long-term care services in the community. Institutionalization can be postponed or prevented when the elderly or disabled live in settings that are accessible to those with physical impairments and safe for those with mental impairments and where assistance with daily activities is available.

Assisted Living

Assisted living is generally defined as any residential setting that provides a continuum of health care services, as well as other social support services, within the residence. Assisted living may be board-and-care homes with additional services, residential units owned by and adjacent to nursing homes, congregate housing settings that have added services, housing built for the purpose of assisted living, or Continuing Care Retirement Communities (CCRCs). Ownership may be either nonprofit or for-profit, the latter including chains of varying sizes. Most often, assisted living facilities are complexes of individual apartments that are targeted to private-pay populations.

Because of state variations in definition, sponsorship, size, physical environments, target populations, admission and retention practices, and service and staffing requirements, it is difficult to know the exact number of assisted living residences. Estimates in 1993 ranged from 30,000 to 40,000, serving an estimated 1 million older persons (American Association of Homes and Services for the Aging [AAHSA], 1995a).

The typical assisted living resident is a female in the low to mid-eighties who needs assistance with basic living skills (Gulyas, 1995). Assisted living is most often paid for by the residents themselves or their families. There has been no government payment for assisted living although some states have included it in a special Medicaid waiver program. The cost of assisted living can range from several hundred dollars or less to more than $3,000 a month. The rates can range from an all-inclusive monthly fee to separate charges for each service provided. Assisted living residences are regulated by states, which vary in the requirements for licensure, staffing, physical design, and resident characteristics (Gulyas, 1995).

Board-and-Care Homes

Board-and-care homes is a broad category of housing that covers adult foster care homes, sheltered care facilities, halfway houses, and adult homes. They provide rooms, meals, help with ADLs, and some degree of protective oversight. Depending on the state, services may include supervising the use of medications by residents and linking residents to community services. In 1994 there were approximately 41,483 licensed homes with about 666,127 beds (Harrington & Swan, 1995). The residents pay for services themselves or receive Supplementary Security Income (SSI) to help pay for the facility (Kane & Kane, 1987). Board-and-care residents are both elderly people who need assistance with dressing and bathing due to physical and mental impairment and younger people who have mental impairment and cannot function without supervision. However, some residential settings do not admit people who use wheelchairs, are incontinent, cannot transfer from the bed to a chair, or have cognitive impairments. Also, if people develop these disabilities, they may have to be transferred to another setting.

Continuing Care Retirement Communities

CCRCs are age-restricted developments offering housing, health and social services, sports facilities, recreational programs, transportation, and social events. There are usually three levels of living available in a CCRC: independent living in unattached houses or apartments, assisted living with services brought into a house or apartment, and nursing home care. As of 1996, 350,000 (a little more than 1%) of elderly people lived in about 1,200 CCRCs. The number of CCRCs increased by 50% during the 1980s and the number is expected to continue to grow through the 1990s.

CCRCs are located in 42 states and the District of Columbia, but 40% are found in five states: Pennsylvania, California, Florida, Illinois, and Ohio. The high costs of these communities make them accessible to only a small proportion of the elderly. In 1993 the entry fee for a one-bedroom apartment ranged from $59,667 to $85,866, with monthly fees from $1,089 to $1,775. The entry and monthly fees for a two-bedroom unit were $88,559 to $125,983 and $1,499 to $1,908, respectively, in the same year. Entry fees can range as high as $176,000 (AAHSA, 1995b). Some CCRCs offer an equity payment plan where the resident owns a condominium or cooperative apartment with a membership arrangement that requires purchase of service and/or health packages. The entrance and monthly fees depend on the amount of services purchased. For example, an extensive agreement might include all support services, including nursing home care should it be needed. In contrast, a fee-for-service agreement would charge for each service (i.e., housekeeping, delivered meals, home health).

The average age of a CCRC resident is 81. As in other types of assisted living, the majority (75%) of CCRC residents are female. Unlike other types of assisted living arrangement and nursing homes, 30% of the residents are living with a spouse (AAHSA, 1995b). Because CCRCs offer the option of independent living in houses and apartments, the younger elderly who are still married find the convenience, activities, and security of CCRCs attractive.

The Smith Family

In the Smith family, both parents work. Mrs. Smith is a dental hygienist at a local dentist office. Mr. Smith is the office manager for a small consulting firm. They have two children, ages 13 and 11. Mr. Smith's father died 2 years ago, and his mother, age 82, now lives with them, as she has become increasingly frail and no longer able to get around completely on her own. In June, Mr. Smith's mother fell in the house when no one was home and broke her hip. She had a total hip replacement, but because of her age and state of frailty will never regain her previous range of motion and now cannot ambulate, even to go to the bathroom, without assistance.

Before Mr. Smith's father retired, he owned a successful car repair shop, and he and his wife were able to live comfortably off the sale of his business until he died. Mr. Smith's mother has too much in assets to qualify for Medicaid. Medicare paid for the immediate post–acute care needs once his mother returned home after surgery but does not pay for ongoing help with things such as bathing, toileting, eating, or moving from bed to chair to watch TV, which are considered unskilled needs. The Smith children are in school all day, and the older child has soccer practice every day after school from 4–6 p.m. Mr. Smith feels that he cannot take time off from work without jeopardizing his job and thinks Mrs. Smith is a better caregiver anyway. The Smith family has some money to spend on hiring a private home health aide but rapidly finds that the cost of private services will eat through the mother's and their savings in 1 year.

Mrs. Smith has therefore had to periodically use her paid time off from work to care for her mother-in-law, and once that ran out, she started taking time without

Case *(cont.)*

pay. She is considering asking her employer if she can reduce her work hours, even though that means less money for the household, because she finds it too difficult to juggle the demands of full-time work, running the house, taking care of her husband and children, and meeting the care needs of her mother-in-law.

Jennifer

Jennifer is a 4-month-old child with a diagnosis of prematurity and multiple developmental delays. She was referred to an early intervention (EI) program for developmentally disabled children by her visiting nurse. Her mother, Annie, is 17 years old, a single mother who dropped out of school when Jennifer was born but has indicated an interest in completing her high school education.

Annie and Jennifer live with Annie's parents, two teenage brothers, and a 4-year-old brother. Her father is disabled. When initially referred to EI, Annie felt depressed and suicidal at her family's lack of support and the baby's condition. A referral from a mobile crisis unit, which provides in-home emergency mental health and crisis services, resulted in Annie's receiving psychotherapy. Her home care service coordinator also assisted her with applying for SSI and Medicaid for Jennifer, learning to ask appropriate questions of Jennifer's medical doctors (she had been hospitalized several times for respiratory distress), and obtaining her own welfare payment and housing. The visiting nurse also referred Annie to a local hospital's Adolescent Medicine Clinic for health care for herself. She was referred to a teen mom program at the Board of Education and will attend the program while her baby is in the nursery at the school.

Jennifer was evaluated and was approved to receive physical therapy, feeding/speech therapy, and special instruction (play therapy). Additionally, approval was given for Annie to attend a weekly parent support group. Ongoing service coordination helps her successfully work through any obstacles that arise regarding Jennifer's or her own service needs.

Charles

At the age of 78, Charles had a stroke that caused him to be paralyzed on his right side and also to partially lose his ability to speak. At the time, he had been living alone because his wife died a year and a half earlier. His daughter lived across the country with her family, and his son was in the air force and traveled all over the world. A neighbor, whom Charles was to drive to the grocery, found him on the back porch when he came by to meet Charles.

Charles was admitted to the local hospital, and after almost 6 weeks in the hospital, he no longer needed acute care but still could not walk without someone supporting him, and he had to communicate by writing. He was ready for discharge from the hospital but still needed intensive rehabilitation. He was transferred to a subacute unit at the local nursing home, where he received physical therapy twice a day, when he was strong enough, and occupational and speech therapy

Case *(cont.)*

once a day. The doctor expected that Charles would eventually be able to walk with a walker or cane and be able to speak again, although not as clearly as before the stroke. It was clear that Charles could not return to his independent lifestyle. Neither of his children was in a position to take care of him, so the social worker looked for appropriate residential services.

After he had reached his maximum benefit from intensive rehabilitation, Medicare would no longer pay for Charles to stay in the subacute level at the nursing home. Charles had to pay the $150 per diem rate for a regular nursing home until a longer term residence could be arranged and Charles regained more of his physical strength. After 6 months, the social worker located an assisted living residence that Charles could afford at $800 per month. He had a large room where he moved his favorite chair, TV, and other personal items from his home. He had assistance in dressing and in going to the dining room when he needed it. There were activities, including movies, entertainment, and trips to the baseball game and other places whenever he wanted to participate. His children visited several times a year. Although he could not live completely independently in his own home, Charles was able to afford a place where he could function at his highest level of independence and have privacy and control over much of his life.

Other Housing Options

A variety of other long-term care housing options exist beyond assisted living. These include home equity conversion, ECHO housing, home maintenance programs, and shared housing. Combined, these housing alternatives comprise a relatively small part of long-term care housing services. Almost 1.5 million elderly receive some type of federal housing assistance. This may be in the form of public housing, rent subsidies and vouchers, or special housing projects (U.S. Department of Housing and Urban Development, 1996). A widely recognized shortage of federally subsidized housing for the elderly has left over 1 million elderly households in need of priority housing assistance, defined as housing for those paying over 50% of their income for rent or living in severely inadequate housing (USDHUD, 1996).

Current Issues in Long-Term Care

Concerns about how to pay for the present and future demand for long-term care is the major issue that is driving changes in the financing and service delivery of long-term care through (1) reform of the Medicare and Medicaid programs, (2) development of long-term care insurance, (3) integrating acute and long-term care services, and (4) segmenting higher levels of long-term care into subacute services.

Medicare and Medicaid Reforms

Preserving the Medicare program and the services it provides to elderly people has become a controversial political issue. This debate has focused on long-term care because benefits for home health and skilled nursing home care have become the fastest growing part of the Medicare benefit package. Home health benefit expenditures increased from $2.6 billion in 1989 to $16 billion in 1995, an average annual growth rate of 35%. As a percentage of total Medicare spending, home health care grew from 3% in 1989 to 9% in 1995. Nursing home spending was $2.5 billion in 1990, and in 1995 it was $10.3 billion, an average annual growth rate of 33%. Nursing home care as a share of total Medicare benefit payments has increased from 2.3% in 1990 to 5.6% in 1995 (NAHC, 1996).

This is an unintended growth in Medicare spending because Medicare, with deductibles and copayments built in, was designed to finance medical expenses associated primarily with acute conditions, with limited post–acute restorative care for the aged and disabled. For example, Medicare does not cover nursing home stays beyond 100 days annually and requires $95 per day copayment after 21 days. Home health services are limited to medically related services provided by a skilled professional (i.e., nurse, physical therapist), not personal care, and can be received only after discharge from a hospital. The unintended growth in Medicare spending for long-term care is largely a result of an increase in the number of users and visits per user. The annual growth rate in costs has contributed little to the increasing costs.

The increase in volume of users and visits is often attributed to definitional changes made in the late 1980s that expanded eligibility and to changes in services covered under the Medicare home health benefit. Other explanations for the growth include the aging of the population, changes in technology, an increased supply of Medicare home care agencies, and consumer preference for non-institution-based care settings.

Medicare has two parts: Part A and Part B. Part A, Hospital Insurance, is financed through dedicated payroll taxes on employees and their employers. The taxes are placed in the Medicare Hospital Insurance Trust Fund (HITF). The amount in the HITF must cover the outlays for services. Part A covers hospital insurance benefits, home health care, and nursing home care for Medicare beneficiaries. Until the 1997 budget law was passed, it had been projected that at the current spending rate, the HITF would be insolvent by 2002. The budget law included measures to reduce Medicare spending by more than $115 billion and keep it solvent until the year 2007.

Part B, Supplementary Medical Insurance, is financed by general revenues and enrollee premiums, and it covers physician services. Beneficiaries pay a 20% copayment plus a monthly premium of $43.80 and a deductible of $100 in 1997.

Part B is not threatened by insolvency because it can be continually replenished through unlimited drawing down of general tax revenues without limits.

A third component of Medicare funding is the "Medigap" insurance purchased by the elderly to fill in the gaps in services covered under Parts A and B. These are private insurance policies that cover deductibles, copayments, outpatient drugs, and so on and sometimes short stays in nursing homes and limited home health days.

Several proposals have been made to address the possible insolvency of HITF:

1. *Shifting home care services from Part A to Part B so that more home care costs can be covered through general revenues.* This was partially implemented in the 1997 budget law. However, it means that Part B premiums will increase from $43.80 to $67 per month by 2007.

2. *Developing a prospective payment system for nursing homes and for home health care.* For home health care, the Health Care Financing Administration, which is responsible for administering the Medicare and Medicaid programs, has started testing two models of prospective payment systems: a per visit model (testing started in 1994) and a per episode model (started in 1996). Prospective payment for home care was included in the president's budget for FY 1998, with attached savings for Medicare of $14 million. This approach attempts to capture the cost savings from hospital prospective payment for long-term care providers.

3. *Enrolling Medicare beneficiaries in managed care.* In 1996 about 4 million, or 11%, of Medicare beneficiaries were enrolled in managed care plans, largely health maintenance organizations (HMOs). From December 1994 to January 1996, Medicare beneficiaries' enrollment in HMOs grew 41% (HCFA, 1996a). Most Medicare beneficiaries in HMOs are concentrated in just a few states and a few large HMOs. In 1995, California and Florida had 55% of all Medicare HMO enrollees and 6 of the top 10 Medicare HMOs. The primary concern about managed care as a way to reduce Medicare costs is that healthier elderly will be enrolled in managed care plans, leaving the less healthy to rely on the fee-for-service system. If the per capita rate for Medicare enrollees is based on the average cost for all Medicare beneficiaries, managed care plans maybe overpaid because their healthier enrollees' care will cost less than the average beneficiary's cost. Further, one recent study found that elderly and poor chronically ill patients had worse health outcomes in HMOs than in fee-for-service payment systems (Ware, Bayliss, Rogers, Kosenski, & Tarlov, 1996). Yet states like Minnesota and Arizona and demonstration programs to be discussed later in the chapter are showing that managed care can work for certain groups in need of long-term care.

4. *Introducing beneficiary cost sharing, or copayments for home health visits.* This would shift more responsibility to the beneficiary and control the use of services. However, a copayment could be unfair for low-income people and discourage their use of services. People with high incomes often have additional

supplemental insurance (Medigap) that covers copayments and would not feel the direct effects of copayments (Moon & Davis, 1995).

5. *Introducing a "bundled" rate, where one payment would cover all post–acute care including home health, skilled nursing facilities, and rehabilitation.* This is expected to reduce the costs of paying for each service separately, but it is not clear yet which provider would receive the bundled payment.

All of these options are attempts to shift more financial responsibility to the beneficiary through copayments; to the providers through prospective payment, managed care, and bundled rates; and to the states, picking up the gaps in Medicare services through their Medicaid programs. Although 75% of Medicaid beneficiaries are poor children and adults, only about one third of the program's expenditures are for this group. Two thirds of Medicaid expenditures are for older people and persons with disabilities. Of the expenditures for the elderly and disabled, one third pays for long-term care, two-thirds of which is for nursing home care (Weiner, Sullivan, & Skaggs, 1996).

Medicaid eligibility requires that individuals be impoverished before benefits begin. If they have assets above a certain level, elderly or disabled persons must use their income and assets until they meet state income eligibility requirements for Medicaid (a process called "spend down"). Given that nursing home stays cost about $40,000 a year, many elderly persons use their assets and can meet the income requirements as soon as they begin to incur nursing homes expenses. For example, a study of nursing home residents in 1990 showed that 31% of nursing home residents who were admitted as private-pay patients eventually spent down to Medicaid (Weiner et al., 1996).

It is not surprising, therefore, that many elderly who need community or home-based services over years or who must enter a nursing home face impoverishment within only weeks. Some people also spend down to Medicaid eligibility by using services in the community. Often the elderly who spend down would otherwise not qualify for any form of public assistance (U.S. House of Representatives, 1987). As Vladeck (1983) has stated, "Medicaid-reimbursed nursing home services have thus become the largest 'welfare' benefit available to formerly middle-class individuals and their families" (p. 360).

Like the proposals for Medicare reform, managed care is also seen by the states as a way to reduce their spending on long-term care. The main problem with this is that states have targeted women and children in the Aid to Families with Dependent Children (AFDC) program for managed care. This is largely a young, healthy population. There is little experience in bringing the long-term care population into managed care and make it as cost-effective as for younger groups.

Several legislative vehicles exist for forming new managed care programs (Kaiser Commission, 1995):

1. *Section 1115 of the Social Security Act—"demonstration" waivers.* These waivers permit the secretary of the Department of Health and Human Services to waive rules that normally govern federal Medicaid payments for covered services and populations. The only requirement of the waiver is that the demonstration be budget-neutral, meaning the state cannot have greater Medicaid spending than there would have been without the waiver. Recently, this waiver is being used by states to restructure their Medicaid programs (HCFA, 1996b).

2. *Section 1915(b) of the Social Security Act, or what is known as "freedom of choice" waivers.* Under Section 1915 of the Medicaid statute, the secretary has the authority to waive the Medicaid freedom-of-choice provision in order to allow states to mandate managed care enrollment. This has increased enrollment in Medicaid programs (HCFA, 1996b).

3. *Section 1915(c) demonstrations involving home- and community-based waiver systems, specifically for long-term care.* These waivers give states flexibility in developing services (i.e., adult day programs, homemaking, transportation) as alternatives to placing Medicaid-eligible people in nursing homes. The costs of these services cannot exceed the cost of care for identical people in a nursing home. There are 200 home- and community-based waiver programs in effect, serving 250,00 people. All states except one have at least one such program (HCFA, 1996b). Although almost every state has applied for a waiver, the programs are for people with long-term care needs. Very little is happening in long-term care using waivers, and activity in this area has remained at a low level so far.

In addition, at least seven states—Alaska, Connecticut, Minnesota, New York, Florida, New Mexico, and North Dakota—have developed task forces to address new ways to finance and deliver long-term care services. As the federal government continues to reduce Medicare and block grants, the states will increasingly become the focus of long-term care reform (Intergovernmental Health Policy Project, 1996).

Long-Term Care Insurance

Another way that states are seeking to defray the growing costs of long-term care is to encourage private responsibility through purchase of long-term care insurance. Although long-term care insurance has been available since the late 1970s, only a few companies offered long-term care coverage before 1986, when approximately 125,000 policies were in force (General Accounting Office, 1988). By 1990, almost 2 million policies had been sold, with over 125 insurance companies marketing the policies. However, only 4% of the elderly population had purchased a policy in that year. In 1995 a survey by the Health Insurance Association of America (HIAA) estimated that 3.5 million long-term care policies had been purchased by individuals (HIAA, 1995). If growth continues at the current 15%–20% per year, less that 20% (5–6 million) of the elderly will have policies by the year 2000 (Cohen, Kumar, & Wallack, 1993).

The average annual premium for policies sold by the leaders in the market was $2,137 if bought at age 65 and $6,811 if bought at age 79 (Coronel & Fulton, 1995). Studies have estimated that only 10% to 20% of the elderly can afford this expense (Weiner, 1996a).

Because of the expense of premiums a high percentage of policyholders let their policies lapse before they receive any services. Insurers report that about 20% of long-term care insurance policies are expected to lapse during the first year of policy ownership. The projected lapse rate within the five years of policy ownership was 50% for five large insurance companies. The General Accounting Office (1993), which conducted the study, concluded: "By the time policyholders may need nursing home benefits, many will have let their policies lapse and will no longer have their long-term care coverage" (p. 2).

Another major drawback in private long-term care insurance is that most policies pay a fixed benefit, ranging from $25 to $100, that is not adjusted for inflation. In each year after the purchase of the policy, the benefit will pay for a smaller part of the actual cost of care. Furthermore, there are major differences in the definition of covered nursing facilities, length of time benefits are paid, coverage, and eligibility for benefits.

An analysis of long-term care insurance options by Rivlin and Weiner (1988) found the most optimistic projection to be that only one quarter to one half of the elderly will be able to purchase or will want to purchase policies by 2018. There will continue to be a need for public financing to pay for most long-term care, particularly for the low- and middle-income elderly, despite the increased availability of private policies.

Dual Eligibility Initiatives/Integrated Systems of Acute and Long-Term Care

As states and the federal government grapple with their fiscal challenges and as they seek to control growth in spending on the Medicare and Medicaid programs, some states are looking at alternative ways of structuring the delivery of care. Specifically, several states are seeking waivers to integrate acute and long-term care for the approximately 5 million people nationwide who are dually eligible for Medicare and Medicaid benefits, meaning they qualify for both Medicaid and Medicare benefits. Nearly all elderly Medicaid beneficiaries and approximately one third of Medicaid beneficiaries with disabilities are dually eligible (Fralich et al., 1995).

Integration of acute and long-term care refers to two things, not necessarily present in so-called integration models: financial integration—the pooling of financial resources for both acute and long-term care services into one funding stream (Wiener & Skaggs, 1995); and service delivery integration—coordination of acute and long-term services. Currently, there are three examples of approaches to integrating acute and long-term care services: Social Health Maintenance Organizations (SHMOs), On Lok Program of All-inclusive Care for the Elderly (PACE), and the Arizona Long-Term Care System (ALTCS) program.

There are nine PACE demonstration sites that replicate the original PACE demonstration site, the On Lok Senior Health Services Program in San Francisco. The Omnibus Reconciliation Act of 1990 authorized the expansion of the PACE project to up to 15 demonstration sites. Like the SHMOs, PACE programs provide a continuum of acute, long-term, and social services; but unlike the SHMOs, PACE programs target the frail elderly who are at risk for admission to nursing homes. Most of the participants are eligible for both Medicare and Medicaid. Funding comes from pooled Medicaid and Medicare funds for dually eligible participants and premiums paid by people who are eligible for Medicare only. Demonstration sites receive a capitated rate in return for providing and contracting for all acute and long-term care services (Weiner, 1996c).

The Program of All-Inclusive Care for the Elderly (PACE)

• Who is cared for at the PACE sites?

Almost all the PACE clients are eligible for both Medicaid and Medicare, which means they meet both the age requirement for Medicare eligibility (65 or over) and have sufficiently low income levels to qualify for Medicaid. They are people who are eligible to receive care in a nursing home but choose to be cared for in the community. They are typically frail and elderly and have some degree of limitation in conducting activities of daily living.

• What services do they receive?

They receive primary medical care, rehabilitation, and other supportive services on site at adult day health centers (ADHCs) that serve as the central setting for all PACE programs. They also utilize inpatient hospital services, nursing home care, skilled home health care, and homemaker or personal care services, that are not provided at the ADHCs. The care of each client is managed by an interdisciplinary team of providers, including physicians, nurses, social workers, and therapists, and the ADHC is the hub around which service delivery is organized and integrated. Clients visit the sites an average of 10 to 15 times a month. The sites also provide some meals and an opportunity for social interaction.

PACE *(cont.)*

> • How is PACE different?
>
> Three main features of PACE make it unique in long-term care: (1) Medicare and Medicaid funding is integrated into one stream, and payment to providers is capitated (i.e., a fixed amount is set) so that they bear financial risk for the care they provide; (2) all health care services are coordinated and integrated through ADHCs; (3) case management is provided through interdisciplinary teams.

The SHMO model was developed at Brandeis University in the early 1980s and has four demonstration sites operating around the country. The SHMOs enroll Medicare beneficiaries with a broad range of functional ability and financial status. SHMOs link Medicare primary and acute services with long-term care into a single benefit package. The main difference between SHMOs and HMOs is the inclusion of long-term care services.

The ALTCS program began in 1989 and is part of the Arizona Health Care Cost Containment System (AHCCS), a demonstration project that finances medical services for the Medicaid-eligible population through prepaid contracts with providers. ALTCS incorporates long-term care services into the AHCCS program. Its goal is to provide long-term and acute services through a managed care system to older people and people with disabilities. Under this model, the state contracts with one entity, in most cases the county government, to serve as the intermediary, the program contractor, who receives a monthly fixed payment per enrollee from ALTCS and in turn arranges for the provision of the necessary services. Because this is strictly a Medicaid program, the contractors are expected to bill Medicare for covered services provided to those who are dually eligible for Medicare. In this sense, the ALTCS model is an integrated approach to care delivery but not a financially integrated model (Weiner, 1996b).

A fourth project testing integration is the Minnesota Long-Term Care Options Project, now in its beginning phases of operation. This program is targeted to Medicare and Medicare-eligible people only, and participants must be at risk for institutionalization. This program coordinates acute and long-term care. The funding comes from pooled Medicaid and Medicare funds paid as a capitated rate to managed care networks that managed the provision of care. Minnesota is the only state that has received Medicare waivers, outside of the PACE sites.

Most Medicaid-managed long-term care service programs have been developed separately from primary and acute programs. They have also been limited primarily to people who meet the criteria for nursing home admission. Examples are the ALTCS, the Wisconsin Partnership Program, and the New York Evaluated Medicaid Long-Term Care Capitation Program.

The ones under way that would integrate all Medicaid and Medicare for mixed groups of people, including those with long-term care needs, are Minnesota and Massachusetts senior care organizations and the Colorado Integrated Care and

Financing Project. These programs are still in the experimental stage, and the true integration of payment streams is as yet in its beginning phase.

Subacute Care Services

Subacute care, although not a new term, has come to represent a new movement in health care. In the past it was used to describe hospitalized patients who failed to meet established criteria for a medically necessary acute stay. Now it is used to describe a level of care—skilled care for patients with complex needs, who are typically high-need Medicare patients. This level of care has been provided historically by nursing homes, home care providers, rehabilitation facilities, and hospitals as patient needs required it. Subacute care now has come to hospitals as rising health care costs and changing demographics make it a cost-effective alternative to inpatient acute care.

The impetus behind the development of subacute care is related to (1) the decreasing inpatient lengths of stay resulting from prospective hospital payment and the pressures to discharge patients earlier—subacute along with home care help to keep patients in the hospital system until the next hospitalization is needed; (2) Medicare reimbursement of subacute care on a cost basis; hospital inpatient care is paid prospectively, so there are higher profit margins attached to subacute care, and Medicare provides an additional payment to providers who care for patients with a greater skill need; (3) consumer preference for noninstitutional care, which has encouraged hospitals and nursing homes to add on or refurbish existing facilities so that subacute settings are more homelike.

Subacute care is controversial. It is an area that some people believe is an emerging, exciting area of health care, whereas others believe it is "old wine in new bottles." The government does not recognize it as a separate kind of care. There is also no consensus that this patient population is different from traditional nursing home residents and traditional postacute-care patients. Nor is there consensus on what subacute care is, beyond that it applies to patients whose care needs lie somewhere between acute hospital care and nursing home care. And whether or not there are true cost savings to merit further development of this kind of care remains in dispute. So far, studies of subacute care do not bear out claims of cost savings. But given the movement in the market toward capitation and the emphasis on cost reduction, many providers are willing to try to better delineate patient populations and to provide service in lower-cost settings as a way to remain financially viable.

Summary and Future Direction

Demographic and technological trends are causing a rapid increase in the need for long-term care services as the number of elderly and those with chronic conditions steadily climbs. These changes are occurring at a time when there is a serious question as to whether federal and state governments will be willing to provide sufficient resources to meet the growing need for services. At present, long-term care services are unevenly distributed and in short supply. Moreover, many individuals and their families must experience personal and financial hardship to get needed services. Private long-term care insurance falls far short of providing any financial relief for most people. Due to the emphasis on institutional long-term care services over the years, community-based services are spottily funded and uncoordinated. Supportive housing, a key component on the continuum of long-term care, is in scarce supply and can be out of the financial reach of people with moderate and low incomes. The influx of large numbers will further stress a long-term care system already lagging behind in its ability to meet existing needs.

Unfortunately, debate about the future of long-term care is narrowly focused on financing issues, not on finding a coherent approach to financing and delivering services to people with chronic conditions. Proposals under consideration center on ways to shift funding away from tax-supported programs to increase the out-of-pocket funding by individuals or restrict payments to providers of care through managed care and prospective payment. Even the efforts to integrate acute and long-term care are another way to reduce costs, although this should also result in better organization and coordination of services. The interest in subacute care is a response of providers in need of new revenue sources to offset their inability to cover their costs.

The debate should be expanded to fully explore and analyze options for developing the capacity to improve care to the chronically ill. These options would address the following issues:

- Changing Medicare and Medicaid financing so that payment mechanisms create incentives for chronic care and integrate hospital, home care, adult day care, assisted living, and nursing home care and shift their payment incentives away from hospitalization as the core of the program.
- Further discussion of the advantages and disadvantages of private insurance as an alternative to expanding Medicare to a more comprehensive chronic care system.
- Incentives that encourage states to plan for the future need for long-term care services and develop strategies for improving the supply and distribution of the full continuum of long-term care services through public-private partnerships.
- Options for developing, through recruitment of new workers and retraining of the existing heath workforce, sufficient numbers of qualified professionals and nonprofessionals to deliver the full range of high-quality long-term care services needed.

The current debate, with its narrow focus on financing, might lead to politically expedient answers that help the federal and state budgets in the short term but will fail to identify the resources required to do the job of developing a system of long-term care services. If this challenge is not accepted, it will not be possible to meet the needs of the rapidly growing number of people whose lives are limited by chronic conditions.

Mini-Case Study

Pleasant View Nursing Home is a not-for-profit, 240-bed nursing home in a suburb of a large midwestern city. It was built in 1967 and has been providing good-quality nursing home care during those years to a middle-class community. However, it has been steadily losing patients to the home health services of the nearby community hospital and to a geriatric day program that recently was opened by church-sponsored residential development. The occupancy rate dropped to 82% during the past year. Although they tried to maximize the number of privately paying patients, these patients had been choosing the new service options in the community, leaving the nursing home with Medicaid as the payer for 70% of the patients. Recently, a large managed care company had approached the nursing home with the proposal that it become part of a provider network in the area. Recognizing that the survival of the nursing home was threatened and uncertain about the new changes in the health care system, the board of directors has contacted you as a candidate for executive director to develop a vision for the nursing home and return it to a viable and vital community resource. What information about the population, community, state and local governments, providers, and Pleasant View Nursing Home would you want to know before you accepted this position?

Discussion Questions

1. Why is the demand for and cost of long-term care difficult to predict?
2. What barriers do the elderly and chronically ill face when trying to obtain long-term care services?
3. Why are social and housing services, in addition to health services, important to the continuum of long-term care?
4. What are the major gaps in long-term care services and financing?
5. What are the advantages and disadvantages of managed care for long-term care?
6. What are likely to be the main influences on long-term care policy in the future?

References

American Association of Homes and Services for the Aging, *Assisted Living*. Washington, DC: Author, 1995a.

American Association of Homes and Services for the Aging, *Continuing Care Retirement Communities.* Washington, DC: Author, December, 1995b.

Blustein, J., Schultz, B. M., Knickman, J. R., Kator, M. J., Richardson, H., & McBride, L. C., "AIDS and Long-Term Care: The Use of Services in an Institutional Setting," *AIDS and Public Policy Journal, 7*(1), 32–41, 1992.

Cohen, M. A., Kumar, N., & Wallack, S. S., "New Perspectives on the Affordability of Long-Term Care Insurance and Potential Market Size," *Gerontologist, 33*(1), 105–113, 1993.

Congressional Budget Office, *Policy Choice for Long Term Care.* Washington, DC: Author, 1991.

Coronoel, S., & Fulton, D., *Long-Term Care Insurance in 1993, Managed Care and Insurance Report.* Washington, DC: Health Insurance Association of America, 1995.

Fishman, P., Von Korff, M., Lozano, P., & Hecht, J., "Chronic Care Costs in Managed Care," *Health Affairs, 16*, 239–247, March/April 1997.

Fralich, J., Riley, T., Mollica, R., Snow, K. I., Carr, D. J., & McDonough, S., *Reducing the Cost of Institutional Care: Downsizing, Diversion, Closing, and Conversion of Nursing Homes.* Portland, ME: National Academy for State Health Policy, 1995.

General Accounting Office, *Long-term Care for the Elderly* (HRD-89-4). Washington, DC: Author, 1988.

General Accounting Office, *Long-term Care Insurance: High Percentage of Policyholders Drop Policies* (GAO/HRD-93-129). Washington, DC: Author, 1993.

Graves, N., & Bechtel, R., *Across the States 1996: Profiles of Long-Term Care Systems* (2nd ed.). Washington, DC: American Association of Retired Persons, 1996.

Gulyas, R., *AAHSA's Position on Assisted Living.* Washington, DC: American Association of Homes and Services for the Aging, 1995.

Harrington, C., & Grant, L. A., "The Delivery, Regulation, and Politics of Home Care: A California Case Study," *Gerontologist, 30*(4), 451–461, 1990.

Harrington, C., Swan, J. H., Bedney, B., Carrillo, H., Keo de Wit, S., & Curtis, M., *1994 State Data Book on Long Term Care Program and Market Characteristics.* San Francisco: Department of Social & Behavioral Sciences/University of California-San Francisco, 1995.

Health Care Financing Administration, *1996 Statistics at a Glance: Growth in HCFA Programs and Expenditures* (HCFA Publ. No. 03394). Washington, DC: Author, 1996a.

Health Care Financing Administration, *Medicaid Waivers.* Washington, DC: Author, 1996b.

Health Insurance Association of America, *Who Buys Long-Term Care Insurance?* Washington, DC: Life Plans, Inc., 1995.

Hoechst Marion Roussel, Inc., *Managed Care Digest Series/Institutional Digest.* Kansas City, MO: Author, 1996.

Institute for Health and Aging, *Chronic Care in America: A 21st Century Challenge.* Princeton, NJ: The Robert Wood Johnson Foundation, 1996.

Institute of Medicine, *Improving the Quality of Care in Nursing Homes.* Washington, DC: National Academy Press, 1986.

Intergovernmental Health Policy Project, "Preparing for an Aging America: States Tackle Long-Term Care Reform," *State Health Notes, 17*(242), 1, 1996.

Kaiser Commission, *Report of the Kaiser Commission on the Future of Medicaid*. Washington, DC: Author, 1995.

Kane, R. A., & Kane, R. L., *Long-Term Care: Principles, Programs and Policies*. New York: Springer Publishing Co., 1987.

Kane, R. L., "The Evolution of the American Nursing Home," in R. H. Binstock, L. E. Cluff, & O. Von Mering (Eds.), *The Future of Long-Term Care: Social Policy and Issues* (pp. 148–168). Baltimore, MD: Johns Hopkins University Press, 1996.

Levit, K. R., Lazenby, H. C., Braden, B. R., Cowan, C. A., McDonnell, P. S., Sivarajan, L., Stiller, J. M., Won, D. K., Doham, A. M., & Stewart, M. W., "National Health Expenditures, 1995," *Health Care Financing Review, 18*(1), 175–214, 1996.

Meltzer, W., *Respite Care: An Emerging Family Support Service*. Washington, DC: Center for the Study of Social Policy, 1982.

Moon, M., *Long-Term Care in the United States*. Washington, DC: The Urban Institute, 1996.

Moon, M., & Davis, K., "Preserving and Strengthening Medicare," *Health Affairs, 14*(4), 31–46, 1995.

Murtaugh, C. M., Kemper, P., & Spillman, B. C., "The Risk of Nursing Home Use in Later Life," *Medical Care, 28*(10), 952–962, 1990.

National Association for Home Care, *Basic Statistics on Home Care*. Washington, DC: Author, 1993.

National Association for Home Care, *Basic Statistics on Home Care*. Washington, DC: Author, 1996.

Rivlin, A. M., & Wiener, J. M., *Caring for the Disabled Elderly: Who Will Pay?* Washington, DC: The Brookings Institution, 1988.

Scruggs, D., *Dare to Discover: The Future of Continuing Care Retirement Communities*. Washington, DC: American Association of Homes and Services for the Aging, 1995.

Strahan, G. W., *An Overview of Nursing Homes and Their Current Residents: Data from the 1995 National Nursing Home Survey*. Hyattsville, MD: USDHHS, Centers for Disease Control and Prevention, National Center for Health Statistics.

U.S. Bureau of the Census, "65+ in the United States," in *Current Population Reports, Special Studies* (pp. 6–9). Washington, DC: U.S. Government Printing Office, 1996.

U.S. Department of Housing and Urban Development, *Rental Housing Assistance at a Crossroads: A Report to Congress on Worst Case Housing Needs*. Washington, DC: USDHUD, Office of Policy Development and Research, 1996.

U.S. House of Representatives, Select Committee on Aging, *Long-Term Care and Personal Impoverishment: Seven in Ten Elderly Living Alone Are at Risk* (Comm. Pub. No. 100-631). Washington, DC: U.S. Government Printing Office, 1987.

U.S. Senate Special Committee on Aging, *Nursing Home Care: The Unfinished Agenda*. Staff Report, Washington, DC: U.S. Government Printing Office, May 21, 1986.

Vladeck, B., *Unloving Care: The Nursing Home Tragedy*. New York: Basic Books, 1980.

Vladeck, B., "Nursing Homes," in D. Mechanic (Ed.), *Handbook of Health, Health Care and Health Professions*. New York: Free Press, 1983.

Ware, J. E., Bayliss, M., Rogers, W., Kosinski, M., & Tarlov, A., "Differences in 4-Year Health Outcomes for Elderly and Poor, Chronically Ill Patients Treated in HMO and Fee-for-Service Systems," *Journal of the American Medical Association, 276*, 1039–1047, 1996.

Weiner, J., *Can Medicaid Long-Term Care Expenditures for the Elderly Be Reduced?* New York: Commonwealth Fund, 1996a.

Weiner, J. M., "Managed Care and Long-Term Care: The Integration of Financing and Services," *Generations*, 47–52, Summer, 1996b.

Weiner, J. M., & Skaggs, J., *Current Approaches to Integration of Acute and Long-Term Care Financing and Services*. Washington, DC: American Association of Retired Persons, 1995.

Weiner, J. M., Sullivan, C. M., & Skaggs, J., *Spending Down to Medicaid: New Data on the Role of Medicaid in Paying for Nursing Home Care*. Washington, DC: American Association of Retired Persons, 1996.

9

Mental Health Services

Steven S. Sharfstein, Anne M. Stoline, and Lorrin M. Koran

Learning Objectives

1. Describe general types of mental disorders.
2. Describe types of treatment for mental disorders.
3. Identify highlights in the development of the U.S. mental health care system.
4. Identify key mental health professionals and their roles in the system.
5. Analyze trends in use over time of the various settings for mental health care.
6. Identify financing differences between general medical and mental health care.
7. Describe key legal issues in mental health care.

Topical Outline

Overview—definition of mental illness, cost of care, current issues
Forms of mental disorders
Prevalence of mental disorders
Treatments and services for the mentally ill
Historical development of the U.S. mental health care system
Mental health personnel
    Psychiatrists
    Psychologists
    Social workers
    Registered nurses
Trends in mental health care delivery
Settings for mental health services
Insurance coverage for mental disorders

Differences between general medical and mental health care
Economic myths surrounding mental health care
Medicare
Medicaid
Legal issues in mental health care
Current issues

Key Words: Mental disorder, mental health care, public psychiatric hospital, deinstitutionalization, mental health professional, managed care, involuntary treatment.

Who is mentally ill? The precise boundaries for the concept of mental disorder are not clear and are influenced by philosophical, social and cultural considerations. This is also true for the concepts of physical disorder and notions of health versus disease. Every society includes individuals who present behavioral or psychological deviancy significant enough to qualify for a definition of mental illness, although the definition of "significant" in this context can vary widely. These syndromes can be associated with painful emotional symptoms or can present as an impairment in ability to think, remember, or concentrate. Such syndromes can also significantly increase the potential for general medical illness, pain, disability, and even death. The causes of mental disorders may be biological, developmental, psychological, environmental, or combinations of these. The important boundary line surrounding the definition of mental illness is the person's level of distress and dysfunction that is expressed primarily through a behavioral syndrome.

Given the scrutiny under which the mental health service sector operates, surprisingly little recent data are available for national estimates of its costs. In fact, 1991 is the most recent year for which data are available. In that year, expenditures for mental health services were estimated at $71 billion, including $58.7 billion for mental disorders, $9.3 billion for alcohol abuse, and $2.9 billion for drug abuse. Services for mental disorders alone accounted for about 8% of the nation's expenditures for health care. At nearly $161.1 billion, indirect costs of mental disorders (including drug and alcohol abuse) in 1991 totaled more than twice the direct treatment costs. Indirect costs of mental disorders ($71.7 billion) resulted from lost wages due to illness or premature death, productivity losses for individuals incarcerated due to conviction related to a psychiatric disorder, and value of time spent by family members of those with psychiatric conditions. Indirect costs of alcohol abuse ($65 billion) and drug abuse ($24.4 billion) result from adverse health effects, accident-related injuries and fatalities, homicides, suicides, fetal alcohol syndrome, productivity lost by addicts, their incarceration due to drug-related crimes, costs incurred by the victims of those crimes, and costs associated with AIDS contracted through intravenous or prenatal exposures (National Foundation for Brain Research, 1992; Rupp, Gause, & Regier, in press). Although dated, these dollar costs have undoubtedly since risen and can only begin to suggest the magnitude of human suffering caused by mental disorders and substance abuse.

Like the general health care sector in the mid-1990s, the mental health care sector is experiencing pressures for cost containment. Through preferred provider organizations and other managed care entities, insurance companies are negotiating with psychiatrists to accept lower reimbursement for their services. The federal government, while maintaining its exemption of psychiatric hospitals and inpatient units from Medicare's prospective payment system, which uses diagnosis related groups, continues to research prospective payment methods for psychiatric inpatient care as well. Another cost-control strategy increasingly employed by Medicare is encouraging enrollment by its beneficiaries in health maintenance organizations (HMOs) and other capitated and managed care entities. Partly in hopes of lowering fees for psychotherapy, state legislatures are acceding to the lobbying of psychologists and other nonmedical psychotherapists to allow them direct access to third-party reimbursement without physician supervision. In a number of states (e.g., New York and Maryland) this is already the case. As policymakers encourage competition to stimulate efficiency, safeguarding the quality of care is a concern that must not be forgotten.

Despite great progress in the past 40 years, the delivery of mental health care, like the delivery of general medical care, is beset by many difficulties. First, the pluralistic service delivery system includes poor coordination with other human service systems (e.g., general medicine, legal, education, and welfare). In the public sector, states take an uneven approach to planning, evaluation, and regulation. Budgetary constraints limit services. In both the public and private sectors, continuity of care and insurance coverage are fragmented. Mental health personnel and community-based treatment programs are in short supply. This problem is likely to be exacerbated by the recent decline in the number of applicants to psychiatry residency programs. The social stigma attached to mental patients (Domenici, 1993; Rabkin, 1974) and public apathy toward their suffering also hamper care. These factors combined lead to inequitable access to care based on geography, class, and diagnosis.

Further complicating the situation, many mental disorders can only be ameliorated, not cured, and require long-term management by experienced clinicians to maintain optimum symptom control. When people with mental illness are also affected by poverty and racism, delivering adequate services to them becomes a most formidable task. All of these factors contribute to the major public health problem of delivery of continuous care for the chronically ill, many of whom have been discharged over the past three decades from long-term psychiatric institutions to ill-prepared communities. The public health problem of homeless people, especially those individuals with schizophrenia and/or substance abuse, rivals today's other major medical crises such as the AIDS epidemic.

The challenge is to find ways to diminish these difficulties at the dawn of a new century. To help the reader analyze this challenge and develop responses to it, this chapter will discuss the forms of mental disorder, the kinds of mental health care, the history of that care in the United States, the prevalence of mental disorders, the mental health labor force, the delivery of services, insurance coverage, and legal issues. (Although generally included in the category of mental conditions, data for services for substance abuse diagnoses are omitted in many of the following sections.)

Forms of Mental Disorders

The American Psychiatric Association published its first edition of the *Diagnostic and Statistical Manual of Mental Disorders* in 1952. In late 1993 the fourth edition of the *Diagnostic and Statistical Manual of Mental Disorders* (DSM-IV) was released (American Psychiatric Association, 1994). The manual currently includes more than 450 conditions and their subtypes, grouped in 17 categories. The culmination of more than 4 years of effort, the DSM-IV includes newly recognized diagnostic entities and reorganizes former diagnostic categories to take account of discoveries in recent years regarding the cause, natural history, and treatment responsiveness of many forms of mental disorder. This diagnostic manual undoubtedly will be revised again as the research that informs practice grows and the validity of the diagnostic categories is further improved. The 17 major diagnostic classes in the DSM-IV are:

1. Disorders usually first diagnosed in infancy, childhood, or adolescence (including intellectual, behavioral, emotional, physical, and developmental disorders).
2. Delirium, dementia, amnestic, and other cognitive disorders.
3. Mental disorders due to a general medical condition not elsewhere classified (including catatonic disorder and personality change when due to a general medical condition).
4. Substance-related disorders (including alcohol, drugs, and tobacco).
5. Schizophrenia and other psychotic disorders.
6. Mood disorders (conditions with manic, depressive, or mixed symptomatology).
7. Anxiety disorders (including phobias, posttraumatic stress disorder, and obsessive-compulsive disorder).

8. Somatoform disorders (physical symptoms suggesting physical disorders but without organic findings).
9. Factitious disorders (disorders deliberately simulated by the individual for psychological gain, excluding malingering because it aims at environmental gains).
10. Dissociative disorders (including psychogenic amnesia).
11. Sexual and gender identity disorders (including desire and arousal disorders).
12. Eating disorders.
13. Sleep disorders (including insomnia and nightmare disorders).
14. Impulse control disorders not elsewhere classified (including pathological gambling and kleptomania).
15. Adjustment disorders (maladaptive reactions to psychosocial stress).
16. Personality disorders (enduring, maladaptive patterns of relating to, perceiving, and thinking about the environment and oneself that cause significant impairment in social or occupational functioning or subjective distress).
17. Other conditions that may be a focus of clinical attention (including malingering, bereavement, and adult antisocial behavior).

Although a few mental health professionals believe all conditions usually described as mental disorders are nothing more than social myths (Szasz, 1961), the reasoning and evidence to the contrary are powerfully convincing (Kendall, 1975; Moore, 1975; Murphy, 1976). Thus, it is all the more important to accurately differentiate the constellations of thoughts, feelings, and behaviors that constitute clinical conditions from those that do not.

Prevalence of Mental Disorders

Epidemiological studies of the prevalence of mental disorders have encountered the same problems as have analogous studies of physical diseases: deciding what constitutes a "case," establishing operational diagnostic criteria, and choosing a method of case finding.

The largest, most carefully conceived and executed study of the epidemiology of mental disorders was carried out from 1980 to 1982 by the National Institute of Mental Health (NIMH) Epidemiological Catchment Area (ECA) program. The ECA program grew out of one of the recommendations of the 1978 President's Commission on Mental Health. A reliable structured interview, the *Diagnostic Interview Schedule (DIS)*, incorporating *DSM-III* diagnostic criteria for 32 mental disorders, was administered by trained interviewers to a random sample of nearly 20,000 people in five U.S. cities. After the initial interview (Wave 1), when possible, the subjects were interviewed again 1 year later (Wave 2). Results of extensive analysis of these data suggest that the 1-year total prevalence rate of the mental and addictive disorders included in the *DIS* is 28.1% for the adult U.S. population (Regier et al., 1993). The 1-year prevalence of the most common disorders recorded were phobias (10.9%), any alcohol disorder (7.4%), and dysthymia (5.4%). (Dysthymia is one form of depressive disorder.) More recent data show similar results. A 1990–1992 study of more than 8,000 persons selected to represent the U.S. population found a 12-month prevalence of 18 mental disorders of 27.7% (Kessler et al., 1994).

Various researchers have tracked the number of people seeking care annually for mental and addictive disorders. Estimates generally fall in the range of one third of all persons with diagnosable conditions who receive care in the general medical or specialty mental health sectors. Other persons may consult clergy, social welfare agencies, voluntary support networks or self-help groups (Narrow, 1993; Regier et al., 1993; Rupp et al., in press).

These numbers suggest that only about one in five persons suffering from a mental or addictive disorder receives any treatment from a mental health professional. The percentage does vary by diagnosis. It is reassuring, although not surprising, that a higher percentage of those with severe and persistent mental illnesses receives care more frequently than the average affected person. For example, almost two thirds of people with schizophrenia receive treatment each year, as do more than 40% of those with mood disorders, compared to only one fifth of those with anxiety disorders and 15% with other conditions. The overall low numbers likely reflect a variety of factors, including lack of insurance coverage, other financial barriers to treatment, and lack of motivation to seek care. The latter may be due to stigma, lack of insight into one's dysfunction (e.g., dementia, schizophrenia), lack of distress, hopelessness regarding potential for improvement (e.g., alcohol and drug addiction), and other psychological barriers to treatment. Some diagnosable conditions (e.g., a phobia of snakes) may not warrant treatment (e.g., for urban dwellers). Nevertheless, mental health professionals are concerned by the low numbers of people receiving treatment each year compared to potential need, and continually search for ways to decrease barriers to care.

The data that follow focus on the mental health sector of the U.S. health care delivery system. As noted above, however, only about one in five people who are afflicted with a mental disorder receives care in this sector. Most prescriptions written in the United States for psychotropic medications are written by primary care providers, and many persons with subtle forms of psychiatric distress or dysfunction present first to a generalist for care. Thus, training primary care providers to recognize and treat mental disorders and establishing better linkages between the general health sector and the mental health sector are vital to improving the overall quality of mental health care (Kessler et al., 1994; Narrow, 1993).

Treatments and Services for the Mentally Ill

The term *mental health care* encompasses diverse preventive, therapeutic, and rehabilitative activities. Preventive mental health care aims at promoting mental health in general and preventing the occurrence of specific mental disorders. The first objective is difficult to attain because it is vague: few people agree on exactly what mental health is. The second preventive aim has met with some success: such disorders as syphilitic dementia and pellagrinous psychosis, for example, now rarely occur. Efforts to prevent childhood mental disorders through prenatal care, neonatal screening, childhood immunization, adequate nutrition, and preschool education are receiving increased study. But primary prevention of schizophrenia, mania, depression, and other mental disorders remains beyond our capabilities (Langsley, 1985).

Therapeutic mental health services include individual, family, and group psychotherapies; expressive interventions such as art therapy and psychodrama; medications; and electroconvulsive therapy. Psychotherapies rely primarily on structured conversation aimed at changing a patient's attitudes, feelings, beliefs, and/or behaviors. The therapist's procedures vary across schools of psychotherapy and with the nature of the patient's problem. Cognitive therapy, for example, focuses on the primacy of thoughts—the patient's cognitive world—in the creation and maintenance of distress and dysfunction. The therapist teaches the patient to examine negative assumptions and to challenge those assumptions through new ways of talking to himself or herself and new patterns of interaction with others. These shifts both within individuals and in their relationships create a brighter outlook. A behavior therapist assists the patient to stop a destructive behavior such as alcohol or drug use, binge eating or other eating disorder symptoms, compulsive hand washing, or other symptoms of obsessive-compulsive disorder (OCD). The therapist helps the patient to identify triggers to the behavior, find alternative coping strategies for that trigger, and interrupt the symptom cycle. Action is emphasized over understanding of the symptoms.

In psychoanalytic therapy, understanding is emphasized as a precursor to meaningful change. The psychoanalyst uses structured conversation techniques, including encouragement of the patient to speak aloud all thoughts ("free association"), and selective interpretations of the patient's verbalizations or associations to bring about change. Some therapists use hypnosis during psychotherapy sessions. Most forms of psychotherapy, however, have much in common (Frank & Frank, 1991). Expressive therapies uncover and explore patients' feelings through professionally guided creative exercises using drama, painting, sculpture, dance, and other modalities. Medications are used to treat a variety of disorders, including psychotic, mood, anxiety, cognitive, and impulse control disorders.

Most drugs effective in treating mental disorders have been available for less than 40 years. These include phenothiazines, butyrophenones, and the new serotonin/dopamine receptor drugs for treating schizophrenia and other psychiatric disorders; tricyclics, hetercyclics, selective serotonin reuptake inhibitors, and certain receptor-blocking drugs for treating depression, panic attacks, and OCD; lithium, valproic acid, and carbamazepine for bipolar (formerly termed manic-depressive) disorders; and benzodiazepines for treating anxiety states (Schatzberg & Nemeroff, 1995). Nonmedication treatments include electroconvulsive therapy (ECT), which is effective for certain forms of depression, schizophrenia, and mania and was introduced in 1938 (Fink, 1979).

Psychosurgery (neurosurgery performed in an effort to treat a mental disorder) was widely used to treat schizophrenia in the late 1940s and early 1950s. The treatments of choice were prefrontal lobotomy and topectomy (removal of large amounts of cortical tissue). Today psychosurgery is used rarely for treatment (e.g., only in refractory cases of OCD and very rarely for neurological conditions of chronic severe pain disorder and uncontrolled epilepsy). Modern techniques permit highly controlled placement of lesions in specific brain regions (Grebb, 1995).

Research advances in the basic sciences include elucidation of the fundamental roles played by the serotonin and norepinephrine neurotransmitter systems in modulating moods and anxiety symptoms. Such knowledge paved the way for synthesis of compounds that affect these neurotransmitter receptors. For example, a new class of antidepressants that selectively affects the serotonin system has been developed in recent years. These drugs, including fluoxetine, fluroxamine, sertraline, and paroxetine, have low side-effect profiles and are safe and effective, not only for severe to moderate depressions but also for OCD, panic disorder, social phobia, bulimia, and milder depressions. Preliminary studies suggest that they may have some efficacy in the impulse control disorders as well. Similar advances have been made in pharmacologic treatments of the addictive disorders, such as agents that selectively affect opiate receptors to modulate the effects of heroin and other opiate drugs in the brain (Schatzberg & Nemeroff, 1995).

Rehabilitative mental health care includes occupational therapy, social skills training, and reeducation aimed at helping the patient return to normal living patterns. It may begin inpatient setting with patient self-government activities and social activities and can progress through transitional settings such as halfway houses, group homes, or supervised apartments. Rehabilitative care is employed primarily with patients recovering from psychoses, drug addiction, or alcoholism.

In part due to expansion of the NIMH mission in the area of research and neuroscience, our knowledge of brain functional anatomy, pathophysiology, and activity patterns in disease states continues to increase rapidly. Private-sector research, particularly by pharmaceutical manufacturers, is adding to the knowledge base as well. Our growing understanding of the brain and the frequent introduction of new treatments for mental disorders makes psychiatry one of the most exciting areas in medicine today.

Brief History of Mental Health Care in the United States

The mentally disordered in colonial America were treated slightly better than their European counterparts: fewer were tortured, burned, hanged, or drowned as witches. (The Salem witch trials of 1691–1692, during which 250 persons were tried and 19 executed, were an exception, not the rule.) Throughout the colonial period most mentally ill people were kept at home or wandered from town to town, where they were lodged in jails or almshouses (workhouses). This remained the general pattern until the 1840s (Shryock, 1947).

In the early 1800s the Quakers and American physicians exposed to European psychiatry took the position that mental illness was treatable and urged the use of kind and sympathetic methods. Partly as a result, a few mental hospitals were opened where "moral treatment" (combining work, recreation, education, and kind but firm management) was predominant (Bockoven, 1972). Violent patients, however, were segregated in separate wards, and in most of the country, mentally disordered paupers and Blacks were sent to workhouses and jails (Mora, 1975). In 1841 an alliance of professionals and reformers began lobbying legislatures for improved care. Reformers, led by Dorothea Dix, encouraged states to build hospitals specifically for the care of the mentally ill. Many mental hospitals then were built, usually in rural areas because the countryside was believed to provide refuge from noxious urban and familial influences.

Despite the reformers' successes in getting state mental hospitals, the quality of care in these hospitals often did not achieve a high level. Financial incentives to move large numbers of individuals from local almshouses to state asylums led to outright neglect and custodial care. This was fostered by the overcrowding of the mental hospitals with criminals, alcoholics, vagrants, and the poor; by a tendency to build larger institutions to keep per capita expenditures down; and by an increasing pessimism regarding the curability of mental disorders. Because mental hospitals were located away from population centers, the dismal conditions within them were easily ignored for a time. Although some improvements were made during the late 1800s, significant changes through implementation of standards and accreditation procedures were not achieved until well into the 20th century.

At the beginning of this century, mental health care was primarily hospital-based, and biological approaches to mental illness dominated etiological theories and applied treatments. During World War I, however, an understanding of the psychological and social contributions to the cause and treatment of mental disorders were forcibly brought home to professionals and the public alike. Thousands of men were rejected for military service because of what were understood even then to be "psychoneuroses." When, during the conflict, war neuroses ("shell shock") accounted for a large proportion of psychiatric casualties, psychiatrists saw that situational stress could precipitate a mental disorder in "normal" individuals as well as in those with "psychopathic constitutions." Military psychiatrists learned to apply psychological and social techniques to treat war neuroses and return soldiers to the front (Strecker, 1947), lessons that psychiatrists carried back into civilian life.

Between 1910 and World War II, Freud's psychoanalytic theory gradually came to dominate psychiatric training, outpatient care, and popular views of the nature of the human mind. Freud categorized childhood development into the oral, anal, phallic, latent, and genital phases. According to this theory, psychiatric distress and dysfunction is caused by conflicts originating in one or more of these phases of childhood development. Psychoanalysis did little, however, for severely disturbed individuals who, for the most part, often received nothing more than custodial care in poorly funded, sparsely staffed, biologically oriented state institutions. In the 1930s renewed hope for these severely disturbed patients was raised by the discovery of new biological treatments, including insulin coma, drug-induced convulsive treatments, electroconvulsive therapy, and psychosurgery. The Federal Public Works Administration added more than 60,000 beds to state and local mental institutions during this period.

World War II again focused public attention on mental disorders: 1.75 million men were rejected for service because of mental or emotional disturbances, and a large number of veterans returned home with emotional problems. In 1946, Congress passed the National Mental Health Act, which established the NIMH and gave new federal support for mental health services, training, and research. Yet the outpatient sector was tiny, and most inpatient treatment still took place in state institutions marked by deplorable conditions. Partly to compensate for limited professional personnel, institutions and outpatient clinics began to use group psychotherapy, which allowed one professional to treat many patients at once.

By the mid-1950s the number of persons hospitalized in state and county mental hospitals reached its peak of 559,000. At the same time, however, effective drugs for treating schizophrenia and mania were discovered (e.g., reserpine and chlorpromazine). These drugs replaced insulin coma and psychosurgery and allowed many patients to behave more rationally in institutions, to leave them, or to avoid hospitalization entirely. By reducing symptoms sufficiently to permit patients to leave hospitals, effective drug treatment indirectly created the need for halfway houses and other forms of aftercare.

In 1955, Congress established the Joint Commission on Mental Illness and Health, representing 36 organizations, to examine the nation's mental health care. The commission's 1961 report, *Action for Mental Health*, concluded that half of the patients in the state mental hospitals were not receiving active treatment. The commission's recommendations set the stage for the emphasis on community mental health care that marked the 1960s. It recommended establishing one fully staffed community mental health clinic per 50,000 citizens, limiting the bed complement of large psychiatric hospitals to a maximum of 1,000, and encouraging the use of community-based, short-term inpatient care.

In the 1960s, Congress, backed by President John F. Kennedy, passed legislation implementing the commission's recommendation. It also continued to expand financial support to the NIMH for psychiatric and behavioral science research, psychiatric education in medical schools, and residency training of psychiatrists. Additional effective drug treatments for mental disorders were introduced, including benzodiazepines for anxiety disorders, tricyclic and monoamine oxidase-inhibiting drugs for depressions, and lithium for bipolar affective disorders. Behavior therapy became popular for treating certain psychological conflicts and behavior disorders, and researchers began to demonstrate the effectiveness of various psychotherapies (Bergin, 1971; Foley & Sharfstein, 1983; Smith & Glass, 1977).

The creation in 1965 of Medicare and Medicaid (Titles VIII and XIX of the Social Security Act; see chapter 12) helped transfer some of the costs of caring for the chronically mentally ill to the federal treasury. Federal welfare support (Social Security Disability Income) and food stamps provided a minimal level of economic support for patients with chronic mental illness who were discharged from state hospitals. Unfortunately, the necessary networks of community medical, mental health, and human service agencies called for by congressional legislation were inadequately organized and severely underfunded, leaving large gaps in services and professional personnel to care for those who were deinstitutionalized.

The early 1970s saw a decline in federal support for mental health research and training and slow growth in funding for community mental health services. Under President Jimmy Carter presidential interest in mental health was renewed. In 1977 he established a President's Commission on Mental Health, with Mrs. Carter as honorary chairperson. The commission's 1978 report included an extensive review of the magnitude of the nation's mental health problems and of the resources available to meet them. Detailed recommendations were made for increasing outpatient services for chronic patients, improving access to care for underserved groups (children, minorities, rural citizens, and the aged), improving insurance coverage for mental health services, increasing public understanding of mental disorders, protecting patients' rights, and expanding the knowledge base through increased federal support of research (President's Commission, 1978).

The passage of the Mental Health Systems Act of 1980 was a significant accomplishment designed to implement many of the recommendations of the Carter Commission. However, with the election of Ronald Reagan in 1980, a new mood pervaded political views on the role of government, and the Mental Health Systems Act was never implemented (Foley & Sharfstein, 1983).The decade of the 1980s was a period of very significant reductions in all areas of national domestic spending, especially at the federal level. This led to, among other things, increasing numbers of Americans on the poverty rolls, cutbacks in programs for the poor, and an increase in the number of homeless persons. At the same time there appeared a new public health menace—the AIDS epidemic. Indeed, the major public mental health problem in this country became the mentally ill homeless. They often wandered the streets, hallucinating, rummaging through garbage, and sleeping on grates. This issue, more than others, has received attention through legislative hearings, the media, and public outcry. It resulted from the release of thousands of patients from state facilities and the imperfect psychiatric technology that can help patients by ameliorating the acute phase of psychosis but does not provide a long-term cure. Patients have been enrolled in underfunded community mental health programs, but when they discontinue treatment and relapse, they are readmitted to hospitals for short-term stays—a cycle dubbed the revolving door syndrome of psychiatric care.

The desire for minimal government prevailed throughout the 1980s and early 1990s, until President Clinton's election campaign. The campaign was based on a number of domestic policy issues, health care prominent among them. Clinton's election in 1992 reflected another shift in national mood, as many Americans became dissatisfied enough with the health care system to support major reform. Soon after his inauguration, he assembled a task force on national health reform, appointing his wife, Hillary Rodham Clinton, as chair of the task force. Vice President Gore's wife, Mary Elizabeth (Tipper), a strong ally of the mentally ill, rallied behind parity coverage of mental illnesses, as did Senator Domenici (Domenici, 1993). Clinton's health care reform proposal was released in September 1993 and generated a stormy congressional debate. The proposal fell victim to political infighting and strong lobbying by special interest groups, and no reform was ratified. The president himself subsequently moved to the "less government" side of the equation.

Because citizens with major mental illnesses are not an effective political lobbying group, the current coalition of former patients, dedicated professionals, and inspired reformers such as Mrs. Gore came together to maintain the momentum of reform. Congress has tended to move incrementally toward creating equal coverage for mental illness treatment, for example, by passing a bill requiring parity in lifetime limits in 1996. Although national reform was not implemented and is not likely in the foreseeable future, these efforts have reinvigorated our society's long-standing moral commitment to care for its disabled and vulnerable citizens. Such efforts continue—small regulatory steps signifying a major victory against stigmatization.

Mental Health Personnel

Many types of professionals serve patients and clients in the mental health sector, including psychiatrists and other physicians (particularly internists and family practitioners), psychologists, social workers and registered nurses. In addition, services are provided by vocational rehabilitation counselors, occupational therapists, teachers, and other health workers such as licensed practical nurses. In 1992, NIMH surveys identified 585,972 filled staff positions in 5,498 U.S. mental health facilities, of which 432,866 were patient care staff. The distribution of these employees is shown in Table 9.1. More than one half (52%) were professional patient care staff; 21% were other patient care staff with less than a baccalaureate degree; and one quarter were administrative, clerical, and maintenance staff. Combining part-time and full-time staff into full-time-equivalent (FTE) staff, 29% of FTE staff were employed in state and county mental hospitals (Center for Mental Health Services, 1996).

Psychiatrists

Psychiatrists are physicians with 4 years of postgraduate training. The American Board of Psychiatry and Neurology (ABPN) develops and maintains criteria and

TABLE 9.1 Number of Full-Time Equivalent Positions in Mental Health Facilities by Staff Discipline: United States, 1988

Staff discipline	All facilities	Percentage
Professional patient care staff	305,988	52.2
Psychiatrists	22,803	3.9
Other physicians	3,949	0.7
Psychologists	25,000	4.3
Social workers	57,136	9.7
Registered nurses	78,588	13.4
Other mental health professionals: B.A. and above (e.g., vocational rehabilitation counselors, occupational therapists, teachers)	102,162	17.4
Physical health professionals and assistants (e.g., dentists, dental technicians, pharmacists, dietitians)	16,350	2.8
Other patient care staff	126,878	21.7
All other staff (administrative, clerical, and maintenance)	153,106	26.1
Total	585,972	

Source: Center for Mental Health Services, 1996.

standards for accredited training programs and their graduates. For example, the first (or internship) year after medical school must include at least 6 months of training in internal medicine and neurology. The 3 subsequent years of specialized training in psychiatry form the *residency*, after completion of which a physician may practice independently in this specialty.

Approximately 10% of all psychiatrists have undergone additional years of education and training, including part-time didactics, a personal psychoanalysis, and supervision of their treatment cases, before being certified as psychoanalysts by a psychoanalytic institute. (Social workers and psychologists can also become certified as psychoanalysts.) Psychoanalysts base their treatment of patients on the psychological model of the mind, embedded within psychodynamic theory. This theory was developed by Freud and has been modified and adapted for clinical use by his followers and by practicing psychoanalysts. It is a long-term form of therapy requiring four to five hourly sessions per week, generally with the patient lying on a couch and the therapist out of view. Analysis of the patient's thoughts and interpretation by the analyst is intended to allow the patient to understand his or her conflicts, and bring about life-enhancing changes.

Psychiatrists may subspecialize in several areas within the field, and accredited training is available in several subspecialty areas, including forensics, child and adolescent care, geriatrics, and the addictions. Such subspecialty training in psychiatry requires additional years of training after completion of the residency.

Psychiatry is a diverse specialty, providing the opportunity to use a variety of treatments (e.g., psychotherapy, pharmacotherapy), practice in many settings (e.g., hospitals, offices, community clinics, and in the patient's home via mobile treatment teams), and care for various populations and for those with a variety of conditions. Some psychiatrists prefer general practice; others enjoy a clinical emphasis on a particular population, setting, or condition. Most psychiatrists divide their time between several part-time settings. This variety generates fluidity in psychiatrists' professional activities. The revolution in psychopharmacology over the past three decades has vastly increased the psychiatrist's therapeutic armamentarium.

Between 1970 and 1994 the number of psychiatrists in the United States grew from approximately 23,300 to nearly 43,300, including those in training. Both the American Medical Association (AMA) and American Psychiatric Association (APA) capture substantial information about psychiatrists working in the United States through annual surveys. Their data provide yearly snapshots of the number and specific activities of U.S. psychiatrists; the most recent data were compiled from their 1994 surveys (AMA, 1995; Center for Mental Health Services, 1996). Review of survey responses over time reveals manpower trends and changes in treatment emphasis, health care organization and delivery modes catalyzed in recent years partly by shifts in payer willingness to reimburse for care in particular settings.

Results of the latest surveys indicate that office-based practice was the primary professional activity of about two thirds of clinical psychiatrists. About one third of clinical psychiatrists were hospital-based, and about 8% of all active psychiatrists worked primarily in administration, teaching and research (Olfson, Pincus, & Dial, 1994). These numbers reflect a substantial shift of psychiatrists out of hospitals and into office settings that has occurred in the last decade, paralleling the shift of patient care from inpatient to outpatient settings.

Like other physicians, psychiatrists are unevenly distributed geographically. In 1996 the number of psychiatrists per 100,000 population ranged from a low of 4.6 in Mississippi to a high of 25.8 in Massachusetts (although the District of Columbia reported the highest overall rate at 50.9) (Center for Mental Health Services, 1996). Within states, psychiatrists are more concentrated in urban areas (American Psychological Association, 1995; Koran et al., 1979). Unfortunately, the same counties that lack psychiatrists also lack other providers of mental health services (e.g., psychologists and family physicians) (Olfson et al., 1994).

Psychologists

Psychologists are nonmedical professionals who may have either a master's or a doctoral degree in one of many kinds of psychology, including experimental, social, general, or clinical (Rodnick, 1985). Only psychologists trained in clinical psychology programs must have supervised patient contact as part of that training. Yet because most states license individuals generically as psychologists, any psychologist, regardless of training, can open a private psychotherapy practice. All 50 states plus Washington, DC, and Puerto Rico regulate licensure and the scope of practice of psychologists. Psychology applicants in all states are required to have either a PhD or a master's degree in addition to 3–5 years of work experience.

In 1995 approximately 70,000 psychologists (of whom over 82% held doctoral degrees) were providing mental health services in mental health facilities, schools, community agencies, and private practices. In that year approximately three quarters of all psychologists provided direct patient care. Office or clinic practice was the primary professional setting of over one half of psychologists caring for patients. About 12% practiced primarily in hospitals, 14% in educational and academic settings. According to the American Psychological Association Research Office, in 1996 one third of all active psychologists provided care in independent practices. Psychologists working in mental health facilities carry out psychotherapy, diagnostic testing, research, teaching, administrative duties, and consultation to other human service agencies.

Social Workers

Social work is a broad field of human service that focuses particularly on the impact of the environment on an individual. Matters of interest include family and other relationships, conditions at home and work, need for financial assistance through government programs, and other life circumstances. Some social workers are clinically trained to diagnose mental disorders and/or provide various types of psychotherapy. Social workers may have a bachelor's, master's, or doctoral degree in social work, although an advanced degree is encouraged for those doing clinical work. Social workers' licensure and scope of practice are regulated in all 50 states. Psychiatric social workers bring community health and welfare agency resources to bear on their patients' problems; provide care in diagnostic and therapeutic roles; offer consultation to human services agencies; and, to a lesser degree, engage in research, teaching, and administration.

The National Association of Social Workers (NASW) is the primary professional organization for social workers, and approximately 50% of U.S. social workers are members (Center for Mental Health Services, 1996). Based on the education level and professional activity of its 152,000 members, the NASW estimates that there were 189,000 clinically trained social workers in the United States in 1996 (Center for Mental Health Services, 1996). Approximately two thirds of social workers undertake some professional activity in a mental health setting (Ginsberg, 1995). The NASW estimates that social workers provide more than half of the mental health counseling in the United States.

In 1996 the primary work setting was a hospital for 19% of social workers, individual or group practice for 27%, and social service agencies for 16%, with the remainder in a variety of other settings (Center for Mental Health Services, 1996). Compared to previous years, the data indicate a shift of social workers out of hospitals into outpatient settings; this change reflects the influence of managed care policies, which preferentially reimburse outpatient care.

Registered Nurses

Registered nurses (RNs) are the largest group providing professional care in mental health facilities. In 1992, 78,588 full-time-equivalent RNs provided care in U.S. mental health organizations (Center for Mental Health Services, 1996). The role of the psychiatric nurse includes assessing patient health status; supervising patient interactions on the inpatient unit; administering medications; planning, administering, and supervising others in somatic treatments; helping patients with activities of daily living; and providing individual, group, or family therapy.

Scope of practice is regulated by the states. Several important classifications include certified clinical nurse specialist, certified specialists in psychiatric mental health nursing, and the growing group, nurse practitioners. These titles require graduate education, clinical practice with supervision, and successful completion of a written exam.

Delivery of Mental Health Services

As described above, from the mid-19th century to the mid-20th century, psychiatric services in this country were primarily based in long-stay institutions supported by state governments, and patterns of practice were relatively stable. Over the past 45 years, remarkable changes have occurred. These changes include a reversal of the balance between institutional and community care, inpatient and outpatient services, and individual and group practice.

Deinstitutionalization, or the discharge of thousands of individuals from the large state hospital system, has occurred over the past three decades and has had a significant impact on the mental health care delivery system. At the peak of public asylum psychiatry in 1955, 559,000 Americans were hospitalized in state and county mental hospitals. Now, long-stay residents in state mental hospitals number well under 80,000, and the total bed capacity is only about 93,000 (Redick, Witkin, Atay, & Manderscheid, 1996). In 1955 three of four patient care episodes took place in state hospitals, one of four in community settings. Today, three of four patient care episodes occur in community settings, only one of four in inpatient settings (and less than 10% of these are state hospital beds) (Redick et al., 1996). The shift of care to community-based settings began in the public sector, although community settings remained dominant in comparison to the private sector. This private sector's bed capacity increased in the 1970s and 1980s, including psychiatric units in nonfederal general hospitals, private psychiatric hospitals, and residential treatment centers for children. Substance abuse centers and child and adolescent inpatient psychiatric units grew particularly quickly in the 1980s, as investors recognized their profitability. However, growth of the inpatient private mental health sector recently has plateaued, whereas the number of outpatient and partial treatment settings has sharply increased (Redick et al., 1996).

In the past quarter century outpatient services have grown dramatically. The rate of additions to outpatient care more than doubled between 1969 and 1992, from 578 to 1,181 per 100,000 population. Most of this service growth occurred in community mental health centers in the 1970s, in nonfederal general hospitals in the 1980s, and in multiservice mental health organizations in the 1990s (Redick et al., 1996).

These changes have occurred as a result of a number of forces, not the least of which was a change in the legal environment in the 1960s, when patients' rights suits established the principle of providing treatment in "the least restrictive setting" (Kaufman, 1979). Further, social psychiatrists had established the deleterious effects of long-term institutional care, that is, the so-called social breakdown syndrome. The development of effective psychiatric medications ameliorated patients' behavioral symptoms and allowed discharge into the community. The increased proportion of the population with private insurance coverage for psychiatric services also has stimulated utilization. Probably the most significant factor in spurring the discharge of patients from state hospitals, however, was financing. With the enactment of federal Social Security entitlements—Medicare, Medicaid, Supplemental Social Security—it became advantageous for states to discharge patients into nursing homes or to a variety of board-and-care-type settings and utilize new federal dollars to deal with state fiscal concerns. As long as patients remained in state institutions, they were not eligible to have their care paid for by federal funds. With the passage of Medicaid (Title XIX) in 1965, patients who moved into the community or into long-term care institutions that were not designated as caring for mental illness exclusively could be supported through that program, which provided a 50% federal subsidy. In 1972, with the creation of the Supplemental Social Security Income system (Title XVI), patients discharged from hospitals could have federal payments made for board-and-care home service and other group living arrangements and for their daily support and also have Medicaid coverage for their treatment costs. This cost shifting from state to federal coffers further encouraged the emptying of state facilities (Foley & Sharfstein, 1983).

Admissions to state mental hospitals and the number of psychiatric beds located in general hospitals increased dramatically during this same period. Most admissions, however, were actually readmissions, as hospitals experienced a "revolving door," with the same patients admitted for multiple acute stays, and lengths of stay became progressively shorter. Further, nursing homes became a substitute for state mental hospitals and assumed a major responsibility for long-term mental illness care. One estimate in the late 1980s placed three quarters of a million Americans with chronic mental illness in nursing homes (Goldman & Manderscheid, 1987). Most of these patients suffer from behavioral disturbances or inability to care for themselves due to dementia (including Alzheimer's disease), head injury, or other physical illness. Other patients, however, have other psychiatric diagnoses, such as schizophrenia or bipolar disorder, that require extended stays. For example, epidemiologic catchment area (ECA) data suggest that approximately 20,000 of the patients admitted to nursing homes in 1 year suffered from schizophrenia or a mood disorder (Narrow, 1993). Although many of these patients likely also suffer from functional impairments rendering them unable to care for themselves independently, it is unfortunate that most patients with mental disorders receive a custodial level of treatment in nursing homes, even though most would probably benefit from more active treatment.

Decline in the use of state hospitals has had negative effects. Many patients—likely more than a million—have been discharged into communities that are ill-prepared to provide the therapeutic and rehabilitative services they need, such as halfway houses, aftercare programs, sheltered workshops, and psychosocial rehabilitation (Belcher & DiBlasio, 1990; Robertson & Greenblatt, 1992; Torrey, 1988). Some of these patients have become homeless wanderers, shifted from the back wards to living on the streets. Many patients now reside in unlicensed and uninspected board-and-care homes that do not offer or arrange for active treatment (Lamb, 1979).

The deinstitutionalization of the mentally ill presents major policy challenges in this era of managed care and therapeutic success. With the progress in psychopharmacology, many patients can do well in noninstitutional settings as long as they take their medications and follow through on their outpatient psychosocial treatments. However, many patients do not comply with either their psychopharmacological or psychosocial regimen, leading to relapse and the need for acute interventions. What is left of the health reform movement in the mid-1990s has shifted from the national to the local level. The plight of the homeless mentally ill presents a major public health challenge.

The Settings for Mental Health Services

The number of organizations providing specialized mental health services rose 83.1% between 1970 and 1992, from 3,005 to 5,498. The number of private psychiatric hospitals also grew substantially, from 150 in 1970 to 475 in 1992, the great majority being part of investor-owned, for-profit medical chains. Costing less to build and operate per bed than general hospitals, psychiatric hospitals are an attractive source of profits for these corporations. On the positive side, corporate management may stimulate innovation, drive down costs via competition, create psychiatric hospitals where none exist, and through marketing reduce the stigma associated with mental health care. On the other hand, these hospitals are less tolerant of nonpaying patients than are tax-supported or charity-supported hospitals, and they may be somewhat less responsive to specific community needs than are locally controlled hospitals. Whereas in 1981, 16 states had no hospital of this kind, by 1992 only Hawaii, Iowa, and North Dakota were without private psychiatric hospitals. Between 1970 and 1992 the number of beds in private psychiatric hospitals and psychiatric units of general hospitals increased by 69,000 (from 26,700 to 95,700, over 250%) (Redick et al., 1996).

Although the number of VA medical centers grew from 115 to 162, their bed capacity shrank from 51,000 to less than 23,000, and the number of state and county mental hospitals also decreased (310 to 273) during the same period. The total number of psychiatric beds for all organizations decreased by nearly one half, and almost all of this decrease can be attributed to reductions in state and county mental hospitals, which decreased their bed counts from 413,000 in 1970 to 93,000 in 1992, a reduction of 77%. As a result, state and county mental hospitals accounted for only about 34% of all psychiatric beds in 1992, compared to 79% in 1970 (Redick et al., 1996).

Reflecting the decline in public sector capacity, nonfederal general hospital psychiatric units have become the most common site of inpatient mental health admissions (45% in 1992), followed by private psychiatric hospitals (22%) and state and county psychiatric hospitals[*] (13%) (Redick et al., 1996). In addition to the admissions to general hospital psychiatric units recorded by NIMH, there are many admissions of patients with psychiatric diagnoses to medical/surgical units in general hospitals that go unrecorded (Kiesler & Sibulkin, 1984). The private and general hospital inpatient psychiatric sector provides acute, short-term psychiatric care. Reflecting treatment advances today, most inpatient units provide crisis intervention and aggressive psychopharmacologic management of symptoms. When patients are stabilized enough to be cared for in less intensive settings, they are discharged for aftercare in a partial hospitalization or other outpatient setting. Both public and private payers reimburse these short-term stays, although utilization review is intense and pressure is high to discharge patients as soon as they are out of crisis. The potential patient volume is large because this sector can serve both the recurring illness flares of the chronically mentally ill and the sporadic episodes occurring in the general population.

State and county hospitals, on the other hand, may be returning to their original role—that of providing asylum for disabled patients who cannot function in their communities. Not everyone responds to today's treatments. Patients who do not improve quickly in a private-sector setting often are transferred for long-term care to a public hospital. Today these are usually patients with treatment-resistant schizophrenia or severe mood disorders or those with chronic cognitive impairment who are dangerous to themselves or others. If adequately funded, public hospitals can serve patients with special treatment and rehabilitative needs, such as chronically ill patients with no families or social supports, patients with severe substance abuse conditions (particularly those with associated cognitive impairment), and patients chronically dangerous to themselves or others.

Despite the drop in resident population, state and county mental hospitals face a number of problems. Fiscal restraint leaves budgets inadequate for high-quality clinical programs. State hospitals must deal with high readmission rates because of insufficient capacity in publicly supported aftercare services. For-profit hospitals have not designed services nor do they currently have the appropriate financial incentives to meet the needs of the severely and persistently mentally ill. As in the general health care sector, if the full range of services is to be provided to all those in need, a new social consensus must be reached regarding who will pay for those who cannot themselves pay for care. Neither for-profit nor nonprofit hospitals can shoulder this burden without realistic sources of revenue (Sharfstein & Stoline, 1992; Sharfstein, Stoline, & Goldman, 1993).

---

[*]Admission data reveal different demographic and diagnostic profiles between patients admitted to public and private sector facilities, reflecting sources of payment as well as historic responsibilities.

Residential treatment centers (RTCs) for emotionally or psychiatrically disturbed children provide inpatient services to children under 18 years of age. Although their focus ranges from personality and behavioral disorders to severe psychoses, RTCs do not attempt to treat all serious mental disorders of children. The programs and physical facilities of RTCs are designed to meet patients' daily living, schooling, recreational, socialization, and routine medical care needs. Because a large number and variety of staff are required, costs are high. Treatments include milieu therapy, psychotherapy, behavior modification, psychotropic medications, and special education. In 1992 there were 497 RTCs, with a resident population of 28,000 (Redick et al., 1996). The lack of coordination between the mental health care, general health care, juvenile justice, education, foster care, and child protective service sectors creates both severe discontinuities and, rarely, redundancies in service delivery for children and adolescents. Improved service coordination is a major focus of reform efforts in the 1990s.

Day hospital or day treatment programs occupy one niche in the spectrum of mental health care settings. Although some provide services 7 days per week, many programs provide services only Mondays through Fridays. Day treatment patients spend most of the day at the treatment facility in a program of structured therapeutic activities and then return to their homes until the next day. Day treatment services include psychotherapy, pharmacotherapy, occupational therapy, and other types of rehabilitation services. These programs provide alternatives to inpatient care or serve as transitions from inpatient to outpatient care or discharge. They may also provide respite for family caregivers and a locus for rehabilitating or maintaining chronically ill patients. Some programs specialize by age group or diagnosis, such as geriatric programs or those for patients with chronic psychotic conditions.

The number of day treatment programs has increased in response to pressures to decrease lengths of hospital stays and the increased number of patients discharged from psychiatric facilities only partially recovered and requiring additional care. Reflecting these changes in treatment style, the number of partial care episodes increased from 78,000 to 544,000 between 1969 and 1992 (Redick et al., 1996).

Despite this impressive growth, expansion of day treatment services has been slowed by the widespread failure of many private insurance policies to cover this treatment modality. Only recently have third-party payers been convinced of the cost-effectiveness of this treatment setting. Medicare has covered this service since 1987, and other plans have gradually followed suit. In rural areas, long travel times continue to impede the use of day treatment. As private insurers continue to ratchet down service availability, an emerging managed care trend is reimbursement of "intensive outpatient treatment," comprising daily visits for medication management and a limited number of therapeutic groups. This mode of treatment, of course, costs less than a full-day treatment program.

Psychiatric halfway houses are nonmedical residential facilities that provide room and board in a homelike atmosphere for psychiatrically disturbed individuals who cannot live independently but who can work or occupy themselves productively during the day if given some support and supervision. Most are 15- to 25-bed facilities with in-house staff who usually provide supervision, medication, and support. Where they exist, halfway houses allow patients a graded transition from the extreme dependency of hospital life to the full responsibility of independent living. Admission to a halfway house may also be used to prevent hospitalization. Despite these advantages, however, residential neighborhoods usually resist their establishment because most patients in halfway houses are not fully recovered. Because residence in a halfway house is usually not covered by insurance, there are far fewer than are needed.

If one adds the growth characteristics enumerated above to the growth in mental health personnel, one can see that the mental health system, in the words of our modern corporate managers, "has expanded and diversified its portfolio." Indeed, expenditures by mental health organizations rose from $3.29 billion in 1969 to $30 billion in 1992, an almost 10-fold increase. However, when measured in constant (i.e., noninflated) dollars, the increase was only 1.5-fold. In 1992 state and county mental health agency expenditures accounted for 27% of the total, followed by private psychiatric hospitals with 18% and general hospital psychiatry services with 18% (Redick et al., 1996). Of course, funding sources vary considerably by type of organization and by location within the country.

Insurance Coverage for Mental Disorders

The provision of insurance coverage for mental health care has always lagged behind the insurance provisions for other medical care. Differences in insurance for psychiatric versus other conditions arose in the 1920s and 1930s, when hospitalization insurance was first written. Inpatient treatment for mental disorders then occurred largely in state-funded mental hospitals or in private mental hospitals used primarily by the wealthy; thus, there was not a broad-based demand for such coverage. Although treatments and treatment settings have changed, rising health care costs, the absence of strong consumer demand for mental health coverage and insurers' continuing fear of the potential cost of this coverage have maintained the differences between medical and mental health care insurance.

Reflecting these factors, only 13% of the payment for mental disorders treatment comes from private insurance dollars, compared with 28% for general medical care. States continue their traditional provision of a safety net for those uninsured and underinsured for psychiatric illness. As a result, states and local governments pay 28% of the costs of mental health care while paying only

14% of the costs of other medical treatments (National Advisory Mental Health Council, 1993).

Today psychiatrists treat approximately twice the proportion of patients with no health insurance as do other physicians, although virtually all individuals with private health coverage have some provision for inpatient psychiatric treatment included in the benefit package. This coverage usually is not equal to the inpatient coverage for other conditions, and recent trends reveal a shrinking percentage of plans offering parity between psychiatric and medical/surgical hospitalization benefits. The limitations on psychiatric inpatient benefits include limitations on days of care and separate dollar limits, including fixed dollar caps on an annual or lifetime basis.

For outpatient care, although the vast majority of those with insurance has some coverage, this coverage is often quite restricted. Typical limitations include lower visit limits, higher copayment charges, higher deductibles, and separate dollar caps. In this era of cost control, mental health outpatient coverage has been further curtailed in a number of plans.

Psychiatric care will not be covered adequately by insurance until the myths surrounding it are addressed. Some myths are economically based, reflecting concern that psychiatric coverage opens insurers up to a bottomless pit of patient demand for services. In fact, much work has been done by economists who study the assumption that the use of psychiatric benefits differs markedly from other health insurance benefits. Examples follow of studies that disprove the hypotheses upon which prejudicial benefit design is based.

The first myth is that costs of psychiatric treatment are uncontrollable and unpredictable. Experience contradicts this hypothesis. In one study of this question the Blue Cross Blue Shield Federal Employee Health Benefits Program (FEHBP) had no limits on mental health coverage from 1967 to 1981, aside from the same deductibles and copayments as for general medical care. After the initial jump in costs immediately following the introduction of broader psychiatric benefits between 1967 and 1969, mental health care accounted for a stable 7.2% to 7.7% of the total benefits paid from 1970 to 1981 (Sharfstein, Muszynski, & Myers, 1984).

In 1971 the Rand Corporation undertook a major study of health insurance that enrolled 7,500 persons at six sites across the country in 14 different insurance plans. Patient copayments ranged up to 95%, with a maximum annual dollar expenditure of $1,000 per family (Brook et al., 1983). The study found that expenditures for mental health care constituted only about 5% of the total health care costs for all insurance plan enrollees. Depending on copayment levels, between 7.1% and 9.6% of the population studied used mental health benefits, including visits to general practitioners and internists. In comparison, recall that the NIMH Epidemiological Catchment Area study reported mental illness prevalence rates of 28.1% of the population (and included only a portion of all mental disorders) (Myers et al., 1984). Only a small percentage of the patients in the Rand study (0.4%) saw clinicians more than 40 times a year (Brook et al., 1983). This study and others underscore the stability over time of costs for mental health care under insurance (Krizay, 1982; Wells, Manning, Duan, Ware, & Newhouse, 1982).

Many of the restrictions on insurance coverage for psychiatric care appear to stem largely from concern about the costs of long-term custodial care or intensive psychotherapy. The standard treatment regimen for intensive psychotherapies involves a minimum of three therapy sessions per week. Within the FEHBP, which placed no restriction on the annual number of outpatient visits for more than a decade, the number of persons receiving intensive psychotherapeutic treatment ranged from 0.9% of all psychiatric outpatients treated in 1971 to 1.1% of those treated in 1973. The cost for treatment of this population during the same period ranged from 8.7% to 10.3% of the total cost of physicians' treatment of mental disorders (Sharfstein & Magnas, 1975).

Data from the 1987 National Medical Expenditure Survey indicate that expenditures for outpatient psychotherapy provided by mental health professionals and medical providers other than psychiatrists accounted for about 8% of outpatient medical care costs. Outpatient psychotherapy accounted for only 5.7% of private insurance and patient expenditures (Olfson & Pincus, 1994).

Another myth is that mental health care costs are unstable because liberal coverage encourages unnecessary and excessive use. Supporters of this view cite data such as these: 9% of outpatient users of mental health care in the Blue Cross Blue Shield FEHBP accounted for 45% of the total cost (Sharfstein & Taube, 1982). That someone with insurance may be more likely to initiate medical care and, once under care, be more likely to opt for more extensive treatment is not a phenomenon limited to mental health care. Insurance encourages utilization of all physician services. The Rand study, for example, reported that 1% of users of medical care in their 7,500-person sample accounted for 28% of the total expenditures (Wells et al., 1982).

A third myth is that mental health care is not cost-effective. This myth is a carryover from the years preceding development of effective psychiatric treatments, when most treatment was custodial instead of curative. Today treatments that are either curative or that markedly improve functioning are clearly cost-effective. For example, considering costs and benefits from a broad societal perspective, the introduction of lithium for the treatment of bipolar psychoses produced a conservatively estimated 10-year savings of $4.2 billion ($2.9 billion in unexpended treatment costs plus $1.3 billion in productivity gains) (Reifman & Wyatt, 1980). In addition to the evident analogies between medical management of psychiatric and nonpsychiatric conditions, a body of evidence suggests that expenditures for psychotherapy produce savings elsewhere in the economy through increased employee productivity, reduced absenteeism, and lower costs for other medical care.

A final myth is that psychiatric treatment cannot be accountable to insurance carriers. However, utilization review (UR) in the form of peer review is now widely and easily available and has become the cornerstone of psychiatry's accountability to payers and consumers. Although the financial savings in some UR programs are negligible and opponents of these strategies point to their negative impact on confidentiality and the doctor-patient relationship, managed care strategies are likely to remain in the near future an integral component of third-party payers' ongoing search for ways to control their expenditures for mental health care. The need to evaluate the effects of managed care arrangements on patients' access to care and the outcomes of care is acute (Pincus, Zarin, & West, 1996).

These numbers suggest that other factors are at work in the persistent disparity between psychiatric coverage and general medical coverage. The belief that patients are to blame for their own problems and/or that they can use force of will to overcome symptoms certainly contributes to payers' reluctance to create parity in benefit design. A general societal stigma, composed of fear, misunderstanding, and distrust, reinforces such policy decisions.

Medicare

The general benefits and costs of Medicare, a federal program that uses the Social Security system to insure some health care costs of individuals aged 65 and over and disabled individuals regardless of age, are described in chapter 3. Under Part A (hospitalization insurance), benefits for inpatient treatment in a psychiatric hospital are limited to 190 days in a lifetime. Only 150 of these days (90 benefit-period days plus 60 lifetime-reserve days) can be used in any one benefit period. Benefits for psychiatric care in a certified general hospital or extended-care facility are the same as for any other form of medical care. This provision has increased the use of general hospitals to provide psychiatric care for the elderly.

Under Part B (supplementary medical insurance), benefits for physicians' inpatient care for mental illness are the same as for other illnesses; that is, they are not limited. One hundred home visits are also covered and may be provided by mental health agencies. Benefits for physicians' outpatient care for mental illness initially were limited to 50% of the charges or $250, whichever was less. Congress expanded the outpatient psychiatric benefit in Medicare as part of the Budget Deficit Reduction Act of 1987. Outpatient benefits were increased in two stages over a 2-year period to $2,200 annually, with a 50% copayment; subsequently, benefits were expanded to equal those of general medical conditions (i.e., the benefit cap was eliminated). This quadrupling in benefits, in effect, kept the outpatient psychiatric benefit on a par with inflation since 1965. Benefits were expanded for partial hospitalization, which was established as a reimbursable service. Perhaps most significantly, all limits and special copayments were removed for "the medical management of psychopharmacologic agents" for Medicare beneficiaries. Thus, "medical management of psychiatric conditions" is now covered on par with outpatient treatment for other medical illnesses, that is, with a 20% copayment and no visit or dollar limits.

During the passage of the Kennedy–Kassebaum Health Care Reform Bill in the spring of 1996, the U.S. Senate approved an amendment to require employer-based health plans to provide coverage of mental health services and to do so "without imposing treatment limitations or financial requirements if similar limitations or requirements are not imposed on coverage for services of other conditions." Equal coverage for mental and physical conditions under insurance, termed "parity," has been a goal of advocates for many decades. The amendment that actually passed prohibits different treatment of mental health care and physical health care in terms of lifetime caps and annual reimbursement ceilings. The final version of the bill allows plans to continue to place annual day and visit limitations on covered services and/or to use higher levels of cost sharing for mental health care than for other services. Yet the bill certainly was a historic first step, a more comprehensive approach toward equal coverage (Frank, Koyanagi, & McGuire, 1997).

The introduction of managed care creates a new context for public and private insurance of mental illness. Managed care used information systems, control of referrals and other gatekeeping, expert utilization review, and financial incentives to constrain use and costs of care. Managed behavioral health care companies now cover the majority of Americans who have insurance and have fueled a continued shift from more expensive inpatient settings to less expensive outpatient alternatives and shorter episodes of both inpatient and outpatient care. As managed care reduces costs, parity becomes a less expensive proposition for payers (Sharfstein, 1996).

Medicaid

Medicaid is a combined federal and state program that covers certain health care costs for eligible persons with incomes falling below stated levels. This program is discussed in detail in chapter 11. Eligibility standards and covered health care services vary from state to state. Although no restrictions by diagnosis are permitted, states can and have limited the amounts of covered mental health care using methods similar to those found in the private sector. Professional reimbursement rates usually fall well below prevailing private sector rates.

In an effort to gain control over the cost of the Medicaid program and to integrate the funding of Medicaid with other public funding, many states have turned to "managed Medicaid." The privatization of public programs has led to a shift in management from state authority to the private, for-profit managed care industry. This experiment is just beginning in several states (e.g., Massachusetts and Tennessee), and its success is yet to be determined.

Legal Issues

"Mental health" encompasses the entire realm of the individual's psychological and social functioning. As a result, legal issues closely interrelate with psychiatric ones. Psychiatrists are often expected to perform a social control role by hospitalizing and treating potentially dangerous patients. At the same time, the criminal side of the legal system is concerned with punishment for wrongdoing, the civil side with the adjudication of noncriminal disputes between private parties or a private party and government, and the protection of civil rights and liberties. It is not designed for the treatment of illness. Patients have individual legal rights, but when their judgment is impaired, what is their right to treatment or to nontreatment? When their judgment is impaired by a mental disorder, who decides which is more important—freedom or health? These questions continue to be debated, both within the medical and legal professions and between them.

Legal issues receiving substantial judicial attention in the past few decades have included commitment procedures, the right to treatment, the right to refuse treatment, and the insanity defense in criminal proceedings. More recently, patient-therapist relationships and utilization review procedures have been subjected to judicial and legislative scrutiny (Mills, Sullivan, & Eth, 1987; Sederer, 1992). A few landmark cases touching on these issues are described below.

Civil commitment to a mental institution deprives a mentally ill person of liberty in exchange for treatment. The grounds for civil commitment vary between states, but most require that the individual be both mentally ill and dangerous to self or others (with criteria for "dangerous" varying from state to state); some states allow civil commitment of individuals who are "gravely disabled," meaning unable because of mental disorder to provide for their own basic needs such as food and shelter. In the 1970s and early 1980s the criterion for dangerousness often required a specific act or that the danger be "imminent." In the past decade a number of states, reacting to public concerns sparked by isolated acts of violence by mentally ill individuals, have dropped requirements for a recent specific act or for imminence, and some have revised commitment statutes to allow the involuntary hospitalization of a mentally ill individual who would substantially deteriorate without hospitalization (Zeman & Schwartz, 1994). Nonetheless, the increased stringency of commitment statutes and case law decisions that began in the 1960s has contributed to the increased numbers of homeless individuals because many are chronically mentally ill but fail to meet the criteria that allow commitment (Cohen, Putnam, & Sullivan, 1984; U.S. Conference of Mayors, 1996).

In the past 30 years, civil commitment has been affected not only by legal changes in the criteria for commitment but also in the procedures surrounding commitment, the duration of commitment, and the committed individual's rights. In a 1978 case, *Addington v. Texas*, the U.S. Supreme Court determined that the standard of evidence for civil commitment should be "clear and convincing evidence" (about 75% certainty) rather than the standard of "beyond a reasonable doubt" (about 90% to 95% certainty) that applies in criminal proceedings. The Court sought to balance a patient's rights with his need for treatment under the doctrine of *parens patriae* (the state's ability and duty to protect the disabled) and the state's need to protect others by means of its police powers. Federal judicial rulings have reduced the length of time a person can be committed by physicians without judicial review, abolished indeterminate states during which the patient cannot initiate discharge of release, and required due process guarantees for longer-term commitments (Appelbaum & Gutheil, 1991; Simon, 1992).

The civil and personal rights of committed and voluntary mental patients have been given increasing statutory recognition. These rights include the right to communicate with persons outside the institution; to keep clothing and personal effects; to practice religion freely; to receive independent psychiatric examination; to manage or dispose of property; to retain licenses, permits, or privileges established by law; to enter into contracts; to marry; and to sue and be sued (McGarry & Kaplan, 1973).

The Mental Health Law Project, sponsored by the American Civil Liberties Union Foundation, the American Orthopsychiatric Association, and the Center for Law and Social Policy, engages in litigation and consults with legislatures and mental health organizations to help secure these and other patient rights. Because of this attention to procedures and rights, seriously disturbed individuals are being given more humane care. Conflicts remain, however, involving patients' rights to liberty, their need for care or treatment, and the state's interests in protecting their welfare and in preventing harm to others (Roth, 1979).

A constitutional right to treatment for involuntarily committed patients was first recognized by a court in *Wyatt v. Stickney* in 1972. In that case, guardians of involuntarily committed patients sued the Alabama mental health commissioner, charging that inadequate care was rendered in a state mental hospital. A federal district court judge agreed that patients had a right to treatment that included the right to certain standards of care. With the aid of internists and psychiatrists who served as consultants, he defined these standards to include individual evaluation, active treatment, minimum staffing ratios, detailed nutritional and physical standards, and compensation for work performed. But the judgment had certain limitations. It did not apply to voluntary patients, and it set no penalty for noncompliance.

Since 1980 the right to treatment has been expanded by actions of the Civil Rights Division of the U.S. Department of Justice (Geller, 1994). Acting under authority granted by the Civil Rights of Institutionalized Persons Act of 1980, the Civil Rights Division has won consent decrees that, for example, markedly improve the staffing ratios established under *Wyatt v. Stickney*. Where the earlier decree required a ratio of 6 physicians or psychiatrists to 250 patients, a 1991 consent decree (*U.S. v. Hawaii*) requires 16. Where *Wyatt v. Stickney* required a total of 100 registered nurses, licensed practical nurses, and aides, the 1991 decree requires 272 (Geller, 1994).

The right of committed patients to refuse treatment is not widely recognized. Committed patients are deprived of their liberty in exchange for treatment that is presumably in their best interests; to allow them to refuse it would seem contradictory. On the other hand, the state's coercive power must be restrained to prevent capricious application. Committed patients usually are regarded as legally incompetent to decide whether to accept particular treatments, although exceptions are made for electroconvulsive therapy and psychosurgery in a few states on the grounds that these treatments may harm patients or change them irrevocably. In most states a committed patient's only grounds for refusing medications is religious principle, recognized by the Second Circuit Federal Court of Appeals in *Winters v. Miller* in 1971. These grounds for refusing were then recognized by the U.S. Supreme Court in the same year.

In Massachusetts, Colorado, and New York, however, committed mental patients can refuse treatment, except in narrowly defined emergencies, unless they are found incompetent by a judge. If a patient is found incompetent, the judge will decide "whether the patient, if competent, would have consented to the administration of antipsychotic drugs" (Gutheil, 1985, p. 213). This patient's rights approach to right-to-refuse-treatment situations has been more characteristic of state than federal courts. Federal courts have tended to limit the right to refuse treatment to situations in which the treatment is not prescribed appropriately and have left this determination to professionals, often independent psychiatrists (e.g., *Jamison v. Farabee*, 1983, discussed below) or multidisciplinary boards (Hoge et al., 1994). There is some evidence that the patient's rights approach, with the requirement of judicial review of committed patient's objections to clinical decisions to treat, may have adverse effects (e.g., disruption of the treatment setting with consequences for other patients and increased use of seclusion and restraints for the objecting patients) (Hoge et al., 1990).

In California the 1983 decision by the Federal District Court for the Northern District of California in *Jamison v. Farabee* established a review process when a treating psychiatrist wishes to use neuroleptic (antipsychotic) medication to treat an involuntary patient who has refused medication or who cannot give informed consent. Rather than resorting to judicial review, as in Massachusetts, Colorado, and New York, the California decision requires an outside psychiatrist to examine the patient and the clinical records and then to approve or deny use of the medication.

That involuntary treatment is not limited to psychiatric settings is often forgotten. Nonpsychiatric physicians on medical and surgical units of general hospitals use or prescribe restraints, psychoactive and other medications, intravenous fluids, and nursing care for patients who have refused these treatments (Appelbaum & Roth, 1984).

The invocation of an insanity defense during John Hinckley's trial for the attempted assassination of President Reagan stimulated great public and professional interest in this difficult area of law. Although this point of intersection between psychiatry and the law episodically receives great public attention, the intersection points discussed earlier affect far greater numbers of citizens.

The growth of managed care has engendered an increase in utilization review in the forms of prior approvals and concurrent reviews of the necessity of care. When such reviews lead to a denial of care, who bears responsibility for adverse patient outcomes? Judicial decisions, in *Wickline v. State of California* and *Hughes v. Blue Cross of Northern California*, for example, are establishing the principles that health care payers can be held responsible when patients are harmed because medically necessary care was not provided, that review procedures must be diligent, and that physicians are obligated to pursue appeal procedures when they disagree with a reviewer's decision to deny benefits and believe the patient may be harmed (Sederer, 1992). As of 1992, 19 states had enacted legislation regulating utilization review procedures. Provisions enacted in one or more states require, for example, clinically trained reviewers, open availability of the review criteria, accessibility of the reviewers to both physicians and patients, and a well-defined appeals process (Sederer, 1992). Undoubtedly, the conflicts between clinically motivated and fiscally motivated decisions and decision makers will provide material for judicial and legislative action for many years to come.

Several well-publicized cases in the 1980s and early 1990s focused public attention on physical relationships between patients and their therapists (Appelbaum & Jorgenson, 1991). Several states have passed legislation or are considering bills invoking criminal penalties for such relationships, for which therapists are held responsible. The APA modified its code of ethics to reflect a stricter standard of behavior. This controversial issue is likely to remain the topic of legal and professional debate for some time.

Current Issues

Mental health care has grown and diversified, particularly over the past 40 years, as psychopharmacologic treatment has made possible the shift away from long-term custodial institutions, and psychosocial treatments continue the process of care and rehabilitation in community settings. Large state hospitals have been supplemented and in many cases supplanted by psychiatric units in general hospitals, new outpatient clinics, community mental health centers, day treatment centers, and halfway houses. Treatment has become more effective and specific, based on our growing understanding of the brain and behavior. Recent advances in the biological and behavioral sciences continue to improve opportunities for diagnosing, treating, and preventing mental disorders (Institute of Medicine, 1984).

Now that we have many effective treatments with which to manage psychiatric symptoms and to support patients in rehabilitation, our challenge becomes the optimum allocation of resources and effective treatments to those patients. Resources are limited, so priorities for care must be established and choices made. Managed care has come to mental health care and will not disappear soon. More extensive education of general physicians regarding mental disorders and their treatments is needed. We must improve our ability to triage and match patients' needs with appropriate care. Other key features of cost containment include an emphasis on alternatives to inpatient settings, with continued development of a continuum of care as an approach to the care, treatment, and rehabilitation of those with serious and persistent mental illness. In this vein, more day treatment programs, home visits, psychosocial rehabilitation programs, and residential group homes are needed (Schreter, Sharfstein, & Schreter, 1997).

Much progress has been made in recent years in increasing efficiency in the health care system, but legitimate concern exists that the system has been pushed too far in the direction of cost control, to the detriment of patient care. We must rethink issues of access, quality, and cost for mental health and substance abuse treatment, with an intensive, public debate about the best way to satisfy the myriad mental health care needs of the U.S. population. A result of this process should be replacement of our two-tiered public/private system with one tier. This will require dedicated effort by policymakers at national, state, and local levels, but is essential if we are to develop an accountable and fair system for all Americans. There is reason to hope for success if medical professionals, payers, and policymakers move beyond entrenched partisan positions to reach consensus on approaches that balance reasonable costs with adequate care. The growth in our knowledge base and opportunities for new discoveries provide reasons for continued optimism and hope. Further converting this promise into reality is the next challenge for mental health services at the dawn of the 21st century.

Mini-Case Study

You are governor of a small island, population 100,000. There is no mental health care system in place. The inhabitants of this island are U.S. citizens, thus U.S.

Mini-Case Study *(cont.)*

epidemiologic data regarding prevalence of mental disorders is applicable to your island as well. How might you use the information in this chapter to design a fair, cost-effective mental health system?

Discussion Questions

1. Why is it important to consider the indirect costs of mental disorders and substance abuse?
2. What are the general criteria for labeling a condition a mental disorder?
3. What factors contribute to the discrepancy between prevalence of mental disorders and extent of their treatment?
4. How did the two-tier system of care for the mentally ill develop, and what perpetuates this discrimination today?
5. What factors might create competition among mental health professionals?
6. How does stigma surrounding mental disorders contribute to the financial pressures facing today's U.S. mental health care system?

References

American Medical Association, Department of Data Survey and Planning, Division of Survey & Data Resources, *Physician Characteristics and Distribution in the U.S.* (1995–96 edition). Chicago: AMA Press, 1995.

American Psychiatric Association, *Diagnostic and Statistical Manual of Mental Disorders* (4th ed.). Washington DC: Author, 1994.

American Psychological Association, Research Office, *Profile of All APA Members: 1995.* Washington, DC: Author, 1995.

Appelbaum, P. S., & Gutheil, T. G., *Clinical Handbook of Psychiatry and the Law* (2nd ed.). Baltimore: Williams and Wilkins, 1991.

Appelbaum, P. S., & Jorgenson, L., "Psychotherapist-Patient Sexual Contact after Termination of Treatment: An Analysis and a Proposal," *American Journal of Psychiatry, 148,* 1466–1473, 1991.

Appelbaum, P. S., & Roth, L. H., "Involuntary Treatment in Medicine and Psychiatry," *American Journal of Psychiatry, 141,* 202, 1984.

Belcher, J. R., & DiBlasio, F. A., *Helping the Homeless: Where Do We Go from Here?* Lexington, MA: Lexington Books, 1990.

Bergin, A. E., "The Evaluation of Therapeutic Outcomes," In A. E. Bergin & S. L. Garfield (Eds.), *Handbook of Psychotherapy and Behavior Change.* New York: Wiley, 1971.

Bockoven, J. S., *Moral Treatment in Community Mental Health.* New York: Springer Publishing Co., 1972.

Brook, R. H., Ware, J. E., Jr., Rogers, W. H., Keeler, E. B., Davies, A. R., Donald, C. A., Goldberg, G. A., Lohr, K. N., Masthay, P. C., & Newhouse, J. P., "Does Free Care Improve Adults' Health?" *New England Journal of Medicine, 309,* 1426–1434, 1983.

Center for Mental Health Services, *Mental Health, United States, 1996*, ed. R. W. Manderscheid & M. A. Sonnenschein (DHHS Publication No. [SMA] 96-3098). Washington, DC: U.S. Government Printing Office, 1996.

Cohen, N. L., Putnam, J. F., & Sullivan, A. M., "The Mentally Ill Homeless: Isolation and Adaptation," *Hospital and Community Psychiatry, 35*, 922–924, 1984.

Domenici, P. V., "Mental Health Care Policy in the 1990s: Discrimination in Health Care Coverage of the Seriously Mentally Ill," *Journal of Clinical Psychiatry, 54*(Suppl.), 5–6, 1993.

Fink, M., *Convulsive Therapy: Theory and Practice*. New York: Raven Press, 1979.

Fink, P. J., & Weinstein, S. P., "Whatever Happened to Psychiatry? The Deprofessionalization of Community Mental Health Centers," *American Journal of Psychiatry, 136*, 406, 1979.

Foley, H. A., & Sharfstein, S. S., *Madness and Government: Who Cares for the Mentally Ill?* Washington, DC: American Psychiatric Press, 1983.

Frank, J. D., & Frank, J. B., *Persuasion and Healing: A Comparative Study of Psychotherapy* (3rd ed.). Baltimore: Johns Hopkins University Press, 1991.

Frank, R. G., Koyanagi, C., & McGuire, T. G., "The Politics and Economics of Mental Health Charity Laws," *Health Affairs, 16*(4), 108–119, 1997.

Geller, J. L., "The Right to Treatment," in R. Rosner (Ed.), *Principles and Practice of Forensic Psychiatry*. New York: Chapman and Hall, 1994.

Ginsberg, L., *Social Work Almanac* (2nd ed.). Washington, DC: National Association of Social Workers Press, 1995.

Goldman, H. H., & Manderscheid, R. W., "Chronic Mental Disorder in the United States," in R. W. Manderscheid & S. A. Barrett (Eds.), *Mental Health, United States, 1987* (DHHS Publication No. ADM 87-1518). Washington, DC: U.S. Government Printing Office, 1987.

Grebb, J. A., "Psychosurgery," in H. I. Kaplan & B. J. Sadock (Eds.), *Comprehensive Textbook of Psychiatry* (6th ed., pp. 2140–2144). Baltimore: Williams and Wilkins, 1995.

Gutheil, T. G., "Rogers v. Commissioner: Denouement of an Important Right-to-Refuse-Treatment Case," *American Journal of Psychiatry, 142*, 213, 1985.

Hoge, S. K., Appelbaum, P. S., Lawlor, T., Beck, J. C., Litman, R., Greer, A., Gutheil, G., & Kaplan, E., "A Prospective, Multi-center Study of Patients' Refusal of Antipsychotic Medication," *Archives of General Psychiatry, 47*, 949–956, 1990.

Institute of Medicine, *Research on Mental Illness and Addictive Disorders: Progress and Prospects*. Washington, DC: National Academy Press, 1984.

Kaufman, E., "The Right of Treatment Suit as an Agent of Change," *American Journal of Psychiatry, 136*, 1428, 1979.

Kendall, R. E., "The Concept of Disease and Its Implications for Psychiatry," *British Journal of Psychiatry, 127*, 305, 1975.

Kessler, R. C., McGonagle, K. A., Zhao, S., Nelson, C. B., Hughes, M., Eshleman, S., Wittchen, H., & Kendler, K. S., "Lifetime and 12-month Prevalence of DSM-III-R Psychiatric Disorders in the United States: Results from the National Comorbidity Survey," *Archives of General Psychiatry, 51*, 8–19, 1994.

Kiesler, C. A., & Silbulkin, A. E., "Episodic Rate of Mental Hospitalization: Stable or Increasing?" *American Journal of Psychiatry, 141*, 44–48, 1984.

Koran, L. M., Sox, H. C., Marton, K. I., Moltzen, S., Sox, C. H., Kraemenr, H. C., Imai, K., Kelsey, T. G., Rose, T. G., Levin, L. C., & Chandra, S., "Medical Evaluation of Psychiatric Patients: 1. Results in a State Mental Health System," *Archives of General Psychiatry, 46*, 733–740, 1989.

Krizay, J., "Federal Employees' Experience as a Guide to the Cost of Insuring Psychiatric Services in the Various States," *American Journal of Psychiatry, 139*, 866, 1982.

Lamb, H. R., "The New Asylums in the Community," *Archives of General Psychiatry, 36*, 129, 1979.

Langsley, D. G., "Prevention in Psychiatry: Primary, Secondary, and Tertiary," In H. I. Kaplan & B. J. Sadock (Eds.), *Comprehensive Textbook of Psychiatry* (Vol. 1, 4th ed.). Baltimore: Williams and Wilkins, 1985.

McGarry, A. L., & Kaplan, H. A., "Overview: Current Trends in Mental Health Law," *American Journal of Psychiatry, 130*, 621–630, 1973.

Mills, M. J., Sullivan, G., & Eth, S., "Protecting Third Parties: A Decade after Tarasoff," *American Journal of Psychiatry, 144*, 68–74, 1987.

Moore, M. D., "Some Myths about 'Mental Illness,' " *Archives of General Psychiatry, 32*, 1483, 1975.

Mora, G., "Historical and Theoretical Trends in Psychiatry," in A. M. Freedman, B. J. Sadock, & H. I. Kaplan (Eds.), *Comprehensive Textbook of Psychiatry* (Vol. 2, 2nd ed.). Baltimore: Williams and Wilkins, 1975.

Murphy, J., "Psychiatric Labeling in Cross Cultural Perspective," *Science, 191*, 1019, 1976.

Myers, J. K., Weissman, M. M., Tischler, G. L., Holzer, C. E., Leaf, P. T., Drauschel, H., et al., "Six-month Prevalence of Psychiatric Disorders in Three Communities," *Archives of General Psychiatry, 41*, 959, 1984.

Narrow, W. E., "Use of Services by Persons with Mental and Addictive Disorders: Findings from the National Institute of Mental Health Epidemiologic Catchment Area Program," *Archives of General Psychiatry, 50*, 95, 1993.

National Advisory Mental Health Council, "Health Care Reform for Americans with Severe Mental Illness: Report of the National Advisory Mental Health Council," *American Journal of Psychiatry, 150*, 1447–1465, 1993.

National Foundation for Brain Research, *"The Cost of Disorders of the Brain.* Washington, DC: Author, 1992.

Olfson, M., & Pincus, A., "Outpatient Psychotherapy in the United States: 1. Volume, Costs and User Characteristics," *American Journal of Psychiatry, 151*, 1281–1288, 1994.

Olfson, M., Pincus, H. A., & Dial, T. H., "Professional Practice Patterns of U.S. Psychiatrists," *American Journal of Psychiatry, 151*, 89–95, 1994.

Peterson, B. D., West, J., & Pincus, H. A., Kohout, J., Pion, G. M., Wicherski, M. M., et al., "An Update on Human Resources in Mental Health," *Mental Health, United States, 1996*, 168–204, 1996.

Pincus, H. A., Zarin, D. A., & West, J. C., "Peering into the "Black Box": Measuring Outcomes of Managed Care," *Archives of General Psychiatry, 53*, 870–877, 1996.

President's Commission on Mental Health, *"Report to the President—1978* (Vols. 1–6). Washington, DC: U.S. Government Printing Office, 1978.

Rabkin, J., "Public Attitudes toward Mental Illness: A Review of the Literature," *Schizophrenia Bulletin, 10*, 9, 1974.

Redick, R. W., Witkin, M. J., Atay, J. E., & Manderscheid, R. W., "Highlights of Organized Mental Health Services in 1992 and Major National and State Trends," in *Mental Health, United States, 1996*, 90–137, 1996.

Regier, D. A., Narrow, W., Rae, D., Manderscheid, R. W., Locke, B. Z., & Goodwin, F. K., "The De Facto U.S. Mental and Addictive Disorders Service System: Epidemiologic Catchment Area Prospective 1-Year Prevalence Rates of Disorders and Services," *Archives of General Psychiatry, 50*, 85–94, 1993.

Reifman, A., & Wyatt, R. J., "Lithium: A Brake in the Rising Cost of Mental Illness," *Archives of General Psychiatry, 37*, 288, 1980.

Robertson, M. J., & Greenblatt, M., *Homelessness: A National Perspective*. New York: Plenum Press, 1992.

Rodnick, E. H., "Clinical Psychology," in H. I. Kaplan & B. J. Sadock (Eds.), *Comprehensive Textbook of Psychiatry* (Vol. 1, 4th ed.). Baltimore: Williams and Wilkins, 1985.

Roth, L. H., "A Commitment Law for Patients, Doctors and Lawyers," *American Journal of Psychiatry, 136*, 1121, 1979.

Rupp, A., Gause, E. A., & Regier, D. A., "Rese   ᵃᵗⁱᵒⁿs of Cost of Illness Studies for Mental Disorders," *British Jour

Schreter, R., Sharfstein, S. S., & Schreter, S.   *Dollars: The Continuum of Mental Health Services*.   Psychiatric Press, 1997.

Sederer, L. I., "Judicial and Legislative Respons   *rican Journal of Psychiatry, 149*, 1157–1161, 1992.

Sharfstein, S. S., "Models of Managed Mer   ales & S. C. Yudofsky (Eds.), *Practical Clinical Stra   and Anxiety Disorders in a Managed Care Environme   an Psychiatric Association, 1996.

Sharfstein, S. S., & Magnas, H. L., "Insuring   *erican Journal of Psychiatry, 132*, 70, 1975.

Sharfstein, S. S., Muszynski, S., & Myers, E., ...   *chiatric Care: Update and Appraisal*. Washington, DC: American Psychiatric Press, 1984.

Sharfstein, S. S., & Stoline, A. M., "Reform Issues for Insuring Mental Health Care," *Health Affairs, 11*, 84–97, Fall 1992.

Sharfstein, S. S., Stoline, A. M., & Goldman, H. H., "Psychiatric Care and Health Insurance Reform," *American Journal of Psychiatry, 150*, 7–18, 1993.

Sharfstein, S. S., & Taube, C., "Reductions in Insurance for Mental Disorders: Adverse Selection, Moral Hazard, and Consumer Demand," *American Journal of Psychiatry, 139*, 1425–1430, 1982.

Shryock, R. H., "The Beginnings: From Colonial Days to the Foundation of the American Psychiatric Association," in J. K. Hall, G. Zilboorg, & H. A. Bunker (Eds.), *One Hundred Years of American Psychiatry*. New York: Columbia University Press, 1947.

Simon, R. I., *Clinical Psychiatry and the Law* (2nd ed.). Washington, DC: American Psychiatric Press, 1992.

Smith, M. L., & Glass, G. V., "Meta-Analysis of Psychotherapy Outcome Studies," *American Psychologist, 32*, 752–760, 1977.

Strecker, E. A., "Military Psychiatry: World War I: 1917–1918," in J. K. Hall, G. Zilboorg, & H. A. Bunker (Eds.), *One Hundred Years of American Psychiatry*. New York: Columbia University Press, 1947.

Szasz, T. S., *The Myth of Mental Illness*. New York: Hocker-Harper, 1961.

Talbott, J. A., *Contemporary Social Issues and Decisions That Will Affect the Future Practice of Psychiatry*. Unpublished manuscript, 1985.

Talbott, J. A. (Ed.), *State Mental Hospitals: Problems and Potentials*. New York: Human Sciences Press, 1980.

Taube, C. A., Goldman, H. H., & Salkver, D., "Medicaid Coverage for Mental Illness: Balancing Access and Costs," *Health Affairs, 9*, 5–18, 1990.

Torrey, E. F., *Nowhere to Go: The Tragic Odyssey of the Homeless Mentally Ill*. New York: Harper & Row, 1988.

United States Conference of Mayors, *The Continued Growth of Hunger, Homelessness, and Poverty in America's Cities: 1986*. Washington, DC: Author, 1996.

U.S. Department of Health and Human Services, *The Registered Nurse Population: Findings from the National Sample Survey of Registered Nurses, March 1992*. Washington, DC: U.S. Government Printing Office, 1994.

Weiner, B. A., "Supreme Court Decisions on Mental Health: A Review," *Hospital and Community Psychiatry, 33*, 461–464, 1982.

Weiner, R. D., Fink, M., Hammersley, D. S., Small, I. F., Moench, L. A., & Sackheim, H., *The Practice of Electroconvulsive Therapy: Recommendations for Treatment, Training, and Privileging*. Washington, DC: American Psychiatric Press, 1990.

Wells, K. B., Manning, W. G., Jr., Duan, N., Ware, J. E., Jr., & Newhouse, J. P., *Cost Sharing and the Demand for Ambulatory Mental Health Services*. Santa Monica, CA: Rand Corporation, 1982.

Zeman, P. M., & Schwartz, H. I., "Hospitalization: Voluntary and Involuntary," in R. Rosner (Ed.), *Principals and Practice of Forensic Psychiatry*. New York: Chapman and Hall, 1994.

10

Health Maintenance Organizations and Managed Care

Anthony R. Kovner

Learning Objectives

1. Identify why HMOs and managed care have developed as they have in the United States.
2. Distinguish the differences between managed and traditional health care delivery.
3. Describe what purchasers want and expect from HMOs in performance.
4. Distinguish between group, staff, and IPA HMO models.
5. Identify what the HMO premium goes to pay for.
6. Analyze how HMOs are changing, the pros and cons of organizing health care through HMOs, and variations in HMO performance.

Topical Outline

What purchasers want
Historical development of managed care
HMO organizational structure
HMO statistics and characteristics
Some prototype HMOs
The HMO premium and where does it go
Forces compelling and constraining change in HMOs
    Regulators

Large purchasers
Competitors
Hospitals
Physicians
Members/advocates
Current issues
Efficiency: Do HMOs cost less?
Appropriateness: Do they encourage too little care?
Value added: Do they add sufficient value relative to cost?
Externalities: Do they pay their fair share for medical evaluation and research
and to provide care to the uninsured?

**Key Words: HMO, managed care, health plan, prepayment, capitation, pre-
ferred provider organizations, point of service plans, IPA model, group model,
staff model, premium.**

Managed care is any health services arrangement in which a contract for both
the services and the payment is created between a provider and a purchaser
(usually an employer or a government agency) on behalf of a group of consumers
or members (Hodge, 1996). This is a fundamental departure from the traditional
direct contractual relationship between a patient and a provider for services.
Managed care organizations (MCOs) are health care systems under which a broad
scope of medical services is provided for a fixed amount of money, negotiated
in advance. This chapter focuses on health maintenance organizations (HMOs)
as one model of managed care. The chapter is divided into sections, as follows:
what purchasers want, historical development of managed care and HMOs, HMO
organizational structure, HMO statistics and characteristics, where the HMO
premium goes, forces compelling and constraining change in managed care, and
issues in managed care (see for a taxonomy of MCOs Weiner and DeLissavoy, 1993).

What Purchasers Want

A distinguishing characteristic of the American health care system is that services
are largely purchased by organizations on behalf of individuals rather than by
individuals themselves. These purchasers include Medicare (see General Accounting Office, 1996), Medicaid, and employers. Of course, not all Americans are
represented by large purchasers of health services. Not all poor people are eligible

for Medicaid, and not all employers offer health insurance to their employees. Moreover, not all purchasers are effective purchasers, and what insurance they offer is highly variable with regard to benefits, cost to the employee, and allowable choice.

Purchasers have been dissatisfied for a long time with the value they have been getting for the health benefits they purchase. Less dissatisfied perhaps are employees whose pay would probably have been higher if the cost of health benefits had not increased so much. Cost and quality of medical care has been a primary concern of many purchasers (Boland, 1993). The cost has been too high relative to any differential improvements in health status, and the quality has been highly variable. Since about 1990 more purchasers have begun to believe that they can intervene to do something about high costs and uneven quality.

For example, the Xerox Company gives its employees standard comparisons of health plan performance to help them choose among a limited number of plans approved by the company. The information provided includes, for example: years of operation, numbers of HMO members, percentage of eligible Xerox employees enrolled, premium changes over 3 years, and the percentage of HMO total premium revenues spent on medical care. Xerox also informs employees as to whether the HMO has been accredited by the National Committee for Quality Assurance (NCQA), an industry-sponsored MCO that reviews HMO performance in the following six areas: quality improvement, physician credentials, members' rights and responsibilities, preventive health services, medical records, and managing the use of care. Xerox has established a "centers of excellence" program for hospital care, helping ensure that patients have access to hospitals that have more than the average experience with complex procedures and have documented evidence of better outcomes. As of 1996, 35,846, or 75.9%, of Xerox beneficiaries were HMO enrollees. Xerox spends over $302 million per year on health care (Xerox Health Link, 1995).

The Health Care Financing Administration and various other agencies of the federal and state governments have similar intentions with regard to Medicare and Medicaid beneficiaries and their own employees enrolled in MCOs (Etheredge, 1995). But of course, these kinds of concerns and priorities are not shared by all purchasers and employers. Further, many of them, particularly small employers, do not even provide health insurance as a benefit to their work force. There are 40 to 60 million Americans, most of whom work, who lack any health insurance and millions of other Americans whose insurance coverage is less adequate than that provided by Xerox, Medicare, or Medicaid.

HMOs, previously called prepaid group practices, were developed in the first place often by employers seeking to provide health care to employees in remote locations, where there were few, if any, physicians and hospitals. For example, the Kaiser Corporation did so when it was building dams in the western United States prior to World War II. Given a major boost (and their current name) during the Nixon administration (1969–1974), HMOs have become popular and prevalent because they aim to control annual cost increases to employers and purchasers and to improve quality. Questions have been raised regarding the extent to which HMOs control costs, as purchasers are concerned with total (rather than merely HMO) health benefits costs. Even as HMO costs hold steady, total costs may increase if healthier individuals join the HMOs while the oldest and sickest employees remain with traditional health insurance coverage. Questions have also been raised as to the quality of care provided by HMOs, although it is acknowledged that this may vary among HMOs, even as it varies among providers who do not treat HMO patients.

An HMO combines financing mechanisms and a delivery system under the control and direction of a single management entity—the health plan. HMOs provide a broad scope of benefits to a voluntarily enrolled population for a prenegotiated and fixed periodic premium payment (Shouldice, 1991). What differentiates HMOs from traditional arrangements for health care delivery are the following factors: (1) the combining of the financing and delivery systems under a single organizational entity, (2) a broad scope of benefits, (3) usually a voluntarily enrolled population (this is not the case if an employer offers only one HMO plan to its employees), (4) prepayment, (5) an organized provider system, and (6) the assumption of financial risk by the HMO. The purchaser enters into a contract with the HMO under which the HMO agrees to provide the purchaser's employees or beneficiaries with a broad scope of benefits for a prenegotiated sum. The HMO assures benefit availability to employees of the purchaser over a designated period even if the population should require more health services than anticipated because of, for example, unexpected occurrences of diseases or changes in utilization patterns or because the HMO has to hire more providers than anticipated.

Other forms of managed care besides HMOs are as follows: (1) direct contracts by purchasers with providers who do *not* assume risk, such as preferred provider organizations (PPOs contract with selected providers who, in exchange for a guarantee of patient care volume, provide health services at a discount); (2) point of service (POS) plans, which combine features of an HMO with the provider selection flexibility of a PPO (in most cases, as in an HMO, the POS member selects a primary care physician, who has the primary responsibility for managing the patient's care; however, members are permitted to seek care from outside the POS network and pay higher deductibles and co-insurance); and (3) administrative-services-only products. Under this last arrangement, the employer bears the financial risk for the cost of services. The HMO bills the employer on a discounted fee-for-service basis for medical services, a fee for "renting" a provider network (many or one specialty such as mental health or behavioral medicine) and for using the HMO's quality management and utilization review program. As more employers have enrolled in POS plans and PPOs, HMOs have expanded their offerings to cover services provided outside the plan. According to Gabel (1997), today most HMOs do not view themselves as HMOs but as MCOs that offer an array of managed care plans. Nearly three quarters of American workers with health insurance now receive that coverage through an HMO, a PPO, or a POS (Jensen et al., 1997).

This chapter focuses on HMOs (rather than PPOs or managed care plans) as the most important and more "managed" care product. Other managed care products, such as PPOs, will be covered in other chapters (for flows of funds, see chapter 3, "Financing for Health Care," and for organization of physicians, see chapter 7, "Ambulatory Care").

Historical Development

In 1932, the national Committee on the Costs of Medical Care recommended the linkage of group practice to prepayment for health services, even as it opposed compulsory health insurance that would, in its view, furnish a medical service limited in scope and deficient in quality (MacLeod, 1993).

The roots of managed care began with the plantation owners, lumber and mining firms, and railroads that provided health services to attract and to retain workers (Friedman, 1996). A key innovative approach to providing health care for workers was developed by the Kaiser corporations and Sidney Garfield, MD, who suggested capitating (paying one amount per each insured for the year) the workers on the 1930s Grand Coulee Dam project in eastern Washington. The experiment was so successful that, when large numbers of workers joined the Kaiser shipbuilding business in Oakland, California, during World War II, the Kaiser Foundation Health Plan was established.

Under the program, the Kaiser Health Plan and the Kaiser Foundation Hospitals (one entity) contract with the Permanente medical groups. Each Kaiser Plan enrolls members, maintains records, collects the premium payments from employers, markets the plan, and contracts with each Permanente medical group. The hospitals corporation provides all facilities, and the Permanente medical groups recruit physicians, who, after a probationary period, become partners (Brown, 1983).

An early HMO pioneer was Michael Shadid, whom Emily Friedman (1996) calls the father of health care cooperatives. Dr. Shadid proposed a prepaid hospital–physician cooperative in Elk City, Oklahoma, the first such organization in the United States. Shadid influenced the consumers who founded the Group Health Cooperative of Puget Sound in Seattle in 1945, an HMO in which physicians are directly salaried by the plan.

The San Joaquin Foundation for Medical Care was established in 1954 as the first association of independently practicing physicians (IPA) in the nation. It was developed by the county medical society when a local union proposed to invite Kaiser-Permanente to establish a clinic for union members. Local physicians established the foundation to provide comprehensive physician services for a fixed capitation rate without forming a group practice. At the same time, the physicians maintained the principles of fee-for-service practice and free choice of physician (Luft, 1981).

The passage of the federal HMO Act in 1973 and its amendments enabled managed care plans to increase in numbers and expand enrollments financed by grants, contracts, and loans. After the passage of the HMO Act, strong support for the HMO concept came from business and government, to decrease costs and encourage free-market competition with only limited government intervention (MacLeod, 1993).

The Federal Employees Health Benefits Program, which went into operation in 1960, covers more than 10 million federal employees and retirees and their dependents and is the largest employer-sponsored health benefits program in the United States today. The federal Office of Personnel Management pays a portion of the premium, and the employee or annuitant is responsible for the remainder. The government contribution has historically been set at 60% of the average premium of the two high-option, government-wide plans, the two largest employee organizations, and the two largest comprehensive plans (Michaels & Rinn, 1993).

Many HMOs are owned by insurance companies. But they are also owned by cooperatives, nonprofit organizations, hospitals, and doctor groups. For example, in the early 1990s, the Mullikin Medical Centers in California (subsequently merged into MedPartners/Mullikin) put together within a very short time the second largest medical group practice in the state of California ("Physician equity model," 1993). Characteristic of this model of HMO, which gains access to HMO contracts for physicians, is the ability of physicians to share risk and reward through shared ownership. A parent company of stockholders owns the health plan and the hospital and contracts with medical groups and the IPAs for management services. The physicians own stock in every entity. With this organization in place, Mullikin could enter into HMO contracts that pay capitation for both hospital and physician services. Then, within the organization, capitation income can be deployed to create profitability in the medical groups or fund the capital and operating needs of the hospital ("Physician equity model," 1993).

The for-profits have been growing rapidly in large part because of their advantages over nonprofits in securing large amounts of capital. This is true even though some states, such as Minnesota, prohibit for-profits from operating in other states (Gabel, 1997). In 1996, Aetna Life and Casualty Company, one of America's leading insurers, paid $8.9 billion for an independent for-profit HMO, U.S. Healthcare. This was the first big acquisition by an insurer of a company involved in the noninsurance part of the health care business. It was also the

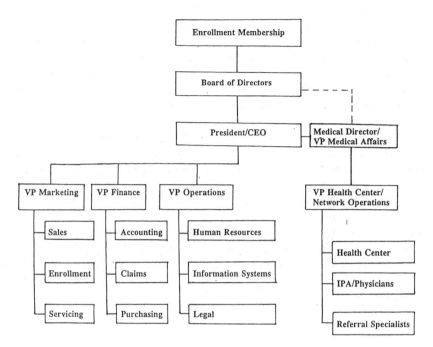

FIGURE 10.1 Typical HMO table of organization.

biggest takeover the health management sector has ever seen. Together the two companies manage health care services for 23 million people, one in every 11 Americans. More than 10 million of these people are members of managed care plans ("Aetna and U.S. Healthcare," 1996).

HMO Organizational Structure

There are five main elements of HMOs: purchasers, plans, hospital providers, medical providers, and members (as shown in Figure 10.1). Purchasers pay plans and/or providers who furnish medical care to members. Each of these five groups can be organized in different ways. The main HMO organizational elements are the plans and the providers. It is possible, of course, but not typical, for either purchasers or member organizations to own and operate plans, usually through separately owned corporations set up for this purpose. For example, in many large cities and in some states, hospital organizations have sponsored "Healthfirst" plans, which are then "sold" to their employees and to others on a voluntary or other basis. Member organizations such as consumer cooperatives have also sponsored their own plans, such as the Group Health Cooperative of Puget Sound.

The more common HMO models are local integrated health systems or national/regional HMOs, which have three main components: plan, hospital, and physicians. Monies from the purchaser can go to any of the three component groups, to some combination of two, or to all acting together in joint partnership. In large national/regional HMOs there is often a geographic layer of organization as well. In this case, an HMO's organizational structure may be decentralized, for example, into nine regions of the United States. Each has a plan, hospitals, and a physician organization (and there may be, as well, national "advisory" organizations within the HMO, such as a council of all the plans, and/or all the hospitals, and/or all the physicians.) What makes running an HMO different from a hospital or group practice are the following additional organizational functions: sales and enrollment, membership relations (from service to health education), risk management, organization and management of clinicians or providers as a network, and enhanced and more sophisticated information systems. These functions may be carried out in part by hospitals and group practices, but they form main organizational elements in any HMO. The three main HMO components are described below.

The Plan

The plan is owned by a corporation (not-for-profit, for-profit, or government), by physicians, and/or by hospitals. The plan is generally responsible for contracting with and marketing health services to employers and other payers and for relations with members. The plan must also comply with government regulations and assume or contract out some or most of the risk of insuring members. The plan is responsible for contracting with providers to deliver all required health services and monitoring provider performance.

The Hospitals

Hospitals may be owned by the plan, or the plan can contract for hospital services. For organizational purposes, hospital facilities may be grouped with all other HMO facilities, including physician group practice centers.

The Physicians

There are three main ways of organizing HMO physicians: (1) the IPA model, (2) the group model, and (3) the staff model. More than one of these ways can be used in the same HMO. When the models are used together, this is sometimes called a fourth model, the network model (Vogel, 1993). Gold et al. (Gold, Hurley, Lake, Ensor, & Berenson, 1995) conclude that hybrid HMO models are common, and the differences among the types of HMOs are less extensive than is commonly assumed.

Under the IPA model, the health plan contracts with an association of physicians, usually a separate legal entity. The physicians maintain their own offices and practices, seeing HMO and non-HMO patients side by side. Advantages of this type of model are that it doesn't require a large capital investment and that individual physicians perceive that they have more autonomy. Yet they are able to compete with physicians organized under the group and staff models (Shenkin, 1995).

In the group model, a health plan contracts with independent multispecialty medical group practices, that only see HMO patients. The advantages of this arrangement include deeper commitment of physicians to the plan (because it is the source of all their patients), economies of scale that act to lower unit costs, and one-stop shopping for the plan members. Disadvantages are the large capital investment required for group facilities and a limited choice of physicians for plan members. An emerging type of group model is the physician equity model (Mullikin is an example, subsequently acquired by MedPartners), under which a for-profit group of physicians itself is the HMO.

The staff model is the third type of HMO method for organizing physicians. In this model the plan provides both management and medical functions. The physicians are plan employees. Advantages of this model include legal simplicity, simpler administration, and perceived greater control over physician behavior. Disadvantages include difficulty in recruiting (many physicians see this model as unduly restricting their practice and autonomy), high start-up costs to hire physicians and guarantee salaries, and limited choice of physicians for a similarly sized membership.

HMO Statistics and Characteristics

As of January 1, 1996 (see Table 10.1) there were 630 HMOs in the United States, with 59,090,989 members. This included 628 HMOs serving 52,464,445 "pure" (non-point-of-service) enrollees, and 291 HMOs serving 6,043,422 "open-ended" (point-of-service) enrollees. These figures represent vast growth in about 20 years. In 1975 (see Figure 10.2) there were fewer than 100 HMOs, with under 10 million members and no point-of-service plans. Three hundred sixty-six of the HMOs follow the IPA model; 41, the group model; and 19, the staff model. The rest are mixed models. Over 80% of members are enrolled in either IPA or mixed models.

TABLE 10.1   Plan Characteristics for Pure HMO Products as of January 1, 1996: Enrollment and Number of HMOs

Characteristics	Total members	Percentage of total	Total HMOs	Percentage of total
All HMOs	52,464,445	100	628	100.0
Model type				
Staff	734,265	1.4	19	3.0
IPA	21,745,717	41.4	366	58.3
Network	3,388,604	6.5	62	9.9
Group	9,373,947	17.9	41	6.5
Mixed	17,221,912	32.8	140	22.3
Size/pure enrollees				
Less than 5,000	184,230	0.4	107	17.0
5,000–14,999	884,708	1.7	91	14.5
15,000–24,999	1,370,255	2.6	70	11.1
25,000–49,999	4,587,664	8.7	125	19.9
50,000–99,999	6,943,111	13.2	97	15.4
100,000 or more	38,494,477	73.4	138	22.0
Age				
Less than 1 year	229,195	0.4	57	9.1
1–2 years	1,276,697	2.4	81	12.9
3–5 years	1,696,061	3.2	30	4.8
6–9 years	10,672,506	20.3	161	25.6
10 years or more	38,589,986	73.6	299	47.6
Region				
Northeast	3,540,176	6.7	38	6.1
Mid-Atlantic	8,333,819	15.9	73	11.6
South Atlantic	7,283,212	13.9	116	18.5
East South Central	1,451,188	2.8	36	5.7
West South Central	3,309,149	6.3	65	10.4
East North Central	7,683,890	14.6	129	20.5
West North Central	2,359,069	4.5	52	8.3
Mountain	3,064,731	5.8	54	8.6
Pacific	15,439,211	29.4	65	10.4
Federal qualification				
Not qualified	16,781,999	32.0	350	55.7
Qualified	35,682,446	68.0	278	44.3
Tax status				
Nonprofit	21,443,363	40.9	171	27.2
For profit	31,021,082	59.1	457	72.8

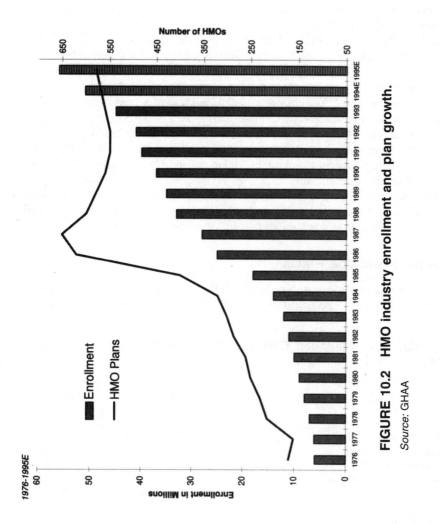

FIGURE 10.2 HMO industry enrollment and plan growth.

Source: GHAA

289

The nation's largest HMOs, ranked by pure enrollment as of January 1, 1995, accounted for 35.5% of the industry's pure enrollment. These same HMOs, ranked by open-ended enrollment, accounted for 62.4% of the industry's open-ended enrollment (Interstudy, 1995). The ten largest plans had 80.5% managed care enrollment of all plans (Table 10.2) (Thorpe, 1997).

Slightly under one half (47.6%) of HMOs have been in operation for 10 years or less, but over 73% of HMO members are enrolled in plans that have been in existence for 10 years or more. Among nine regions in the country, the largest HMO membership (15.4 million) is in the Pacific region, and the largest number of HMOs are in the East North Central (129) and the South Atlantic (116) regions. Less than half (44.3%) of HMOs are qualified by the federal government as meeting their voluntary national standards; 457, or 72.8%, of HMOs are for profit, and they have 59.1% of total HMO members. This compares with nonprofit enrollment in the remaining 27.2% of HMOs, with 40.9% of total enrollment (Interstudy, 1996). Percentage of enrollment by state varies widely as shown in Figure 10.3. As of 1995, 35.3% of California's population was enrolled in HMOs and only 0.2% of Mississippi's (*Journal of Accountancy*, 1996).

Some Prototype HMOs

Descriptions of some prototype HMOs follow. These have been chosen because they are large and successful as of 1996. They include the Kaiser Permanente

TABLE 10.2 Managed Care Enrollment of the Ten Largest Plans, 1995

Plan	Enrollment (millions)	Cumulative enrollment (%)
Blue Cross	8.5	15.7
United Healthcare	6.7	28.1
Kaiser Permanente	6.7	40.6
Aetna/U.S. Healthcare	·5.7	51.1
Prudential	4.7	59.8
Cigna	3.9	67.0
PacifiCare/FHP[a]	3.6	73.7
Humana	2.1	77.6
Health Systems[b]	1.8	80.9
All other plans	10.3	100.0
Total all plans	54.0	100.0

[a]Data reflect PacifiCare's buyout of FHP; prior to acquisition, each plan enrolled approximately 1.8 million subscribers.
[b]Health Systems is involved in merger discussions with Foundation Health Plan.
Source. Sanford C. Bernstein and Co. 1996 and *Interstudy* 1996.

Medical program, Group Health Cooperative of Puget Sound (prior to the recent merger with Kaiser Permanente), and Humana.

Kaiser Permanente Medical Program

In 1996 the Kaiser Foundation Health Plan cared for 7.49 million enrollees with 9,396 physicians and annual revenues of $13.2 billion. Kaiser Permanente is a national program located in 16 states. Kaiser (the hospital and health plan) and Permanente (the medical groups) work as partners to provide prepaid medical care. The number of members served by the 12 Kaiser Permanente Medical Groups range from 55,000 to 2.5 million.

The Kaiser Permanente Medical Program pursues the implementation of seven basic principles of form and function, which were developed in the 1930s by Dr. Sidney Garfield. These include preventive care and health promotion, joint physician responsibility for program management and effectiveness, prepayment, multispecialty group practice, organized facilities and service, voluntary enrollment and consumer choice, and nonprofit auspices (Kissick, 1994).

Group Health Cooperative of Puget Sound

As of 1995, Group Health Cooperative of Puget Sound (Washington) was a recognized leader among staff-model HMOs. Its enrollment approached 500,000, and it employed more than 750 full-time-equivalent physicians and other medical staff and almost 900 full-time-equivalent staff nurses, who provided health services at 30 primary care or family care medical centers, five specialty medical centers, two hospitals, an inpatient-care center, and a skilled nursing facility. Revenues for 1992 were $854 million.

Humana

Headquartered in Louisville, Kentucky, Humana is a for-profit corporation that as of 1995 provided health care services to 3.8 million members (Humana, 1996). Humana offers plans to seniors, Medicaid recipients, individuals, and more than 100,000 small and large businesses. It offers a full array of managed care health plans: HMOs, preferred provider organizations, and administrative-services-only plans. Most Humana medical services are provided by IPAs, the most common form of HMO (see Table 10.1). At Humana, physicians are employed neither by the HMO (as at Group Health of Puget Sound) nor by a medical group contracted with by the HMO (as at Kaiser-Permanente). Rather, most physicians

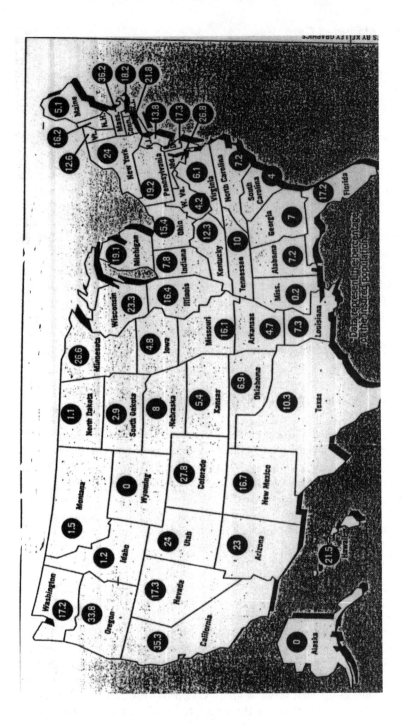

FIGURE 10.3   Data represent the percentage of the insured population.

Source: *Journal of Accountancy*, March 1996, p. 20.

provide services to members as part of their individual contracts with the Humana HMO, of the IPA type, while still seeing their fee-for-service patients.

In 1995 operating revenues were $4.7 billion. Humana acquired a health insurance company in 1995, adding 1.3 million new members, and was chosen by the Department of Defense to provide health care to approximately 1 million military beneficiaries in the southeastern United States. All four Humana health plans inspected by the National Committee for Quality Assurance (NCQA) were accredited. Humana sold off its hospitals in 1993. As of January 1, 1995, Humana had 1,753,600 HMO members in 16 plans.

The HMO Premium and Where It Goes

According to InterStudy (1996) average monthly commercial HMO premiums in 1995 were $384 for families and $140 for individuals (a traditional plan). Corresponding amounts for an open-ended plan were $389 for families and $147 for individuals.

As shown in Figure 10.4, a purchaser pays 100% of the premium to a health plan. This premium is divided into three parts: the hospital, the physicians, and the health plan. These three parts may be paid to separate organizations or to one organization. Around 1992 in California, for example, the typical premium was divided by plans among the three parts as follows: hospital (30%–33% of the premium), physicians (30%–33% of the premium), and health plan (35%–40% of the premium). Typically, the money was paid by the purchaser to the HMO that contracted for hospital and physician services. Hospitals can be paid on a capitation, per case, or per diem basis covering the following: all inpatient hospital costs, such as supplies, pharmacy, room charges, and diagnostics; reinsurance premiums; and administration. Typically, reinsurance to cover adverse cost experience much higher than anticipated is contracted out by the plan to insurance companies specializing in reinsurance.

The physicians' services premium covers all outpatient services, inpatient physician services, all outpatient imaging, all outpatient lab and diagnostic services, durable medical equipment, home health care, reinsurance premiums (for physicians' services), and administration. Physicians may be paid according to a fee schedule or on a capitation basis.

The premium part for the health plan was divided up into five major categories (with percentage of the full premium shown in parentheses): pharmacy (7%); out-of-area allocation (covering services for patients as needed in a different geographical location than that served by the plan, 6%); administration (12%–14%), which includes enrollment, marketing, sales, and licensing expenses; broker commissions (4%–7%, to sell policies to small employers and individuals); and profit (6%).

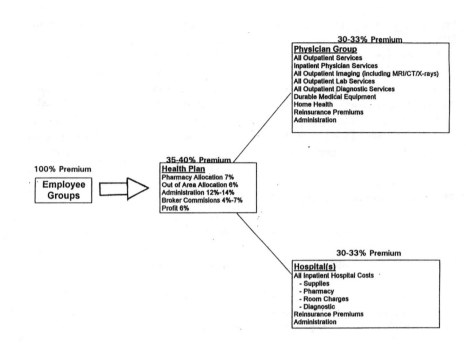

FIGURE 10.4   Division of HMO reimbursement (California, 1992).

Forces Compelling and Constraining Change in Managed Care

Some of the stakeholders pressuring change in managed care include the following: government regulators, large purchasers, competitors, hospitals, physicians,
and members/consumer advocates. What follows is a discussion of what it is
that these stakeholders want from managed care, approaches they are taking to
achieve such objectives, and likely responses from HMOs (and other managed
care organizations).

Regulators

Regulators are interested in cost, quality, and access. Government is a large
purchaser as well as a regulator. With regard to populations other than Medicare,
Medicaid, and the indigent, government regulates HMOs largely as other businesses are regulated. The government wants to see to it that minimum standards

of quality are met and that laws applicable to other businesses—from labor relations to environmental pollution—are followed by HMOs. Government has intruded into the management of HMOs under the protection of quality banner.

For example, government has mandated that HMOs provide certain benefits, such as mental health care, or that HMOs provide certain services, such as 2 days of hospitalization for a mother delivering a child. Government has also regulated HMOs with regard to disclosure, for example, how physicians are paid and what incentives are offered. HMOs respond to regulation differently depending on competitive consideration, either regarding other MCOs or relative to other providers who "do not manage care." For example, HMOs have definite interests regarding the amounts of insurance reserves required by the plans under state insurance regulations.

Large Purchasers

Large purchasers, like regulators, are interested in cost, quality, and access to care for their members. Purchasers want to make sure that premiums are appropriate and that HMOs are not making excess profits "at their expense" by, for example, charging the same rates for younger, healthier populations as they would if those enrolled were older and sicker than the average population. Large purchasers are interested in obtaining the best—excellent care and service for the money—rather than in merely seeing that HMOs meet minimal standards of access and quality. Purchasers pursue these ends through economic bargaining, either alone or as part of larger employer coalitions.

HMOs must be careful in tailoring services to the preferences of each employer. For example, certain populations have higher preferences for using mental health services, or because they are more dispersed, they may require multiple centers to assure adequate access to primary care. Large HMOs have well-developed marketing departments and large advertising budgets. They attempt to develop brand loyalty among customers and to document HMO value added relative to alternative providers.

Competitors

Competitive strategies of health plans are typically linked to lower prices, higher quality or better service, or to some combination of these three parameters. One HMO may adopt different strategies for different purchasers, for example, emphasizing health assessments for the elderly Medicare population and health prevention services (e.g., for weight loss and alcoholism) to a commercial client whose population is youthful, highly paid, and in a stressful industry, such as advertising. HMOs will typically use advertising that focuses on general, mood-creating associations, using persons in the ads with perceived high status who are plan members, or on the qualities or attractiveness of a plan's health providers, such as physicians.

Hospitals

In attaining their objectives, hospitals are conflicted regarding a posture toward HMOs. On the one hand, given a national average of 40% hospital bed overcapacity, hospitals are seeking HMO business to keep beds full; given the buyer's market, HMOs are driving the prices paid to hospitals below those that some hospitals can accept. Some hospitals alternatively are trying to form their own HMOs, but typically they lack the capital and management skills to be successful at this. The most common hospital strategy, given the environment, is to merge with other hospitals under the presumption that if all or most or the best hospitals in a given area are under one ownership, this strengthens that ownership's bargaining position with HMOs.

Merged hospitals are attempting to create what are called integrated delivery systems, which are a continuum of health services, including hospital, nursing home, ambulatory care, and hospice (see chapter 6, "Hospitals," for further discussion). But hospitals have been constrained in integrating clinical services because they remain loosely aligned with their affiliated physicians. Although hospital CEOs say aligning with physicians is their top priority, many do not want, for example, to add more physicians to their governing boards. Many hospital systems have integrated human resources, financial and materials management, strategic planning, information systems, managed care contracting, and risk management. HMOs are more successful than hospitals in developing integrated clinical systems because their large size permits the capital investment in information and medical management systems and because they have more formalized organizational relationships with fewer numbers of physicians.

One way for hospitals to enhance their bargaining position is to attempt to secure by legislation, economic advantages vis-à-vis HMOs which they have been unable to obtain in the marketplace. Hence, hospitals have attempted to compete with HMOs by forming provider groups that under special state or federal legislation can provide capitated care without having to maintain large financial reserves, as do insurance companies under state insurance regulation (National Health Policy Forum, 1996).

Physicians

As a compelling and constraining force, physicians can be categorized as generalists and specialists. These two groups view HMOs quite differently. As with hospitals, there is an oversupply of specialists, who are at a disadvantage, therefore, in economic bargaining with HMOs. Generalist physicians, in contrast, are greatly desired by HMOs as they are the key to containing health care costs by educating patients and limiting referrals. HMOs are interested in full-time commitments from such physicians and have been able, in large part, either to hire them at higher salaries than previously required or to develop more or less exclusive arrangements with them. What generalist physicians like about HMOs are the regular hours and coverage and support arrangements. What they dislike about HMOs are constraints on their autonomy, both in terms of how they practice medicine and of where they spend their time.

Members/Consumer Advocates

What members want from HMOs is high-quality services at reasonable access and limited cost. HMOs have adapted to consumer preferences by developing out-of-network options so that members can go outside the HMO network to obtain services from certain physicians and yet have these services reimbursed by the HMO. Typically, members pay much more out of pocket than if they had received services within the HMO physician network. Those members who are seriously ill have expectations from HMOs that differ from those of the normally healthy membership, and their concerns are mirrored and advanced by consumer advocate groups. Such groups argue for regulatory safeguards, as many HMOs are unprepared to care appropriately for members with special health problems, such as mental health or HIV-AIDS; try to avoid enrolling such persons; and exclude coverage for needed member services, such as brain surgery, which are typically costly and about which expert physicians have differences of opinion as to medical appropriateness, given the cost.

HMOs and Other Managed Care Organizations

The HMO response to traditional indemnity financing is to offer a price to the purchaser of only 80% of the traditional price and at the same time achieve a bottom line profit that is 50% greater than that of the traditional indemnity insurer (Hodge). This private reduction comes typically from three sources—reductions of about one-third each in payments to specialists, drug suppliers, and hospitals. Given the lack of concentration in the American health care market (the largest provider, United Healthcare has less than 4% market share, compared with, for example, General Motors' over 50% of the market for automobiles), the logical HMO (and PPO and POS) strategy is to use current profits and capital to expand market share so that, as markups inevitably decrease, they will be more than made up for by volume.

Current Issues

Some current issues, circa 1998, involving managed care and HMOs include the following questions: Does provision of medical care by HMOs cost any less than that provided by traditional and other providers? To what extent do HMOs and managed care encourage too little care for members? Do health plans and insurers add sufficient value (over that provided by doctors and hospitals) to justify 33%–40% of the health plan premium? To what extent should HMOs and managed care share in the financing of medical education, research, and the cost of serving the uninsured?

Efficiency

To evaluate whether or not HMOs are more or less costly than traditional fee-for-service medicine, one would have to compare care for patients/members who have similar health status and demographics in terms of health outcomes for a given amount of money spent taking care of them. We do not currently have this information (Bernstein & Bernstein, 1996). What we do know is that HMOs are 10%–15% less costly than fee-for-service medicine, as HMOs enroll healthier people. Experts have hypothesized that HMOs should be less costly as they are paid a capitated rate in advance, with the HMO "making more money" to the extent that members use fewer hospital and physician services (we are assuming that members were using "too many" of these services prior to enrolling in an HMO). Critics counter that HMOs provide fewer services than does fee-for service medicine, some of which members do need (Larson, 1996); that is why they are less costly (total costs) and cost less (the unit costs).

Appropriateness

To what extent do health plans exclude or expel doctors for ordering tests or consultations the health plans deem unnecessary? If the same doctors who overused services under fee-for-service underuse services under capitation payment, what should government or purchasers or members do about it? As of 1996, twenty-eight states have banned so called drive-through maternity care, in which hospitals send mothers home less than 48 hours after they give birth, and 13 states have barred insurers from refusing to pay for what turn out to be "unnecessary" emergency department visits (when chest pains, for example, are traced to stomach upset, not a life-threatening heart attack).

In addition, six states guarantee a patient's right to go directly to certain types of specialists without first getting approval from a primary care physician, or "gatekeeper" (Bodenheimer, 1996). HMO apologists would argue in rebuttal that there are good and bad HMOs as there are good and bad physicians in fee-for-service private practice. Knowledgeable purchasers buy health care from HMOs that provide quality care; knowledgeable workers work for organizations that want the "best" care for their employees at reasonable cost. Government can require disclosure regarding HMO performance, and its responsibility to protect the public is at least as great as that of assuring safe cars or a safe workplace.

Value Added

There are two issues here: (1) how much of the HMO premium dollar should go to the "plan" rather than to providers (or be refunded to purchasers or members); and (2) how much money are plans and top HMO managers entitled to make. These issues are intertwined with similar arguments about the American capitalistic society—how much profit are firms entitled to make, under what circumstances, and how much money are managers entitled to be paid? In either case should it be what the "traffic will bear"? Isn't that the capitalistic way of life? Is health care any different because it is more important to people, more of a life-or-death service, and more difficult for consumers to judge?

These issues require extensive discussion for proper analysis. Health plans often take 35%–40% of the HMO premium, which is spent on pharmacy allocation, out-of-area allocation, administration (enrollment, marketing, sales, licenses), broker commissions, and profit. Assuming greater market competition and more knowledgeable purchasers in larger numbers, we can assume that, in the future, profits will tend to be squeezed—unless purchasers are willing to pay more for health care provided by HMO X or Y because they are convinced that they will be getting greater value for the money in terms of quality of care, better health outcomes, better service, or better perceived service. Some HMO executives have made as much as $10 million a year in salary and bonus and much more than that as a result of increases in the stock prices of the HMO. Salaries, bonuses, and stock gains are higher in industries where much less of the purchasing dollar is from public funds (40% in health care). Does that make health care different enough to limit salaries or profits? You decide.

Externalities

Traditionally, medical education, medical research, and health care for the uninsured have been substantially financed by dollars paid for service, largely to hospitals. HMOs have no short-term interest in paying for noncontracted activities out of the dollars with which plans pay for medical care services. If those dollars are not replaced, there will be cuts in medical education and research, and access to care will be further limited for those lacking health insurance. Kassirer (1995) argues that market-driven care is likely to "cripple academic health centers, handicap the research establishment, and expand the population of patients without health care coverage" (p. 52). But is this the responsibility of HMOs or of government and the general citizenry? There are at least three opinions about expenditures in these areas: (1) HMOs should pay their fair share; (2) government or someone else should foot the bill for medical education, research, and health care for the uninsured; (3) less money should be spent on such activities. Again, there is no current consensus on how these issues can best be resolved.

Summary

HMOs are growing rapidly and taking advantage of new technology and the information revolution to begin to manage care more effectively. And they are beginning to sell their services in the marketplace based on claims to be able to provide medical care of higher quality at a lower price; that is, compared with traditional stand-alone medical and hospital providers, even when paid by PPOs at discounted rates. The next phase of the managed care revolution promises to be improved health care outcomes giving more value to the purchaser per expended dollar for health care. This will be accomplished under the direction of primary care providers influencing patient behavior and use of hospital and specialist services. Organizational forms and allocation of the premium dollar will further evolve accordingly.

Mini-Case Study
HMOs Reward High-Quality Health Care: What Do You Think?

The American Health HMO, with over 2 million members in six midwestern states, rewards physicians who score well on four cost and quality scales with bonuses that range from 12.5% to 25% of the HMO's average capitated payment to the physician. The capitation of physicians who don't meet standards is cut down to 25% below their average capitated payment.

The quality measures involve chart reviews, patient satisfaction surveys, patient turnover rates, and physician compliance with prevention protocols. There are five reimbursement categories, and scores are reevaluated every 6 months.

No physician scores in the lowest category. Physician offices with a high percentage of plan members seem to score highest.

Discussion Questions

1. What are the reasons that HMOs have developed in the ways that they have in the United States?
2. What do purchasers expect from HMOs, and do they get it?
3. What are the chief models regarding how physicians are organized and relate to HMOs?
4. How is the HMO premium divided up? Do you think this is appropriate?
5. How are HMOs changing and why? What are the strengths and weaknesses of HMOs from the consumer's point of view?

References

"Aetna and U.S. Healthcare: Yet More of the Same Medicine," *The Economist*, April 6, 1996.

Bernstein, A. B., & Bernstein, J., "HMO and Health Services Research: The Penalty of Taking the Lead," *Medical Care Research and Review, 53*(Suppl.), 18–43, 1996.

Bodenheimer, T., "The HMO Backlash: Righteous or Reactionary?" *New England Journal of Medicine, 335*, 1601–1603, 1996.

Boland, P., *Making Managed Healthcare Work*. Gaithersburg, MD: Aspen, 1993.

Brown, L. D., *Politics and Health Care Organization: HMOs as Federal Policy*. Washington, DC: Brookings Institution, 1983.

Etheredge, L., *Reengineering Medicare: From Bill-Paying Insurer to Accountable Purchaser: Research Agenda Brief*. Washington, DC: Health Insurance Reform Project, George Washington University, 1995.

Friedman, E., "Capitation, Integration and Managed Care," *Journal of the American Medical Association, 275*, 957–962, 1996.

Gabel, J., "Ten Ways HMOs Have Changed during the 1990s," *Health Affairs, 16*(3), 134–145, 1997.

General Accounting Office, *Medicare: Federal Efforts to Enhance Patient Quality of Care* (GAO/HEHS-96-20). Washington, DC: Author, 1996.

Gold, M. R., Hurley, R., Lake, T., Ensor, T., & Berenson, R., "A National Survey of the Arrangements Managed-Care Plans Make with Physicians," *New England Journal of Medicine, 333*, 1678–1683, 1995.

Hodge, M. H., "Health Care and America's Rolling Depression," *Health Care Management Review, 21*(3), 7–12, 1996.

Humana, *First Quarter Report*. Louisville, KY: Author, 1996.

InterStudy, *Competitive Edge: Industry Report 5.2*. Excelsior, MN: Author, 1995.

InterStudy, *Competitive Edge: Industry Report 6.2*. Excelsior, MN: Author, 1996.

Jensen, G. A., Morrisey, M. A., Gaffney, S., & Liston, D. K., "The New Dominance of Managed Care: Insurance Trends in the 1990s," *Health Affairs, 16*(1), 125–136, 1997.

Journal of Accountancy, March 1996.

Kassirer, J. P., "Managed Care and the Morality of the Marketplace," *New England Journal of Medicine, 333,* 50–52, 1995.

Kissick, W. L., *Medicine's Dilemmas.* New Haven, CT: Yale University Press, 1994.

Larson, E., "The Soul of an HMO," *Time,* 45–52, January 22, 1996.

Luft, H. S., *Health Maintenance Organizations: Dimensions of Performance.* New York: John Wiley, 1981.

MacLeod, G. K., "An Overview of Managed Health Care," in P. Kongstvedt (Ed.), *The Managed Health Care Handbook* (2nd ed.). Gaithersburg, MD: Aspen, 1993.

Michaels, J. L., & Rinn, C. C., "The Federal Employees Health Benefit Program and Managed Care," in P. Kongstvedt (Ed.), *The Managed Health Care Handbook* (2nd ed.). Gaithersburg, MD: Aspen, 1993.

National Health Policy Forum, *Issue Brief: Trends in Health Network Development: Community and Provider Initiatives in a Managed Care Environment,* No. 690. Washington, DC: George Washington University, 1996.

"The 'Physician Equity' Model," *Integrated Healthcare Report,* September 1993.

Shenkin, B. N., "The Independent Practice Association in Theory and Practice: Lessons from Experience," *Journal of the American Medical Association, 273,* 1937–1942, 1995.

Shouldice, R. G., *Introduction to Managed Care.* Arlington, VA: Information Resources Press, 1991.

Thorpe, K. E., "The Health System in Transition: Care Cost and Coverage," *Journal of Health Politics, Policy and Law, 22*(2), 344, 1997.

Vogel, D. E., *The Physician and Managed Care.* Chicago: American Medical Association, 1993.

Weiner, J. P., & DeLissavoy, G., "Razing a Tower of Babel: A Taxonomy for Managed Care and Health Insurance Plans," *Journal of Health Politics, Policy and Law, 18*(1), 75–103, 1993.

Xerox Health Link, *HMO Performance Report.* Rochester, NY: Xerox, 1995.

III

SYSTEM PERFORMANCE

Part III, "System Performance," provides a cross-sectional view of the health care system, focusing on different functional characteristics such as regulation, governance and management, quality improvement, access to care, cost containment, and ethical issues. For example, hospitals and nursing homes are regulated by government, owned by different sectors such as government, and both non-profit and for-profit corporations, focus on different critical indicators in measuring the quality of care, face different access and cost containment challenges and are affected by different ethical questions ranging from the cost of care that is or is not effective to the amount of voice in the operation of the facility that should be given to nursing home patients and their families.

In chapter 11, Brecher describes the different levels of government and principal agencies at each level of government that have roles in health care services. He describes the activities of governments as financers and purchasers of health care, as direct providers of care, and as regulators of care. He explains the causes of change and variation in government roles, to include major changes in federal policy and sources of variation in state policies. Brecher concludes with a discussion of current issues for government, including the expansion of coverage for the currently uninsured, regulating private insurance, and planning for and financing graduate medical education.

A. R. Kovner, in chapter 12, first defines what governance is and then describes who owns health care organizations and how their goals differ, for example, contrasting church and investor ownership of HMOs or nursing homes. He outlines the roles of governing boards in nonprofit health care organizations and identifies desired board competencies. Kovner explains the changing role and function of the board of directors in health care organizations, and the role of hospital boards in relating to independent medical staffs. Kovner identifies current issues in governance to include: what are preferable ownership patterns for health care organizations? How should nonprofit board performance be improved? To what extent should the autonomy of health care organizations be limited by government? And, what should be the extent and nature of organizational accountability to those served and potentially served? The second part of chapter 12 focuses on managers in health care organizations, what do they do, how they are trained, and how they contribute to organizational performance and how this can be measured. Kovner identifies current issues in the management of health care organizations to include: what should managers do in these organizations? Is their compensation too high relative to that for other health care workers? How should managers be trained? And, how can management performance be improved?

In chapter 13, Weitzman is concerned with improving the quality of health care. First, she defines quality and explains how quality is measured, focusing on the structure, process, and outcomes of care. She explains how data are used to measure quality, how these data are obtained and by whom. Next she discusses organizational considerations in promoting quality and quality improvement mechanisms. These include licensing, accreditation and certification, quality improvement organizations, malpractice limitations, and financing approaches. Weitzman explains implementing quality improvement through the continuous quality improvement (CQI) framework.

An important aspect of quality of care is the access of different groups in the population to different elements of health care. Such access is widely variable, in part due to variable health insurance coverage, but also for other reasons, as Billings explains in chapter 14. First he discusses the economic barriers to care, to include under-insurance and other limitations of coverage. He then explains the impact of these economic barriers both on patients and on the health care delivery system. Billings goes on to review the noneconomic or quasi-economic barriers to health care. These include race/ethnicity, culture/acculturation/language, gender, education, and resource availability/performance. He uses examples to demonstrate these influences, such as how barriers to primary care services can result in increased utilization of other health care services, particularly more costly hospital care. He concludes by discussing governmental approaches to improve access, starting with the failure of the Clinton health plan and continuing to discuss state initiatives, innovations, and their limitations.

In chapter 15, Thorpe reflects on the history of cost containment in health care and presents what might be future directions. He describes demand side distortions and supply side factors that have accounted for health care expenditure growth. Government has responded to such growth with a variety of initiatives including limits on hospital inputs, regulating the utilization of medical care, and hospital rate setting. Thorpe discusses the successes and failures of such initiatives and of others such as the growth of managed care, the growth and subsequent decline in all-payer rate-setting programs, and the reform of physician reimbursement. He concludes by pointing out that new technologies and practice patterns account for up to 90% of the growth in health care expenditures, reemphasizes that innovations in medicine have been nothing short of remarkable, increasing life expectancy and its quality. Spending over 13% of our gross national product on health care may simply reflect social preferences to direct limited resources to health rather than to other areas. At the center of the debate over the growth of health care is "whether the same level of health care could be purchased for less." Thorpe thinks that it can, but at issue is what are the appropriate interventions made by whom (and what are all the positive and negative results of such interventions) in reaching the desired outcomes.

Part III concludes with Hofmann's chapter 16, "Ethics in Health Care Delivery." Hofmann attempts to assist the reader in identifying some of the tensions between organizational and community priorities, presenting guidelines for organizations to serve the public and compete in an ethical manner. He reviews the bright and dark sides of managed care because of conflicting incentives and outlines steps to minimize ethical liabilities. Hofmann confronts the painful dimensions of downsizing in health care organizations and makes suggestions as to how managers and owners of these organizations can demonstrate ethical sensitivity. Hofmann recognizes the current and future dilemmas of medical rationing as Americans can never have sufficient medical care resources to meet all our needs and expectations. Hofmann concludes by reemphasizing how organizations and their stakeholders can promote ethical behavior, specifying the value of an ethics audit and the requirements of ethical behavior.

11

The Government's Role in Health Care

Charles Brecher

Learning Objectives

1. Differentiate among the levels of government and the roles of government.
2. Describe the current roles of the federal, state, and local governments in the United States.
3. Analyze the factors causing change in the governments' roles and variation in roles among states and localities.
4. Identify current controversies over the governments' roles and options being considered.

Topical Outline

Key questions and concepts
   Levels of government
   Roles of government
Description of current government activities
   Governments as financers and purchasers
   Governments as direct providers
   Governments as regulators
Causes of change and variation in government roles
   Major changes in federal policy
   Sources of variation in state policy
Current issues
   Expanding coverage among the currently uninsured

Regulating private insurance
Planning for graduate medical education

Key Words: **Government, regulation, federalism, Medicare, Medicaid, health departments, Food and Drug Administration, Health Care Financing Administration, Department of Veterans Affairs, Indian Health Service, ERISA (Employment Retirement and Income Security Act).**

The government is a major force shaping health care in the United States. As of 1995 it spent over $456 billion annually, or more than $46 of every $100 spent on care; it employs at least 1 million people to deliver health care directly; and it regulates individual and institutional private providers by determining who shall be entitled to deliver medical care and what the standards for that care shall be. Without an understanding of what government does, and why, one would be ignorant of an important part of what happens in health care.

This chapter provides an introductory perspective on the nature of the government's role. The first section identifies the key questions to be addressed and presents some concepts essential for answering them. The second section describes the functions governments perform, and the third analyzes why government health care policies change. The final section identifies current issues relating to what government's role ought to be in the future.

Key Questions and Concepts

In light of the vast and diverse nature of government activities, some particular perspective should be chosen for considering the role of the public sector. Three distinct but not mutually exclusive approaches to the subject can be taken.

The first is descriptive. It asks simply, what is the government's role? Much of this chapter will be devoted to answering that question.

A second approach seeks to go beyond knowing what government currently does to understanding what causes government to act in certain ways. It asks, why does government do certain things? It is based on a recognition that government activities vary among units of government (the U.S. public-sector role differs markedly from that of Great Britain) and over time (the public sector role today in the United States is markedly different from what it was at midcentury).

A third approach considers not what is but what might be. It asks whether the government's role conforms to some normative standard of what is a desirable set of public activities. Because reasonable individuals differ over what is the best role for government, the answers to this question vary widely. Yet it is possible to reach some judgments after making explicit the value assumptions that underlie them.

The next three sections of this chapter examine these three types of questions in successive order. But to answer them in a sophisticated fashion, it is necessary to use a few key concepts. One set relates to the fragmented nature of American government; a second set relates to the multiple possible roles government can play.

Multiple Governments

In the United States there is no single government; rather there are multiple governments with distinct roles in a federal system. The nation has one national government entity but 50 states and 84,955 units of local government within the states (see Table 11.1). Not all these units are involved in health care, but many are. The federal government and virtually all the states play some role in health care financing and delivery. Of the local governments, many of the 3,043 counties and some of the larger cities are involved in health care activity, and most of the 14,422 school districts also have some health education and health delivery functions.

The federal nature of American government has important implications for how the key questions identified above are answered. Descriptive questions must be answered separately for each level of government; the answers to causal

TABLE 11.1 Governmental Units in the United States, 1992

Type of government	Number of units
U.S. government	1
State governments	50
Local governments	84,955
County	3,043
Municipal	19,279
Township	16,656
School district	14,422
Special district	31,555

Source: U.S. Department of Commerce, Bureau of the Census, *1992 Census of Governments*, Vol. 1, Table A, p. vi (Washington: U.S. Government Printing Office, 1993).

questions may vary among units of government; and normative arguments about the proper role for government must specify not just what *government* should do but which *level of government* should do it.

Potential Roles

In any sector of society, including health care, government activity can be considered along three dimensions—financing (or purchasing), delivery, and regulation. The extent of government activity can vary along each dimension, and units of government most active on one dimension need not be active on another. Moreover, the same roles are played in varying degrees by the private sector.

Government financing of an activity typically takes the form of levying a tax to raise funds and then appropriating the funds to purchase or provide the service. However, financing can be separated from delivery. Tax funds can be used to purchase care provided by the private sector or to pay the salaries of civil servants employed to provide care directly. As will be seen, American governments follow both courses. It is also worth noting that governments can provide care without financing it. Governmental units established to provide care can and do operate without appropriations of tax dollars; they can "earn" revenues from private purchasers or from insurance programs sponsored by other organizations. Examples of such arrangements in health care include those local public hospitals that operate without direct governmental subsidies.

Regulation is the setting of standards for those engaged in the delivery of care. Regulations include licensing of occupations as well as facilities, setting standards for the process of care, and imposing restrictions on capital investments. The extent to which governmental entities engage in each form of regulation varies, as do the particular standards they set.

It is worth noting that these roles are not unique to the public sector. Obviously, private individuals and firms engage in the financing and delivery of care; they also engage in regulation. Private insurers set standards for receipt of payment and engage in utilization review; private health maintenance organizations (HMOs) set standards for practice by their physicians and monitor utilization. Thus, there is tremendous potential variation in the way in which roles are divided both between the public and private sectors and among units of government within the public sector.

What Are the Governments' Roles?

The key concepts of federalism and multiple potential roles can be combined to create a framework for describing governments' roles. As summarized in Table 11.2, the federal government plays a major role in financing and purchasing health

TABLE 11.2 Summary of Governments' Major Health Care Roles

	Financing/ purchasing	Delivery	Regulation
Federal	Large role through Medicare and Medicaid; other categorical programs	Operates facilities for veterans and Native Americans	Sets standards for Medicare providers; determines what drugs and devices may be sold; sets standards for employee fringe benefits under ERISA
State	Funds Medicaid, mental health, medical education and public health programs	Operates mental hospitals, health departments, and medical schools	Regulates insurance industry; licenses facilities and personnel; establishes health codes
Local	Subsidizes public hospitals; funds local health departments	Operates county and municipal hospitals; operates local health departments	Establishes local health codes

services, serves as a direct deliverer only for selected specialized populations, and engages in some significant regulation. The states show tremendous variation in their roles, but an aggregate summary is as follows: they play a substantial role in financing and purchasing; they are important direct providers of mental health and professional education services; they vary widely in regulatory activity but typically license providers, set standards for insurers, and are otherwise the dominant source of restrictions on the private sector. Similarly, local governments vary in their health activities, but they typically provide relatively little funding, especially for general medical care, and establish few local regulations. However, many cities or counties operate hospitals and clinics to ensure access to care for poor residents. This summary description provides an introduction to a more detailed analysis of the ways in which government units perform each role.

Governments as Financers and Purchasers

More complete information about the public sector's financial role is presented in Table 11.3. In 1995 (the most recent year for which data were available at

TABLE 11.3   National Health Expenditures, Selected Years, 1965–95

Expenditures	1995	1990	1985	1980	1975	1970	1965
Amount (in billions)							
Total	$988.5	$697.5	$419.0	$248.1	$132.7	$75.0	$41.9
Private	532.1	413.1	244.0	142.9	76.4	47.2	30.9
Public	456.4	284.3	175.0	105.2	56.3	27.8	11.0
Federal	328.4	195.8	123.1	71.0	37.0	17.7	5.5
State and local	128.0	88.5	52.0	34.2	19.3	10.1	5.5
Percentage distribution							
Total	100.0%	100.0%	100.0%	100.0%	100.0%	100.0%	100.0%
Private	53.8	59.2	58.2	57.6	57.5	63.0	73.8
Public	46.2	40.8	41.8	42.4	42.5	37.0	26.2
Federal	33.2	28.1	29.3	28.6	27.9	23.6	13.2
State and local	13.0	12.7	12.4	13.8	14.5	13.5	13.0

Source: Data for 1985 and earlier from Health Care Financing administration, U.S. Department of Health and Human Services, press release November, 18 1988; data for 1990 and 1995 from Katharine R. Levit et al., "National Health Expenditures, 1995," *Health Care Financing Review, 18*(1), 175–214, 1996.

the time of writing), government was the source of over 46% of all expenditures for health care. Within the public sector the federal government played the largest role, accounting for over two thirds of all government spending on health care.

The trend in governments' financing role is a sharp increase from the early 1960s to the mid-1970s and relative stability since. In 1965 government accounted for just 26% of health care spending, but by 1975 the figure was 42%. It remained at about that level through most of the 1980s but subsequently grew to exceed 46% in 1995. The stability and latest modest increase in *share* of funding has occurred in the context of rapid increases in total spending, causing the absolute amount of public spending to rise dramatically. Between 1980 and 1990 public spending jumped from $105.2 billion to $284.3 billion, or 170%; from 1990 to 1995 the increase was another $172.1 billion to $284.3 billion, or 60%.

Much of the public spending is accounted for by two programs—Medicare and Medicaid. The passage of these two programs in 1965 and their subsequent implementation explains much of the trend in government spending. Nonexistent in the early 1960s, these two programs accounted for $317.1 billion in spending in 1995, or 69% of the government total.

Medicare is a two-part program designed to help pay the medical care costs of the elderly. (Certain disabled individuals also have been made eligible.) Part A covers most hospital and some nursing home care; part B covers physician care and some other out-of-hospital services. Part A benefits are financed primarily through a payroll tax; Part B is financed through a combination of federal general fund appropriations and premiums paid by elderly enrollees. Both parts are administered by the federal Health Care Financing Administration (HCFA), a division of the Department of Health and Human Services.

Medicaid is a joint federal-state program to pay for medical care of the indigent. The federal legislation authorized the federal government to reimburse states for the cost of providing such care. In the years following enactment in 1965 most states established such a program, with Arizona being the last to do so in 1982. Until passage of federal welfare reforms in 1996, eligibility was linked to receipt of public assistance and to federal poverty thresholds for certain children, with states able to expand eligibility to others at their discretion. States must provide certain basic services, including hospital care, family planning, skilled nursing care, and physician services; they have the option of receiving federal reimbursement for additional services. Benefit structures vary widely because of the extent to which states include the optional benefits and because states' provision of the mandatory services vary, for example, in the number of days of hospital or nursing home care covered and the rate at which the states pay for the benefits. Thus, in effect, Medicaid is 50 different programs having different eligibility criteria and different benefit structures. The share of the population with income below the federal poverty threshold and enrolled in Medicaid varied from 91% in Rhode Island to just 28% in Nevada. The average cost per beneficiary was $7,162 in New York, compared to $2,381 in Mississippi (Liska & Obermaier, 1995).

Both Medicare and Medicaid are modeled on private insurance programs. Few of the benefits are provided directly by government agencies; most are purchased from private vendors. Medicare Part A pays hospitals directly at rates established by the federal government. (The basis for setting the rate was shifted from per diem to per admission in 1983.) Part B pays physicians directly if they agree to accept government-established fees or reimburses patients for the established amounts if they choose to pay the provider directly. Medicaid only pays providers directly, but the basis for setting rates varies widely among the states. Some states have adapted the Medicare payment standards; others have established less generous rates; still others have been imaginative in designing innovative payment schemes to encourage more efficient delivery. In the mid-1990s, states were increasingly turning to capitation payment mechanisms and mandatory enrollment in HMOs as a way to restructure their Medicaid programs (U.S. General Accounting Office, 1995a).

Because the states have so much discretion in designing their Medicaid programs, it is important to note that the aggregate spending figures cited earlier understate the role of state governments. Although they raise less than half of the $133.1 billion of Medicaid expenditures, state governments substantially control the entire sum, including the federal portion. In this sense the states control expenditures amounting to about one third of all public expenditure for health care.

The benefit structures of the Medicare and Medicaid programs strongly influence the distribution of government spending among different types of health care services. Although 46% of the total, government spending is under 32% of spending for physician services and over 61% of hospital expenditures. The relatively generous payment for hospital care by Medicare and the heavy use of hospitals by the elderly makes government the predominant source of hospital revenues. In contrast, the more uniform use of physician services among age groups and the less generous role of Medicare in paying for the elderly's doctor bills leaves the bulk of physician services paid for from private sources. More than half (58%) of all nursing home care is paid for by government, and Medicaid is the dominant source of public funds. It accounts for 47% of nursing home expenditures, compared to Medicare's 9%. The restrictions on eligible nursing home care under Medicare, which limit it to conditions causing an acute hospital stay, have kept its share of nursing home payments in check.

Governments as Direct Providers

In assuming a strong role in financing health care, governments have typically followed an insurance model and avoided operating medical care facilities and employing physicians and other providers. However, there are important exceptions to this pattern. Each level of government has assumed responsibility for delivering either certain types of care or more comprehensive care to a specific subset of the population.

Over the years the federal government has selected three population groups for which it funds and delivers services: veterans, Native Americans, and merchant seamen. The medical care program operated by the federal Department of Veterans Affairs (VA) is one of the largest health delivery systems in the world. With an annual budget of about $17 billion, the VA employs 191,000 people to operate 173 hospitals, 401 ambulatory care clinics, 133 nursing homes, and other facilities. It is, in one observer's words, "an anomaly in a capitalist country . . . a tax-financed agency that delivers care directly through salaried physicians and government-owned facilities" (Iglehart, 1996, p. 140).

The VA program evolved through a special congressional concern for veterans of the armed services. In addition to providing pension and cash disability benefits, Congress sought to provide veterans' health care. Like hospitals generally, the VA's hospital system initially grew as an extension of homes for the aged and disabled. Homes were authorized for indigent and disabled Civil War veterans, and after World War I this system was expanded to include a separate hospital system. After World War II the system was dramatically expanded and integrated with more advanced medical science and practice through a program of affiliations with medical schools. In 1965 nursing home benefits were broadened, and the system was expanded accordingly, although much VA nursing home care is purchased from the private sector rather than provided in VA-operated facilities (Congressional Budget Office, 1984).

Initially, VA medical care benefits were limited to those persons who developed conditions during their wartime service. A 1924 law broadened eligibility to include those who suffer from a condition likely to have been linked to military service even if it did not require treatment or become evident until later. Subsequently, any veteran who testified he was unable to pay for care became eligible, and in 1970 benefits were extended to any veteran past age 65 regardless of income or nature of condition. The aging of World War II and Korean War veterans and the extension of benefits to all veterans over age 65 has and will continue to markedly increase the number of people eligible for VA care.

However, the VA system is not based on an insurance model with benefits funded as an "entitlement." Instead, each year Congress appropriates a fixed sum to the VA for provision of care to its constituents. To live within its budget, the VA has established priorities for deciding who should receive what. The priority system has become complex, making distinctions based on whether or not the veteran has a service-related condition, his or her household income, and the type of service required. A General Accounting Office report (1996c) recently observed, "the complex eligibility provisions that have developed over many decades are often ill-defined and confusing—which ultimately creates frustration for veterans and VA staff" (p. 6). In 1991 an advisory commission questioned how adequately the VA could continue to perform its mission without changes in structure and financing, as well as a revised priority system (Commission on the Future Structure of Veterans Health Care, 1991). In 1995 the VA's undersecretary for health presented a plan for reform that relies on restructuring facilities into 22 integrated service networks; its implementation will require congressional cooperation and is uncertain.

A second group to whom the federal government provides care directly are Native Americans living on reservations. In 1996 the federal Indian Health Service (IHS), a division of the Department of Health and Human Services (HHS), spent about $2.2 billion to provide care for approximately 1.4 million of the nation's 2 million American Indians. The agency operates 37 hospitals, 64 health centers, and numerous other clinics (Indian Health Service).

Federal involvement in health care for Indians dates from the early 1800s, but the current program traces its origins to the Snyder Act in 1921. It provided a relatively open-ended authorization, which was used by the Bureau of Indian Affairs in the Department of the Interior. The Bureau gradually expanded its commitment, and in 1955 a separate unit to provide care to Indians was established within the Public Health Services (PHS). Significant new funding and staff followed the Indian Health Care Improvement Act of 1976.

Because there is no "mainstream" system serving Native Americans living on reservations, the need for a separate federal system seems self-evident. However, there are efforts to integrate the IHS facilities into the larger medical system through referrals. Because many of the IHS facilities are necessarily in rural areas and have low volume, they often refer cases to other providers for specialized care. In addition, the 1976 legislation gave tribal governments the right to assume responsibility for operating IHS facilities. Tribes wanting to do so can contract with the IHS for operation of hospitals and clinics. In 1996, 12 hospitals, 116 health care centers, and numerous other clinics were managed by tribes under these contracts and grants. The IHS seems committed to promoting tribal self-determination, and the policy of tribal management of health facilities is consistent with this goal.

A third federal delivery system, that for merchant seamen, has been largely dismantled. The federal responsibility in this area dates from the 1798 act creating the Marine Hospital Service. Subsequently, responsibilities of care for foreigners in quarantine were added, and in 1889 a separate quasi-military personnel system, known as the commissioned corps, was established within the federal PHS. To provide this care, separate PHS hospitals were constructed. However, after World War II the PHS expanded its responsibilities in other areas, including research on and control of communicable diseases. The PHS hospitals became vestigial organs as the need for care of seamen and foreigners declined. Eventually, budgetary pressures led to either the closure of the PHS hospitals or their transfer to private control. However, the commissioned corps of the PHS remains a group of federal employees who engage in health care activities. Few provide direct personal care; they primarily work in communicable disease control.

Despite its disengagement from delivery of personal health care, the PHS remains a federal agency within HHS. It operates the National Institute of Health, a major source of funding for extramural and intramural research. Its Centers for Disease Control and Prevention are the nation's major source of intervention in control of communicable diseases; its Food and Drug Administration (FDA) regulates food, cosmetic, and medicinal products; its Health Resources and Services Administration and its Alcohol, Drug Abuse, and Mental Health Administration have as their major activities the distribution to states and to private organizations of federal grant funds to expand the capacity of the health care system.

In summary, in recent years the federal government has restricted its role as direct provider at the same time that it has expanded its commitments as a financer and purchaser. The PHS hospitals have been eliminated; the IHS is relying more on private contracting and management by tribal organizations; the VA also is increasing its reliance on private purchase of care, although it remains strongly committed to maintaining a separate delivery system.

State governments are involved in the direct provision of medical care in three important ways: the operation of state mental hospitals, the conduct of medical education, and the maintenance of state (or often combined state and local) health departments. States' roles in the provision of mental health services dates from the late-19th century movement to characterize insanity as a medical or mental condition requiring treatment rather than confinement in either poorhouses or prisons. The reformers successfully encouraged state governments to create mental institutions, usually in remote areas, where the ill could be removed from sources of stress and receive available treatment. However, the facilities were often underfunded and eventually became notorious "snake pits," providing only minimal treatment and low-quality food and shelter. The poor conditions, together with the availability of drug treatment in the 1950s, led to a movement toward deinstitutionalization.

The initial impetus for deinstitutionalization was accelerated in the 1960s through expanded federal financial resources for alternative modes of care or at least residence. The federal Community Mental Health Centers Act in 1963 funded outpatient care in facilities located closer to patients' previous homes; the Medicaid and Medicare programs funded psychiatric care and nursing home care for many previously supported in state facilities by state appropriations; the federal Supplemental Security Income program, passed in 1972, provides direct cash benefits for the aged and disabled that have permitted many persons to reside in private homes rather than be placed by their relatives in state institutions (Clarke, 1979). As a result of these medical and policy changes the population in state mental hospitals dropped from 558,000 in 1955 to under 76,000 in 1993 (American Hospital Association, 1994).

Despite the shrinkage, state mental hospitals remain major institutions in the American health care system. In 1993 these 211 hospitals accounted for 85,647 beds. Their budgets totaled over $7 billion, and they employed about 155,000 workers (American Hospital Association, 1994). These hospitals are often a major source of employment within state government, and their historic location in small communities often makes them a dominant source of employment for communities with little other major economic activity. As a result of related political pressure, as well as a serious need to upgrade the facilities, employment at state mental hospitals has not shrunk at a pace anywhere near that of their bed capacity.

A major problem associated with the deinstitutionalization of the mentally ill has been a lack of corresponding investment in outpatient care for those sent home or not admitted. States have tended to rely on local government to provide the outpatient care and have not typically shifted resources to the localities to assist them in meeting the expanded need. There is poorly planned, poorly coordinated, and poorly supervised outpatient care for many of the mentally ill. As a consequence, they too often end up on the streets, homeless and unmedicated. The extent to which the states have themselves or in cooperation with localities undertaken a system of outpatient mental health services varies widely. In some states efforts to design and implement such a system remain a major policy failure (Blum & Blank, 1989).

States are also important supporters of medical education, and because medical education has a significant clinical component, states have been required to become involved in direct delivery of general medical care. In the 1992 academic year, state and local appropriations exceeded $2.8 billion and comprised nearly 10% of total revenues for all medical schools. State governments, through their public university systems, sponsor 73 of the nation's 125 medical schools (Krakower, Ganem, & Jolly, 1996). Often the state medical schools have a general hospital attached to them, also operated by the state.

These state general-care hospitals typically combine two roles. They provide medical students access to patients, and they provide the medical school faculty a place to admit private patients. The two roles are sometimes quite divergent; the patients with whom medical students obtain clinical training are typically poor and dependent on the state subsidy to the hospital for their access to care; the faculty's private patients are often commercially insured, and their fees provide the faculty with a significant source of private income. In some instance the two roles are performed satisfactorily at the same facility, but often the state's general hospitals serve only one of these functions. Where it is primarily a source of clinical experience for students, the medical school typically lacks an affiliation with a large voluntary hospital; where it is primarily a source of income for faculty, the medical school typically has an affiliation with another hospital (often public) that has a large patient volume, but the faculty do not use that facility as the preferred site for their private patients.

State health departments are another area of direct government provision. In this area it is often difficult to distinguish state from local efforts. The relations between state and localities in structuring a public health department are often complex; some states establish subunits that are identified as local entities, whereas others primarily fund local governments to conduct activities. However, in some areas the combined network of state and local health departments provides a significant volume of medical care along with engaging in regulatory and other public health activities. The personal care delivery is typically oriented to maternal and child health, vaccination and other communicable disease control activity, and treatment for chronic conditions. Although sometimes available to all citizens, the state health department services are more typically targeted to low-income residents (Davis & Millman, 1983).

Health departments provide these services directly because they believe the services would not otherwise be available. Even when other agencies or programs fund services, there may not be adequate delivery capacity available in a community in the private sector. Reluctance or an inability of private practitioners to treat indigent (even Medicaid-enrolled) patients with multiple disabilities or psychiatric or substance abuse problems, as well as the need to have outreach services for many poorly educated potential patients, often justifies continued health department provision of personal services.

The major remaining form of government involvement in direct delivery of care is local governments' operation of general care hospitals. The last comprehensive examination of these hospitals in the late 1970s found that they comprised over one third of all community hospitals, nearly one quarter of all community hospital beds, and 28% of such hospital outpatient department visits. Moreover, they account for a major share of health professions' education, including a disproportionate share of graduate medical education (Commission on Public General Hospitals, 1978). A more recent effort to examine the significance of these hospitals by the National Association of Public Hospitals found that its 100-member hospitals accounted for disproportionately large volumes of residency training, outpatient services, care of AIDS patients, care for the uninsured, and trauma care (Gage, Burch, Fagnani, Camper, & Andrulis, 1994).

The most troubled and widely publicized of these public institutions are those located in the nation's largest cities. A mid-1980s survey found that 48 of the 100 largest cities had a local public hospital and another 23 had a state government hospital (Altman, Brecher, Henderson, & Thorpe, 1989). These urban public hospitals are often characterized by political controversy because of their staffing and financing arrangements, but they play a major role in providing care to the urban indigent. Cities with public hospitals were found to provide more care to the uninsured poor than did cities without such hospitals, although private hospitals did somewhat increase their uncompensated care in areas that lacked a public hospital (Thorpe & Brecher, 1987).

Governments as Regulators

The authority to regulate private behavior is inherent in the sovereignty of government and is not derived from the public sector's role as financer. Government legally can call the tune even when it does not pay the piper. In its role as regulator of otherwise private behavior, the government is generally seeking to protect the consumer. Because private individuals have little basis on which to determine if a seller of medical goods or services is competent and honest, the government sets standards for such providers. Many government regulatory activities derive from this distinct legal authority.

The leading example of federal regulation intended to protect consumers in otherwise private transactions is the role of the FDA. This agency's authority dates from the 1906 Pure Food Act, enacted in response to scandals arising from the unsanitary methods used to produce some food products (Grabowski & Vernon, 1983). Regulatory authority was extended to drugs and cosmetics by 1938 legislation, this time in response to the death of more than 100 children due to a drug company's use of a toxic chemical in creating a liquid form of sulfanilamide. The FDA was given authority to set standards that pharmaceuticals must meet before being marketed.

Important amendments to the law were passed in 1962, again following large-scale tragedy. Only limited testing of the sedative thalidomide had been done before it was used in the United States and more widely used in Europe. However, its use among pregnant women led to the birth of deformed babies. The well-publicized tragedy led Congress to establish extensive requirements for premarket testing of drugs.

The standards for drug testing that the FDA now administers are a source of controversy. It is believed that they provide little or no additional protection over the prior 1962 standards, but they add substantially to the cost of developing new drugs and the time required before they can be widely used (Statman, 1983). As a result, the United States often lags behind other countries in the use of new drugs. Also, American pharmaceutical firms are at a disadvantage in developing new products. The spread of AIDS and a consequent sense of urgency in developing treatments for AIDS produced additional pressures to alter the extensive premarket requirements (Panem, 1988). In 1991, amid much controversy, the FDA permitted more widespread use of a previously experimental drug used in AIDS treatment and thereby set a precedent for more rapid use of other experimental drugs (Arno & Feiden, 1992).

Another form of consumer protection regulation is the licensing of health care practitioners and facilities. This licensure activity is conducted by state governments. The scope of state licensure authority varies, but virtually all states require that physicians, nurses, optometrists, chiropractors, and podiatrists meet state standards to obtain a license before practicing in that state. Some states recognize the licenses granted by other states in order to facilitate mobility among professionals, but this is not always the case.

Although the principle of licensure as a form of consumer protection is well established, its practice by state governments has been criticized on two grounds (Begun, 1981). First, the standards are not well enforced. The record of state agencies in locating and disciplining practitioners who violate professional standards is poor. Relatively few licenses are revoked each year despite evidence of more widespread professional misconduct. Second, licensing sometimes seems to protect the "turf" of selected professionals and thereby thwarts more effective delivery of care. Physicians have been accused of using state laws to prevent nurses, physician assistants, and optometrists from assuming broader responsibilities in delivery of care. Reforms designed to make state licensing efforts more effective include the appointment of more consumers and nonphysicians to the state boards that set and enforce licensing standards.

State government regulation of the insurance industry is another example of consumer protection efforts. Initial public regulation of the insurance industry was intended to protect consumers from firms, particularly life insurance firms, that might sell policies and then disappear with the premium income before paying benefits. To protect consumers, firms were required to establish reserves for future benefit payments and meet other standards.

These regulatory requirements have been applied to private health insurance as well. In addition, most states have extended their scope of regulation to include minimum benefit standards. These requirements were initially designed to protect consumers from believing they were well protected when benefits were actually very poor. Thus, minimum numbers of days of hospital inpatient coverage and other standards were set for health insurance products. This concept has been extended by some states to require the inclusion of certain types of benefits, such as chiropractic services, and minimum periods of postpartum care or to prohibit certain types of exclusions, such as alcoholism treatment (General Accounting Office, 1996b).

Federal government regulations established for participation in Medicare and Medicaid programs in some ways complement state regulations and in other ways expand the scope of government regulations. The complementary nature of the two types of activity is evident in the standards set by the federal government for providers; they generally defer to state licensing requirements and recognize physicians, hospitals, and other providers licensed by a state as eligible.

The federal government has also relied on state governments to implement its regulatory program for hospital capital investments. Between 1974 and 1986 the federal government required that a hospital or nursing home receive approval from a state planning agency before making a major hospital investment in order for that capital expense to be reimbursed by Medicare and Medicaid. The federal government abandoned this form of regulation in 1986, but some states continue to regulate the capital investments of providers within their borders despite the absence of federal requirements to do so and of federal funds to underwrite the effort. Both the aborted federal programs and the continuing state programs are justified not on grounds of consumer protection but on grounds that excessive capital investment, especially in hospital bed capacity, leads to unnecessary costs that will be financed by government funds and by private consumers through higher insurance premiums.

Federal Medicare and Medicaid regulations also work independently of state governments. A particularly dramatic example was the requirement that hospitals and nursing homes desegregate in order to be eligible for funds under the programs. When the legislation passed in 1965, many facilities in the South remained racially segregated, and there were no state laws prohibiting this. The federal requirements for racial integration of hospitals (for patients and medical staff) were widely perceived as helping to speed overall integration in the South.

Yet another type of relationship between federal and state regulations has arisen between the national Employee Retirement and Income Security Act (ERISA) of 1974 and state efforts to regulate health insurance. Passed with the primary intention of regulating employer fringe benefits in order to protect workers' pension assets, ERISA has been interpreted as preempting state regulation of employers' behavior with respect to group purchase of health insurance. Although states still can regulate insurance companies, ERISA prevents state (as opposed to federal) regulation of employer activities. This has two important policy implications.

First, it prohibits states from mandating that employers provide their workers with health insurance. (The state of Hawaii has a unique exemption because it had such a law when ERISA was passed.) Consequently, state efforts toward this end, such as a Massachusetts initiative in 1988, took the form of "play or pay" arrangements that did not directly mandate coverage but instead levied a tax on those employers who did not provide health insurance meeting minimum standards.

Second, ERISA effectively exempts from state regulation and state insurance taxation employers who choose to "self-insure." Recent estimates are that fully 44 million individuals, or about 17% of the population, are covered by self-insured employers, and therefore their coverage is not subject to any state regulation regarding benefits and other features. The use of self-funded plans is increasing, with enrollment estimated to have grown about 6 million between 1988 and 1993; in the later year about 46% of all employers with more than 100 workers provided insurance through a self-funded plan (General Accounting Office, 1995b).

To establish some standards for ERISA-covered plans and to supplement states with lax regulations the federal government has begun to establish some standards for health insurance. The Consolidated Omnibus Budget Reconciliation Act (COBRA) of 1985 required employers to offer laid-off employees the right to purchase continued health insurance coverage through the employer's group plan. The Portability Act of 1996 limited insurers' ability to refuse coverage based on preexisting conditions and their ability to deny coverage to workers changing jobs. Additional federal legislation in 1996 required that plans provide minimum hospital stays of 48 hours for normal deliveries and 96 hours for C-section deliveries and established parity for mental illness and physical illness with respect to certain benefits. These relatively recent federal efforts to regulate insurance are a new and potentially important development in the relationship between federal and state governments.

Causes of Change and Variation

The previous section illustrates that governments' roles change over time and vary among places. In the past quarter-century major new federal programs have been enacted and significantly modified several times; the practices of states and localities in financing and delivering services and in regulating providers vary widely. For example, as noted, Medicaid is in many ways 50 different state programs rather than a single, uniform national program.

Explaining change and variation in government activity is a major focus of political science, and political scientists have applied their conceptual tools to the analysis of health policy. Two types of theoretical explanations can be categorized as the Marxist approach and the interest group (or pluralist) approach (Marmor, 1983). Both theories see change arising from conflict within society, but they differ over the sources of those conflicts. Marxists see the conflicts as essentially economic and as between two inherently hostile economic groups (or classes)—those who own means of production (capitalists) and those who work for them (labor). The public sector is seen as serving the interests of capitalists in the United States and other non-Communist nations. Fundamental change can occur only after violent revolution places control of the government in the hands of the laboring class. Pending such revolutionary change, reforms are made by the ruling capitalist class only as necessary to appease workers and to ensure peaceful compliance with government rules that serve capitalist interest.

Interest group theory sees conflict arising from a more diverse set of interests than only economic positions. Individuals perform multiple social roles and may belong to numerous social groups. Those groups have diverse interests, and their efforts to promote their particular goals through government action draws opposition from other groups. The groups and their competing interests have many different sources besides economic class, including place of residence, ethnic identity, religious beliefs, and occupational roles. Decisions of government are seen as shaped by the relative influence different groups bring to bear on elected officials (Truman, 1960).

In American society variations of interest group theory have proved more useful than Marxist theory for explaining change and variation. The emergence of a large "middle class" with substantial influence and income derived from service as opposed to capital-intensive manufacturing industries, the effectiveness of elections in promoting the interests of labor organizations as well as middle-class citizens, and the concentration of social and economic problems among an "underclass" that is largely outside the world of regularized work have reduced the relevance of classic Marxist theory and led its revisionists to adopt modifications that closely approximate variations of interest group theory. Thus, the concept of changing or different balances of influence among competing groups is a more useful conceptual framework for analyzing American health care policy.

Changes in Federal Policy

From a broad perspective, the development of federal health care policy can be analyzed over time in four distinct periods. Prior to 1960 the federal government avoided large-scale participation in the financing of personal health care services; from 1960 to the mid-1970s the federal role expanded rapidly; from approximately 1975 to 1992, the federal role was relatively stable, with some efforts at contraction; the election of President Clinton in 1992 was followed by an unsuccessful effort by his administration to alter American health care dramatically, and the nation remains in a period during which major problems are unresolved as a result of a political stand-off among competing groups.

These shifts in policy can be related to broad shifts in patterns of interest groups' influence. In the first two periods the same types of groups were active, but their relative influence shifted; the third period was associated with the partial withdrawal of one type of interest and the emergence of a new, influential group. The current phase is related to the emergence of additional new influential groups.

For much of this century national health care politics was primarily a battle between proponents of national health insurance and its opponents (Marmor, 1973). Proponents included many working Americans who promoted their cause through union political activity. Their cause was championed by the Democratic Party. Opponents were many physicians and other providers, including hospitals, that feared the consequences of government involvement in their income flow; private insurance companies that feared a loss in their market for health insurance; and business organizations that feared the tax burden associated with a government funding program.

Until 1960 the opponents were highly successful. Efforts to include a health insurance program in the original 1935 Social Security Act were dropped by President Roosevelt because he feared that the strong physician opposition to it would jeopardize the entire program. Post–World War II efforts to add national health insurance to the nation's Social Security system by President Truman led to a large-scale, well-funded campaign against it by the American Medical Association and organizations representing businesses. The victory of a Republican in the 1952 presidential election led to an eight-year period of little action or prospect for change in federal health care policy.

The presidential election of 1960 saw a revival of interest in federal efforts. This time the Democrats, supported by labor organizations, advocated hospital insurance for the elderly only, rather than immediate enactment of a universal system. The Democratic presidential candidate won, but the legislation that emerged from Congress reflected major compromises with more conservative legislative leaders. The Kerr-Mills Act of 1961 established a program to pay for the medical expenses of the poor elderly that was closely linked to joint state-federal welfare programs rather than a broader program linked to federal Social Security.

The landslide victory of the Democrats in the 1964 national elections made possible the passage of broader legislation. The 1965 amendments to the Social Security Act added Titles 18 and 19, Medicare and Medicaid. As described earlier, these programs provide relatively comprehensive health insurance for the elderly and opportunities for states to create relatively extensive programs for the indigent.

In response to the initial success of Medicare, the opponents, including physicians and many business leaders, changed their position on national health insurance. By 1974, Democrats and Republicans in Congress appeared to have reached agreement on programs that would cover all Americans through a combination of Medicare for the elderly, a more uniform national version of Medicaid for the poor, and mandatory employment-based insurance for others (Rivlin, 1974). However, the impending impeachment of President Nixon diverted congressional attention, and improved prospects for the Democratic Party in the 1976 elections undermined the compromise and ended the immediate prospects for enacting national health insurance at that time.

From the mid-1970s to 1992, federal efforts focused on controlling the rising cost of Medicare and Medicaid rather than expanding their scope. This shift was first evident in 1972 with the creation of utilization review organizations for the programs. The federal Health Maintenance Organization Act of 1973 sought to promote the development of these organizations because they were viewed as cost-saving delivery mechanisms. The health-planning legislation of 1974 established a system of regulation for capital investments also intended to promote efficiency.

The election of a Democrat to the White House in the 1976 elections did not lead to renewed pressure for national health insurance. Instead, President Carter sought to create an effective mechanism for controlling hospital costs before expanding government financing of the industry. However, his 1977 proposal for a national system of price controls for hospitals was defeated in Congress through strong lobbying efforts by the hospital industry. Initiatives taken to redefine the administration's position after this defeat never came to fruition but did lead to the exploration of greater emphasis on competition among providers as a means for cost control.

The triumph of conservative Republicans in the 1980 national elections and the reelection of President Reagan in 1984 gave greater energy to efforts to curb spending under Medicare and Medicaid, as well as virtually all other domestic programs. Health policy, like most domestic policy, became a subtheme of budget policy. Expenditure reductions for Medicaid were sought through measures that limited growth in federal reimbursement to states and that gave states greater freedom in structuring their programs. States pursued some of these options and innovated in designing new ways to pay providers to encourage efficiency, but the states relied on other policies as well. Specifically, states reduced enrollment in the program by failing to adjust Medicaid income eligibility limits for inflation. As a result, the share of the poor covered by Medicaid nationwide fell from 74% in 1979 to just 59% in 1984 (Holahan & Cohen, 1986).

Reagan administration efforts to curb Medicare spending led to the institution of a new prospective payment system in 1983. This changed the basis on which Medicare pays hospitals from cost reimbursement based on average per diem costs to a national price system that establishes standardized rates for different categories of hospital admissions. Under the new system the federal government has been able to curb Medicare benefit payment growth and better control expenditures under Part A.

The apparent success of the prospective payment system for hospitals led to new efforts to revise the payment system for physicians. Rapid increases in Medicare Part B expenditures led to a freeze on physician fees in 1984 and 1985 (Holahan & Etheredge, 1986). With the recognition that a freeze was not a viable long-term policy, Congress created a Physician Payment Review Commission in 1986. The commission made recommendations for a new system for paying physicians in 1989. Legislation establishing a national fee schedule and expenditure targets for Medicare was adopted that year and became effective in 1991. The intention is to slow the rate of growth in Part B spending and to narrow disparities in income among physician specialties (Smith, 1992).

The shift in emphasis of federal policy from a period of expansion in federal financing to one of cost control was linked to changes in patterns of interest group influence. In the initial two periods, the battles were largely between groups seeking expansion of federal policy and those opposed; the dormant period of 1935–60 resulted from stronger influence by the opponents; the expansion from 1960 to 1974 represented greater influence by the proponents. However, the post-1974 shift to cost control saw a new actor become prominent and develop new relations with the old opponents.

The new actors in federal health politics were bureaucrats administering the federal programs. Lodged in the Health Care Financing Administration and the Office of Management and Budget, these professionals administer programs on behalf of taxpayers. They bargained with providers in a pattern political scientist Lawrence Brown (1985) called "technocratic corporatism." Professionals hired by the government interact with representatives of provider organizations to shape health policy. This pattern was evident in the creation of the prospective payment system in 1982 and in the revisions of physician payments under Medicare in 1989. Health care politics in this period of cost containment were battles between professionals representing taxpayers and the providers of services (Smith, 1992).

The period of contraction in health care politics was checked to some extent by the emergence of a consumer interest group other than labor unions. The most influential new consumer group is the elderly—Medicare beneficiaries—represented by the powerful American Association of Retired Persons (AARP). Although founded in the 1950s, the AARP grew rapidly in the 1980s to have a membership of over 27 million and an annual budget of $185 million by 1987

(Kosterlitz, 1988). Because its members have direct economic dependence on the federal government through cash Social Security benefits as well as Medicare, they vote in national elections at high rates and give great attention to domestic policy positions, including health care issues.

The influence of the AARP was evident in the passage of the Medicare Catastrophic Coverage Act of 1988 and its repeal a year later. At a time when budget deficits were leading to expenditure reductions for most federal programs and when tax increases were politically unacceptable, Congress nonetheless passed a program that extended benefits at an added annual cost projected at $10.6 billion. The new benefits were passed largely due to the effective lobbying efforts of the AARP. However, in a compromise with the Reagan administration, the AARP agreed to phase in the new benefits and finance them with higher premiums and a new surcharge on the personal income tax liability of the elderly. When the elderly began to pay the price before receiving all the benefits, many objected loudly. Especially disgruntled were the wealthier elderly, who paid more income tax, and they are a key segment of the AARP's membership. As a result, in 1989, with the AARP's tacit consent, the catastrophic benefits were repealed in exchange for dropping the higher taxes (Rovner, 1995).

The start of the current phase of federal health policy was marked by President Clinton's unsuccessful effort at national reform. Clinton sought to address the dual problems of a large segment of the population's being either uncovered or at risk of losing their coverage and of rapidly rising costs. His solution was to revamp the way in which services are purchased and delivered.

The Clinton proposal, called the Health Security Plan, would have restructured the health care industry by creating two new types of entities: health alliances and certified health plans. Alliances would have been state-created bodies serving as large-scale purchasers of health care. Most individuals would purchase their care through an alliance. Alliances would accept bids from competing plans. The certified plans would offer a nationally established benefit package for a fixed premium. The plans would guarantee the benefits and have arrangements with hospitals, physicians, and other providers to deliver the care. Individuals could choose from among several plans with which their alliance had negotiated arrangements.

The Health Security Plan would have assured services to virtually all residents, including most of those now uninsured. This would have been accomplished financially by requiring employers to pay a new tax typically equal to 7.9% of their payroll expenses, a figure close to the average current cost of private group health insurance premiums. The employer payments would be supplemented by federal payments to subsidize the cost of coverage for the unemployed. In addition, because the new plan would replace Medicaid, states would be required to make payments approximately equal to their current expenditures for Medicaid. The benefit package for all those enrolled, including those formerly in Medicaid or uninsured, would be equal, permitting its proponents to assert, "The Health Security Plan guarantees every American and legal resident health coverage that can never be taken away."

The plan also proposed to use regulatory authority to guarantee cost-containment objectives. Its intent was to have the price competition among plans keep premiums charged to alliances low, presumably by encouraging efficiency within the plans' operations. However, if these market forces did not curb growth in premiums, a federal agency would set and enforce caps on the rate of premium increases. Under certain conditions, health alliances would not be permitted to pay premium increases above the capped rate.

Politically, President Clinton counted on support from a potentially broad set of interest groups. Consumers, including organized labor, would be attracted by the guarantee of secure health insurance coverage; large employers would be attracted to the potential for cost control and slower rates of increase in health insurance costs; providers, including physicians and hospitals, would be drawn to the new coverage for those now unable to pay for care themselves and who represented both a financial drain on providers and a national embarrassment in a moral sense. However, opposition from other quarters emerged and carried the day. Small businesses not providing health insurance objected to the new employer mandate, arguing that the tax would drive them out of business or force them to lay off low-wage workers. Pharmaceutical firms and other health care suppliers feared the consequences of the strong cost-control measures; demand for their products, existing and under development, would be curbed by the enforcement of caps on premiums. Insurance companies objected that the health alliances would replace them and their workers, effectively eliminating a major industry. Finally, partisan Republicans feared that giving the new president credit for a major expansion of the Social Security system would undermine their chances for electoral success in future national elections (Johnson & Broder, 1996). The opposition took their case to the public with television advertisements. Their commercials and other efforts played upon public fear of government involvement in the choice of physicians and the potential for limitations on benefits due to cost controls (Skocpol, 1996). The result was a clear defeat for major health care reforms in 1994 and was followed by a round of congressional elections, featuring unusually low voter turnout, in which Republicans achieved dramatic gains (Schick, 1995).

Variations in State Policy

The substantial variation in health care activity among the states is related to three sets of factors: levels of economic development, general political culture, and patterns of interest group activity. The first two are general state characteristics; the third is distinct for the health care arena.

Studies of a wide range of state policies have demonstrated that states with higher levels of income and urbanization tend to spend more per capita and generally follow an expanded government role (Gray, Jacob, & Vines, 1983). This generalization applies to health care. However, the relationship between economics and state government activity is influenced by political forces. The degree of party competition in states, the division of responsibility between states and their localities, and the balance of political values among citizens between moralistic and traditionalist values have been found to be important influences on state expenditure levels for a variety of services, including health.

Finally, the nature of interest group activity also shapes state health policy. The principal competing interests within state capitols typically are provider groups, business groups concerned with tax levels, local government officials involved in financing or delivering care, and more recently, state employees analogous to the federal "technocrats." However, the relative influence of these groups and the resulting policies vary widely among states.

The different patterns of state health politics are illustrated by important decisions for state Medicaid programs during the 1980s in Arizona, California, and New York. Arizona was the last state to establish a Medicaid program, a decision not reached until 1982 (Brecher, 1984). The absence of a program was largely due to sentiment among conservative business interests; they felt state taxes should not be increased to finance health care for the poor; rather this should be either a private concern or one of local governments. The pressure to change this policy came from local government officials, who faced great difficulty in financing local programs when statutory limits were placed on local revenues from the property tax. To obtain federal aid for care for the indigent, the local officials successfully pressured the state legislature for a Medicaid program. Health care provider groups played little role in shaping the program, which mandated enrollment in capitation programs.

In California the same interests interacted differently. California established a relatively generous Medicaid program early, and its expenditures increased rapidly. The program was supported by local officials and health care providers with little opposition. However, a state budget crisis in the early 1980s led to major reforms, in which the business community played a strong role. The reforms changed the way the state pays hospitals for its Medicaid enrollees, with the intention of lowering payments to hospitals, and altered the distribution of financial responsibility between the state and localities for care to the indigent in a way that obliged localities to do more. These changes resulted from business interest intervention in a policy area previously left largely to the localities and the providers. As one observer put it,

With the passage of this remarkable legislation, the relationship among interest groups, units of state and local government, and private medical care systems were changed, perhaps permanently. The California Medical Association and the California Hospital Association, previously undisputed winners of the legislative game, had been crowded off the board by pressures from the budget, by the newly activated business coalitions, and by the insurance companies. (Bergthold, 1984, p. 213)

In contrast, Medicaid reforms in New York in the 1980s were more responsive to providers'—particularly hospitals'—concerns (Brecher, 1986). In 1975, in response to state and local budgetary pressures, New York began tight regulation of prospective payments to hospitals. The hospitals did not respond with necessary expenditure reductions and soon faced severe operating deficits. After several years of such deficits, many hospitals were facing contraction or bankruptcy. In response, the state established a new payment system that included extra revenues for hospitals providing care to the uninsured poor. This substantially improved the financial position of the providers (although it did little to improve coverage for the uninsured poor). Providers obtained additional concessions after the federal government switched Medicare to a prospective payment basis. The state abandoned its waiver under Medicaid in order to permit hospitals in the state to participate in the new federal program because the state hospital association had calculated that members' revenues would be greater under the new federal system than under the continued state-controlled system (Thorpe, 1989).

A more recent study covering Medicaid programs in the early 1990s compares New York and California with respect to nursing home policy, home care policy, hospital policy, and managed care policy. It finds that the substantially higher spending in New York is due to the different roles played by technical experts employed in the executive branch. In California these staff members had significant independent discretion to design cost-effective policies; in contrast, in New York they were restricted by the strong influence of providers and other interest groups working through the legislature and the governor's office. In the author's words,

The study suggests that variation in Medicaid spending is due in large part to variations in bureaucratic discretion. California officials have significant discretion to implement a cost-control agenda. . . . The bureaucracy in New York operates in a very different political environment. Medicaid politics in New York is fragmented, decentralized, and pluralistic. Purchaser groups, labor leaders, and consumer advocates all exercise significant political authority. (Sparer, 1996, p. 193)

As these examples suggest, a state's health policy is shaped by more than the state's level of economic development. Competition among state bureaucrats, local officials, providers, business groups, and others leads to a wide range of compromises. Within the federal system, states respond to these competing pressures in different ways, with widely differing benefits for the interests represented as well as for the low-income consumers who are often unrepresented at the bargaining tables.

Current Issues

The political competition among interest groups produces divergent policies among states and localities and leads to a steadily changing set of federal policies. This section identifies three issues currently being debated at the federal level and the policy options that different groups are pursuing—expansion of health insurance coverage to the uninsured, the source and type of government regulation of private health insurance, and the government's role in determining the size and specialty mix of the physician workforce.

Expanding Coverage among the Currently Uninsured

Many Americans view the fact that about 40 million of their fellow citizens lack health insurance as a serious problem about which the federal government ought to take some action. Yet the failure of President Clinton's health care reform proposals in 1994 illustrate the difficulty in designing a politically acceptable plan.

The perceived desirability of changes in governments' roles, such as those proposed in the Clinton plan, is a function of individual values relating to equity and efficiency. Proponents of the plan and other reforms like it attach a high value to its promotion of equity by extending coverage to almost all residents. In addition, advocates argue that the plan would promote efficiency by curbing the rate of growth in national health expenditures through its combination of competitive pressures and regulatory authority.

Opponents of the plan see its threats to efficiency as outweighing its equity gains. They argue that the required employer contributions would be a burden to employers of low-wage workers and would destroy many low-wage jobs. Some firms would no longer be able to compete at the higher labor costs and would go out of business. They also argue that the federal capping of premiums and regulation of benefits will have adverse effects. Limiting premiums is believed to lead to slower innovation in the development and deployment of new lifesaving technology, leading to an undermining of the U.S. position as a leader in advancing high-technology medicine. Similarly, the regulation of benefits may be used to slow the availability of new procedures that emerge and new devices that are developed.

The current and future Congresses will have to wrestle with how to balance these competing values. Given the demonstrated ability of opponents of comprehensive reforms aimed to make coverage universal and to impose strict cost controls to block change, future initiatives will necessarily be less ambitious. Advocates for change are likely to pursue one or more of three avenues at the federal level.

First, reforms such as those in the 1996 Portability Act can make health insurance available to a broader segment of the population. Federal regulation of employers and insurers can oblige them to make health insurance available to those who might otherwise be excluded and to help them gain access to group purchasing, which lowers the cost from individual or community-rated premiums. Because such measures do not involve direct expenditures by government, they engender less opposition than do tax-supported subsidies to help the uninsured pay for care. At the same time, however, such reforms are inherently limited in how far they can extend coverage to the uninsured because they do little to address the problem of affordability for low-income households.

The two approaches to public subsidies for care that have some chance of gaining public support focus on the unemployed and on children. President Clinton has proposed helping to finance premiums for temporarily unemployed workers who qualify for COBRA coverage but cannot afford the necessary premiums. A program to support continuation of employer-linked coverage for those who become unemployed may prove a feasible next step in extending coverage, especially if a future recession increases concerns over unemployment and the loss of health insurance it may cause.

Uninsured children are another group for whom it may prove possible to muster public support. It is estimated that about 10 million children are uninsured, and various proposals have been developed to reduce this figure significantly (General Accounting Office, 1996a). Political support is feasible because the costs are relatively low; most children are healthy, and average expenditures for their care are relatively low. This makes it fiscally easier to finance broader coverage. If a low price tag can be combined with a general sympathy for children (as opposed to low-income adults), then this may prove an achievable incremental step in dealing with the inequities in the current system for providing health care to Americans.

Regulating Private Insurance

Most insured Americans are covered by a private policy purchased either individually or through their employers. As noted earlier, it has long been recognized that government ought to regulate the nature of these private insurance polices, but the source of that regulation and its content are currently a matter of controversy.

Historically, insurance regulation was almost exclusively a function of state government. And the states performed this function with widely varying degrees of effort and competence. A 1993 survey found that the number of staff states devoted to health insurance regulation ranged from 1 to 153, and 14 states had no actuary on staff or under contract to work on health insurance (General Accounting Office, 1993).

The federal government entered this arena indirectly through ERISA, which established federal jurisdiction over employer-sponsored insurance plans and restricted the states' regulatory authority over employer-based benefits. However, the federal government was not aggressive in setting strict standards for the plans it regulated, and the major impact of ERISA was only to prevent the more active state governments from imposing new standards (and taxes) on employer-sponsored plans.

The rise of commercial managed care plans and their tight cost-control practices revived a movement within several states to use their regulatory authority to better protect consumers. Mandatory benefits and other quality standards were enacted in many states. The most widely publicized example was the legislating of minimum standards for length of stay for the delivery of newborns to prevent so-called drive-through deliveries. By 1996 fully 29 states had such laws or regulations (Declerq & Simmes, 1997).

The federal government entered the arena of benefits regulation with legislation mandating minimum lengths of stay in 1996. Congress and the president apparently found it attractive to establish standards because it responds to popular consumer concerns and requires that added costs be paid through private premiums rather than tax dollars, yet the action was based more on anecdotes in the press than on objective analysis of the appropriateness of different lengths of stay and their impact on outcomes for mother and child. Also, as noted, a majority of states had already enacted similar rules.

In early 1997, President Clinton, meeting an election campaign pledge, appointed the national Advisory Commission on Consumer Protection and Quality in the Health Care Industry. Congress and the president will be looking to this commission to identify policies for regulating insurance and establishing quality-reporting standards to guide consumers. Among the difficult issues facing the commission are how to divide authority between the federal government and the states and where to set the limits on appropriate mandatory benefits. Although some consumer protection is essential, private plans also need the freedom to innovate in their practices if cost-containment and efficiency gains through competition are to remain possible.

Planning for Graduate Medical Education

The nation's physician supply is now widely criticized as being too large, growing too rapidly, and being maldistributed both geographically and among specialties.

This is not primarily the result of an expansion of undergraduate medical schools in the United States; instead, it results almost entirely from a great expansion in the number of residency positions offered for graduate (i.e., specialty) medical education at teaching hospitals and the filling of these positions by persons who have received undergraduate medical education at schools located in other countries. From 1988 to 1993 the number of residents in the country's hospitals jumped from 82,791 to 102,335, with those trained at foreign medical schools accounting for almost one quarter of the group in the later year compared to 14% in 1988 (Congressional Budget Office, 1995).

So far, the governments' role in graduate medical education has been restricted almost exclusively to financing. Through the Medicare program, the federal government provides significant funding (over $6 billion annually in 1995) to hospitals based on the number of residents they train. Some state Medicaid programs also provide additional funding to hospitals sponsoring residencies. In effect, government has created financial incentives for hospitals to expand their scale of graduate medical education.

A major controversy is arising over whether these government policies should continue and how they might be changed. Opponents to continued generous and relatively unconditional public funding argue that the amounts should be restricted and that more conditions should be imposed on hospitals. Proposals include capping or reducing the total amount now spent on graduate medical education and setting limits on the number of residency positions eligible for public funding in each specialty. One proposal would establish a national trust fund for graduate medical education, with money drawn from all sources of medical care financing—Medicare, Medicaid, and private insurance—and distributed by a national board on the basis of their selection of the number, specialty mix, and location of residency positions that best meet national needs. The intention is to produce a future physician supply that is better matched to the population's needs and to save taxpayer dollars.

Opponents to expanding the government's role beyond financing to include planning to meet population needs question the ability of a government body to accomplish the intended goal. They argue that it is not possible to predict accurately and objectively the country's future physician requirements and that it is unfair for government to restrict opportunities for both citizens and foreign students to enter medical careers when this is not the practice for other professional careers, such as law.

The different points of view each have powerful representation in Congress. In the coming legislative sessions some change is likely to emerge that reaches a compromise among those seeking to maintain a large, high-quality, and autonomous graduate medical education capacity at existing academic medical centers, those seeking to limit public spending for this purpose without necessarily imposing more conditions on the funding, and those seeking to establish some form of public planning for the nation's future physician supply.

Mini-Case Study

New York City has a large HHC. There are too many hospital beds. There are problems in access to care. The mayor has been prevented from selling hospitals. What are some of the problems and issues city hospital ownership raises for various levels of government? What should be done to improve the situation? Respond from the viewpoints of the governor, a union leader, and taxpayer and user advocates.

Discussion Questions

1. What is and should be the role of the various governmental levels (federal, state, city, county, and regional) in health care delivery?
2. What changes should be made in Medicare so that the program breaks even? Should benefits be cut and why?
3. Why do Medicaid costs and benefits vary so much from state to state? Should there be such variance?
4. How should care be expanded for the currently uninsured?
5. How should private insurance be regulated?
6. What should government's role be in limiting the number of physicians educated and in practice?

References

Altman, S. H., Brecher, C., Henderson, M. G., & Thorpe, K. E., *Competition and Compassion*. Ann Arbor, MI: Health Administration Press, 1989.

American Hospital Association, *Hospital Statistics* (1994–95 ed.). Chicago: Author, 1994.

Arno, P. S., & Feiden, K. L., *Against the Odds: The Story of AIDS Drug Development, Politics and Profits*. New York: Harper Collins, 1992.

Begun, J. W., *Professionalism and the Public Interest*. Cambridge, MA: MIT Press, 1981.

Bergthold, L., "Crabs in a Bucket: The Politics of Health Care Reform in California," *Journal of Health Politics, Policy and Law, 9*(2), 203–222, 1984.

Blum, B., & Blank, S., "Mental Health and Mental Retardation Services," in G. Benjamin and C. Brecher (Eds.), *The Two New Yorks*. New York: Russell Sage Foundation, 1989.

Brecher, C., "Medicaid Comes to Arizona," *Journal of Health Politics, Policy and Law, 9*(3), 411–425, 1984.

Brecher, C., "Progress in New York State Hospital Payment Policy," *Bulletin of the New York Academy of Medicine, 62*(1), 115–123, 1986.

Brown, L. D., "Technocratic Corporatism and Administrative Reform in Medicare," *Journal of Health Politics, Policy and Law, 10*(3), 579–600, 1985.

Clarke, G. J., "In Defense of Deinstitutionalization," *Milbank Memorial Fund Quarterly, 57*, 461–479, 1979.

Commission on the Future Structure of Veterans' Health Care. *The Price of Freedom is Visible Here*. Washington, DC: U.S. Department of Veterans Affairs, 1991.

Commission on Public General Hospitals, *Readings on Public General Hospitals*. Chicago: Hospital Research and Educational Trust, 1978.

Congressional Budget Office, *Veterans Administration Health Care: Planning for Future Years*. Washington, DC: Author, 1984.

Congressional Budget Office, *Medicare and Graduate Medical Education*. Washington, DC: Author, 1995.

Davis, E. M., & Millman, M. L., *Health Care for the Urban Poor*. Totowa, NJ: Rowman and Allanheld, 1983.

Declercq, E., & Simmes, D., "The Politics of 'Drive-Through Deliveries:' Putting Early Postpartum Discharge on the Legislative Agenda," *Milbank Memorial Fund Quarterly, 75*, 175–202, 1997.

Gage, L. S., Burch, C. C., Fagnani, L., Camper, A. B., & Andrulis, D. P., *America's Urban Health Safety Net*. Washington, DC: National Association of Public Hospitals, 1994.

Grabowski, H. G., & Vernon, J. M., *The Regulation of Pharmaceuticals*. Washington, DC: American Enterprise Institute, 1983.

Gray, V., Jacob, H., & Vines, K. N. (Eds.), *Politics in the American States: A Comparative Analysis*. Boston: Little, Brown, 1983.

Holahan, J. F., & Cohen, J. W., *Medicaid: The Trade-off between Cost Containment and Access to Care*. Washington, DC: Urban Institute Press, 1986.

Holahan, J. F., & Etheredge, L. M., *Medicare Physician Payment Reform: Issues and Options*. Washington, DC: Urban Institute Press, 1986.

Iglehart, J. K., "Reform of the Veterans Affairs Health Care System," *New England Journal of Medicine, 355*, 1407–1411, 1996.

Indian Health Service, Public Health Service, U.S. Department of Health and Human Services, "Indian Health Service Fact Sheet," <http://www.tucson.ihs.gov/9Vision/ThisFacts/htm/> (April 11, 1997).

Johnson, H., & Broder, D. S., *The System: The American Way of Politics at the Breaking Point*. New York: Little, Brown, 1996.

Kosterlitz, J., "Graying Armies," *National Journal*, 664–668, March 12, 1988.

Krakower, J., Ganem, J. L., & Jolly, P., "U.S. Medical School Finances 1994–95," *Journal of the American Medical Association, 276*, 720–724, 1996.

Liska, D., & Obermaier, K., *Medicaid Expenditures and Beneficiaries: State Profiles and Trends, 1984–1993*. Washington, DC: The Urban Institute, 1995.

Marmor, T. R., *The Politics of Medicare*. Chicago: Aldine, 1973.

Marmor, T. R., *Political Analysis and American Medical Care*. New York: Cambridge University Press, 1983.

Mechanic, D., "Correcting Misconceptions in Mental Health Policy," *Milbank Memorial Fund Quarterly, 65*, 203–230, 1987.

Panem, S., *The AIDS Bureaucracy*. Cambridge, MA: Harvard University Press, 1988.

Rivlin, A. M., "Agreed: Here Comes National Health Insurance," *New York Times Magazine*, July 21, 1974.

Rovner, J., "Congress' 'Catastrophic' Attempt to Fix Medicare," in T. E. Mann & N. J. Ornstein (Eds.), *Intensive Care: How Congress Shapes Health Policy*. Washington, DC: American Enterprise Institute and the Brookings Institution, 1995.

Schick, A., "How a Bill Did Not Become a Law," in T. E. Mann & N. J. Ornstein (Eds.), *Intensive Care: How Congress Shapes Health Policy*. Washington, DC: American Enterprise Institute and the Brookings Institution, 1995.

Skocpol, T., *Boomerang: Clinton's Health Security Effort and the Turn against Government in U.S. Politics*. New York: W. W. Norton, 1996.

Smith, D. G., *Paying for Medicare: The Politics of Reform*. New York: Aldine de Gruyter, 1992.

Sparer, M., *Medicaid and the Limits of State Health Reform*. Philadelphia: Temple University Press, 1996.

Statman, M., *Competition in the Pharmaceutical Industry*. Washington, DC: American Enterprise Institute, 1983.

Thorpe, K. E., "Health Care," in G. Benjamin & C. Brecher (Eds.), *The Two New Yorks*. New York: Russell Sage Foundation, 1989.

Thorpe, K. E., & Brecher, C., "Access to Care for the Uninsured Poor in Large Cities: Do Public Hospitals Make a Difference?" *Journal of Health Politics, Policy and Law*, 12(2), 313–324, 1987.

Truman, D., *The Governmental Process*. New York: Alfred Knopf, 1960.

U.S. General Accounting Office, *Health Insurance Regulation: Wide Variation in States' Authority, Oversight and Resources* (HRD-94-26). Washington, DC: Author, 1993.

U.S. General Accounting Office, *Medicaid: Spending Pressures Drive States toward Program Reinvention* (HEHS-95-122). Washington, DC: Author, 1995a.

U.S. General Accounting Office, *Employer-Based Health Plans: Issues, Trends and Challenges Posed by ERISA* (HEHS-95-167). Washington, DC: Author, 1995b.

U.S. General Accounting Office, *Health Insurance for Children: Private Insurance Coverage Continues to Deteriorate* (HEHS-96-129). Washington, DC: Author, 1996a.

U.S. General Accounting Office, *Health Insurance Regulations: Varying State Requirements Affect Cost of Insurance* (HEHS-96-161). Washington, DC: Author, 1996b.

U.S. General Accounting Office, *VA Health Care: Issues Affecting Eligibility Reform Efforts* (HEHS-96-160). Washington, DC: Author, 1996c.

12

Governance and Management

Anthony R. Kovner

The organization of managerial work in HCOs
Current management issues
   Who should be in charge of HCOs?
   How much should be spent on management?
   Accountability of managers to "owners"

Key Words: **Governance, governing boards, accountability, organizational performance, managerial skills, managerial performance.**

Put simply, governance in health care organizations (HCOs) is the system for making important decisions, and management is the group responsible for implementing these decisions. Increasingly, health care is being provided by large organizations in which governance is differentiated from management. In smaller physician groups and nursing homes, the owner-managers may often govern, manage, and also provide care.

This chapter has two parts. The first, on governance, defines what governance is, describes who owns health care organizations, outlines the competencies governing boards should have, specifies distinctive characteristics of for-profit and nonprofit boards, and discusses current governance issues. These include what are the preferable ownership patterns; what should be the extent of organizational (HCO) autonomy, and how HCOs are to be held accountable to users. The second part of this chapter, on management, reviews the contribution of managers to the performance of HCOs, describes how managerial work is organized, and discusses management issues, such as who should be in control of HCOs, how much should be spent on the management process, and the accountability of managers to HCO "owners."

Governance

Governance is direction, control, and exercise of authority. Authority is the power or admitted right to command or act. The difference between governance and authority is that governance describes who has power and how it is exercised, whereas authority explains the bases for such power. Governance may be dominated by a few individuals or by many; it may be exercised in an authoritarian or in a democratic way. Those who govern have the final say and are accountable for HCO performance.

How the several stakeholders of an HCO view its governance depends on the particular interests of each. An HCO may be viewed as existing primarily to satisfy those who use its services, those who own or work in the organization, or some combination of both. Those who govern make decisions that affect organizational performance or, by not making decisions, allow others to influence HCO behavior. HCOs are dependent on the resources they require to achieve their purposes and survive. Such resources include patients, clinicians, facilities, and legitimacy. Governance influences the supply of resources as well as their allocation. It also influences the futures of those who work in HCOs and are served by them.

Level of Analysis

HCOs are defined as organizations directly providing health care. By this definition, a hospital, a nursing home, or a group practice is included but not a pharmaceutical company, a governmental regulatory agency, or a consumer advocacy group. There are several levels at which the behavior of HCOs can be analyzed. Decisions are made by the national government that affect the behavior of local HCOs. For example, the Medicare legislation of 1965 provided those covered by it with a higher level of financing compared with that of other age groups. General hospitals provided older Americans with more inpatient service per capita than they had previously done. The outcome was, in essence, determined not by each general hospital but by the elected representatives of the American people, who would now have government collect and reimburse more adequately for inpatient services provided to the elderly than had been done prior to enactment. Decisions affecting HCOs are also made at the level of the clinician or the consumer. For example, registered nurses may choose to work in a home care agency or in a nursing home, and patients may choose to enroll in competing health plans, such as United Health Care or US Healthcare.

In this chapter, governance will be examined at the level of the HCO, rather than that of regulators or customers. Within the HCO the focus is on the level at which policy is determined rather than that at which it is implemented.

Governance and Managers

Although those who govern are supposed to make policy and those who manage are supposed to administer policy, there is no clear-cut boundary between governance and management. In practice, those who manage are often key participants in governance, as they have the necessary time and information to define a problem or limit the policy alternatives. In large part, this is what those who manage are paid to do. On the other hand, because they have the power and the will to do so, those who govern the organization may carry out policy or manage as well. A more useful distinction between governance and management may therefore be the nature of the decisions and their relative importance. Decisions about who governs, the organizational mission, and capital investment for the future are governance, not management decisions. Hiring, scheduling, and coordinating services within departments are typically day-to-day management decisions.

Griffith, Sahney, and Mohr (1995) state that any firm or organization faces four kinds of decisions: what the mission/vision is, how resources are to be allocated, the design of the organization, and how its programs are to be implemented. They also point out that these processes may be considered at a strategic or a programmatic level. For example, at the strategic level, mission/vision can be considered in terms of assessing the environment and developing a strategic plan; at the programmatic level, developing and carrying out a marketing plan or a specific joint venture with another organization. These decisions may also involve governance, as concerned with the scope of services and the generation of resources. Or they may involve management, for example, generating information and motivating workers to carry out policy decisions. Governance also includes decisions about whom the organization provides what services at what price. Management decisions concern carrying out those governance decisions by formulating priority objectives and strategies and then reconsidering objectives and strategies as circumstances change.

Measuring Organizational Performance

Those who own HCOs are typically concerned with organizational performance. This includes defining standards and specifying measures of acceptable performance and hiring, retaining, or firing the key managers who are responsible for attaining organizational objectives. Organizational performance is variously defined by different stakeholders. Employees want higher salaries, clinicians want better equipment, patients want more services provided more conveniently, large purchasers want costs to be contained. Those governing the organization must decide what is acceptable performance and how it is to be measured. If they do not formally decide this, the judgments on performance attainment will be made by individuals and groups working at lower levels in the organization. A most common way to evaluate HCO performance is in terms of financial profitability or market share. Different parts of HCOs obviously may be operating more or less successfully relative to each other or to the organization as a whole.

HCO Ownership

Different sponsors or owners of HCOs govern in different ways and have different goals. Owners of HCOs can include physicians and nurses, cooperatives, government (federal, state, and local), churches, investors and employers, unions, and philanthropists. These groups start an HCO for various reasons. Motives are often mixed. A classification of the main reasons and goals by sponsor is shown in Table 12.1.

A word of explanation about Table 12.1. That a key goal of government is to gain votes, signifies, for example, that a politician running for election claims credit for building a local health facility and "creating" local jobs. Or an archdiocese may seek to attract, retain, and add value to members, for example, by owning and operating a facility that delivers health care according to the values of the church; that is, providing care to the poor or not allowing abortions or birth control services in its hospitals.

Health care organizations in the United States may be owned by for-profit, not-for-profit, and public agencies. There are large investor-owned for-profit hospital corporations and small for-profit home care agencies. There are church-sponsored and non-church-sponsored hospitals and nursing homes. And there are HCOs sponsored by federal, state, and local governments. Which kind of sponsorship makes the most sense varies according to circumstances and the interests of the sponsoring stakeholders. It is not uncommon for the ownership of an HCO to change when the stakeholders' interests change. For example, a church may decide to sell a hospital to a for-profit corporation because the church feels that the monies gained from the sale can be used to benefit its service constituency more than retaining the hospital will and that the for-profit corporation can better attract the capital required to operate the hospital properly.

Governing Boards

In most HCOs, especially general hospitals, HMOs, large group practices, and nursing homes there is a specialized structure such as a board, a group, or a

TABLE 12.1 Governance by Group and by Key Goals

Group	Goals
Physicians and nurses	Profit
Cooperatives	Services to members
Government	Votes
Church	Believers
Employer	Lower costs
Investors	Profit
Union	Jobs
Philanthropists	Prestige

committee that determines policy and makes a substantial number of important decisions for the HCO.

The Legal Basis of the Governing Board

Generally, there is a governing body of designated persons who have legal responsibility for the conduct of an organization. Corporations are required to make such designations as a condition of incorporation by the state in which their home office is located.

HCO bylaws usually outline the purposes of the organization, the composition and duties of the governing board, the requirements for meetings of the board and notice of meetings, the duties and nature of corporate officers and the method of their selection, the nature and purpose of board committees, and how the bylaws can be amended. A physicians' partnership agreement, for example, may typically include the responsibilities of partners, how net income is shared and losses borne, disability provisions, termination of a partner's agreement, and the composition of the executive committee or board and its functions.

The legal powers of the governing board, suggested in a model constitution and bylaws for voluntary hospitals published by the American Hospital Association (1981), are the following:

> The general powers of the corporation shall be vested in the governing board which shall have charge, control and management of the property, affairs, and funds of the corporation; shall fill vacancies among the officers for unexpired terms; and shall have the power and authority to do and perform all acts and functions not inconsistent with these bylaws or with any action taken by the corporation. (p. 11)

These bylaws can be used by any corporation, health care or otherwise, for-profit or not-for-profit.

Although in theory the governing board has the responsibility for making policy for the organization, in practice, the power and function of governing bodies in HCOs vary widely depending, for example, on the HCO's history, key resources required for survival and growth, and the nature of the local power structure. Policy in various areas may be formulated and decided on by different groups or by external organizations. For example, capital funding allocations may be decided by the board of a multiunit organization of which the hospital is only a part, the scope of hospital services decided by the governing board, the nature of clinical education programs decided by professional staff, and, issues of local marketing and community relations decided by management.

The role of the not-for-profit governing board tends to be more ambiguous than that of for-profit boards. In the nonprofit, board members may not even be aware that they are the owners of the HCO. Board members serve for a variety of reasons: community service with fiduciary responsibility, status, access to medical care, or belief that their skills and experience are vital to HCO mission attainment.

Selection of Board Members

The functions and powers of a governing board are influenced by its composition and its method of selecting members. When a hospital or a group practice is first established, the governing board usually consists of the founders, those who are contributing key resources to begin the enterprise. Officers are elected by members of the governing board. In the case of investor-owned institutions, this is done formally by voting of shares. In nonprofit organizations and large partnerships, all full members generally have an equal vote. The board members themselves then select additional members or replacements. Or board members may be chosen from larger corporate bodies whose membership may be self-selected by those making a contribution of a certain sum to the corporation. In consumer-dominated HMOs or neighborhood health centers, some or all of the members may be elected by health plan subscribers or residents of areas served by the organization.

In large HCOs, the majority of board members are typically businessmen, bankers, and lawyers, White males between 50 and 70 years of age. Board composition varies widely by type of control. Unsurprisingly, government and religious hospitals have greater proportions of governmental officials and religious leaders on their boards. For-profit and osteopathic hospitals have a greater proportion of physicians on their boards.

Board members may be "insiders" (HCO managers or clinicians) or "outsiders," chosen for some special expertise, status, or access to resources. The type of person selected will depend in large part on the functions and role of the board. If the primary function of the board is to raise money or to give advice and counsel to the chief executive officer (CEO), then outsiders are more likely to be selected. If the primary function is to decide policy, then the directors should have detailed knowledge of HCO operations and the environment; in that case insiders may be preferred. Governance of hospitals has been dominated by outsider trustees and governance of group practices by insider physicians.

According to Bowen (1994), the principal functions of a board of directors or trustees are as follows:

- To select, encourage, advise, evaluate, and if need be, replace the CEO.
- To review and adopt long-term strategic directions and to approve specific objectives, financial and other.

- To ensure, to the extent possible, that the necessary resources, including human resources, will be available to pursue the strategies and achieve the objectives.
- To monitor the performance of management.
- To ensure that the organization operates responsibly as well as effectively.
- To nominate suitable candidates for election to the board and to establish and carry out an effective system of governance at the board level, including evaluation of board performance.

Except in large, investor-owned HCOs, most board members are not paid for their time. The vast majority of nonprofits do not pay board members. But a great deal of time is required to serve, time that could be spent earning money, and remuneration might force accountability or motivate certain persons to serve. See Pointer and Ewell (1994) for the pros and cons of this issue.

Board Competencies

Chait, Holland, and Taylor (1991) have identified six specific competencies that characterize highly effective boards. These are

- The *contextual* dimension: the board understands and takes into account the culture and norms of the organization it governs.
- The *educational* dimension: the board takes the necessary steps to ensure that members are well informed about the organization, the professions that work in it, and the board's own roles, responsibilities, and performance.
- The *interpersonal* dimension: the board nurtures the development of its members as a group, attends to the board's collective welfare, and fosters a sense of cohesiveness.
- The *analytical* dimension: the board recognizes complexities and subtleties in the issues it faces, drawing on multiple perspectives to dissect complex problems and to synthesize appropriate responses.
- The *political* dimension: the board accepts as one of its primary responsibilities the need to develop and maintain healthy relationships among key constituencies.
- The *strategic* dimension: the board helps envision and shape institutional direction in order to ensure the long-term survival and growth of the organization.

In helping boards become more effective, the competency approach lends itself to measuring baseline performance, developing an intervention program to improve performance, and then remeasuring perceived competencies after the intervention.

We are assuming that (a) the board and the CEO are committed to improving board performance and (b) the board has work of its own to do, rather than merely rubber-stamping proposals of the CEO. The board is costly to the organization in terms of executive time devoted to it and to the process of board decision making in relation to which benefits should be derived. Such benefits to the organization may include fund-raising and selection and evaluation of the CEO, but perhaps most important are development of long-range strategies to focus and improve organizational performance and monitoring of existing strategies and their implementation.

Board Composition, Structure, and Function

Governing boards vary in composition, internal structure, and function. According to an Ernst and Young study (1997), hospital board memberships average about 13 members, although some boards had fewer than 7 or more than 16 members. As noted, the majority of hospital board members are between 50 and 70 years old and are typically predominantly White male businessmen, bankers, and lawyers. Boards usually meet on a monthly basis; some boards meet quarterly. Most boards have committees of two types: standing or permanent committees and special committees, which are discharged on completion of a task. Typical standing committees are executive, finance, nominating, and long-range planning. Nonboard members can serve on these committees. Executive committees usually have the power to act between regular meetings of the governing board.

Appropriate composition, structure, and function depend on environmental and organizational circumstances. The boards of a national for-profit nursing home corporation and a nonprofit academic medical center should not necessarily have the same composition, structure, or function. What makes the most sense in any set of circumstances depends on the mission of the organization and the expected contribution of the board to attainment of that mission.

The Changing Role of the Board

Views of the role of governing boards differ and are changing. More than 40 years ago, Burling, Lentz, and Wilson (1956) stated that a hospital governing board has a responsibility to provide and maintain the hospital to serve a community need according to the wishes of the donor(s). To Umbdenstock (1987) the board must be the "organization's conscience, constantly assessing proposed directions . . . in light of what these steps mean for the implementation of a mission to serve and care for all" (p. 12).

It is easy to say that the board should be concerned with policy and oversight functions and that the staff should be responsible for management and administration (Bowen, 1994). But how this is best worked out in any organization depends on the skills and experience of the board and those of top management and on mutual perceptions and expectations, given the organization's circumstances and history.

Board Relationship to Independent Medical Staff

According to Griffith (1995), in the nonprofit HCO, the governing board "owns" the organization but cannot practice medicine. The independently practicing physicians are appointed to the medical staff by the board and do practice medicine. The CEO is the board's designate on site. The privileges agreement between the attending physicians and the HCO goes as follows: the board participates in implementing and revising the medical bylaws (and there may be some physicians on the board). The medical staff organization develops and enforces the rules as long as the board agrees that these are beneficial (in nonprofits, to the community; in for-profits, to the shareholders). According to Griffith, the compact breaks down if the board does not act vigorously as trustees for community (or shareholder) interests.

Current Governance Issues

Some key current governance issues include the following questions: What are preferable HCO ownership patterns? How should and can nonprofit board performance be improved? To what extent should the autonomy of HCOs be limited? What should be the extent and nature of HCO accountability to those served and potentially served?

Preferable Ownership Patterns

Does it make any difference whether HCOs are owned by government or by for-profit or nonprofit corporations? Does it make enough of a difference to justify tax exemption for nonprofits? Currently, government is the primary owner of facilities that provide long-term mental health care and those that serve veterans, for-profit corporations and partnerships dominate in nursing home and physician practice markets, and nonprofits own most of the short-term community hospitals.

There is insufficient evidence to make categorical statements regarding the effect of the type of ownership per se on the cost or quality of medical care or as to whether the performance of nonprofit HCOs justifies continued preferential tax treatment. Tax exemption applies to income, state, and local taxes. Exempt status makes gifts to the organization tax-deductible for donors and allows the organization access to tax-free bonds. A related issue concerns conversions from nonprofit to for-profit status and their valuation.

Schlesinger, Gray, and Bradley (1996) argue that persons associated with nonprofits respond to different incentives and that nonprofits operate under constraints that are different from those of for-profits. In their empirical study of 225 utilization review organizations (UROs), they found that nonprofit UROs are significantly more likely to engage in grant-funded research and to make public information about their processes for utilization review. The nonprofit UROs also appear more community minded in that they are significantly more influenced by their boards of directors and are more likely to incorporate norms of treatment than for-profits.

Those who argue against for-profit ownership say that for-profits concentrate on providing only those services that are profitable, leaving the not-for-profits and public HCOs to provide services to those who lack adequate health care insurance. A corollary argument is that for-profits build facilities only in expanding high-income communities, leaving nonprofits and governmental HCOs to provide services to the urban and rural poor. Opponents argue that the monies allocated to the shareholders of for-profits can better be reinvested in the delivery of services to those lacking access and that health care is of lower quality in for-profits than in nonprofit or governmental HCOs.

Counterarguments have been made in favor of for-profit ownership. Those in favor say that, even allowing for profit, these HCOs are more efficient because of the profit incentive, and they pay taxes. Consumers should be charged for the costs of the services that they use, rather than overcharging, as nonprofits do, certain consumers because others cannot pay. Moreover, for-profits respond more quickly and more flexibly in meeting community demand, and the quality of care most of them provide is adequate and sometimes higher than that of some similar nonprofits and public HCOs.

Proponents of public ownership argue that their total costs and unit costs are lower, signifying greater efficiency, yet every user gets treated similarly, based on health needs and regardless of income or disease status. They say that the quality of care is not lower than that provided by other HCOs. Those who disagree say that primary emphasis in public HCOs is on keeping costs low rather than on providing adequate health care services. Moreover, government operations are bureaucratic and inflexible, and the quality of care is lower in public HCOs.

Those in favor of nonprofits praise their high quality of care and the high level of community service; those opposed cite their high cost. For specific nonprofits, opponents add that the quality of care is low and the community services nonexistent.

In order to come to any conclusions as to preferred auspices, further research relating ownership to performance must be conducted. To properly carry out such research, it is required that conditions other than ownership, such as the size of the HCO, be held constant. Also required is a greater consensus on what is adequate and effective performance in various HCOs.

Nonprofit Governing Board Performance

What is the value of the nonprofit governing board, and how can the value of the board be increased relative to its cost? This assumes some consensus as to what the nonprofit HCO board is supposed to do. Boards represent an ownership interest that is different from management's interest. Different owners have different values that they seek to maximize. In nonprofit HCOs such values may include improving health services in a community at acceptable levels of cost and quality. In any case, nonprofit boards add value by holding management accountable for results in respect to specified values and by considering longer range HCO futures, again to attain certain objectives and expectations of stakeholders.

Are boards adding enough value, however, given the costs of perpetuating them or the alternatives to not having them? Large government agencies are usually not run by boards but rather by executives with oversight from the legislative branch. The goals of for-profits are usually clear-cut—to make more money, now or over the longer term. Some of the costs of self-perpetuating nonprofit boards include the time it takes for these boards to reach policy decisions, the ineffectiveness of those decisions or a lack of sufficient decisions, and the time and effort it takes for management to staff and provide support to the boards. Costs increase when board members lack the skills and experience to carry out their responsibilities (i.e., hold management accountable) or when boards act to pursue interests conflicting with the purposes of the organization.

Board costs tend to be higher in nonprofit organizations whose accountability lacks the clarity of for-profit firms organized to maximize returns to shareholders. Board costs can be lowered when board members are selected on the basis of relevant skills and experience, when they focus on areas where the boards can add value rather than on micromanaging issues better decided by qualified managers, and when organizational accountability is sharpened because the health services organization faces competitive pressures.

So then, what is the issue? When nonprofit boards do not perform well and lack the will or ability to perform better, what should government or managers or the market do about it? Obviously, where there is healthy competition, the market forces accountability, and how boards add value is of less public concern. Although management should assist the board in carrying out its responsibilities, obviously management should be accountable to the board, as owners, rather than the other way around. Government should at least set the rules for and disclose the performance of health services organizations. Accrediting organizations have similar concerns. Setting the rules includes, for example, establishing personal liability for board members when they have committed a breach of fiduciary duty, as when they pursue self-interest such as gaining secret profits personally or competing with the organization. Disclosing performance includes disclosing information related to board performance—for example, limitations on terms of office, the presence of measurable objectives for the board, and the numbers and types of board members and board committees.

Others have argued that government should set requirements for boards, such as who can serve on nonprofit boards, whether meetings should be open to the public, and establishing quality-of-care committees to review systems of quality of care in HCOs.

The Extent of Organizational Autonomy

To what extent should an HCO be allowed to determine what services to provide to whom and at what price? The autonomy of HCO governing boards has been shrinking since 1960. Federal and state governments have passed legislation, for example, forbidding discrimination against patients who seek admission or persons seeking employment and invalidating a requirement that staff physicians of a voluntary hospital be graduates of a medical school approved by the AMA and be members of the county medical society. Government has removed the exemption of hospitals from state labor laws, specified standards to be met by HCOs in order to be licensed by a state or reimbursed by Medicare, and forbidden construction of hospitals, nursing homes, and related facilities in some states without prior approval by state planning authorities. Limitations on the autonomy of HCOs also include limiting payment for new technology under Medicare and Medicaid; imposing requirements for community services for hospitals to retain not-for-profit status; requiring, in West Virginia, community representation on governing boards; and capping revenues in some states or limiting reimbursement under Medicare (by diagnosis-related groups [DRGs]) to average payments for length of stay regardless of cost. Most recently, some states have required that all Medicaid beneficiaries enroll in managed care plans. Managed care plans have been regulated in some states so that normal deliveries must be covered for a hospital stay of 48 hours, and physicians must be allowed to discuss with patients treatments for which the HMO will not pay.

There is no simple answer to the question of the extent to which HCOs should independently determine what services they offer, what prices they charge, and what population they serve. Too little autonomy for the HCO board will result in withdrawal from leadership positions of high-quality individuals who have been a strength of not-for-profit HCOs. Excessive standardization and centralization of decision making in governmental bureaucracies will result in decreased HCO innovation and eventually in lower productivity. On the other hand, too much autonomy for HCOs may have been responsible, at least in part, for the present situation of uneven age-adjusted mortality and morbidity rates by race and income, overutilization of acute care and underutilization of long-term care, uneven productivity and service, and high cost. One suggestion for appropriate centralization and decentralization is the regionalization of HCOs. Of course, this may be accomplished through the market, as well as by government.

Accountability to Those Served

Whatever the scope of HCO activities and their regulation by government, what should be the extent and nature of organizational accountability to users and potential users of service? Some who advocate more formal accountability argue that this can be assured only by a governing board controlled by consumer representatives. Opponents argue that such control will lead to ineffective decision making at the board level and eventual withdrawal of community resources formerly donated. The opponents ask, furthermore, what evidence there is that the newly chosen representatives will be any more accountable to either users of the service or to the community in general. In what ways would they be more accountable and to whom?

Regardless of the issues at the governing board level, appeal mechanisms should be available for consumers at the level at which services are received, especially in large HCOs. In many HCOs, consumers lack an organized voice when they are dissatisfied, for example, with the manner of the provider, the wait for services, or the explanations they receive about their examination, diagnosis, and treatment plan. Consumers may be told only to seek service elsewhere, or they can sue for malpractice. Consumers who are poor or institutionalized often lack even these unsatisfactory alternatives. Proposals have been made and implemented regarding a variety of appeal mechanisms—the special board committee, the externally appointed ombudsman, the patient advocate—all specialized mechanisms for helping patients who feel that they have been unfairly treated by the HCO. Other, more general responsiveness mechanisms include quality improvement, consumer advisory councils, focus groups and market surveys, and holding the CEO personally accountable for responding to consumer complaints. As with most solutions, there are difficulties in implementing the various mechanisms and limitations to their usefulness. For example, to whom does the consumer appeal if dissatisfied with the response of the appeal mechanisms, which is, after all, a creation of the HCO? Appeal mechanisms may be costly in relation to benefits obtained by the consumer. And there are many aspects of care that consumers (and providers) find objectionable but about which little can be done at the level of the HCO, such as obtaining high-quality accessible ambulatory care for the uninsured. Finally, appeal mechanisms may serve only as buffers that satisfy the occasional vocal complainant but do little to change the system of care that may be the cause of much more unspoken dissatisfaction among many.

Management

Now we shall focus on managers in HCOs—what they do, how they are trained, how they contribute to organizational performance and its measurement—and on management issues, such as what managers *should* do, how much money *should* be spent on the management function, how managers *should* be trained, and how management performance *should* be improved.

The Organization of Managerial Work in HCOs

In simple organizations such as the physician's office, clinicians themselves perform managerial functions such as billing patients or contracting with an outside vendor to bill patients (see Figure 12.1). In a group practice, the hiring, paying, and firing of physicians is done either by the whole group or, generally in the larger group practices, by all or a subset of clinicians who manage and also practice medicine. Other work for the group, such as billing, is supervised by nonclinician managers. In the large hospital or HMO, specialized functional managers support clinician and nonclinician general managers. Such functions include human resources (personnel), finance, information services, and marketing, among others. In multiunit organizations (also called integrated delivery systems), which may include hospitals, nursing homes, group practices, and an HMO, managers of these units may report to divisional managers for a geographical area, such as the northeastern United States. Division managers, in turn, report to managers in corporate headquarters who are accountable to a board of directors. In these large organizations certain management functions are allocated among headquarters, division, and local HCOs. Headquarters functions commonly include legal affairs, construction, capital financing, and corporate public relations. Other functions, such as quality improvement and production standards, may be divided among the three organizational levels.

A newer development in the organization of managerial work in HCOs is product-line management. The large hospital or group practice can be reorganized into several product lines, such as women's health services, emergency care,

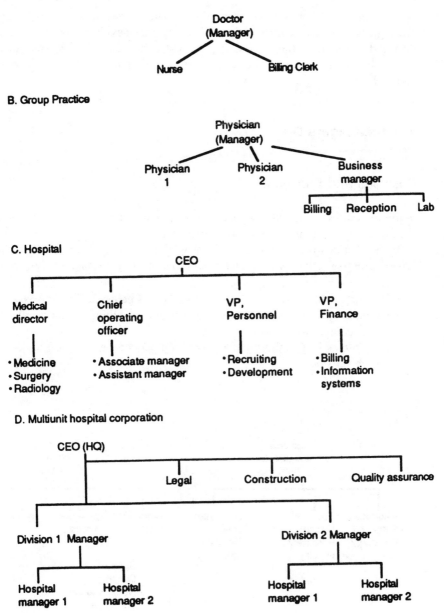

A. Doctor's office

Doctor (Manager)
- Nurse
- Billing Clerk

B. Group Practice

Physician (Manager)
- Physician 1
- Physician 2
- Business manager
  - Billing
  - Reception
  - Lab

C. Hospital

CEO
- Medical director
  - Medicine
  - Surgery
  - Radiology
- Chief operating officer
  - Associate manager
  - Assistant manager
- VP, Personnel
  - Recruiting
  - Development
- VP, Finance
  - Billing
  - Information systems

D. Multiunit hospital corporation

CEO (HQ)
- Legal
- Construction
- Quality assurance
- Division 1 Manager
  - Hospital manager 1
  - Hospital manager 2
- Division 2 Manager
  - Hospital manager 1
  - Hospital manager 2

FIGURE 12.1   Organization of managerial work in HCOs.

cancer care, and rehabilitation services, each with its own manager and budget. The logic behind such reorganization is that these services can be more effectively managed as separate "businesses" than as part of a large HCO. Whether or not this really is so is unproved. (For a comparison with traditional organization, see Figure 12.2.)

What Managers Do

Positions and Functions

A job or position description is one way of looking at the work that managers do. For an example of an HCO position description, see Table 12.2.

Implicit in this job description are managerial functions, each of which comprises a group of activities. Longest (1980) views the basic managerial functions as

- Planning, which involves the determination of goals and objectives.
- Organizing, which is the structuring of people and things to accomplish the work required to meet the objectives.
- Directing, which is the stimulation of members of the organization to meet the objectives.

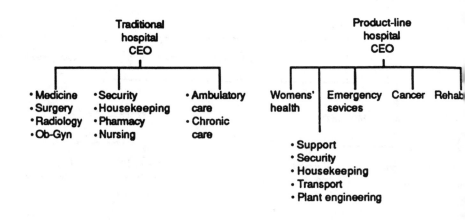

FIGURE 12.2   Traditional versus product-line organization.

TABLE 12.2   Position Description of Operations Coordinator

Reason position exists
　To assist in all operational aspects of the physician hospital organization (PHO). To provide analytical support, maintain PC systems and coordinate various implementation projects.

Reports to
　Executive director, PHO

Duties and responsibilities
　Schedule, coordinate, and maintain minutes for all IPA and PHO board meetings and board committee meetings.
　Prepare written correspondence, including, but not limited to, position papers and research, education and information pieces, and memos and letters.
　Maintain PC files on database, spreadsheet and word processing programs. Possible desktop publishing responsibilities.
　Maintain financial income and expense spreadsheets for preparation of financial statements; maintain bank accounts and perform banking functions; maintain files for budget preparation and presentation.
　Design and produce reports for distribution on IPA and PHO activity.
　Maintain and assist in the analysis of reports from utilization management, HMOs, hospital systems, and IDX to produce data, as needed to analyze PHO performance.
　Maintain, update, and assist in the preparation of reports on IPA membership demographics, finances, and utilization performance.
　Assist in other projects as needed.

Knowledge, skills, and abilities
　Knowledge of managed care reimbursement and operations, working knowledge of physician and hospital reimbursement
　Proficiency in spreadsheet and database applications
　Excellent writing, organization, and presentation skills
　Motivation to initiate/recommend action or research options for problem solving or program enhancement. Ability to follow up appropriately and effectively to affect action.
　Superior interpersonal skills and judgment
　Comfort level with financial issues and accuracy in financial work

Education and experience
　Bachelor's degree in public administration, health care administration, or finance/accounting with health care course work or experience; master's degree preferred
　Managed care experience in finance, analysis, utilization management, contracting, or a combination of the above; experience may be in a hospital, physician group, HMO, or regulatory setting
　Proven organizational or project management experience

- Coordinating, which is the conscious effort of assembling and synchronizing diverse activities and participants so that they work toward the attainment of objectives.
- Controlling, in which the manager compares actual results with objectives to provide a measure of success or failure.

Boyatzis (1995) has developed a model that includes three groups of 22 managerial abilities. These include efficiency orientation, planning, initiative, attention to detail, self-control and flexibility (goal and action management), empathy, persuasiveness, networking, negotiating, self-confidence, group management, developing others, oral communication (people management), and use of concepts, systems thinking, pattern recognition, theory building, technology, quantitative analysis, social objectivity, and written communication (analytic reasoning).

Managerial Roles

Another way of conceptualizing what managers do is in terms of roles, which are aspects of behavior that can be isolated for analytical purposes, such as leading or handling disturbances. Managers settle conflicts, inspire other workers, and represent the organization to outside groups. An individual manager's roles can thus be abstracted. This helps in understanding how managers contribute to organizational effectiveness and the constraints and opportunities they face in their work.

Because of the fragmented authority structure of many HCOs, managers often must lead by persuasion rather than by directive. Leadership is a relational rather than an individual characteristic, and therefore effectiveness as a leader is measured by what followers do rather than by how managers behave. The health care manager, especially in public and voluntary organizations, is constantly involved in testing the positions of others inside and outside the HCO and in confronting the several claimants for organizational resources. The manager must constantly persuade physicians, nurses, and others that the organization has good reasons for not doing what they want to do or the way they want to do it. External regulatory agencies may compel or allow certain actions desired by some claimants. What some claimants want may not be equitable for other parties. Some claimants may demand unequal treatment because the organization is especially dependent on them.

An example of this is the demand by a hospital department head of inhalation therapy, supported by the chief of pulmonary medicine, for an increase in salary beyond the general guidelines for department heads. Either the hospital administrator must deny the request and convince these two individuals that the denial is fair or the administrator must approve the request and convince the other department heads that the increase is fair or at least that the decision was arrived at fairly. If he denies the increase request, the administrator may face trying to persuade the head of inhalation therapy not to leave and the chief of pulmonary medicine not to oppose management.

Kovner (1984) has reconceptualized managerial roles into four sets: motivating others, scanning the environment, negotiating the political terrain, and generating and allocating resources.

Motivating Others. Managers spend a great deal of time recruiting and retaining managerial and supervisory staff and in making decisions about rewards and promotions, work procedures, and development and training. To carry out these activities, they use communications and analytical skills. Managers assist subordinates in doing what is required and in doing what subordinates want to do, within organizational limits. This can be difficult if managers have not recruited their own subordinates.

An example of motivating others is managerial development and training. Managers in new organizations or in new positions in existing organizations must be developed and trained by their supervisors. Such development and training can assist in the subordinate's learning process. Managers can aid those who work with them by identifying the skills that must be learned and the experience that must be acquired for effective job performance. Senior managers can also help those less experienced become more aware of their own values, how they are perceived by others, and how the values of others affect their job performance in their current position in this HCO.

Scanning the Environment. Effective managers scan or search the environment for potential problems and targets of opportunity. Scanning activities include market and product research, long-range planning, and quality benchmarking. The development of management information systems may be essential for effective scanning. In large HCOs scanning activities are usually performed by special units for marketing, quality assessment, development, and planning. In smaller HCOs managers may scan the environment themselves or be assisted by subordinates or colleagues. Information about what similar organizations and managers do is available from journals, books, the Internet, newsletters, and advertisements. Managers attend continuing education and trade association meetings and are part of on-line networks where colleagues and experts communicate about organizational and managerial opportunities and challenges. Managers visit similar organizations to learn at firsthand about possible ways to improve effectiveness and efficiency. Openness to such visits has been a characteristic of public and voluntary HCOs.

Negotiating the Political Terrain. Effective managers maintain trust and build alliances with groups and individuals. A positive political climate contributes to effective decision making and implementation. New managers must find out "who in the organization is doing what to whom." Or put another way, "What is the ball park in which I am playing, who are the players, and what are the rules?" Managers learn the informal power structure by looking and listening. The operative rules are not always easy to ascertain. They vary by organizational setting, and they depend on the issue being discussed. Decision makers involved in modernizing a management information system are different from those who decide to establish a new renal dialysis unit.

Activities the manager undertakes in negotiating the political terrain also include public relations, lobbying, labor relations, influencing decisions made by governing boards and medical staffs, arbitrating between internal units and departments, and making alliances with other organizations.

Generating and Allocating Resources. Effective managers spend a great deal of time analyzing organizational efficiency and finding ways to increase revenues and decrease expenses. In doing this, managers must consider past performance in this organization, present performance in like organizations, and industry standards.

Effective managers attempt to improve financial performance, for example, by streamlining of buying procedures, efficient securing of long-term and working capital, effective maintenance of buildings and equipment, appropriate pricing changes, and coordination of the timing of new construction or renovations. Effective managers try to understand special circumstances as they influence preferences among alternative objectives and strategies, and they listen closely to explanations of and analysis by subordinates and clinicians.

Effective managers continually make decisions about generating and using resources. This occurs as part of the budgetary process and in response to emergency or extraordinary requests. Less tangible resources, such as staff time, must also be allocated, as must resources that may be less amenable to negotiation, such as use of space.

Other ways of looking at what managers do include task specification, skills and experience required, how and where the manager spends his or her time, and managerial beliefs and personalities.

Educating Health Services Managers

How do people learn to be health care managers? Can health care management be taught? Is it a science, an art, a craft, or something of all three? What can best be learned at school and on the job?

Graduate Programs. Graduate education is often required of persons seeking employment as health care managers, particularly in some large HCOs. There are over 250 graduate programs in health care management in the United States today. Such programs are named differently and often related to school auspices or age of the program. Such names commonly include health care or medical care administration or management. Other programs are titled health policy and management, health systems management, or health and hospital administration. Graduate programs in health services management exist now throughout the world, in such cities as Buenos Aires, Athens, London, Warsaw, Nairobi, Melbourne, and New Delhi. As of 1996, 70 American and Canadian graduate programs were members of the Association of University Programs in Health Administration (AUPHA) headquartered in Arlington, Virginia. Twenty-eight of these programs were housed in graduate schools of business or public administration, 16 in schools of public health, and 16 in schools of medicine. Some of these programs are under joint auspices such as business and public health, and some are under other auspices, such as allied health or pharmacy (AUPHA, personal communication, December 19, 1996).

In academic year 1995–96 a total of 6,231 students were enrolled in 72 AUPHA graduate programs; 53% of these students were full-time, 57% were female, and 17% were members of minority groups. In the same academic year, 52% of those applying were accepted. An average of 1,500 to 2,000 students graduate from these AUPHA member programs annually.

As of 1996, 67 of the AUPHA programs had been accredited by the Accrediting Commission on Education for Health Services Administration (ACESHA). ACESHA is sponsored by AUPHA, together with the American College of Healthcare Executives (ACHE), the American Hospital Association (AHA), the American Public Health Association (APHA), the American Medical Association (AMA), the American College of Medical Practice Executives (ACMPE), the American College of Physician Executives (AMPE), the American Organization of Nurse Executives (AONE), the Healthcare Financial Management Association (HFMA), and the Canadian College of Health Services Executives (CCHSE). For accreditation, ACEHSA requires that the curriculum of a graduate program cover the following areas:

- Health status of populations; determinants of health and illness; and factors influencing the use of health services.
- Organization, financing and delivery of health services, drawing on the social science disciplines.
- Development of skills in economic, financial, policy and quantitative analysis.
- Values and ethical issues associated with the practice of health services administration, and the development of skills in ethical analysis.
- Positioning organizations favorably in the environment and managing these organizations for continued effectiveness.

- Development of leadership potential including stimulating creativity, and interpersonal and communication skill development.
- Management of human, capital, and information resources.
- Assessing organizational performance and in particular, methods to assure continuous improvement in the quality of services provided. (ACEHSA, 1994)

In addition to curricular requirements for accreditation, ACEHSA sets criteria in the following areas: program mission, goals, objectives, and evaluation; faculty; research and community service; students and alumni; and resources and academic relationships.

Many graduate programs in health services management include an academic and a practice component, which may involve employment with or without pay for students in HCOs for a period of from 3 to 12 months. Increasingly, 1-year fellowships are being offered by large HCOs to provide additional training to program graduates.

Undergraduate Programs. Undergraduate programs are also offered in health care administration. As of 1995–96, 31 undergraduate programs in the United States were members of AUPHA, and 3,697 students were enrolled in these programs.

Many of the undergraduate programs attempt to produce managers for intermediate-level positions in large HCOs and for higher level positions in smaller organizations. The curriculum offered by the undergraduate programs is generally similar to that offered by graduate programs. Courses that are generally required include introduction to the health care field, economics, health law, management, human resources, financial management, health policy, medical sociology, and quantitative methods.

Continuing Nondegree Education. In addition to graduate and undergraduate programs, there is a great variety of continuing education programs in health services management. They are of various length and cover various subjects, such as shaping an efficient and sustainable physician compensation system or developing a competitive integrated delivery system. Some continuing education programs are offered by the university programs themselves. Others are offered by centers of continuing education that are freestanding or that have been sponsored by professional associations or by corporations that sell equipment and services to health services organizations. Still others are offered by large HCOs.

On the Job. Much of what managers learn about what works in an organization and about how best they can work with clinicians and customers is taught on the job. Most large HCOs have formal orientation programs and offer special training courses on site as well. Managers can learn from others at work how best to write what they mean, how not to always say what they are thinking, and how to more effectively influence others. Superiors, subordinates, and peers can assist managers also in developing agendas and in forming and energizing networks through which to accomplish their agendas.

Managerial Contribution to Effective HCO Performance

HCOs are seldom formally evaluated in terms of preset measurable objectives. Part of the reason is the difficulty of securing agreement among the various parties of interest as to what these objectives should be, who should evaluate performance, and by what methods. Yet the basic problem in public organizations, according to Drucker (1973), is not high cost but lack of effectiveness: "Only if targets are defined can resources be allocated to this attainment, priorities and deadlines be set, and somebody be held accountable for results" (p. 46).

Measuring Organizational Performance

One reason for attempting to specify effective or acceptable organizational performance is to focus attention on "whose organization this is." If performance is acceptable to managers, clinicians, and trustees, does it matter what anyone else thinks? If it does matter, what are others going to do if they find performance unacceptable?

Another reason for developing measures of organizational performance concerns the distribution of organizational resources. To adjudicate claims on resources, questions may have to be raised about the organization's purposes. For example, "How is our HMO doing? How does what we do compare with what our competitors do? How does what we do compare with what our doctors, nurses, trustees, customers, and potential customers think we ought to be doing?"

Prior agreement about standards of performance facilitates agreement on performance evaluation. Otherwise, performance is not measurable in terms such as excellent, acceptable, and unacceptable. Statements such as "The hospital operated at a $100,000 surplus this year, 1% of patients made formal complaints, and our turnover rate in nursing was 15% this year" are uncertain indicators of performance unless they can be related to agreed-upon standards and purposes. The standards of performance for which the organization and its managers are to be held accountable must be made clear in measurable terms and in advance. Of course, targets can be adjusted for fully explained reasons as circumstances change.

Putting Performance Standards into Operation

Standards can be developed regarding performance requirements. Certain standards, such as financial ratios, are easier to quantify than others, such as commitment of clinicians and other workers to organizational performance requirements. Yet commitment can be quantified in terms of nurse turnover and absenteeism rates; employee attitudes, as measured by surveys; and physician commitment, as measured by attendance at quality improvement meetings and contributions to fund-raising campaigns. Whether the effort and cost of implementing such requirements and then measuring performance is "worth it" is, of course, a separate and not trivial question.

In 1978, Griffith argued that guidelines must be developed for hospital performance in the face of national concern about rapidly increasing health care costs. As of 1996 the Foundation for Accountability (FACCT), a new organization measuring quality whose services can be bought by employers purchasing health services from large health plans, was developing criteria for evaluating care in the areas of breast cancer, diabetes, and depression (Belkin, 1996). Diabetes care, for example, can be reviewed to determine whether a health plan individual physician regularly examines a patient's feet to avoid loss of the foot to circulatory complications, regularly checks blood sugar levels, and does annual eye exams to detect problems that can lead to blindness. Using patient questionnaires, laboratory billing records, and test results, an organization such as FACCT can next look at patients' satisfaction and their access to specialists and support services. Finally, they can count results: Are patients able to cope with diabetes and its treatment? How many keep their blood sugar at desired levels? How many can avoid being hospitalized? We are still a long way from the acceptance of a few well-understood measures of health care for diseases—not to mention populations—uniformly available and designed to permit any community to compare itself to other similar populations, by state, region, and the nation as a whole. But perhaps we have finally started down the road toward that goal.

Results of Not Specifying Goals

Not specifying or targeting organizational performance requirements may result in lower levels of performance than would otherwise occur. By not focusing on particular goals and levels of attainment, the organization may fail to perform satisfactorily. Strong members of a coalition may gain more power or resources at the expense of the weak than would have happened if the goals of the weak had been considered formally by all participants.

When performance requirements are not specified and opportunistic interests prevail, long-term survival of HCOs may be threatened or short-term organizational crises may become more frequent and more severe. Not specifying performance requirements favors retention of the present power structure. And as long as the organization can continue to obtain the necessary and appropriate inputs and sell or dispose of adequate quantities of outputs, the status quo will tend to be perceived as a satisfactory level of goal attainment.

The environment that many HCOs will be facing in the next 5 years before and after 2000 is expected to be even more competitive and problematic than that of the early 1990s. Hospitals, medical groups, and health plans are competing and allying with each other to recruit patients and primary care physicians. Clinicians and managers disagree about nurse staffing and functions. Physicians and organizations are in conflict concerning pay and productivity standards. In these circumstances, goal specification may be increasingly perceived by effective HCOs as less costly than direct conflict over limited resources. Evidence of a trend toward goal specification may be found in the startling growth of investor-owned corporations, such as Columbia (and of the large nonprofits who compete with them), many of which have well-developed internal systems specifying performance requirements by division, unit, or department.

Measuring Managerial Contribution

Managers disagree regarding how and whether they should be evaluated and by whom, and it is indeed difficult to isolate managerial contribution to organizational performance. For example, despite substantial managerial contributions, an organization may be floundering because of a hostile environment or poor decisions by previous managers. Or the reverse situation may be occurring; despite little or ineffective managerial contribution, an organization may be growing rapidly or raising quality standards and performance because of lack of competitors, excellent previous manager performance, and excellent physicians and nurses now.

Reasons for Evaluating Managers

Generally, health services managers are evaluated, as are other employees, to improve organizational performance. A manager may be evaluated relative to what he or she has accomplished previously or relative to what managers in like organizations contribute, assuming a correlation between managerial and organizational performance.

Evaluation is a way of communicating to managers how superiors feel about their performance and of learning from managers how they regard superiors' assessments. This can serve as a basis for desired changes in behavior by managers, or it may stimulate superiors to make certain changes that would enable managers to perform as desired. The evaluation process can focus both superiors and managers on the most important organizational objectives for a future time period and can stimulate efforts to generate additional resources necessary to attain goals.

Formal evaluation may not be necessary for a high level of managerial performance or for a high level of satisfaction with managerial contribution by superiors. Nor is formal evaluation of the manager a panacea for effectively adjudicating political conflict, as between board members and physicians. Formal evaluation can avoid misunderstandings about what constitutes satisfactory managerial performance. The process can facilitate specification of managerial performance requirements that are realistic and responsive to organizational constraints and opportunities.

Current Management Issues

Some current issues in HCO management include the following questions: How should managers function in HCOs? Is managerial compensation too high relative to other HCO workers? How should managers be trained? How can management performance be improved?

The Role of HCO Managers

Should HCO managers basically support the work of more or less independent clinicians, or are managers in charge of HCO goal attainment to conclude alliances with other organizations and coordinate the work of the organization? What should be the relationship of line and staff managers in large HCOs? For example, to what extent should a local HMO manager be responsible for marketing relative to the marketing specialists in HMO central headquarters in another state? How should front-line managers best spend their time—attending internal management meetings, improving service quality, or meeting with suppliers and competitors?

Given the increasing size and complexity of HCOs, the manager's job is becoming more important (and more highly paid) and his or her job security less secure. New kinds of managerial jobs are being created in large HCOs, such as risk management specialist, medical service organization (MSO) director, and director of system development. The risk management specialist evaluates the actuarial health risk of a population in support of capitated contract negotiations. The MSO director solicits and negotiates contracts for hundreds of physicians and oversees administrative support across different physician groups. The director of system development leads joint venture discussions and continuously scans the market for merger and acquisition candidates (Advisory Board, 1996).

There is an increasing demand for managers skilled in the production process of health care and in marketing services to different target populations, such as seniors. Often, functional experts operate at the corporate headquarters of large HCOs and set standards that must be carried out corporation-wide. Managers must attend internal meetings focused on strategies to attain organizational objectives and listen to customers, suppliers, and competitors in formulating the objectives and monitoring results.

Managerial Compensation

Do HCOs spend too much money on management relative to provision of care? Do managers make too much money related to their contribution, compared with clinicians, technicians, and nonprofessional workers? How should managers be paid, and to what extent should pay be related to performance?

The reader will get different answers to the above questions from a public hospital CEO, a for-profit HMO manager, a primary care physician, and a unionized dietary worker. Part of the answer relates to what contribution top managers make to organizational performance, and part relates to determinations of what are acceptable profits in a just society. These questions are by no means specific to health care but can be raised about other sectors of the economy as well. For example, some argue that top business executives make too much or too little money and unionized teachers make too little or too much relative to their contributions to their organizations and to society.

High salaries generate newspaper stories, which sometimes lead to new legislation. Chief executive officers of HMOs, who on average earn 62% more than those of other corporations of similar size, are criticized in the press as making multimillion-dollar incomes by denying patients medical treatment. Mergers and takeovers may generate large fortunes; the CEO of U.S. Healthcare received almost $1 billion in cash and stock as part of that company's merger with Aetna insurance company (Bodenheimer, 1996).

Proponents of paying managers more argue that health care is increasingly a competitive sector of the economy as patients are choosing lower-cost and higher-quality HCOs that are managed better. The management function may be generally responsible for keeping costs down and quality high, and managers must be attracted to work in health care as opposed to other sectors of the economy.

In the United States, payment to workers is largely determined by market forces. Markets, of course, are influenced by reimbursement policies of payers, subsidies to suppliers, and governmental licensing of clinicians. What managers earn relative to orthopedic surgeons, family practitioners, nurses, x-ray technicians, nurse's aides, and accountants is largely determined by what HCOs must pay to hire and retain the type of staff they require to perform in variably competitive markets. Hospital and other HCO managers are not licensed; nursing home administrators are licensed in some states. Whether earnings of health care managers are too high, too low, or just right relative to other workers is determined by perceptions of boards of directors, which are often controlled by managers.

Instituting a single-payer system, as in Canada, or nationalizing the system of hospitals and doctors, as in Great Britain, would obviously lower the earnings of managers and decrease competition among HCOs, lowering total system costs. But is that the kind of health care system that most Americans demand?

Training of HCO Managers

Should managers be trained in business or management schools, schools of public health, schools of medicine, or schools of allied health professions? Should managers of hospital and group practices be physicians, lay managers, or nurses with management training?

These questions are hard to answer because of the variability among HCOs and of the management jobs within them. Current trends include a greater supply of physicians relative to demand (hence, more physicians interested in management), increased competition among HCOs, fewer and larger HCOs, and better-trained HCO managers. There is undoubtedly a greater need for training of persons already managing in HCOs than for more schools of management or numbers of graduates from existing programs of health services management.

Health care has been an industry that has chronically underinvested in training for all workers after they have entered the workforce. Increasingly, large HCOs are starting their own training programs, and they are starting to be more involved in the design of training programs for which they contract out. University programs are adapting as well by strengthening relationships with local HCOs, involving students in carrying out projects as if they were management consultants, and doing research that is more responsive to management concerns than to theoretical or disciplinary concerns.

Educational programs in management and for clinicians will be increasingly subject to the same kinds of scrutiny as are hospitals and medical specialists. That is, is much of the educational service offered worth the money that people are paying? Can it be provided more cheaply and yet add more value relative to the jobs graduates will be performing? Can it be purchased in quantity and at a discount? Rapid change will undoubtedly come to the education industry as it has to health care.

Improving Managerial Performance

To what extent does managerial performance in HCOs have to be improved? Why don't more HCOs have a greater capacity for change? Why do they spend so little in training their managers and other employees? Would management performance of HCOs be improved by converting more organizations from governmental and not-for-profit to for-profit auspices?

In some HCOs in the early 1990s, management was transforming organizational performance. The costs of providing care plummeted, the quality of care improved dramatically, and market share grew for the high-performing, well-managed HCOs. So perhaps nothing has to be done to improve management performance, other than to see that the market is allowed to force out ineffective and inefficient firms while the government exercises vigorous oversight to protect the consumer from any market excesses.

Rapid change creates management problems and opportunities. This has been the case in other service industries facing rapid change, such as airlines and banks. Changing power relationships requires owner leadership for effective responses. For-profit business expertise has made a great contribution to some HCOs, particularly in the functional areas such as marketing, finance, information systems, and accounting. Many managers benefit from having an opportunity to reflect on what they do, and many HCOs and other organizations are increasingly structuring reflective opportunities for boards, top management, and physician managers. At management retreats or in special educational programs, managers working together can focus on organizational objectives and how best to attain them.

Disclosure to customers and stakeholders of objectives and their degree of attainment is an excellent way to hold managers' feet to the fire, in terms of improving service, monitoring quality, cutting costs, or restraining managerial compensation. It is the owners' responsibility to assure effective managerial performance. When the owners fail, the customers either try to change things or they seek services elsewhere, and the business fails. This has been the American way, and this has been generally highly regarded by other nations with comparable resources, even as we are criticized as a society for the high preference given to organizational performance relative to community solidarity.

Mini-Case Study

What follows is the mission statement of the Henry Ford Health System of Detroit, Michigan:

> To enable a given population to maximize its present and future health and provide tangible benefit to its community the Health System will provide the

Mini-Case Study *(cont.)*

highest quality service to prevent episodes of illness and provide coordinated episodes of care in a way that satisfies and delights both clients and system staff with efficient use of resources, appropriate facilities and labor capacity, and the financial performance to maintain and improve the above activities, while continuing to support research and education.

Please answer the following questions about this statement of purpose:

1. How should organizational performance at Henry Ford be measured?
2. Why don't all health care organizations have statements of purpose similar to Henry Ford's?
3. What contribution should the board of Henry Ford make to accomplish the statement of purpose?
4. What contribution should the management team of Henry Ford make to the attainment of the statement of purpose?

Discussion Questions

1. What are the advantages and disadvantages of the different forms of ownership of health care organizations?
2. What mechanisms of accountability are most effective for not-for-profit health care organizations?
3. What are some of the ways to measure the performance of health care organizations?
4. What are some of the ways to measure the performance of managers in health care organizations?
5. What skills and experience are required to own and to manage health care organizations?
6. What are some of the ways to improve managerial contribution and to contain the costs of nonclinical services in health care organizations?

References

ACEHSA, *Criteria for Accreditation* (2nd rev. ed.). Arlington, VA: Author, 1994.

Advisory Board Company, *The Rising Tide: Emergence of a New Competitive Standard in Health Care*. Washington, DC: Author, 1996.

American Hospital Association, *Guide for Preparation of Constitution and By Laws for General Hospitals*. Chicago: Author, 1981.

Belkin, L., "But What about Quality?" *The New York Times Magazine*, December 8, 1996.

Bodenheimer, T., "The HMO Backlash—Righteous or Reactionary?" *New England Journal of Medicine, 335*, 1601–1603, 1996.

Bowen, W. G., *Inside the Boardroom: Governance by Directors and Trustees.* New York: John Wiley and Sons, 1994.

Boyatzis, R. E., "Cornerstones of Change: Building the Path to Self-Directed Learning," in R. E. Boyatzis, S. S. Cowen, D. A. Kolb, & Associates (Eds.), *Innovation in Professional Education* (pp. 50–94). San Francisco: Jossey-Bass, 1995.

Burling, T., Lentz, E., & Wilson, R., *The Give and Take in Hospitals.* New York: G. P. Putnam's Sons, 1956.

Chait, R. P., Holland, T. P., & Taylor, B. E., *The Effective Board of Trustees.* New York: Macmillan 1991.

Drucker, P. F., "Managing the Public Service Institution," *The Public Interest, 33,* 46, 1973.

Ernst & Young, *Shining Light on Your Board's Passage to the Future.* Cleveland, OH: Author, 1997.

Griffith, J. R., "Measuring Hospital Performance," *Inquiry, 3,* 1978.

Griffith, J. R., *The Well Managed Health Care Organization* (3rd ed.). Ann Arbor, MI: Health Administration Press, 1995.

Griffith, J. R., Sahney, V. K., & Mohr, R. A., *Reengineering Health Care: Building on CQI.* Ann Arbor, MI: Health Administration Press, 1995.

Hales, C. P., "What do Managers Do? A Critical Review of the Evidence," *Journal of Management Studies, 23*(1), 88–115, 1986.

Kovner, A. R., *Really Trying: A Career Guide for the Health Service Manager.* Ann Arbor, MI: Health Administration Press, 1984.

Kovner, A. R., "Reflections in Health Management Education," *Journal of Health Administration Education, 4*(3), 359, 1986.

Longest, B. B., *Management Practices for the Health Professional.* Reston, VA: Reston Publishing, 1980.

Pointer, D. D., & Ewell, C. M., *Really Governing* (pp. 166–168). Albany, NY: Delmar, 1994.

Schlesinger, M., Gray, B., & Bradley E., "Charity and Community: The Role of Nonprofit Ownership in a Managed Health Care System," *Journal of Health Politics, Policy and Law, 21*(4), 697–752, 1996.

Umbdenstock, R. J., "Refinement of Board's Role Required," *Health Progress, 68*(1), 47, 1987.

13

Improving Quality of Care

Beth C. Weitzman

Learning Objectives

After studying this chapter the student should be able to:

1. Describe the evolution of quality assurance, assessment, and improvement activities in health care.
2. Discuss differing definitions and components of quality.
3. Discuss the implications of various mechanisms for reimbursement and organization of health care delivery on quality.
4. Describe, and give examples, of measures of quality, in regard to structure, process, and outcomes.
5. Describe and assess various sources and methods for gathering information on the quality of care.
6. Critique various mechanisms for assuring, promoting, and improving the quality of care.

Topical Outline

Historical perspective
Definition of quality
   Components of quality
     Competing definitions
     Quality of care vs. quantity of care and their relationship to reimbursement
Measuring quality
   Structure, process, and outcome
   The causal model
   Formulation of criteria and standards

Sources of information
    Administrative data and computerized systems
    The medical record
    Observations of process
    Patient and practitioner interviews
    Methods of assessment
Promoting quality: Assurance and improvement
    Organizational considerations in promoting quality
    Quality assurance mechanisms
      Licensing
      Accreditation and certification
      PSROs, PROS, and quality improvement organizations
      Malpractice litigation
      Economic approaches and the managed care context
    Quality assurance through the CQI framework

Key Words: **Accreditation, certification, continuous quality improvement (CQI), Joint Commission for the Accreditation of Healthcare Organizations (JCAHO), licensing, National Commission on Quality Assessment (NCQA), optimal care, outcomes, overutilization, peer review, process, peer review organizations (PROs), quality assurance, reliability (of criteria), structure, Total Quality Management (TQM), underutilization, utilization review, validity (of criteria).**

> There are differences in the quality of care given by physicians and hospitals. We can measure those differences and that information should be conveyed to the public.

Rarely does a statement provoke as much heated debate as the above issued by Dr. William L. Roper, administrator of the Health Care Financing Administration in 1988 ("US Plans," 1988). But then, few health care issues engender as much controversy as do those concerning the assessment and improvement of the quality of care. Recent changes in health care delivery—especially the move to managed care—have only intensified the debate. Although it is agreed that high-quality health care is desirable, and despite substantial advances in the field, there continues to be much disagreement about its definition, its measurement, and methods for promoting its occurrence.

    Quality-of-care problems are diverse, and as new quality assessment tools have become available new problems have been identified. They include excessive or inappropriate surgery, variable outcomes of surgical procedures, inappropriate diagnosis or treatment of common acute conditions, and excessive or inappropriate use of prescription drugs (Lohr, Yardy, & Thier, 1988). Such problems may be classified as overuse, underuse, or misuse of medical care (Chassin, 1991). Whether one is discussing the relative merits of fee-for-service and capitated payment systems, the increased role of nonphysician providers, or the introduction of new technologies, questions of quality must be addressed.

Historically, there has been surprisingly little concern about the quality of care provided. "Do no harm," taken from the Hippocratic Oath, served as the guiding principle. In recent years, however, quality has been pushed to the forefront of the health care debate. Attempts to reduce health care costs cause many to worry that quality will be jeopardized (Blumenthal, 1996). New circumstances of medical practice, including declining hospitalization, industry consolidation through mergers, and the growth of for-profit plans also raise concern about quality (Gabel, 1997). Our knowledge of methods to measure and improve the quality of care have increased dramatically (Blumenthal, 1996) and have been bolstered by new management models for approaching questions of quality improvement and control in industries other than health care.

This chapter begins with a brief review of the history of quality assessment and assurance. Definitions and methods of measuring quality health care are then explored. This is followed by a discussion of the strategies for promoting the quality of health care services. Throughout the discussion the potential effect of recent changes in health care on quality are highlighted.

Historical Perspectives

> Quality of care is making a comeback.—M. R. Chassin (1996)

It is only within recent decades that the concern with quality has become a focal issue for the health care community. The stage for this discussion, however, was set well over 100 years ago. In the early 1860s, Florence Nightingale helped lay the groundwork for medical care evaluation by suggesting a uniform format for collecting and presenting hospital statistics (Christoffel, 1976). At the turn of the 20th century a Boston surgeon, Dr. Ernest Codman, advocated the collection and evaluation of systematic information on the end results of patient care activities (Christoffel, 1976). Entitled "end result analysis," it was introduced at Massachusetts General Hospital in 1900 and featured a careful analysis of cases for which treatment was unsuccessful. Like many current approaches, end result analysis featured data collection on large numbers of patient outcomes and a recognition that a poor outcome might result from a range of factors. Codman's ideas failed to gain widespread acceptance in the earliest years of the 20th century, a period characterized by rapid gains in medical science, growth in medical professionalism, and limited consumer knowledge.

Despite the initial lack of enthusiasm for end result analysis, one of the foremost agencies for quality assurance, the Joint Commission on Accreditation of Healthcare Organizations (JCAHO), traces its inception back to Codman's original proposal (Roberts, 1987). Dr. Edward Martin believed the American College of Surgeons should be established to introduce and implement Codman's end result ideas. In 1917 the college established and published the *Minimum Standard for Hospitals*, which contained the first formal requirements for the review and evaluation of the quality of patient care. Quality of care in hospitals that participated in the Hospital Standardization Program improved noticeably (Shanahan, 1983). In 1951 the American College of Surgeons joined with the American College of Physicians, the American Hospital Association, the American Medical Association, and the Canadian Medical Association to establish the Joint Commission on Accreditation of Hospitals (JCAH). JCAH's function was to oversee the *Minimum Standards*; by this time over one half of all hospitals in the United States were approved (Roberts, 1987).

In the mid-1970s the JCAH commenced a period of dramatic change in its approach to quality, moving away from retrospective audits toward a standard that stressed "optimal" care through continuous evaluation (Joint Commission, 1991). By the early 1990s, the JCAHO emphasized a system of continual assessment and improvement. During this period, in recognition of the growing diversity of health care provider settings, the JCAH also broadened its scope and in the mid-1980s, became the Joint Commission for the Accreditation of Healthcare Organizations. As the organization of health care has changed, the JCAHO has been recently joined by other accrediting bodies. For example, the NCQA (National Commission on Quality Assessment) accredits state-licensed managed care plans.

During the past few decades, government has also played an increasingly active role in regard to health care quality. With the funding of hospital facilities through the Hill-Burton Act and, more dramatically with the enactment of Medicare and Medicaid in the 1960s, the federal government became a major source of health care dollars. Quality standards for participation in these federal programs were established. By the 1970s, due to the large federal deficit and increasing federal health care expenditures, cost containment and its relationship to quality emerged as key issues in health care (Thurow, 1985). Through the introduction of new initiatives such as utilization review (see next section), emphasis was placed on the elimination of the overuse of medical procedures; overuse occurs when the risks of the service outweigh the benefits (Chassin, 1991). The quest to contain costs, however, raised many new questions and concerns about quality assurance. Government began to take steps to ensure that needed care would not be sacrificed in the name of cost savings. As the mechanism for financing health care shifted from fee-for-service to flat-fee and capitated payments (see chapter 3), the insurance industry became another focus of the government's quality assurance activities. States, for example, began passing legislation to ensure reimbursement for minimum stays for routine childbirth and for procedures such as mastectomies.

Accompanying these changes in the financing and method of payment were equally dramatic changes in the organization and delivery of health care services. Traditionally, the focus of quality assurance programs has been on hospital care both because it is so expensive and because hospitals are more amenable to organizational constraint (Donabedian, 1985). Yet it is care outside the hospital setting that is growing most rapidly. Questions regarding the quality of care in ambulatory and long-term care settings are paramount. Concerns about quality under various organizational arrangements, such as provider networks, are first being tackled.

Definition of Quality

> Quality is in the eye of the beholder.—E. A. McGlynn (1997)

According to *Merriam Webster's Collegiate Dictionary* (7th edition), quality may be defined as "degree of excellence" or "superiority in kind." This concept of quality is certainly not unique to health care. As consumers we must assess the quality or degree of excellence of a broad range of products and services. Whether we are selecting a restaurant, purchasing an article of clothing, or making a reservation with an airline, consumers—like providers—use available information to try to identify the best-quality product, relative to its cost. Yet in few cases is this assessment of quality more difficult to make than in regard to health care. Many have concluded that, given the complexity and diversity of health care services, there is not one quintessential definition of quality but rather several legitimate definitions. Yet planners, managers, policymakers, and purchasers must work from some definition that is consensually accepted before quality of care can be assessed and promoted.

The Components of Quality

In defining *quality*, widely agreed on components do, indeed, exist. Quality care aims to promote, preserve, and restore health; it is delivered in an appropriate setting in a manner that is satisfying to patients. Quality care is achieved when the improvements in health status that are possible are, in fact, realized. It is not an assessment of the state of medical science but rather an assessment of the application of existing knowledge (Donabedian, 1980). Quality has several components, including appropriateness (the right care is provided at the right time), technical excellence (care is provided in the correct manner), accessibility (care can be obtained when needed), and acceptability (patients are satisfied) (U.S. GAO, 1996).

In trying to define and measure precisely what can be called quality care, there is a dilemma or tension between focusing on that which is unacceptable or poor-quality care and that which is optimal or highest-quality care. For many purposes, good-quality care is seen as that which is free of incidence or evidence of poor quality; this is a standard that focuses on minimal requirements for quality. Such definitions are often employed because they are easy to use and measure. In other cases, the definition aims to characterize an optimal or ideal standard of high quality. Often this sort of definition can be difficult to use in a meaningful way. Further, operationalizing the concept of optimal care may be elusive because there can be a wide gap between the actual level of quality that is achieved and the level of quality that is possible (Laffell & Berwick, 1992).

Competing Definitions. Research has indicated that one's role in the health care delivery process is likely to influence how one defines quality. Traditionally, quality of care has been defined by clinicians, primarily in terms of the technical delivery of care: "the application of the science and technology of medicine, and of the other health sciences, to the management of a personal health problem" (Donabedian, 1980, p. 4). From early in the development of medical practice in the United States, and especially since the beginning of the 20th century, society has delegated the establishment of quality standards to the medical profession (Caper, 1988). Peer review—a member of a profession being responsible for assessing the work of colleagues within that same profession—has traditionally been at the center of quality assessment and assurance efforts. The medical profession's peer review efforts have emphasized the scientific aspects of quality; appropriate drug prescription, postoperative infection rates, and accuracy of diagnosis are among the measures of quality that have been used. The physicians' grip on the definition of quality has eroded somewhat in recent years, as both purchasers and patients have become more active in this arena.

In contrast to the physician's emphasis on the technical aspects of care, patients tend to focus on interpersonal aspects of care in assessing quality. Lacking technical expertise, they typically judge the quality of technical care indirectly, by evidence of the practitioner's interest in and concern for their health and welfare (Donabedian, 1985). Also, patients may assume technical competence, especially in university-affiliated settings, and thus assess quality in terms of the interpersonal relations and the amenities of care (Donabedian, 1985). Research has indicated that patients use such indicators as length of visit and the time spent in counseling as indicators of physician merit (Ware, Davies-Avery, & Stewart, 1978). In one study, patients were found to be more satisfied with the care provided by female physicians, who used more of their time with patients to engage them in a partnership than their male counterparts (Bertakis, Helms, Callahan, Azari, & Robbins, 1995). Similarly, hospital quality is often assessed in regard to the care and concern demonstrated by the nursing staff, although consumers appear more likely to choose a hospital if it is affiliated with a medical school (Luft et al., 1990). Of note, different aspects of quality may be of greater or lesser importance to different types of inpatients (e.g., surgical versus medical). For example, in one study satisfaction with nurses mattered a good deal to medical patients, whereas pain control and satisfaction with their rooms were most important to surgical patients (Cleary, Keroy, Karapanos, & McMullen, 1989).

There is a growing appreciation of the importance of client satisfaction and of the interpersonal relationship to medical outcomes. The concept of "customer service" (not a focus of this chapter) has, also, grown in health care.

A significant body of research indicates that the quality of the patient-practitioner interaction may be a major contributor to treatment success, through greater patient compliance with treatment regimens and return for prescribed follow-up care (Cleary et al., 1989; Danziger, 1986; Svarstad, 1986). Further, the viewpoint of patients must be understood because client satisfaction is in itself an important component of the quality of care. Clients' assessments of quality guide them through the competitive market of health care providers. Under emerging managed care arrangements, with their focus on the "gatekeeper," maintaining satisfied patients is critical to providers' economic survival.

In the current era, definitions of quality in health care no longer are left solely to physicians. Administrators, nurses, and other health care personnel tend to emphasize different aspects of quality from that stressed by physicians and patients (Donabedian, 1980). Administrators, for example, tend to focus on the amenities of care, perhaps because this is the area over which they have greatest control. Nurses present something of a middle ground—looking both to indicators of technical competence and interpersonal relations. As health care becomes more of a team effort, and as more nonphysician professionals begin to practice independently, the approach to quality of care must broaden (Lohr et al., 1988). Patients, purchasers, and other providers will increasingly define what is "good" care; for example, the recently organized Foundation for Accountability (FACCT) brings together the voices of payers, providers, purchasers, and consumers to define performance standards for the managed care industry. Further, there is growing recognition of the need to consider quality in terms of the consequences, or outcomes, of care rather than its structure or process of delivery.

Quality of Care vs. Quantity of Care
and Their Relationship to Reimbursement

More care does not necessarily equal better care. Sometimes, however, quality of care may be confused with quantity of care. Consumer ratings of quality do reflect, at least in part, how many services are received (Davies & Ware, 1988). Yet closer examination reveals that although there are times when more care does equal better care, there are also times when more is not only not better but actually worse.

The precise relationship between inputs and benefits is not clear in health care. When the care received by any one patient is insufficient to bring about the potential benefits, the care is clearly poor in quality because of quantitative inadequacy (Donabedian, 1980). Underuse occurs when although the benefits of an intervention outweigh the risks, it is nevertheless not used (Chassin, 1991). Such inadequacy is exemplified by a the failure to complete a vaccination series; more care is needed before the benefits of the intervention can be realized. In the poorest nations, and in some of our own country's most desperate communities, more is almost definitely better (Maxwell, 1985). Further, noting a range of beneficial procedures and approaches that are underemployed, Chassin (1997) argues that underuse is "ubiquitous in U.S. medicine." Where the existing quality of care is low because of the inadequate quantity of care, improving quality may increase costs. Eventually, however, care can become excessive and even harmful; such care is costlier but of equal or poorer quality.

There are many good examples of care that may be simply excessive or unnecessary. Annual Pap smears (Benedet & Murphy, 1985) and routine use of fetal sonograms in low-risk pregnancies (Luthy et al., 1987; McCusker, Harris, & Hosmer, 1988) have been criticized on these grounds. Such care is excessive but carries with it little attendant risk. Costs for unnecessary care are hard to justify; resources could be better spent elsewhere.

There are other situations in which additional care is not only excessive or wasteful, but also harmful. According to some, routine chest and annual dental x-rays are examples of care that is more intensive and expensive yet of poorer quality than protocols with less frequent use. Such "ritualistic" care may appear to be of good quality because additional services are being provided, but it offers no real benefit to the patient and introduces a potential danger to the patient's physical well-being through excessive exposure to x-radiation, for example.

Overuse of many procedures, including some that are highly invasive, has been well documented. In a study of Medicare patients it was found that 17% of angiographic procedures and 32% of carotid endarterectomies were inappropriately performed (Brook et al., 1990); both procedures are associated with a fair degree of risk. In another example, the use of the intensive care unit as a precautionary measure was found to lengthen hospital stays and result in lower patient satisfaction, without any improvement in medical outcomes (Eagle, 1990). Eliminating the use of these unnecessary and potentially detrimental medical procedures and practices would clearly improve the quality of health care.

In addition to unnecessary and excessive care, sometimes care is produced inefficiently. In such cases, reducing the costs of care can be achieved not by reducing the quantity or intensity of care but rather by producing it more efficiently. Substitution of a nurse-practitioner for a physician or the use of ambulatory rather than inpatient surgery are two examples of strategies aimed at maintaining good quality while reducing costs.

The relationship between the quantity and quality of care is of critical importance to policymakers as they decide on the relative merits of various health care reimbursement systems. Theoretically, the incentive structure built into traditional fee-for-service medicine encourages overuse because more money is made when more costly procedures are undertaken. Under capitated and managed care systems, the perceived risk of such systems is underuse. Similarly, fee-for-service medicine is expected to use resources inefficiently, and capitated systems are expected to be more efficient. Emerging evidence is that reality is not so clear as the theory might suggest. "There is little objective information that suggests that patients are greatly disadvantaged in one model of practice versus another" (Ogrod, 1997, p. 86). Underuse exists in both fee-for-service and managed care settings; in fact, some conditions, such as depression and hypertension, are more likely to be treated under managed care than fee-for-service medicine (Chassin, 1997).

Supporters of managed care argue that "by focusing cost-containment efforts on reducing the inappropriate use of health services and avoiding preventable adverse effects, physicians can cut costs and improve quality at the same time" (Chassin, 1996, p. 1062). Although studies to date are reassuring in that they suggest that managed care results in lower costs with equal or better quality, these studies are limited because, for example, they have focused on short-term outcomes (Berwick, 1996a). Very little is known about the effect of specific reimbursement or organizational arrangements on the quality of care (Enthoven & Vorhaus, 1997). Further, there is emerging evidence that the quality of care provided under capitated systems may differ across population groups; whereas average patients fare well under managed care, chronically ill elderly and poor patients show poorer outcomes than those treated under fee-for-service arrangements (Ware, Bayliss, Rogers, Kosinski, & Tarlov, 1996).

Measuring Quality

Structure, Process, and Outcome

Defining what is meant by the term *quality* is only the first step toward assessing the delivery of health care. Appropriate variables must be identified for assessing the degree to which quality is present. Structure, process, and outcome are the three most commonly defined approaches to gathering information on the presence or absence of the attributes that constitute or define quality. Structure has been defined as "the relatively stable characteristics of the providers of care, of the tools and resources they have at their disposal, and of the physical and organizational settings in which they work" (Donabedian, 1980, p. 81). We may view structure as those things that exist prior to and separate from interaction with patients. Structural indicators that are commonly used include board certification for physicians, nurse/bed ratios for hospitals, and availability of laboratory facilities for HMOs. Structure, an indirect measure of quality, is useful to the degree that it can be expected to influence the direct provision of care.

Process concerns the set of activities that go on between practitioners and patient. Process may be seen as the object of assessment. Process measures may be used to assess the quality of the technical management of care (e.g., was the appropriate laboratory test ordered?), as well as the interpersonal aspects of care (e.g., was the medical history taken in a sensitive and caring manner?). Process may be viewed as what is done to patients; outcomes are what happens to them as a result of the intervention(s) (Hogness, 1985). Outcome refers to a change in a patient's current and future health status that can be attributed to antecedent health care (Donabedian, 1980). Outcome measures include mortality rates, postoperative infection rates, and rates of rehospitalization.

The Causal Model. Before we can use structure, process, or outcome measures to assess quality, it is important that we understand something about the relationship among all three. The underlying causal model in most quality assessments is that structure influences the process of care, which in turn has an impact on the outcome of care. In other words, the basis for the judgment of quality is what is known about the relationship between the characteristics of the structure and processes of the care that is delivered and their subsequent impact on the health and welfare of individuals and of society. Most definitions of quality assume that the application of the appropriate process of care will maximize patient outcomes (Lohr et al., 1988). However, the validity or justifiability of this inference must be established; there is considerable disagreement about cause and effect in health care.

Scientific research methods are used to establish the links between particular structures and processes and the desired outcomes, that is to test whether changes in health status (outcome) are really the result of the care given. Are board-certified physicians (structure) more likely to make appropriate use of laboratory tests (process)? And does the appropriate utilization of laboratory tests have a positive impact on patient recovery (outcome)? Do second surgical opinion programs (structure) influence the use of surgery (process)? And does this benefit patient health (outcome)? Once the relationships between structure, process, and outcome are established, we can focus on one area of measurement and have greater confidence that it is, in fact, providing a good indicator of quality.

"Structure . . . is relevant to quality in that it increases or decreases the probability of good performance" (Donabedian, 1980, p. 82). Despite the fact that structure has traditionally been used to measure quality, there is only limited information about the relationship between structure and performance. We know relatively little about when and how structural indicators (e.g., board certification for physicians, bachelor's degrees for nurses, or hospital affiliation) influence the processes and outcomes of care. Structure is, at best, a crude predictor of the quality of care since it can only address general tendencies. Structural indicators are, however, generally easy and inexpensive to access, whereas information on the process and outcomes of care is often unavailable, incomplete, or expensive to obtain. Therefore, in those cases where there is sufficient information to link structural characteristics with health care outcomes, structure can provide an important measure of quality in health care.

When the link between process and outcome has been validated, process indicators become an important tool for assessing and assuring quality in a direct and timely fashion. Another great virtue of process evaluation lies in the broad clinician involvement and education that is a consequence and may subsequently result in improved practices (Blum, 1974).

Too often, however, what is described as high-quality care has not been demonstrated to have much impact on the health status of patients. The Congressional Office of Technology Assessment estimated that only 10%–20% of clinician practices were shown effective by randomized controlled trials (Eddy & Billings, 1988). In other words, too many health care treatments lack scientific evidence of efficacy.

Although the validity of elements of process depends on the contribution of process to outcome, outcomes tend to be inherently valid, because change in health status and patient well-being is the ultimate goal of health care. When high-quality care is delivered, we expect improvement in such outcomes as mortality, morbidity, or social functioning. But before outcomes are used to make inferences about the quality of care, it is necessary to establish that the observed outcomes can be attributed to that care. Intervening factors must be ruled out; were the changes in health really the result of the care that is provided? Would the improvement in the patient's health have occurred without the treatment? Conversely, poor outcomes must not be simplisticly attributed solely to current failures of the health care organization or process (Blum, 1974).

The release of hospital-based mortality rates by the federal government's Health Care Financing Administration (HCFA) has been criticized on these grounds; many argue that there is insufficient evidence to attribute the mortality to poor hospital performance. Rather preexisting health differences among the patients' served (one aspect of structure) may instead be the cause for many of these differences. Although the HCFA had acknowledged that "preventable deaths" would be a more valid indicator of quality of care (Roper & Hackbarth, 1988), they began "to measure the performance of individual physicians by seeing how well their patients do" ("U.S. Plans," 1988, p. 1). However, in 1993, when Bruce Vladeck was appointed administrator of HCFA, he decided to withhold the data because there was "something lacking in the methodology" (*Medicine and Health*, 1993). This debate reminds us that in the absence of strong scientific evidence, the use of health outcomes, such as mortality, as an indicator of quality of care, may be misleading.

Research linking structure, process, and outcomes has improved and intensified. A recent study on the treatment of breast cancer illustrates this work. Mastectomy was contrasted with a treatment protocol that included the less disfiguring lumpectomy combined with radiation. The researchers found that urban and teaching hospitals (structure) were more likely to use lumpectomies (process) and that the use of lumpectomy resulted in similar clinical outcomes (Johantgen, Coffey, Harris, Levy, & Clinton, 1995). In another example, family physicians were found to be less likely than obstetricians to use epidural anesthesia, Cesarean sections, episiotomies, and other interventions with low-risk deliveries, but these differences in the process of care did not result in differences in the clinical outcomes of care (Hueston, Applegate, Mansfield, King, & McClafin, 1995).

Formulation of Criteria and Standards

Whether one decides to approach the assessment of quality via indices concerning structure, process, or outcomes, specific criteria or standards must be formulated. Before we can assess or monitor the quality of care, the abstract construct of quality must be translated into concrete variables, and those variables must be made measurable or "operationalized." Differences in structure, process, or outcome across practitioners, institutions, or regions do not, in and of themselves, indicate the appropriate level or highest quality of care. Rather, these standards must be established through scientific study or consensus.

Measurement is critical to the assessment and improvement of quality, for it is through measurement that we can make precise comparisons of benefits and risks. In selecting appropriate quality measures, note that no single indicator can capture the entire concept of quality or even any major component of it. Indeed, there may be certain aspects of quality that are all but impossible to measure. It is therefore better to use multiple operational definitions or measures that can account for the broadest understanding of quality. For example, in a study comparing costs and benefits of hospice and conventional care for terminally ill cancer patients, a broad range of criteria and measures had to be developed, including measures of pain, symptoms, and activities of daily living, as well as patient and family satisfaction (Kane, Wales, Bernstein, Leibowitz, & Kaplan, 1985). Any single measure would have provided an incomplete and misleading assessment of the quality of care provided.

Furthermore, criteria and standards change over time; this is integral to the philosophy of quality improvement. Whereas an optimal—and therefore, set—level of quality was implicit in earlier work in the field of quality assurance, more recent activities have stressed a changing standard.

In assessing the quality of care, the criteria or measures that are selected must be both valid and reliable. Reliable measures are those that do not fluctuate randomly from one episode of measurement to the next; this is called test–retest reliability. Reliable measures yield the same results regardless of who is making the rating; this is called interrater reliability. As examples, mortality data tend to be highly reliable, whereas psychiatric and social assessments do not.

The validity of a measure concerns how well it really reflects the concept being assessed. A reliable measure is not necessarily a valid one; although mortality data are considered highly reliable, they may be an invalid indicator of quality of care. The validity of a measure may be considered in terms of its correlation or convergence with other measures of the same concept; if several different measures of the same concept all lead to the same conclusions, we can have greater confidence that the individual measures are valid. For example, if we were trying to rate physician performance we might include a review of lab tests ordered, an assessment of the medical histories taken, and a judgment of quality of the medical record; if all three measures led to the same conclusion about the physician's performance, we would have greater confidence about the validity of any one measure. Validity of measures may also be considered in terms of their ability to distinguish between cases that are known to differ and in terms of their predictive power.

The scientific validity of a measure is based on a demonstrated causal relationship, as described above. In the absence of a scientifically demonstrated relationship "normative validity" is often substituted. Normative validity rests on the presence of professional consensus (e.g., agreement among physicians), so it could also be called consensual validity (Donabedian, 1980). In conducting an assessment of the quality of care, process elements are often used when there is general agreement that certain procedures are appropriate for certain situations, even though there is no "scientific proof" of appropriateness (Donabedian, 1980). The problem with relying on measures that have normative validity, compared to scientific validity, is that they can lead to the perpetuation of ineffective process. Similarly, when there is a lack of information linking process to outcomes, there is also a tendency to apply the criterion of potential benefit. In this framework a practice is considered appropriate if it *might* have benefit (Eddy & Billings, 1988). The appeal of the criterion of potential benefit is that it is easy to apply and it deals smoothly with the uncertainty that surrounds many practices. As an example, rather than limit the use of fetal monitors to high-risk deliveries, in some hospitals all pregnancies are monitored because it may be difficult to assess risk and there may be rare cases where otherwise unidentified problems might be found. Unfortunately, the criterion of potential benefit translates easily into "when in doubt, do it."

Clinical Protocols. Growing sophistication in research on the relationship between the structure, process, and outcomes of care, and federal support for this research through such agencies as AHCPR (Agency for Health Care Policy and Research), have made possible the development of clinical protocols, which greatly enhance the scientific basis of medical decision making. Belief in the efficacy of various methods and procedures, and long-held standards, are being subject to scientific scrutiny—often for the first time and often with surprising results. CONQUEST 1.0 (Computerized Needs-Oriented Quality Measurement Evaluation SysTem) was released by AHCPR in 1996. It summarized information on approximately 1,200 clinical-performance measures, developed by a variety of public, private, and not-for-profit organizations, and provided health care organizations the opportunity to use recent research to set standards and monitor the care provided. This increased availability of scientific information for health care decisions holds tremendous promise for the quality of care.

Finally, greater attention is being paid to those criteria, or measures of quality, that are most salient for consumers of care. In reviewing the criteria used to produce managed care "report cards" by HEDIS (the Health Plan Employer Data and Information Set), Hibbard and Jewett (1997) underscored the need to ensure that quality criteria are understood by consumers if they are to be used by consumers. Although consumers indicate that specific quality-of-care information is important in choosing a health plan, most still rely on the advice of their current physician or family and friends in making such a selection (AHCPR, 1996).

Sources of Information

In trying to measure and promote good quality care, one can use computerized administrative records or data may be gathered through interviews, observations, or review of individual records. Data sources and collection methods may be compared in terms of costs, acceptability, reliability, and validity (Gerbert, 1988). Generally, the method becomes more expensive and less feasible if it requires information that is not routinely collected. On the other hand, routinely gathered data may not have quality assessment as its primary focus; the available information may be only an indirect and incomplete measure of quality.

Computerized Administrative Data Systems. Administrative data on health care institutions and providers are regularly compiled by a range of public and not-for-profit agencies. Such administrative data typically represent structural indicators of quality. These measures—number of beds, number of registered nurses, number of board-certified surgeons—have become a routine part of accreditation and certification procedures (discussed in greater detail in the next section).

Routinely collected data on insurance claims, drug prescriptions, and malpractice suits may provide information on the process of care. Their disadvantage is that these data that may represent a narrower view of quality than might be considered optimal. Yet, these data—if properly organized—can permit relatively inexpensive, large-scale quality-assessment activities. Recognizing the potential benefit of such a system concerning malpractice information, a General Accounting Office (GAO) report suggested that "a centralized medical malpractice information system would help identify recurring problems, including problems with individual medical care providers, and focus attention on needed corrective and preventive actions" (Baine, 1987, p. 3). The National Practitioner Data Bank, operated by the Department of Health and Human Services, was opened in 1990. Insurance companies must report information on medical malpractice payments to the Data Bank. Similarly, health care organizations, state medical and dental boards and professional societies are required to report adverse professional actions (such as actions against a practitioner's license). It is a source of data regarding some of the most egregious examples of "bad-quality" care.

The Medical Record. Medical records are the most commonly used source of information on the process of care. Record review or chart audit have been an integral part of many quality assurance and cost containment programs, such as utilization review. Access is the most attractive characteristic of the medical record. The information is routinely gathered; using it for quality assessment involves limited additional expense or time.

Ideally, the medical record provides accurate and detailed information on patient symptoms, on the tests and procedures that were undertaken, and on patient progress. Unfortunately, in reality, medical records rarely reach the ideal standard. They tend to be incomplete. Medical record keeping is local and uses practice-specific terminology; this fragmentation means that information on diagnosis, treatment, and outcome cannot be linked across settings (Lohr et al., 1988). Problems with the medical record are especially acute in ambulatory care settings, where practitioners have been less likely to be subject to institutional constraints. Growing use of computerized systems for maintaining patient records, structured formats for such record keeping, and institutional review for network providers may all enhance the quality of the patient record and therefore make it an improved tool for monitoring the quality of care.

In the case of patients who have died, autopsy reports have been traditionally used to help improve medical practice and assess the quality of care. Was the diagnosis correct? Is there indication that some aspect of the care provided contributed to the cause of death? In recent years, however, the rate of autopsy has dropped and information from those that are performed is not routinely fed back to physicians (Landefeld & Goldman, 1989). As a result, an important source of information on the quality of care may be lost.

Observations of Process. Another method of obtaining data on the process of care is via direct observation. Several studies have been undertaken to observe and in some cases videotape the physician–patient interaction. Because the observation allows actual viewing of the process of care, and the videotape provides a record of that process, it has often been assumed that this method would provide a perfect report of the care provided. Instead, videotaped observations have been found to be difficult to standardize, and time-consuming and costly to make (Gerbert, Stone, Stulborg, Gullian, & Greenfield, 1988). Of even greater importance, recent studies have indicated that the "videotaped observation does not adequately capture the content of visits to the physician in areas of medication regimen, patient signs and symptoms, tests and treatments recommended, and patient education" (Gerbert et al., 1988, p. 530). Finally, there has been limited discussion about the degree to which observation biases the process of care. That is, does a provider (and a patient) change his or her practice style (behavior) when under observation?

Patient and Practitioner Interviews. In addition to chart or record audit and direct observation, information may be obtained by directly interviewing, or surveying, providers and patients. The provider is probably the most accurate source of reported information regarding the process of care (Gerbert et al., 1988). But physician interviews are a very expensive source of information and may not be a good source of information on the nontechnical aspects of care. In contrast, getting information from consumers of care may be no more expensive and, under many circumstances, is less expensive than traditional sources such as the medical record (Davies & Ware, 1988).

There is good evidence that the information reported by patients is valid and reliable. The consumer seems to be able to distinguish poor quality from high-quality care, especially for common problems. Most crucially, the consumer is probably in the best position to rate the interpersonal aspects of care. It has become routine for managed care organizations to survey their members regarding their satisfaction and experience with network providers.

Methods of Assessment

Researchers in the area of quality assessment have developed a broad range of techniques and methods for conducting quality assessments. Overall, methods may be characterized in terms of those that assess the quality of care relative to a positive standard (i.e., what should have been done or what should have occurred) and those that assess it relative to a negative standard (i.e., what should not have been done or what should not have occurred). As an example of the latter, prescription patterns can be especially useful after drugs that are ineffective or hazardous have been identified.

Assessments that focus on unnecessary or inappropriate care can be conducted prospectively (i.e., before care is provided) or retrospectively (after care is provided). For example, if we are interested in using unnecessary surgical procedures as an indicator of poor quality of care, second surgical opinions would provide a prospective quality measure (how often does the second opinion contradict the first physician's recommendation?). Tissue analysis provides a retrospective method of using the same indicator, unnecessary surgery (how often does the tissue analysis indicate that a healthy organ was removed?). Assessments that have focused on the use of inappropriate techniques and interventions have found poor quality of care to be concentrated; that is, a very small percentage of physicians tend to account for a large proportion of poor-quality care delivered (Donabedian, 1985).

Utilization review is another example of quality assessment and assurance that identifies cases of poor quality or inappropriate care. Inappropriate hospital usage may arise from inappropriate admissions, delayed discharges, or extra days during which services are not fully provided (Donabedian, 1985). Rehospitalizations after hospital discharge may be used as an indicator of poor quality, that is, of the patient's being released too quickly.

Promoting Quality: Assurance and Improvement

> The policy discussion about improving quality of care has rarely focused on the question of how to move the entire health care delivery system toward improving quality.—M. R. Chassin (1997)

Measuring or assessing the quality of care does not, unfortunately, result in immediate improvements in that care. Simply defining what is meant by "high-quality" care does not guarantee its implementation. Practice guidelines are established, yet little attention is paid to helping practitioners implement those guidelines (Laffell & Berwick, 1992). Quality-promotion activities—including assurance and improvement—are intended to translate the concepts and findings of quality assessment into programs that will promote the delivery of higher quality care. The rest of this chapter is devoted to methods of controlling and improving the quality of care.

Efforts to encourage the delivery of high-quality care take place at the local and at the national level. They are geared both at individuals and at institutions. Currently, professional associations, health care institutions and organizations, government, private external quality-review associations, consumer groups, managed care organizations, and group purchasers of care all play a role in trying to promote quality care.

Organizational Considerations in Promoting Quality

In order to assure good quality care, we need to know something about changing or modifying the behaviors of providers and the organizations in which they practice. And organizational change creates strains and tensions; it raises conflict between the norms of professional freedom and bureaucratic autonomy (Hetherington, 1982).

Professional autonomy has been one of the most important impediments to health institutions becoming more fully accountable for the care they provide. Physicians have traditionally operated as free agents within the hospital structure. As quality assurance activities have grown and the organization of health care services have shifted away from the independent, solo practitioner, new restrictions and requirements have been imposed on physicians. Resistance is an expected by-product of these changes. In recent years, as the accountability obligations of health institutions have been formalized and the economic imperatives have become explicit, the potential for conflict between institutional goals of self-regulation and survival and the autonomy requirements of clinicians has grown.

Despite resistance and the obstacles posed by the tradition of autonomy, it is possible to improve the quality of care and to hold clinicians and organizations accountable for the care given. Even within the context of a change-resistant environment we know a great deal about the ways in which health care delivery can be shaped or modified. For example, we know that quality-promotion activities are more likely to succeed when professionals have played an active role in developing and administering the regulations. There is also evidence to suggest that, to change physician behavior, information must come from a credible source (e.g., a professional organization) and should be backed with financial incentives

(Ball, 1988). Furthermore, it is easier to change behavior when there is consensus about what constitutes good quality care. In one study, researchers attributed the success of an on-site educational program to reduce inappropriate use of x-ray pelvimetry to the general agreement about the use of this procedure (Chassin & McCue, 1986).

Institutional commitment to change may also play a role in modifying providers' behaviors. Slenker, Coban, and Lind (1985) looked at the impact of establishing procedural guidelines for physicians, nurses, and allied health professionals in the diagnosis and treatment of cancer. Factors contributing to program success were hospital commitment to the program, ready availability of guidelines, and mandatory participation in the educational program. "Practice guidelines, particularly when combined with other methods of communication, such as feedback on performance and education by respected peers, have been shown in randomized trials to improve both the process and outcomes of care" (Chassin, 1996, p. 1061).

Within the continuous quality improvement (CQI) framework (see next section), organizational change must begin with commitment at the very top of the organization (Berwick, 1988). There is recognition that quality improvement requires resources and that the methods of quality measurement must be taught and learned. Finally, the proponents of quality improvement argue that traditional assurance methods, which attempt to identify and discipline an unruly few, are antithetical to true improvement, which must emphasize change in the overall system and its processes. In this model, fear must be replaced by shared commitment and trust.

Quality Assurance Mechanisms

As already noted, regardless of the mechanism for assessment, there are different approaches to trying to ensure high quality of care. Three such approaches, licensing, accreditation, and certification are similar in that they assess an individual's or institution's ability to provide quality care on the basis of meeting established criteria at a particular time. In the past, these approaches aimed to ensure quality by guaranteeing the presence of certain fundamental, structural characteristics of the institution or individual. In contrast, a number of other approaches have attempted to promote quality by reviewing specific instances of provider–patient interaction. These approaches, which have been used by peer review organizations and are typified in malpractice litigation, tend to focus on the processes and outcomes of care.

Licensing. Licensing may be distinguished from all other quality assurance activities because licensing is backed by the force of law. Under the U.S. Constitution the states have been empowered to license both individuals and institutions. That is, the states are permitted to restrict certain activities (e.g., the performance of surgery or a dental exam) to those individuals and institutions it has determined to possess acceptable standards. Numerous health professions and occupations are currently licensed by one or more states, as are a broad array of health care facilities.

In licensing individuals the state enters into a compact with a professional group. The professional group assumes responsibility for controlling the quality of work provided, and the state grants the professional group the right to control entry into that group and, in many cases, to define the content of that work. Some of the occupations that are licensed by all states include medicine, dentistry, pharmacy, nursing, nursing home administration, and podiatry. In some states occupations such as laboratory technicians, midwives, and psychologists are also licensed. Generally, the profession (e.g., nursing) establishes standards based on educational attainment, experience, and performance on a written exam. Once a license is granted, it has been traditionally valid for life; in the absence of egregious conduct licenses are rarely suspended or revoked. Increasingly, however, practitioners are required to participate in continuing education programs in order to maintain an active license.

The use of licensure as a method of ensuring quality is a source of great controversy. There is ample evidence that, rather than protecting the public, licensure protects the professional group and its members from competition and public scrutiny. Licensing makes it difficult to change occupations within the health care sector, or to move from one state to another. For example, as a result of licensing restrictions, the most qualified labor-room nurse may not be able to take responsibility for a baby's delivery. Most significantly, there is little evidence to indicate that the criteria used in licensing actually predict the quality of care to be delivered.

The issues posed by licensing are especially complicated in the case of physicians. Physicians are in an unusual professional position; they do not merely control their own work but are also the dominant professional group throughout the health care arena (Freidson, 1970). This position of professional dominance has, until most recently, effectively shielded doctors from public scrutiny and accountability. Many argue that the public has not been well served by this isolation. Consumers, purchasers, and health care organizations are no longer willing to be silent partners in these health care decisions.

One area of "self-policing" that has received considerable attention is the disciplinary actions of the state medical boards that are responsible for licensure. Although increasing in number, such disciplinary actions continue to be the exception. One study indicated that the number of reprimands and censures had grown. Revocations and suspensions of licenses, however, had remained relatively constant despite an increase in the number of practicing physicians (Kusserow,

Handley, & Yessian, 1987); that is, the rate of suspending licenses had actually decreased. In this study it was also found that most reports to state medical boards were provided by consumers and law enforcement agencies, not by health care professionals, hospitals, or peer review organizations.

Licensing of facilities is usually accomplished directly by a state agency, for example, the state health department. All states license hospitals (short- and long-stay, general, and/or psychiatric), nursing homes, and pharmacies; many also license such facilities as homes for the mentally ill or developmentally disabled (Wilson & Neuhauser, 1987). Certain services, such as ambulances and home health care, are also licensed in some states. Institutional licenses may be granted for a period of 1 or more years. The criteria for licensing typically emphasize structural elements like bed/nurse ratios and the presence of appropriate equipment. Licensing boards for institutions tend to be less completely dominated by providers from the regulated institution than do those for individuals.

Accreditation and Certification. Although licensing is critical to understanding the role of government in the assurance of quality, volunteerism has long been the primary approach to quality assurance in health care (Luke & Modrow, 1983). Voluntary self-regulation is reflected in both accrediting bodies such as the JCAHO and in professional certification boards. Accreditation is limited to institutions, whereas certification applies to individuals.

The basic principles of accreditation are similar to those of licensure; it is assumed that if the institution meets certain standards of physical and organizational structure, then good-quality care will be delivered at that time and will continue into the future. In the case of accreditation, groups of like institutions or organizations with mutual interests come together to set up an organization, establish standards, and proceed to inspect and "accredit" themselves on a periodic basis. Although accreditation is not a legal procedure, there are often strong legal and financial incentives for undergoing accreditation. For example, state education departments will not recognize diplomas from medical schools that are not accredited.

The JCAHO is perhaps the oldest and best known of the accrediting bodies in health care. As already noted, recent changes in the Joint Commission's accrediting standards are reflective of shifts in the approach to quality taken throughout the field. Traditionally reliant on minimal structural standards, in 1966 JCAH's board of commissioners voted to rewrite the standards to raise them from "minimal essential" to "optimal achievable" standards, and in 1975 numerical requirements for audit were established to ensure optimal care (Shanahan, 1983). In 1979 new standards were issued that eliminated the numerical audit requirement and directed hospitals to develop a hospital-wide program that integrated all quality-assurance activities (Roberts, 1987). In 1987 the Joint

Commission embarked on its "Agenda for Change," which represented a refocus-ing of its own standards and greater emphasis on quality improvement through better measures and a system of feedback. In its 1992 *Accreditation Manual for Hospitals*, the "Quality Assurance" chapter was renamed "Quality Assessment and Improvement," symbolizing the JCAHO's full adoption of the CQI model (Joint Commission, 1991).

The NCQA is the accrediting organization for HMOs, as well as the developer of HEDIS. Started in the late 1970s as a creation of the managed care industry, NCQA became an independent body in the early 1990s. Just as the JCAHO came to define what is good quality for hospitals, the NCQA has increasingly become the arbiter of good quality for HMOs. As of 1996, 57% of all HMOs operating in the country had asked for accreditation; compared to the JCAHO process, denials and provisional accreditation were common ("NCQA," 1996). The NCQA accreditation process gives enormous weight to quality improvement indicators (evidence that improvements are being made) and the ongoing monitoring of physician performance.

Accreditation also plays a critical role in medical education. Medical schools are accredited by the Liaison Committee on Medical Education. The American Medical Association and the Association of American Medical Colleges are equally represented on the committee. Separate accrediting bodies review post-graduate medical education and accredit residency programs. Training for other health care occupations also takes place in accredited programs or schools; accreditation is carried out by a range of boards and agencies representing such fields as dentistry, medical technology, and health services administration.

Certification, like accreditation, represents a form of voluntary self-regulation, and although certification is not backed by law, there are incentives that encourage individual practitioners to seek certification. For example, some third-party payers will only reimburse visits to certified social workers. Of great consequence, most hospitals limit privileges to board-certified specialties. Certification uses standards of education, experience, and achievement on examinations to deter-mine qualification. The HCFA requires fee-for-service institutional providers to be certified under the Medicare Provider Certification Program, in which state agencies and private bodies enforce Medicare standards.

A great diversity of health care occupations have certifying bodies. In nursing alone there are 23 different organizations that offer certification in nursing or one of its subspecialties (Scofield, 1988). These include the American Nurses Association, the Oncology Nursing Certification Corporation, and the Association of Operating Room Nurses.

PSROs, PROS, and Quality Improvement Organizations. Profes-sional standard review organizations (PSROs) were established by the 1972

amendments to the Social Security Act. They represented a major step toward institutionalizing peer review of physician care and the quality of care provided outside the hospital setting. The purpose of the law was to involve local practicing physicians in the ongoing review and evaluation of health services covered by Medicare, Medicaid, or the Maternal and Child Health Programs of the Department of Health and Human Services. PSROs were charged with the dual role of quality assurance and utilization review (which had previously been the function of medical staff review committees). Most PSRO activity focused on utilization review rather than on overall quality assurance, and cost containment became the hallmark of the PSRO's own measure of success. Established in 195 geographic areas, the efficacy of PSROs as a tool for quality assurance was limited by physician protectionism, lack of concern for the nontechnical aspects of care, and overemphasis on cost containment.

Peer review organizations (PROs) went into operation in 1984, as the successor to the PSROs. Unlike PSROs, PROs reviewed only Medicare; Medicaid review was left to the states. Limited to one per state, physician-based organizations were given a prominent role in the control of the PROs. Under the PRO system, disciplinary procedures were simplified, and review functions could not be delegated to hospitals. In 1987, PROs were also given responsibility for reviewing HMOs participating in the Medicare program (U.S. GAO, 1991).

PROs were awarded fixed-price contracts that specified, in numerical terms, the results to be achieved. For example, some of the PROs' objectives focused on reducing inappropriate admissions; others focused on reducing admissions overall. Because of the specific nature of the objectives, PROs were given an increased incentive to actually try to change physician behavior. The results, however, were disappointing. A review of medical records for hospitalized Medicare patients found that approximately 18% of them had received below standard care; yet the PRO had found only 6.3% (Rubin, Rogers, Kahn, Rubinstein, & Brook, 1992).

Further, there had been limited follow-through in cases where the PROs had identified weaknesses and made recommendations. For example, the General Accounting Office concluded in 1991 and in 1995 that HCFA was unwilling to enforce compliance with the PRO recommendations for HMOs (U.S. GAO, 1996). "In practice, the central role of PROs has been to prevent the inappropriate use of services primarily through utilization review and to identify individual instances of poor quality for focused remedial efforts or punitive actions" (Wilensky, 1997, p. 78). During the 1990s, however, the focus of PROs began to shift toward patterns and outcomes of care, and toward the promotion of quality-improvement strategies, especially in ambulatory care settings (Wilensky, 1997). consistent with these trends, PROs have been renamed Quality Improvement Organizations.

Malpractice Litigation. Malpractice litigation may also be seen as an approach to quality assurance. Malpractice litigation focuses on extreme cases of poor quality care. Using it as a tool for quality assurance shifts the focus away from frequent but low-cost errors toward infrequent and high-cost ones. Malpractice litigation is not an effective tool for trying to control the overprescription of antibiotic drugs, for example, because the damages accrued to an individual are generally not of the magnitude to instigate a law suit.

Some studies have suggested that malpractice litigation may not be an effective tool for identifying problems in the quality of health care. In reviewing a random sample of patients discharged in New York State in 1984, researchers found that in approximately 1% of the cases there was evidence of an adverse event which was caused by negligence (Localio et al., 1991). Yet malpractice claims were filed in few of these cases; the researchers estimate that only 1.5% of negligent events lead to claims. Given the relative rarity of malpractice claims, only very incompetent physicians could be identified in this way (Rolph, Kravitz, & McGuigan, 1991).

Despite empirical evidence suggesting that malpractice claims are relatively infrequent, malpractice litigation is seen as a growing problem in the United States that has threatened the solvency of some institutions and the practice of some physicians. It is not clear, however, the degree to which the malpractice "crisis" is a function of a more litigious society, excessive profits within the insurance industry, declining patient-provider relations, or the unwillingness of the medical profession to engage in effective quality control, especially in regard to disciplining those physicians responsible for a significant share of practice error.

As already noted, the federal government has become involved in the malpractice debate through the establishment of the National Practitioner Data Bank under the Health Care Quality Improvement Act of 1986. Congress enacted this legislation to (1) moderate the incidence of malpractice, (2) allow the medical community to demonstrate new willingness to weed out incompetents, and (3) improve the base of timely and accurate information on medical malpractice (Waxman, 1987). The act requires hospitals to request information from the Data Bank whenever they are hiring, granting privileges, or conducting periodic reviews of a practitioner (U.S. GAO, 1992). The use of a mandatory national data bank may eventually help to close the loopholes that permitted interstate movement and continued participation in Medicaid and Medicare for practitioners who had been disciplined in a particular state or institution.

Economic Approaches and the Managed Care Context. "The problem with using incentives to shape physicians' behavior is the bluntness of the method" (Berwick, 1996a, p. 1228). Yet this method has become ubiquitous in health care. Third-party payers and managed care organizations have initiated a number of activities that may be viewed as approaches to quality assurance. Although such activities are often primarily concerned with cost containment, they serve a quality-assurance function to the degree that they reduce unnecessary or excessive use of care. Second surgical opinion programs, preadmission review, and DRGs all aim to reduce costs by eliminating unnecessary or excessive care. Employers and unions who must foot the bill for insurance premiums have also begun playing a role in this dual area of cost containment and quality assurance. Most broadly, capitated payments, wherein the provider is paid for the ongoing care of the patient rather than for individual instances of care, may be seen as the strongest economic incentive to eliminate duplication, waste, and unnecessary services.

Unfortunately, there is limited reason to be optimistic about the potential of these cost-containment efforts to enhance quality, especially at the level of the individual provider. Economic solutions seem to have as much impact on appropriate care as they do on inappropriate care (Brook, 1988). Evidence from the RAND Health Insurance Experiment suggests that cost sharing for inpatient and outpatient care reduces the use of effective and presumably needed services about as much as it lowers the use of ineffective or unnecessary services (Lohr et al., 1988). Before cost-containment efforts can be expected to have a positive impact on quality, economic solutions must be coupled with medical solutions. Some argue that medicine must begin to be codified (Brook [1988] calls for a "gourmet cookbook" of practice guidelines) and physicians must be rewarded for appropriate medical practice.

Economic incentives may be more powerful at the organizational level. "Capitation may have a more important and powerful effect on influencing the design of the health care system, than on individual physician decisionmaking" (Berwick, 1996a, p. 1228). To the degree that quality can be improved through a more carefully considered and designed system, managed care may enhance quality. Capitation provides a strong incentive to the organization to maximize the health of its members, and managed care also allows for control of physician practice (Eddy, 1997). As noted earlier in this chapter, the evidence to support the idea that managed care and its economic incentives will result in less costly, higher quality care, remains weak.

Technological Approaches. The growth in sophisticated computer technologies has offered new promise to those concerned with quality assurance. Those who have conducted research on the introduction of new information systems find that they can greatly modify provider practice, improve information dissemination, and prevent individual instances of error. In a study examining the impact of "computer alerts" on individual patient care, Safran, Rind, and Davis

(1996) found that the computer generated prompts to practitioners significantly improved the care of HIV-infected patients and promoted the adoption of practice guidelines. The promise of technology for quality assurance may be more likely to be realized under newly emerging systems of care.

Quality Assurance Through the CQI Framework

> The cycle of action and reflection is enshrined in the lingo of quality improvement.—D. M. Berwick (1996b)

Dramatic shifts in the activities surrounding quality promotion have resulted from the widespread adoption of the CQI paradigm. The thrust of CQI, based on the concepts of Total Quality Management (TQM), is to integrate methods of measurement and assessment with those of change and improvement. The Deming Cycle—plan, do, check, act, and analyze—is named for the creator of TQM (Gabor, 1990). As applied to health care quality, TQM emphasizes the results of care from the patients' point of view (Laffell & Berwick, 1992). CQI uses reliable statistical methods to raise the norm of performance, rather than to weed out "bad apples" (Joint Commission, 1991). The goal is to obtain more uniform, or predictable, results through the analysis of process (Gabor, 1990).

There are six principal ideas underlying this framework (Gabor, 1990). First, quality should be defined by the consumer. Second, variation in the process of care must be understood and reduced. Next, top management must be committed to improvement. The fourth principle states that change and improvement must be continuous; it must be all-encompassing and involve all members of the organization. Fifth, in order to succeed, training and education of all employees must be ongoing. Finally, trying to measure the contribution of individual employees to overall quality is usually destructive to the process of improving it.

Whereas the quality assurance methods discussed above, such as licensure and certification, have traditionally relied on set minimal standards, CQI encourages change and growth. Whereas PROs have relied on punitive actions to enforce their recommendations, CQI requires collaboration, cooperation, and compromise. Quality improvement "does not seek to identify errors in order to assign blame, but instead assumes that faulty systems of care are very often responsible for errors" (Chassin, 1996, p. 1061). The use of sophisticated methods of measurement and statistical analyses are, slowly, becoming the every day tool of managers, who can feed information back to practitioners in order to help them enhance their manner of care. If CQI is to fulfill its promise, the delivery of high-quality care must be the central goal of all players in the health care field. The promise made by CQI is noble. It remains to be seen whether is has the ability to transform the health care delivery system.

Issues

Two broad questions concerning the quality of care remain to be addressed in the coming years. First, who shall define quality of care? Is it, ultimately, the consumers who decide the critical elements of what constitutes good quality? Or, will health care professionals continue to play the lead role? How will differing perspectives—government, insurers, providers, and consumers of care—be reconciled? Will a negotiated definition of quality care satisfy any of the key constituents?

Second, who is, ultimately, responsible for assuring that high-quality care is provided? What role should government play? Is this to be a federal or state responsibility? How will individual institutions and organizations balance their responsibility for ensuring the quality of care against the responsibility of individual health care providers? In a rapidly changing environment, who will make sure that consumers are receiving the best possible health care?

Mini-Case Study

You are the director of human resources for a mid-size not-for-profit social service agency, in a city that is just beginning to experience extensive managed care market penetration. Providing your employees with health insurance is costly. Traditionally, your agency has offered its employees a fee-for-service insurance arrangement, but you have decided to eliminate this expensive option. Instead, you have selected a large managed care company, whose premiums are far lower than your former carrier. You are preparing to make the announcement of this change to the agency staff, but you sense that your employees may be distressed to learn that their health insurance has been changed in this way.

A formal announcement is sent to all staff and a meeting is scheduled to allow for questions and discussion. At this meeting, a well respected worker says, "with the emphasis on cost containment, the quality has got to go down." To what degree are cost containment arrangements compatible with quality care? What information will you use to persuade your employees that your decision will not put their health in jeopardy? What evidence will you use to encourage their support of the managed care arrangement?

Discussion Questions

1. Provide at least two indicators of quality based on structure, on process, and on outcomes. What are their strengths and weaknesses?

2. Can a physician be the "best" if patients are dissatisfied with the care that they receive?
3. In what ways does CQI represent a real shift in the approach to quality assurance?
4. How are quality assurance activities affected by the move away from solo practice medicine?
5. What are the most critical factors to consider in designing a program for quality improvement?

References

"AHCPR and Kaiser Examine Consumers Use of Quality Information," *Agency for Health Care Policy and Research, 199*, 10–11, 1996.

Baine, D. P., DOD Health Care. Statement given by the General Accounting Office before the U.S. House of Representatives Subcommittee on Military Personnel and Compensation, July 21, 1987.

Ball, J. R., Physician Payment: Why Money Doesn't Buy Quality. Paper presented at the Association for Health Services Research, San Francisco, CA, June 27, 1988.

Benedet, J. L., & Murphy, K. J., Cervical cancer screening: Who needs a pap test? How often? *Postgraduate Medicine, 78*, 1985.

Bertakis, K. D., Helms, L. J., Callahan, E. J., Azari, R., & Robbins, J. A., "The Influence of Gender on Physician Practice Style," *Medical Care, 33*, 407–416, 1995.

Berwick, D. M., "Quality Assurance and Measurement Principles: The Perspective of One Health Maintenance Organization," in E. F. X. Hughes (Ed.), *Perspectives of Quality in American Health Care* (pp. 203–210). Washington, DC: McGraw-Hill's Healthcare Information Center, 1988.

Berwick, D. M., "Quality of Health Care, Part 5: Payment by Capitation and the Quality of Care," *New England Journal of Medicine, 335*, 1227–1231, 1996a.

Berwick, D. M., "Harvesting Knowledge from Improvement," *Journal of the American Medical Association, 275*, 877–878, 1996b.

Blum, H. L., "Evaluating Health Care," *Medical Care, 12*, 999–1011, 1974.

Blumenthal, D., "Quality of Health Care, Part 4: The Origins of the Quality-of-Care Debate," *New England Journal of Medicine, 335*, 1146–1149, 1996.

Brook, R. H., *Physician Payment: Why Money Doesn't Buy Quality.* Paper presented at the Association for Health Services Research, San Francisco, CA, June 27, 1988.

Brook, R. H., Park, R. E., Chassin, M. R., Solomon, D. H., Keesey, J., & Kosecoff, J., "Predicting the Appropriate Use of Carotid Endarterectomy, Upper Gastrointestinal Endoscopy and Coronary Angiography," *New England Journal of Medicine, 323*, 1173–1177, 1970.

Caper, P., "Defining Quality in Medical Care." *Health Affairs, 7*, 49–61, 1988.

Chassin, M. R., "Quality of Care—Time to Act," *Journal of the American Medical Association, 266*, 3472–3473, 1991.

Chassin, M. R., "Quality of Health Care, Part 3: Improving the Quality of Care," *New England Journal of Medicine, 335*, 1060–1063, 1996.

Chassin, M. R., "Assessing Strategies for Quality Improvement," *Health Affairs, 16*, 151–161, 1997.

Chassin, M. R., & McCue, S. M., "A Randomized Trial of Medical Quality Assurance," *Journal of the American Medical Association, 256*, 1012–1017, 1986.

Christoffel, T., "Medical Care Evaluation: An Old Idea," *Journal of Medical Education, 51*(2), 83–88, 1976.

Cleary, P. D., Keroy, L., Karapanos, G., & McMullen, W., "Patient Assessments of Hospital Care," *Quality Review Bulletin, 15*(6), 172–179, 1989.

Danziger, S. K., "The Use of Expertise in Doctor–Patient Encounters During Pregnancy," in P. Conrad & R. Kern (Eds.), *The Sociology of Health and Illness.* New York: St. Martin's Press, 1986.

Davies, A. R., & Ware, J. E., Jr., "Involving Consumers in Quality of Care Assessment," *Health Affairs, 7*(1), 33–48, 1988.

Donabedian, A., *Explorations in Quality Assessment and Monitoring (Volume I): The Definition of Quality and Approaches to its Assessment.* Ann Arbor, MI: Health Administration Press, 1980.

Donabedian, A., *Explorations in Quality Assessment and Monitoring (Volume III): The Methods and Findings of Quality Assessment and Monitoring.* Ann Arbor, MI: Health Administration Press, 1985.

Eagle, K. A., "Length of Stay in the Intensive Care Unit: Effects of Practice Guidelines and Feedback," *Journal of the American Medical Association, 264*, 992–997, 1990.

Eddy, D. M., "Balancing Cost and Quality in Fee-for-Service vs. Managed Care," *Health Affairs, 16*, 162–173, 1997.

Eddy, D. M., & Billings, J., "The Quality of Medical Evidence: Implication for Quality of Care," *Health Affairs, 7*(1), 19–32, 1988.

Enthoven, A. C., & Vorhaus, C. B., "A Vision of Quality in Health Care Delivery," *Health Affairs, 16*(3), 44–57, 1997.

Freidson, E., *Profession of Medicine.* New York: Harper and Row, 1970.

Gabel, J., "Marketwatch: Ten Ways HMOs Have Changed During the 1990s," *Health Affairs, 16*, 134–145, 1997.

Gabor, A., *The Man Who Discovered Quality.* New York: Penguin Books, 1990.

Gerbert, B., Validity of Patient Report: A Comparison with Other Methods of Physician Quality Assessment. Paper presented at the Association for Health Services Research conference, San Francisco, CA, June 28, 1988.

Gerbert, B., Stone, G., Stulborg, M., Gullian, D. S., & Greenfield, S., "Agreement Among Physician Assessment Methods: Searching for the Truth Among Fallible Methods," *Medical Care, 26*, 519–535, 1988.

Hetherington, R. W., "Quality Assurance and Organizational Effectiveness in Hospitals," *Health Services Research, 17*, 185–201, 1982.

Hibbard, J. H., & Jewett, J. J., "Will Quality Report Cards Help Consumers?" *Health Affairs, 16*, 218–228, 1997.

Hogness, J. R., "What About the Patient?" *New England Journal of Medicine, 313*, 689–690, 1985.

Hueston, W. J., Applegate, J. A., Mansfield, C. J., King, D. E., & McClafin, R. R., "Practice Variations Between Family Physicians and Obstetricians in the Management of Low-Risk Pregnancies," *Journal of Family Practice, 40*, 345–351, 1995.

Johantgen, M. E., Coffey, R. M., Harris, D. R., Levy, H., & Clinton, J. J., "Treating Early-Stage Breast Cancer: Hospital Characteristics Associated with Breast-Conserving Surgery," *American Journal of Public Health, 85,* 1432–1434, 1995.

Joint Commission on Accreditation of Healthcare Organizations, *An Introduction to Quality Improvement In Health Care.* Chicago: Author, 1991.

Kane, R. L., Wales, J., Bernstein, L., Leibowitz, A., & Kaplan, S., "A Randomised Controlled Trial of Hospice Care," in L. Aiken & B. Kehrer (Eds.), *Evaluation Studies Review Annual* (Vol. 10, pp. 159–169). Beverly Hills, CA: Sage, 1985.

Kusserow, R. P., Handley, E. A., & Yessian, M. R., "An Overview of State Medical Discipline," *Journal of the American Medical Association, 257,* 820–825, 1987.

Laffell, G., & Berwick, D. M., "Quality in Health Care," *Journal of the American Medical Association, 268,* 407–408, 1992.

Landefeld, C. S., & Goldman, L., "The Autopsy in Quality Assurance: History, Current Status, and Future Directions," *Quality Review Bulletin, 15*(2), 42–48, 1989.

Localio, A. R., Lawthers, A. G., Brennan, T. A., Laird, N. M. T., Herbert, L. E., Peterson, L. M., et al., "Relation Between Malpractice Claims and Adverse Events Due to Negligence: Results of the Harvard Medical Practice Study III," *New England Journal of Medicine, 325,* 245–251, 1991.

Lohr, K. N., Yardy, K. D., & Thier, S., "Current Issues in Quality of Care," *Health Affairs, 7*(1), 15–18, 1988.

Luft, H. S., Garnick, D. W., Mark, D. H., Peltzman, D. J., Phibbs, C. S., Lichtenberg, E., & McPhee, S. J., "Does Quality Influence Choice of Hospital?" *Journal of the American Medical Association, 263,* 2899–2906, 1990.

Luke, R. D., & Modrow, R. E., "Professionalism, Accountability, and Peer Review," in R. D. Luke, J. C. Krueger, & R. E. Modrow (Eds.), *Organization and Change in Health Care Quality Assurance.* Rockville, MD: Aspen Publications, 1983.

Luthy, D. A., Shy, K. K., von Belle, G., Larson, E. B., Hughes, P., II, Benedetti, T. J., et al., "A Randomized Trial of Electronic Fetal Monitoring in Pre-term Labor," *Obstetrics and Gynecology, 69,* 687–695, 1987.

Maxwell, R. J., "Resource Constraints and the Quality of Care," *Lancet, 2,* 8461, 1985.

McCusker, J., Harris, D. R., & Hosmer, D. W., Jr., "Association of Electronic Fetal Monitoring During Labor with Cesarean Section Rate and with Neonatal Morbidity and Mortality," *American Journal of Public Health, 78,* 1170–1174, 1988.

McGlynn, E. A., "Six Challenges to Measuring the Quality of Health Care," *Health Affairs, 16*(3), 7–21, 1997.

Medicine and Health, 47(25), 4, June 21, 1993.

"NCQA: Setting the Standard in Setting Standards," *Medicine and Health: Perspectives,* Sept. 2, 1996.

Ogrod, E. S., "Compensation and Quality: A Physician's View," *Health Affairs, 16*(3), 82–86, 1997.

Roberts, J. S., "A History of the Joint Commission on Accreditation of Hospitals," *Journal of the American Medical Association, 258,* 1987.

Rolph, J. E., Kravitz, R. L., & McGuigan, K., "Malpractice Claims Data as a Quality Improvement Tool; II. Is Targeting Effective?" *Journal of the American Medical Association, 266,* 2093–2097, 1991.

Roper, W. L., & Hackbarth, G. M., "HCFA's Agenda for Promoting High-Quality Care," *Health Affairs, 7*, 936–940, 1988.

Rubin, H. R., Rogers, W. H., Kahn, K. L., Rubinstein, & Brook, R. H., "Watching the Doctor-Watchers: How Well Do Peer Review Organization Methods Detect Hospital Care Quality Problems?" *Journal of the American Medical Association, 267*, 2349–3354, 1992.

Safran, C., Rind, D. M., & Davis, R. B., "Effects of a Knowledge-Based Electronic Patient Record on Adherence to Practice Guidelines," *M.D. Computing, 13*, 55–63, 1996.

Scofield, R., "Certification: What Does it Mean?" *Current Concepts in Nursing, 2*(1), 6–10, 1988.

Shanahan, M., "The Quality Assurance Standard of the JCAH: A Rational Approach to Patient Care Evaluation," in R. D. Luke, J. L. Krueger, & R. E. Modrow (Eds.), *Organization and Change in Health Care Quality Assurance.* Rockville, MD: Aspen Publications, 1983.

Slenker, S. E., Coban, C. D., & Lind, D. A., "Increasing Physicians' and Nurses' Compliance with Treatment Guidelines in Cancer Care Program," *Journal of Medical Education, 60*, 847–854, 1985.

Svarstad, B. L., "Patient-Practitioner Relationships and Compliance with Prescribed Medical Regimens," in L. H. Aiken & D. Mechanic (Eds.), *Applications of Social Science to Clinical Medicine and Health Policy* (pp. 438–459). New Brunswick, NJ: Rutgers University Press, 1986.

Thurow, L. C., "Medicine versus Economics," *New England Journal of Medicine, 313*, 611–614, 1985.

U.S. General Accounting Office, *Medicare: PRO Review Does Not Assure Quality of Care Provided by Risk HMOs* (GAO:HRD-91-48). Washington, DC: U.S. GAO Human Resources Division, 1991.

U.S. General Accounting Office, *Practitioner Data Bank: Information on Small Medical Malpractice Payments* (IMTEC-92-56). Washington, DC: U.S. GAO Information Management and Technology Division, 1992.

U.S. General Accounting Office, *Medicare: Federal Efforts to Enhance Quality of Care* (GAO: HEHS-96-20). Washington, DC: U.S. GAO Health, Education, and Human Services Division, 1996.

"US Plans to Rate Doctors Treating Medicare Patients," *New York Times*, June 12, 1988.

Ware, J. E., Bayliss, M. S., Rogers, W. H., Kosinski, M., & Tarlov, A. R., "Differences in 4-Year Health Outcomes for Elderly and Poor Chronically Ill Patients Treated in HMO and Fee-for-Service Systems," *Journal of the American Medical Association, 276*, 1039–1047, 1996.

Ware, J. E., Davies-Avery, A., & Stewart, A. L., "The Measurement and Meaning of Patient Satisfaction," *Health and Medical Care Services Review, 1*(1), 1978.

Waxman, H. A., "Medical Malpractice and Quality of Care," *New England Journal of Medicine, 316*, 934–935, 1987.

Wilensky, G. R., "Promoting Quality: A Public Policy View," *Health Affairs, 16*(3), 77–81, 1997.

Wilson, F. A., & Neuhauser, D., *Health Services in the United States: Second Edition with 1987 Revisions.* Cambridge, MA: L. Ballinger, 1987.

14

Access to Health Care Services

John Billings

Learning Objectives

1. To understand the nature of the access problem
2. To understand the distinction between economic and noneconomic barriers to care
3. To understand the characteristics of the uninsured and the policy implications of those characteristics
4. To understand how access barriers impinge on health
5. To understand how access barriers affect the health care delivery system
6. To understand the range and limitations of options for reform—increasing coverage and reducing barriers to care

Resource availability/performance
An example of the impact of noneconomic and quasi-economic barriers: preventable hospitalizations
Health care reform: improving access
At the federal level: Failure of the Clinton Health Plan and beyond
State initiatives to improve access: innovations and limitations
The future: continuing and emerging issues

Key Words: **Access barrier, noneconomic barreirs, quasi-economic barriers, underinsurance, cost-shifting, resource availability/performance, ambulatory-care-sensitive conditions, safety net, ERISA, pay or play.**

For most of the 20th century the U.S. health care system has struggled in its efforts to assure access to health care services for all Americans. There have been major steps forward. The growth of private employer-based health insurance following World War II, the passage of the Medicare and Medicaid programs in 1965, and the growth of federal programs in the 1970s to expand direct service programs (such as community health centers) for low-income patients helped improve access for many. But the debate surrounding the proposed Clinton health reform plan of 1993 and its subsequent failure (as well as the experience with incremental reforms at the state and federal level before and after the Clinton health reform debacle) illustrate the technical, financial, and political difficulties that are entailed in making further progress.

Access is often viewed as a one-dimensional problem: too many Americans lack health insurance coverage. By this measure, the magnitude of the problem is substantial, with more than 40 million persons estimated to be uninsured in 1996, more than 15% of the U.S. population (U.S. Census, 1997). Moreover, the situation has actually deteriorated over the past 20 years, with the rates of uninsured growing as a result of structural changes in the U.S. economy and rising costs of insurance (that have generally tracked the rapid increases in health expenditures).

The potential impact of lack of insurance on patients is obvious—delaying or forgoing needed care can lead to adverse health outcomes, and the costs of obtaining necessary care can be financially ruinous. The impact of large numbers of uninsured patients on the health care delivery system is also serious, as providers of uncompensated care struggle to subsidize or "cost-shift" to other payers the expense incurred by patients without coverage. These efforts by providers can create structural distortions in the health care delivery system, steering uninsured patients toward "safety net" providers (often hospital outpatient departments or emergency rooms), further increasing the costs of care for these patients, undermining the financial integrity of many institutions, and reinforcing the development of a two-tiered health care delivery system in many communities. With the expansion of managed care and the emergence of stronger market forces in the health care delivery system, these distortions are expected to be exacerbated and the consequences for uninsured patients and their providers to be more severe.

However, the problem of access itself is enormously more complex than simply considering whether or not a patient has insurance coverage. An insurance card alone does not eliminate barriers to access. First, there are issues of what kind of card—the extent and adequacy of the coverage. What is covered? Are outpatient services covered as well as inpatient care? Are prescription drugs included? Mental health and substance abuse services? Long-term care? And what about the levels of copayments and deductibles? Forty million Americans have no health insurance, as many as 29 million are estimated to be underinsured, with levels of coverage inadequate to assure financial access to care (Bodenheimer, 1992; Short & Banthin, 1995). Another important factor is the adequacy of payments to providers made by third-party payers. For example, low payment levels to physicians have historically plagued the Medicaid program (the joint federal/state program to provide coverage for some low-income patients), discouraging participation of many private physicians and limiting where Medicaid patients can receive care (often steering many to institution-based providers).

In addition, patients with an insurance card can also face serious noneconomic or quasi-economic barriers to care that can have a dramatic effect on access, utilization patterns, and health outcomes. Although health care networks and managed care systems seek to overcome the difficulties inherent in navigating the complexities of our fragmented health care system, the delivery of care remains largely disconnected, creating substantial barriers for many users. Moreover, to the extent that the health care delivery system fails to respond to differences in language, culture, health care beliefs, care-seeking behavior, and educational levels, additional impediments to access can be created. These nonfinancial barriers are often aggravated for low-income patients by quasi-economic barriers. Obtaining timely care for a child may require that a parent get off work, forgo wages, arrange child care for siblings, or procure transportation—all of which may be difficult for families with limited resources or those that are socially isolated.

In this chapter the nature and extent of all of these barriers to care are examined. In the next section, economic barriers to care are explored, including an overview of the characteristics of the uninsured, a discussion of problems associated with extent and adequacy of coverage, and examination of the consequences of uninsurance and underinsurance on patients and the health care delivery system. In the section following, noneconomic and quasi-economic barriers to care are described in greater detail, and their impact on utilization patterns and health outcomes are documented. In the final section some of the reforms that have been proposed or are being implemented at the federal and state level are examined, their potential impact and limitations are discussed, and future issues related to access are explored.

Economic Barriers to Care

Who Are the Uninsured?

Although there has been little progress in the past 20 years in expanding health coverage in the United States, the characteristics of the uninsured population have been studied extensively. The first step in most efforts to examine the problem of access to care, especially at the state and local level, is the appointment of a task force to study the problem; the next step is typically the hiring of a consultant who documents the number of uninsured and their characteristics. From these analyses has emerged a description of the uninsured that suggests much about the causes of the problem and the requirements of any efforts to expand coverage.

First, it is important to note that the level of uninsurance among the elderly is very low (less than 2%), reflecting the impact of the Medicare program that provides almost universal coverage for Americans age 65 and over. Although there are important limitations in coverage for the elderly and some noneconomic or quasi-economic barriers for this population (discussed below), the Medicare program has done much to reduce barriers to access for the elderly.

Among the nonelderly (see Table 14.1), the highest rates of uninsurance are among the young adult population (ages 18–29). The higher rates among these age groups reflect two important factors: the historical dependence on employer-based coverage for private insurance in the United States and the impact of the federal/state Medicaid program. In contrast to most Western industrialized societies, the United States has relied predominantly on employers to provide coverage for the nonelderly workers and their families. Accordingly, when employers fail to provide or offer insurance to their workers or when an individual becomes unemployed, the risk of becoming uninsured increases enormously. Although some initiatives have attempted to make nongroup coverage more affordable, the cost of individual coverage is prohibitive for most persons without coverage, especially low-income workers or the unemployed. Accordingly, the higher rates of uninsurance among young adults reflect, in part, their higher rates of unemployment, as well as their recent entry into the workforce (often with lower wage, part-time jobs and in sectors where employer-sponsored health coverage is commonly not provided).

TABLE 14.1 Nonelderly Population Without Health Insurance Coverage by Demographic Characteristics, 1996 Current Population Survey

Characteristics	Percentage of total uninsured	Percentage of uninsured within categories
Male	53.5	21.0
Female	46.5	17.0
Total	100.0	17.4
Under 18	24.3	13.8
18–20	6.2	23.2
21–24	11.2	32.3
25–34	23.2	23.1
35–44	17.7	16.7
45–54	10.4	13.3
55–64	6.9	13.4
Total	100.0	17.4
White	54.3	13.4
Black	16.9	22.4
Hispanic	23.4	35.0
Other	5.4	20.3
Total	100.0	17.4
< 100% poverty level	27.6	33.0
100–149%	16.8	32.8
150–199%	14.9	27.3
200–399%	27.7	14.4
400+	13.0	6.7
Total	100.0	17.4

Sources: EBRI, 1997; and U.S. Bureau of the Census, 1997.

Young adults also often have difficulty establishing eligibility for Medicaid coverage. Although there are substantial differences among state Medicaid programs (the federal government sets only minimum requirements), eligibility for the program is limited to low-income persons who fall into one of the following eligibility categories: children, elderly, blind/disabled, pregnant women, single parents, or unemployed parents (in some states). Employed parents or childless adults simply cannot become eligible for Medicaid regardless of income (unless they become blind, disabled, or pregnant), although some states provide coverage though state-financed programs (home relief, medical indigency, etc.) for some of these noncategorically eligible individuals. The targeted nature of the Medicaid program is also reflected in the lower rates of uninsurance among children (categorically eligible) and women (more likely to be single parents or to become eligible through pregnancy).

The overwhelming majority of the uninsured have some attachment to the workforce. About 85% of the uninsured live in households where the family head has been employed during the past year (EBRI, 1997). Accordingly, the problem of uninsurance is typically not due to unemployment but either to the failure of an employer to offer insurance or to the refusal of coverage by an employee (e.g., where cost-sharing of the premium is unaffordable to the employee). The highest rates of uninsurance are in the retail, service, construction, and agricultural sectors, with much higher rates among small employers (and the self-employed). Low-wage earners (incomes less than $10,000 per year) represent more than half of the working uninsured and have rates (30.6% uninsured) more than 10 times greater than high-income workers (2.8%). See Table 14.2.

Rates of uninsurance also differ significantly among states. For example, less than 10% of the nonelderly are uninsured in Connecticut and Minnesota, whereas rates in Louisiana, Texas, and Oklahoma are above 25%. This variation reflects differences in the structure and health of local economies as well as in the breadth of coverage in the states' Medicaid programs. In addition to the categorical requirements noted above for Medicaid coverage (children, aged, blind/disabled, etc.), there are also minimum income standards for eligibility. These standards are set by the states and have been historically tied to welfare payment levels,[1] again with huge differences among states (e.g., eligibility limited to incomes below $2,280 for a family of three in Louisiana, compared with $6,972 in Connecticut).

Although there are uninsured persons across all income groups and sectors of the economy, the profile of the typical uninsured person might be a young adult in a low-wage job working for a small employer in the retail/services sector of the economy. Accordingly, any realistic solution to the problem of uninsurance cannot be dependent on the uninsured themselves to provide significant support for coverage—more than half of the uninsured earn less than $10,000 per year, and 85% earn less than $20,000 (EBRI, 1997). Requiring employers to provide coverage is often proposed by policy analysts and is an attractive option, but the uninsured tend to be in the weakest sectors of the economy, among smaller employers and with very low wage levels. Adding insurance coverage would represent a large percentage increase in labor expense for these employers, and the perception of potential financial impairment will undoubtedly continue to foster strong political resistance to "reform" among these groups. The intractable

---

[1]Recent federal reforms have broken this link and given states somewhat more flexibility in setting eligibility standards.

TABLE 14.2   Nonelderly Workers Age 16–84 Without Health Insurance Coverage, Current Population Survey, 1996

Characteristics	Percentage of total uninsured	Percentage of uninsured within industry category
Self-employed	13.1	25.1
Government	5.9	7.1
Agriculture	4.0	36.4
Construction	8.3	31.3
Manufacturing	11.9	13.2
Retail	23.1	26.0
Finance/insurance/real estate	2.6	8.3
Services	24.0	18.0
Other	7.0	14.5
Total workers	100.00	17.6
Self-employed	13.1	25.1
Total wage and salary workers	86.9	16.8
Public sector	5.9	7.1
Private sector	81.0	18.7
Fewer than 10	21.9	32.7
Ten–24	13.6	27.6
25–99	13.6	20.3
100–499	10.4	15.3
500–999	3.6	13.0
1,000	17.8	11.6
Total workers	100.0	17.6
Under 5,000	11.5	38.5
5,000–9,999	10.6	29.9
10,000–14,999	12.9	33.8
15,000–19,999	11.8	29.8
20,000–29,999	19.0	24.4
30,000–39,000	12.1	16.6
40,000–49,999	7.1	11.0
50,000 and over	15.1	6.9
Total workers	100.0	17.4

Sources: EBRI, 1997; and U.S. Bureau of the Census, 1997.

nature of this problem is likely to get worse, not better—small employers in the services and retail sectors are where much of recent job growth has occurred, suggesting that continued economic expansion of the type experienced in the past decade holds little promise for any improvement.

Underinsurance and Other Limitations of Coverage

An insurance card does not always assure financial access to care. Private insurance often has serious limitations on coverage, excluding mental health services, preventive care, long-term care, or other important health services. Most individual plans and many group plans have exclusions or waiting periods for preexisting conditions, restrictions that bar coverage for illnesses or conditions that existed at the time of enrollment. These limits, of course, affect patients most in need of coverage, exposing millions of Americans with medical problems or chronic diseases to substantial financial risk if they change jobs. Many plans also lack adequate coverage for catastrophic illnesses, with maximum lifetime benefit limits too low to cover the costs of serious illness or accident. Moreover, virtually all private insurance plans, even most managed care plans, have some form of copayment or deductible. These devices are intended to discourage frivolous utilization and to help reduce premium costs (by shifting some expenses to the patient). However, they also can have the effect of discouraging patients from seeking needed preventive care (such as immunizations, Pap smears, mammograms, etc.), especially lower income patients most sensitive to out-of-pocket costs (Lohr et al., 1986).

Although almost 97% of Americans over age 65 have Medicare coverage, the program has substantial patient cost-sharing provisions and serious gaps in coverage. The deductible is more than $700 for hospital care and $100 for outpatient care, with substantial copayments (20%) also required in many cases. Moreover, Medicare provides no coverage for prescription drugs and has substantial restrictions on long-term care (only 2% of nursing home costs of the elderly are paid by Medicare). As a result of these limitations in coverage, Medicare is estimated to pay less than 50% of the total costs of health care for the elderly (Greenbook, 1995). Many elderly have supplemental coverage for some of these expenses ("Medigap" plans), either through their employer/retirement plan or by purchasing such coverage directly. However, more than 20% of the elderly (35% of low-income elderly) have no supplemental coverage, exposing them to serious financial risks and potentially creating substantial barriers to access (U.S. House of Representatives, 1996).

Low-income elderly (and elderly patients who exhaust all of their financial resources on health care costs) qualify for Medicaid coverage along with the other low-income categorical eligibles discussed above (children, disabled, single parents, etc.). Medicaid coverage is generally very comprehensive, covering most services (including drugs and long-term care) and having few restrictions or copayments. However, the program, which is jointly funded by federal and state governments and administered at the state level, has been plagued by serious problems of provider nonparticipation. Although hospitals historically have been guaranteed payment levels that were reasonably related to costs (pursuant to the Boren Amendment repealed in 1997), physician payments are set by state administrative agencies that have struggled to cope with staggering increases in Medicaid program costs. Not surprisingly, payment levels for physicians and other noninstitutional providers have often been set below market rates. For example, in New York, the office-based physician payment rate for an "intermediate office visit" is $11, a level unchanged since the mid-1980s.

Not surprisingly, many physicians elect not to participate in the program, even in competitive markets with a potential oversupply of physicians. As a result, Medicaid card holders (both elderly and nonelderly) often experience barriers in seeking a source of care, and many are effectively restricted to institution-based providers (emergency rooms, hospital outpatient departments, or large community-based clinics) that have an explicit mission of assuring a safety net for these patients.

The Impact of Economic Barriers to Care

Economic barriers to health care access can have an impact both on patients (their utilization of services and health status/outcomes) and on the health care delivery system itself. As the numbers of uninsured/underinsured continue to grow and pressures of managed care and the influence of market forces on the health care system intensify, the consequences of impediments to access are likely to become more severe.

For patients, the impact of lack of insurance can be profound. Uninsured patients are less likely than the privately insured to have a usual source of care (24% vs. 8%). Among patients with health problems, uninsured patients are more likely to have had no physician visits during a 12-month period than are those with private insurance (22% vs. 9%) and have had fewer average number of physician contacts (9.1 vs. 14.8)—and these differences persist even after adjusting for socioeconomic status among the insured and uninsured (Millman, 1993).

The impact of coinsurance on utilization is also significant. The Rand Health Insurance experiment documented substantially lower rates of ambulatory utilization among patients with significant levels of copayments and deductibles, especially among lower income patients (Lohr et al., 1986). While one goal of coinsurance is to discourage frivolous utilization, lower rates for preventive services (such as immunizations for children or screening tests for cervical cancer for adult women) were documented among low-income patients with cost-sharing plans, suggesting that these barriers to care affect other utilization as well (Lurie et al., 1987).

The lack of insurance can also affect hospital utilization. Uninsured patients are more likely to be admitted for preventable or avoidable conditions, such as asthma, diabetes, cellulitis, or other infections (Billings & Tiecholz, 1990). Moreover, once admitted, uninsured patients have been found to receive fewer resources and procedures than insured patients (Weissman & Epstein, 1989; Yergan, Flood, Diehr, & LoGerfo, 1988). For example, in one study, hospitalized uninsured patients were found to have substantially lower rates for common diagnostic tests (colonoscopy, endoscopy, coronary arteriography, etc.) and for costly surgical procedures (bypass surgery, joint replacement, eye surgery, etc.), even after controlling for sociodemographic and diagnostic case-mix factors (Hadley, Steinberg, & Feder, 1991).

Although it is difficult to document the effect of insurance status on health status and health outcomes (especially long-term effects) because the lack of insurance tends to be somewhat episodic (with individuals going on and off of insurance periodically), substantial differences for the uninsured have been observed. Following cutbacks in California's MediCal program in response to the state's property tax revolt in the early 1980s, a substantial number of low-income patients lost coverage. In the 2-year follow-up period after losing coverage, researchers documented serious deterioration in blood pressure levels among hypertensive patients, compared with patients who remained in the program (Lurie, 1986). The Rand Health Insurance Experiment also documented that, among low-income patients with vision, blood pressure, and other health problems, insured patients with free care had better vision, better control of blood pressure levels, and lower overall risks of dying than did patients whose plans had substantial cost-sharing provisions (Brook et al., 1983).

In other studies, uninsured mothers have been found to begin prenatal care later and to have fewer total visits than do privately insured mothers (Braveman, Egerter, Bennett, & Showstack, 1991), and uninsured newborns have been shown to have more adverse outcomes than do babies with insurance (Braveman, Oliva, Miller, Reiter, & Egerter, 1989). Uninsured women have also been found to present with later-stage breast cancer than do privately insured patients and have lower survival rates (49% higher risk of death among uninsured patients) (Ayanian, Kohlker, Toshi, & Epstein, 1993).

Most dramatically, overall mortality rates for uninsured patients have also been shown to be higher than for those with insurance. In a study of a national cohort of patients between 1971 and 1987, uninsured patients were found to have a 25% increased risk of dying during the study period, even after adjusting for differences in sociodemographic characteristics, general health status, and health habits (Franks, Clancy, & Gold, 1993).

Although the cost of no insurance and underinsurance in human terms is high, there is also a serious impact on the health care delivery system that can affect all patients. First, distortions in utilization patterns can increase total costs for the health care delivery system. While lack of insurance promotes underutilization, it also has the effect of steering uninsured patients to providers who are willing to provide care regardless of ability to pay. These providers tend to be institution-based providers, such as hospital outpatient departments, emergency rooms, and community-based clinics. As noted above, Medicaid patients also tend to be heavy utilizers of care in these settings, partially due to low rates of participation by office-based physicians (Cohen, 1989). Costs in these institution-based settings are often higher, therefore increasing total costs for the health care delivery system.

Potentially more pernicious are the financial disequilibriums these utilization patterns can create for providers. Providers serving large numbers of uninsured patients (such as hospitals and clinics in low-income areas) must cover the costs of unreimbursed care to these patients. These same providers usually serve substantial numbers of Medicaid patients as well, and although payment levels are typically more generous than those for office-based physicians, costs of care for Medicaid patients often exceed reimbursement rates, which may be subject to arbitrary payment limits and restrictions. These expenses can either be cost-shifted to other payers (by raising charge levels for these payers sufficiently above actual costs to provide enough revenue to cover unreimbursed expenses), or providers can seek government or private subsidies. Although some states have established elaborate pooling systems to offset some of these costs and many publicly operated providers receive direct subsidies, in most jurisdictions providers are dependent on the "cost shift."

In the bygone days of cost-based reimbursement from public payers and charge-based payments from private insurers, "cost shifting" was often an effective strategy. However, in the current era of fixed fee schedules, ratcheted-down DRG payments, and price negotiation by managed care providers, market forces make this approach less viable. Raising charges in a price-competitive market can mean loss of market share, as managed care plans steer their patients to facilities with lower charges, making "cost shifting" even more difficult as the base of paying patients shrinks and even larger increases in charges are required to shift costs. The wholesale movement of Medicaid patients into managed care plans that has begun in most states is likely to further exacerbate this situation for many providers because this once relatively reliable payer base may be subject to erosion and price bargaining.

Although the failure of some hospitals in this competitive environment is viewed by some as an effective means of reducing the huge oversupply of hospital beds in many communities, the impact of hospital closures and provider failures on access to care for low-income patients may be serious. The providers most at risk are those with the highest levels of care to vulnerable populations. With the loss of these traditional safety net providers, it is not clear that these patients will be assured access to needed care from the remaining providers, who may be located farther away and who have previously avoided provision of care to these patients.

Noneconomic or Quasi-Economic Barriers to Care

Is an Insurance Card Enough?

The importance of adequate insurance coverage in assuring access is obvious—an insurance card opens doors and can help assure viability of providers serving these patients. But it is also becoming increasingly apparent that other factors can have an enormous influence on the ability of many patients, especially vulnerable populations, to obtain needed care and on how these patients utilize the health care delivery system.

The impact of uninsurance on health outcomes and utilization was documented above; however, in many of these studies it was possible to analyze Medicaid patients separately from the uninsured and privately insured. For example, rates of preventable hospitalizations for Medicaid patients were below those of uninsured patients but were still found to be almost 75% higher than insured patients (Billings & Teicholz, 1990). Incidence of late detection of breast cancer and survival rates for the cancer among the uninsured and Medicaid patients were found to be comparable (Ayanian et al., 1993), and pregnant women on Medicaid had rates of late initiation of prenatal care and average total prenatal care visit rates similar to those of uninsured mothers (Braveman, 1993).

For these patients, insurance coverage (in the form of a Medicaid card) failed to eliminate all barriers to needed care. The problems of provider participation and low reimbursement rates noted above undoubtedly contributed to these poor outcomes, but the special problems faced by vulnerable populations in dealing with any system, let alone the complexities of our fragmented health care delivery system, undoubtedly continued to create impediments to timely and effective care for many. These noneconomic and quasi-economic barriers are just beginning to be explored and better understood, but clearly must be addressed to assure more effective utilization of the health care delivery system by those with and without insurance coverage.

Race/Ethnicity

Large and persistent differences in health status, utilization, and outcomes among racial and ethnic groups are well documented. Black and Hispanic/Latino populations have been shown to be less likely to have a usual source of primary care and to have fewer physician visits, higher rates of no or late prenatal care, lower rates of immunizations and screening tests, and worse self-reported health status. Large racial differences have also been documented in rates for infant mortality, low-birthweight infants, late-stage diagnosis of cancer, and mortality from all causes (Council on Ethical and Judicial Affairs, 1990; Millman, 1993).

While many studies and databases do not account for differences in income, insurance status, education, or other important variables, there is a growing body of research that attempts to control for some or all of these factors, suggesting that minority status itself is an important determinant of utilization and health outcomes. For example, after adjusting for differences in insurance coverage, minority adolescents were found to be less likely to have a usual source of primary care and to have fewer annual physician contacts and lower levels of continuity of care (Lieu, Newacheck, & McManus, 1993). Among children enrolled in managed care plans, minority status was linked to lower rates of utilization, even after controlling for differences in health status (Riley, Finney, & Mellits, 1993).

In other research that could adjust for insurance coverage differences, African Americans with end-stage renal disease have been found to be 50% less likely to receive kidney transplants, and those ultimately receiving surgery had been on waiting lists significantly longer than nonminority patients (Gaston, Ayres, Dooley, & Diethelm, 1993). Similarly, among patients with coronary artery disease, Black patients have been found to receive fewer angiographies and to have lower rates of coronary artery bypass surgery, controlling for insurance status and disease severity (Johnson, Lee, Cook, Rovan, & Goldman, 1993; Wenneker & Epstein, 1989).

Similar differences in rates for invasive cardiac procedures have also been observed for Hispanic/Latino populations (Carlisle, Leake, Brook, & Shapiro, 1996). A study of patients with bone fractures, visiting a trauma center emergency room, found that non-Hispanic Whites were more than twice as likely to receive pain medication as were Hispanic patients, even after accounting for patient differences in injury severity, pain assessment, insurance status, gender, and language (Todd, Lee, & Hoffman, 1994; Todd, Samaroo, & Hoffman, 1993). Other studies have documented additional differences among Hispanic/Latino subgroups, with Mexican American, Puerto Rican, and Cuban American populations experiencing different rates of no usual source of care, no preventive care, and no physician visits (Council on Scientific Affairs, 1991).

Large racial/ethnic disparities in utilization have also been observed within the Medicare program. African American beneficiaries have fewer physician visits and lower rates of preventive care, such as influenza immunizations. African Americans with Medicare coverage also have lower rates for many diagnostic procedures (such as CT scans, barium enema x-rays, mammography, etc.), surgical procedures (coronary bypass, prostatectomy, hysterectomy, orthopedic surgery, etc.), and other services (Friedman, 1994). Even within the Veterans Administration hospital system, White veterans have been shown be significantly more likely than Black veterans to receive coronary surgery (Whittle, Conigliaro, Good, & Lofgren, 1993).

Of course, there are many potential explanations for these differences in utilization, outcomes, and health status associated with race/ethnicity. In research controlling for factors such as socioeconomic status, education, disease incidence/prevalence, illness severity, resource availability, and even insurance coverage can be extraordinarily difficult, and interpretation of these research findings must be tempered by recognition of these methodologic limits. However, these differences by race/ethnicity are substantial and persistent across numerous studies using a variety of research designs. But even isolating race as the determining factor in these differences leaves much unknown. The impact of overt or latent racial or cultural bias at all levels of the health care delivery system cannot be discounted. However, further research is required to understand more about the factors that contribute to or mediate any bias and to identify how patient preferences (e.g., in weighing risks and benefits of medical intervention), care-seeking behavior, and attitudes toward the health care delivery system affect utilization and outcomes.

Culture, Acculturation, and Language

The effect of culture and acculturation on health care use and outcomes is not well understood. It is often hypothesized that cultural barriers may contribute to lower or less optimal utilization patterns by Hispanic/Latino and Asian immigrant populations in the United States. These barriers can involve a broad range of potential problems, including social isolation, distrust of Western medicine, unfamiliarity with the U.S. delivery system, differences in concepts of disease and illness, alternative care-seeking behaviors, perceptions of provider disrespect, fears about immigration status, or simply language difficulties.

Several studies have attempted to evaluate how increased acculturation (as measured by English language proficiency or preference, degree of ethnic identity, etc.) tends to ameliorate these impediments to access. Some studies have documented an increase in utilization among more acculturated or assimilated populations (Chesney, Chavira, Hall, & Gary, 1982; Wells & Feinstein, 1988); whereas others have found no independent effect (Markides, Levin, & Ray, 1985; Marks, Solis, Richardson, & Shelton, 1987). This research is limited by the difficulty of assessing levels of acculturation. One of the better designed studies suggests that language proficiency may be either the best indicator of acculturation or the most important component of these cultural factors in facilitating access. In that study, better language skills resulted in more use of preventive services such as physical exams, cancer screening, and dental checkups (Solis, Marks, Garcia, & Shelton, 1990).

Of course, acculturation itself may create new problems and new barriers. For example, many immigrant families have stable family structures, including strong intergenerational ties. To the extent these relationships become more attenuated in urban America, the ability to cope with the requirements of managing a health condition or chronic disease may be impaired.

Gender

Less research has been conducted on gender-related barriers to health care. However, similar differences in rates of procedures have been documented, with female end-stage renal disease patients less likely to receive a kidney transplant than male patients (Held, Pauly, Bovberg, & Saltvatierra, 1988; Kjellstrand, 1988). Women have also been shown to have lower rates of cardiac surgery than men (Udvarhelyi et al., 1992), although these differences were not associated with higher mortality for women (raising an important issue about whether access to more surgical care is always beneficial). Another study documented that among men and women with comparable smoking habits and medical conditions, women were less likely to receive diagnostic screening tests for lung cancer (Wells & Feinstein, 1988).

Again, the impact of patient preferences and attitudes toward risk and benefits when considering surgical and diagnostic procedures requires further study to understand their influence on utilization rates. However, there are three emerging lines of research that underscore the potential seriousness of gender-related impediments to health care for women. First, it is well established that women have historically been systematically excluded from clinical trials for new drugs and procedures (Cotton, 1990a, 1990b). The impact of bias in medical research is not yet fully established, but the potential is obvious. To the extent that medical practice is based on findings of medical research (a matter of some debate), many practitioners may be reluctant to prescribe medications or recommend surgical or diagnostic procedures that have not been fully tested for women. Accordingly, access to newly emerging drugs and technologies may be delayed for women and resource utilization patterns significantly altered. But the corollary also raises serious concerns: when care provided to women is based on research that has been generalized from gender-biased studies, it may in fact be inappropriate, creating impediments to optimal medical care for women.

A second body of research has begun to document how physician gender can affect practice patterns and utilization rates of care for women. For example, in one study of preventive care it was documented that women patients of female physicians were more than twice as likely to receive cervical cancer screening tests (Pap smears) and 40% more likely to receive mammograms than women whose physicians were male (Lurie et al., 1993). Again, although the full impact of how differences in physician gender can influence the care provided to female patients has not yet been determined, the potential for serious barriers to needed health care services for female patients is large. While the number of female physicians is growing (13.7% of medical school entrants were women in 1971 compared to 42.7% in 1997), only 21.2% of physicians in current practice are female (American Medical Association, 1996).

Finally, the continuing politicization of the abortion issue has meant that many women do not have access to family planning, abortion counseling, or abortion services. There are explicit restrictions on use of Medicaid funds for these services, and many religion-affiliated providers simply do not offer such services. Moreover, the aggressive tactics of many antiabortion groups have achieved some of the intended effects, deterring many providers from offering these services and discouraging many women from seeking care. Medicaid and provider restrictions tend to affect low-income patients disproportionately because they are likely to have fewer alternatives, but the chilling affect of politicization of abortion-related care affects access for all women (Henshaw, 1995; Mathews, Ribar, & Wilhelm, 1997; Rosenblatt, Mattis, & Hart, 1995).

Education

As with other indirect barriers to health care, it is difficult to isolate and quantify the effect of education on health care utilization and outcomes. However, parental education deficits have been shown to be associated with delayed entry to care (Guendelman & Schwab, 1986), lower levels of well-baby and other preventive services (Short & Lefkowitz, 1992), and lower overall use by their children (Newacheck, 1992; Newacheck & Halfon, 1986). Differences in education have also been linked to lower rates of breast cancer screening even after adjusting for a broad range of economic and sociodemographic factors (Lantz, Weigers, & House, 1997). In another study, Medicaid patients with limited education were found to be less likely to use preventive services, have greater difficulties following medical regimens, miss more appointments, and seek care later in the course of an illness (Weiss, 1994).

A growing body of research has begun to document the impact of "functional health literacy," or the ability to use reading, writing, and computational skills in typical everyday patient situations, such as reading prescription labels, following diagnostic test instructions, or understanding treatment directions. Because 40 million Americans are estimated to be illiterate and another 50 million marginally literate (Kirsch, Jungeblut, Jenkins, & Kolstad, 1993), the potential impediments to timely and effective care are serious. In a study conducted in two public hospitals, 42% of patients could not understand directions for taking medication on an empty stomach, 26% could not comprehend information on an appointment slip describing the scheduled follow-up visit, and more than 25% could not follow instructions for preparing for a gastrointestinal radiological exam. Overall, almost 30% of patients using the facilities were determined to have inadequate functional health literacy and another 14% to have only marginal levels (Williams et al., 1995).

Of course, illiteracy and educational deficits are not a medical problem. However, to the extent that the health care delivery system fails to recognize and to develop mechanisms to respond to these patient limitations, access to care and health status will continue to be impaired for millions of Americans.

Resource Availability and Performance

The supply of health care resources has obvious implications for access. In remote rural areas the absence of a primary care practitioner, an obstetrician/gynecologist, or even a hospital can have a serious impact on the ability of area residents to obtain timely care (Kindig & Ricketts, 1991; Nesbitt, 1990). In urban areas, supply issues are often more complex. There are huge, well-documented differences in physician supply across and within communities (Cooper, 1995; Grumbach et al., 1995; Politzer, Harris, Gaston, & Mullan, 1991), with some central city areas having serious shortages of practitioners.

However, the issue for access is availability of providers, not supply. Many large urban hospitals (and their associated medical office buildings) are located in or near lower income neighborhoods, but this proximity does not assure access. Although many hospital outpatient departments accept patients without restrictions on ability to pay (or charge on a sliding-fee schedule), this is certainly not necessarily the case for the privately practicing physicians clustered nearby. Moreover, the low Medicaid reimbursement rates for physician visits noted above discourage many of these physicians from participating in the Medicaid program, creating potential barriers even for Medicaid card holders. Therefore, while a simple physician-to-population ratio for the areas surrounding these hospitals would suggest a sufficient supply, the reality is likely to be less satisfactory for low-income residents of the areas because a substantial portion of the supply is simply not available to them.

Not surprisingly, many studies of physician supply fail to find a clear-cut relationship between the level of local physician supply in an area and the adequacy of access for area residents (Grumbach, Vranizan, & Bindman, 1997). However, other research examining the impact of expansions of availability (e.g., the opening of a primary care clinic serving insured, Medicaid, and uninsured) has documented improvements in reducing barriers to care among clinic users (Orr, Charney, & Straus, 1988), but better designed research is required to strengthen our understanding of the link between expansions in availability and improvements in access.

There is also very little known about the performance of the primary care delivery system and access to care. Clearly, a more efficient provider that can serve more patients has the potential to reduce barriers in its service area. But more important, providers can also have a dramatic impact by creating care delivery approaches that reduce many of the indirect barriers to care discussed above (eliminating language barriers, reducing wait times, developing a culturally sensitive environment, using telephone consultations more effectively, developing more effective compliance techniques for chronic disease patients with literacy problems, etc.).

In the more competitive environment that has begun to emerge for middle-class medicine, patient satisfaction has become the focus of many health care delivery systems as they struggle to attract and maintain their patient base. These developments have spawned a mini-industry of researchers and consultants attempting to assist providers in becoming more responsive to this new world. A parallel effort targeted at understanding the indirect barriers to care for low-income patients and helping safety net providers better adapt their care delivery approach to these needs is not yet on the horizon.

One Example of the Impact of Noneconomic and Quasi-Economic Barriers: Preventable Hospitalizations

As illustrated in many of the studies described above, the impact of noneconomic and quasi-economic barriers on utilization patterns and health status can be substantial, in many cases resulting in fewer visits or procedures and often contributing to poor health outcomes and increased mortality. A growing body of analysis has also begun to explore how barriers to primary care services can result in increased utilization of other health care services, such as more costly hospital care (Billings, Anderson, & Newman, 1996; Billings et al., 1993; Bindman et al., 1995; Weissman, Gatsonis, & Epstein, 1992).

This research is based on the simple premise that timely and effective primary care can often (1) prevent the onset of an illness (e.g., congenital syphilis, pertussis, tetanus, etc.), (2) control a condition before it becomes more acute (e.g., ear infections in children, urinary tract infections, dehydration, etc.), or (3) manage a chronic disease or condition to help reduce the chances of a serious flare-up (e.g., asthma, diabetes, congestive heart disease, hypertension, etc.). To the extent that barriers of any kind exist for ambulatory-care services and a patient delays or is unable to obtain care, an illness or condition may deteriorate beyond control in an outpatient setting, resulting in the need for hospitalization for effective management.

By analyzing hospital admission rates for diagnoses related to these conditions, referred to as ambulatory care sensitive (ACS) conditions, researchers have documented huge differences in rates among areas (see Table 14.3). Areas with

TABLE 14.3 Preventable/Avoidable Hospitalizations, ACS Admissions/1,000, Age < 65, 1990

MSA	All zip/FSA/areas		
	ACS admissions per 1,000	Association with income (Rsq)	Ratio low income/high income
Boston	11.84	0.581	2.58
Buffalo	8.90	0.840	2.92
Jersey City/Bergen/Passaic	13.20	0.675	3.21
Los Angeles	10.34	0.518	2.09
Miami	10.90	0.371	1.58
New York City	15.16	0.663	3.13
Newark	14.48	0.827	3.51
Oakland	8.90	0.674	2.55
Orlando	10.29	0.557	2.36
Portland	6.85	0.586	2.59
Rochester, NY	8.21	0.734	2.95
San Diego	7.15	0.756	2.64
San Francisco	8.55	0.633	3.70
Seattle	6.92	0.606	2.32
Tampa/St. Petersburg	9.63	0.513	2.05
Hamilton	7.25	0.409	1.58
Ottawa	7.43	0.672	1.79
Toronto	7.38	0.103	1.39

Source: Billings et al., 1996.

high ACS rates have been found to have higher levels of self-reported barriers to access than do low ACS rate areas (Bindman et al., 1995). Moreover, these differences have been found to be strongly associated with area income, with more than 80% of the variation in admission rates among zip codes in some communities being explained by a single variable, the percentage of low-income persons living in an area. Admission rates for ACS conditions in low-income areas on average have been found to be 2.5 to 3.5 times higher than more affluent areas, with individual zip code rates in some low-income neighborhoods as much as 20 times higher than rates in high-income zip codes in the same community. See Figures 14.1 and 14.2 illustrating these differences.

Of course, not all admissions for these ACS conditions are preventable. However, the extraordinarily high rates among low-income areas and the strong association between area rates and the level of poverty suggest that significant barriers to primary care exist in most low-income areas. Insurance coverage is

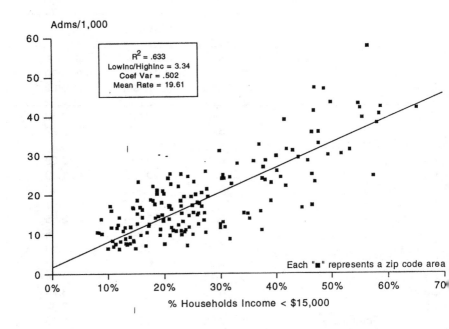

FIGURE 14.1   New York City: Ambulatory-care-sensitivity (ACS) admission, ages 0–64 (1995).

Source: SPARCS, UHF, NYU Health Research Program.

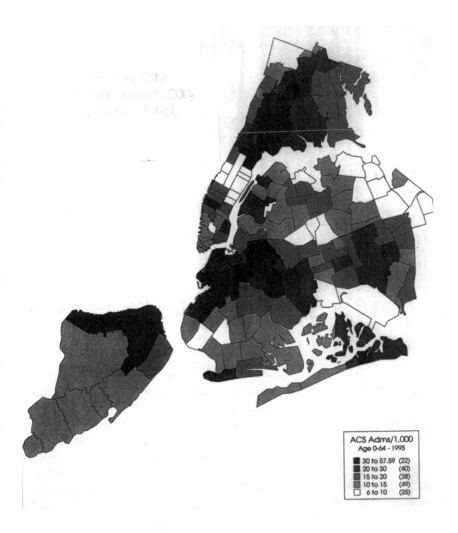

FIGURE 14.2 New York City: ACS admissions/1,000, ages 0–64 (1995).

Source: SPARCS, UHF, NYU Health Research Program.

undoubtedly an important factor—differences in rates among Canadian urban areas (with universal insurance coverage) have been found to be significantly lower than those for U.S. urban areas (Billings et al., 1996). See Table 14.3. Nevertheless, lack of insurance coverage is unlikely to be the sole or even

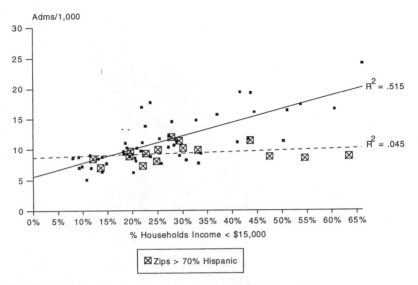

FIGURE 14.3   Dade County (Miami): ACS admissions age 0–64 (1990).

predominant cause for the disparities documented in most U.S. urban areas, as the overwhelming majority of low-income patients admitted for ACS conditions in these studies had Medicaid coverage. The impact of the noneconomic and quasi-economic barriers discussed above is undoubtedly substantial. A low-income patient who has no regular source of care, who is dissatisfied with available providers (because of long wait times, language difficulties, or lack of cultural sensitivity), or who has difficulties arranging child care, getting off work, or simply coping with problems associated with illness is clearly at significant risk of delaying or not getting needed care.

The potential relationship between these noneconomic factors and access is illustrated by the findings for ACS admission rates in Miami. Although like most U.S. urban areas, Miami has significant concentrations of poverty and minority populations, the difference in ACS admissions rates between low- and high-income areas is much smaller (only about 1.6 times higher in low-income areas), and the association between area rates and income is also lower ($R^2 = .371$, indicating only 37.1% of variation is explained by income). This lack of a large difference between low- and high-income areas was particularly evident among Cuban-American zip codes [Figure 14.3], where admission rates were virtually identical regardless of area income ($R^2 = .045$). In fact, in the other non-Latino zip code areas, the association was comparable ($R^2 = .515$) to other U.S. metropolitan areas (Billings et al., 1996). These data offer some promise that the noneconomic and quasi-economic barriers to care that appear to exist for other low-income populations in U.S. urban areas are not insurmountable. However, further research is needed to help sort out the impact of various factors such as family and social structure of the Cuban-American immigrant population, their health status and care-seeking behavior, and the organization and performance of the primary care delivery system serving this population (including a substantial cadre of Cuban-American physicians who also left Cuba).

The extent and nature of some of these indirect barriers to care are illustrated in a study of patients hospitalized for ACS conditions in New York City (Billings, Mijanovich, & Blank, 1997). In interviews after hospital admission and medical stabilization, 60.9% of low-income patients reported that they had received no care prior to the admission, and another 17.4% had received care only in the emergency room (compared with 31.4% of higher income patients receiving no care and 5.8% with only emergency room care). More than half of low-income patients reported that they had delayed or not obtained needed care (compared to about one fourth of higher income patients). The leading explanations for delay or the failure to obtain care among low-income patients were not directly related to the costs of care (the overwhelming majority had Medicaid coverage) but rather to a range of social and quasi-economic problems reflecting the difficulties encountered by low-income patients and their families in their daily lives and in negotiating the complexities of the health care delivery system. Over 25% of adult patients indicated they were "too nervous or afraid," "too busy with other things," or simply "not up to going," reflecting serious ambivalence about the health care delivery system. Substantial numbers also reported difficulties arranging child care, problems with transportation, concern about having to wait too long, uncertainty about where to go, or apprehensions that providers wouldn't understand their needs. See Table 14.4.

These nonfinancial barriers to timely and effective care are substantial and serious. It is clear that successful interventions to facilitate timely and effective care will have to do more than simply provide the uninsured with an insurance card. Part of the solution will involve making the health care delivery system more responsive to the unique needs of low-income patients. It will require development of a care delivery system that recognizes that low-income patients are struggling with many other aspects of their lives (as well as their health care problems). These patients are "busy with other things" and do have difficulty getting off work or arranging child care. Longer clinic hours, home visits, and special outreach may be required for effective care management and delivery. But many of these problems are also beyond the immediate reach of the health care delivery system and necessarily will require that social service, education, and other programs become more responsive to the needs of these populations.

TABLE 14.4   Type of "Access" Problems Reported by Low-Income Patients Hospitalized for Preventable/Avoidable Conditions

	Percentage of low-income patients with "access" problems who reported type of reason		
Reason for problem	Age 6 mos–17 yr	Age 18–64 yr	All ages
Not up to going	5.1	36.1	29.2
Too nervous or afraid	10.2	33.8	28.6
Unable to free time to get care	8.1	27.2	22.9
Had to wait too long to get appointment	20.3	20.4	20.4
Problems with child care	32.8	14.3	18.2
Costs too much	13.8	18.1	17.2
Unable to keep medical appointment	7.4	20.2	17.1
Couldn't fill prescription	16.4	16.9	16.8
Transportation difficulties	19.3	15.8	16.5
Didn't know where to go to get care	8.6	13.8	12.7
Not sure provider would understand needs	22.4	9.1	12.2
Care not available when needed	11.3	12.1	12.0
Denied care	13.4	9.7	10.6
Didn't like place usually get care	17.2	7.9	9.9
Lose pay/trouble getting off work	12.1	6.0	7.3
Language problem	1.8	4.7	4.3

Note: Percentages total more than 100% because some patients indicated multiple reasons.

Source: Hospitalized Patient Interview Survey, United Hospital Fund.

Health Care Reform: Improving Access

At the Federal Level: Failure of the Clinton Health Plan and Beyond

In 1992 public support for some form of national health insurance reached a 40-year high of 66%. During the presidential election that year voters ranked health care as the third most important issue facing the nation, after the economy and the federal budget deficit. By the time President Clinton took office in 1993 the issue had risen to second place, with 90% of Americans indicating they believed there was a crisis in health care (Blendon, Brodie, & Benson, 1995).

The new president responded by appointing a task force that developed a proposal for a "Health Security Act" in the fall of 1993. Several key components of the complex plan addressed access issues head-on. The plan would assure coverage with a comprehensive benefits package for almost all Americans. The elderly would continue to be covered by Medicare (although the coverage was to be expanded to include prescription drugs and expanded long-term care benefits for the severely disabled), and the plan excluded undocumented immigrants and prisoners. However, coverage for everyone else would be provided through competing plans offered through "health alliances" to be formed at state and substate levels to administer enrollment, collect premiums, and pay participating health plans. Large employers (5,000+ employees) could opt out of the alliance system but would be required to offer comparable coverage from an array of competing plans and would be assessed a 1% payroll tax to support medical education and care for low-income, high-cost individuals insured in the regional alliances.

Almost all employers were to be required to offer coverage to all of their employees and dependents and pay for 80% of the average premium costs. Premium subsidies were to be provided for small employers and for low-income workers. Medicaid coverage would be provided through the alliances (state and federal funding for these patients would be maintained at prior levels), and unemployed workers would also obtain coverage through the alliances (with premium subsidy support based on income). Employer and individual premiums would be community rated (i.e., cost the same regardless of health status of those being insured), although payments to plans would be risk adjusted to account for differences in health status of plan enrollees. The restructuring of the health care marketplace by inducing competition among competing health plans was expected to help control health costs, but there was also a mechanism to impose caps on premiums if costs began to rise more than expected.

The proposal included other provisions to help reduce barriers to access. Expanded funding was to be provided for public health services and for programs to support "essential" community providers. This latter group included so-called "safety net" providers (such as community-based clinics), which have traditionally provided care to uninsured and Medicaid patients. The support for these entities was intended to assure continuation of important services such as patient outreach programs and to ease the transition to a more competitive health care environment that was expected to be spawned by competing managed care plans.

The Clinton health plan avoided any new broad-based taxes to support the coverage expansions and premium subsidies but rather relied on a combination of funding sources such as mandated employer contributions, Medicaid/Medicare savings (lower provider payments), assessments of large employers who opted out of alliances, and an increase in the tobacco tax. The expected costs of the program ($300+ billion by 2002) would be offset by these program savings and new revenues, making the plan budget neutral, at least on paper.

Of course, the plan failed. Large employers never supported the proposal, even though they were exempted from many of its requirements and the approach had promise of eliminating their financing of the cost-shift for uninsured patients embedded in their current premiums. Small employers were strongly opposed to the mandate coverage, although many would have been insulated from some of its effects by premium subsidies. Insurance companies strongly resisted the proposal, perhaps concerned that not all would survive in the competitive managed care environment contemplated by the approach of the alliances. Conservatives saw further encroachment of government into health care, with the complex system of quasi-governmental alliances and premium caps. Many liberals were concerned that the plan did not go far enough or had discomfort with the concept of managed competition. Virtually everyone had reservations about the numbers—was it really possible to create such a huge expansion of coverage and restructuring of the system without large amounts of new revenue?

The net effect of the failure of the Clinton plan has been to virtually extinguish comprehensive health reform from the national public policy debates. Only 5% of voters in the 1996 elections indicated that reforming health care was a top issue for the new administration (Blendon et al., 1995). Not surprisingly, the focus at the federal level has largely returned to consideration of incremental reforms and cost control. In 1996 the Kennedy-Kassebaum proposal was enacted to assure greater portability of insurance coverage when an employee changes jobs (an important issue for many middle-class workers but having only small effect on the 40 million uninsured). The 1995–1997 budget battles between congressional Republicans and President Clinton have focused primarily on how much savings can be extracted from Medicare and Medicaid. In fact, the Balanced Budget Act of 1997 includes Medicare/Medicaid reductions of almost $140 billion (mostly from reduced payments to providers), an amount comparable to the $190 billion savings contemplated by the Clinton health plan. Of course, these savings are now targeted for budget deficit reduction, whereas in 1993 the monies were intended to expand coverage for the uninsured and to broaden Medicare benefits.

However, two important features of the Balanced Budget Act of 1997 address access issues more directly and also provide a strong indication about the probable locus of near- and medium-term health reform activity. First, the Balanced Budget Act gives states greater flexibility in the administration of Medicaid programs. Many states have begun to examine strategies to use managed care more effectively for Medicaid patients and/or to expand coverage to populations who are ineligible for Medicaid (because of the categorical requirements noted above). These initiatives have historically required a discretionary federal waiver, an uncertain process that usually caused substantial delay and inevitably entailed limitations on state initiatives. Under the new law, states are not required to obtain waivers for many of these reforms. Although there are concerns that states may abuse this new flexibility, it will also undoubtedly encourage even greater state-level activity and innovation.

The Balanced Budget Act also included $24 billion to provide coverage for some of the estimated 10 million uninsured children in the United States. Again the action will be at the state level, with funding distributed to states based on the number of low-income uninsured children in the state, adjusting for differences in wages and the cost of health care. States can use the funding, which must be matched with local support (up to 35% depending on current Medicaid match rates), to expand Medicaid coverage for children up to 200% of the poverty level or to create new programs targeted at providing coverage for low-income uninsured children. Up to 15% of the funding can be used for direct service programs (community-based clinics) and outreach services.

Although assuring the financial integrity of the Medicare trust fund is likely to reemerge soon, and there will inevitably be further tinkering with the Medicaid and Medicare program, the Balanced Budget Act of 1997 signals a clear shift of health reform debate and activity to the states. Many states attempted to cope with these problems in the 1980s, and new approaches are again being considered at the close of the 1990s. In the following section these activities are examined and their strengths and limitations explored.

State Initiatives to Improve Access: Innovations and Limitations

The level and character of state activity to improve access have gone through several cycles and iterations over the past 15 years as federal activity has gone up and down and as various state approaches have been tried and sometimes abandoned. However, most of the activities or proposed approaches fit into one of the following major categories: (1) initiatives to stimulate or facilitate voluntary action by employers or individuals to purchase insurance, (2) efforts to coerce employers to provide coverage ("pay or play" approaches), (3) support of direct services for uninsured (e.g., community-based clinics), and (4) purchase of coverage for targeted uninsured populations (with or without federal assistance).

Many of the initial efforts in the 1980s focused on coping with the apparent failure of the insurance market for small employers where rates of uninsurance were observed to be high (see Table 14.2 above). Because of the inherent high marketing costs for small employers and the difficulties of spreading risks for small groups, it was believed that new products had to be developed that could lower premiums for small employers. Attempts were made to stimulate development of larger groups or cooperative purchasing pools that could centralize marketing and spread risks, giving small employers some of the advantages of larger employers and reducing premiums by 10%–20%. Although some of these areitiatives were successful (Jacobson, Merritt, & Bartlett, 1994), most faced the difficult problem that for many small employers any premium was perceived as too much, and a relatively small number of small employers previously not providing coverage opted to purchase care from the pools.

Many states also established pools for high-risk individuals who could not get coverage in the private market because of their health status or history of high utilization. These programs have historically tended to reach only a small number of individuals. Without significant subsidies, the premiums for individuals using these pools are typically very high and beyond the means of many most in need. Second, the overwhelming majority of uninsured individuals lack coverage not because it has been denied for health reasons but because their employers simply do not offer coverage and the individual insurance market is beyond their means (the majority of uninsured workers are in low-wage jobs).

These voluntary efforts have met with only limited success, but more coercive approaches have not fared well either. The approach considered by many states has been a "pay-or-play" strategy, where employers who do not offer coverage to their employees ("play") are assessed a tax ("pay") sufficient to support state-sponsored plans for uninsured workers. The goal is to either induce employers to offer insurance plans to their employees or raise enough revenue to finance state-subsidized plans for employees of firms not offering coverage.

These approaches have faced two major obstacles: legal challenge and political feasibility. The legal challenge relates to the federal Employee Retirement Income Security Act of 1974 (ERISA), which has been interpreted to preempt state law in regulation of state employee benefit plans. To the extent that the pay-or-play requirement is interpreted as a mandate to provide coverage, it may be subject to legal challenge. The political obstacle is obvious—small employers strongly oppose the approach, even when subsidies or exemptions for new and very small employers are included. Of the several states that have considered or even initially legislated some variant of pay or play, none has actually fully implemented the approach.

Initiatives to support direct services for the uninsured, such as community-based clinics, have generally fared better. The financial support typically goes to publicly operated facilities or in some cases to not-for-profit entities. Financing can come from general tax revenue, earmarked taxes (e.g., sales tax add-ons, tobacco and alcohol taxes, etc.) or assessments on providers (usually hospitals). The smaller scale of these initiatives makes them more politically feasible but also limits their reach.

The area that has generated the most interest at the state level is the last category, efforts to purchase coverage for targeted groups of the uninsured. In the 1980s this typically involved expansions of Medicaid coverage to include all optional categorically eligible groups and to raise income eligibility thresholds to take advantage of federal matching funds. Many states have also elected to use state funds to purchase coverage for very low-income single adults and childless couples who cannot become categorically eligible, individuals who are often on local general assistance welfare rolls. State funds also have been used to provide coverage for children or pregnant women who are above the maximum income thresholds. In the 1990s several states have used the Section 1115 waiver process to expand Medicaid coverage to these groups, who would otherwise not be categorically eligible or who are above income eligibility thresholds. These Section 1115 waiver coverage-expansion initiatives attempt to avoid increasing total costs of the Medicaid program (a requirement of the waiver) by use of managed care or provider payment limits (e.g., Tennessee) or by cutting the services covered by the program (e.g., Oregon). While the provisions in the Balanced Budget Act of 1997 provide federal support for state initiatives to expand coverage for children, these state initiatives will undoubtedly continue to expand.

Although many of these state initiatives in health care reform hold significant promise, it is also important to recognize their limitations. First, most are narrow in scope. Even more recent initiatives to expand coverage typically reach a relatively small portion of the uninsured. Of the 14 states with the most developed initiatives, only 5% of the total uninsured have been reached to date. Because of the targeted nature of these initiatives (children, pregnant women, etc.), even if they reach their enrollment goals, only about 20% of the uninsured will receive coverage assuming current numbers of uninsured and no dropping of coverage to take advantage of the new programs (Lipson & Schrodel, 1996). See Table 14.5. Moreover, the focus on children and pregnant women, although important and politically understandable, tends to overlook the more serious problems of lack of insurance among the adult population who often experience the most serious barriers to access.

State initiatives are also often hindered by limits on revenue sources. The economic growth of the mid-1990s has relieved some of the budget woes at state and local levels, pressures to cut taxes and limit spending that have been at the center of federal policy debates actually began at the state level and are felt even more acutely at the local level. Accordingly, general tax revenues are seldom a viable or reliable source, and initiatives are often dependent on a more limited potential revenue base of "sin taxes" (tobacco and alcohol excise taxes), earmarked sales taxes, or complicated provider assessments. In addition, as the implications of recent federal budget reductions for welfare and Medicaid begin to be felt at the state level, state budget problems are likely to deteriorate.

The potential for revitalization at the state level of approaches aimed at employers (such as the pay-or-play option) also seems remote. In an environment where states perceive it to be important to maintain a climate that is attractive to business, putting burdens on local employers that are not present in competing or nearby states may be unrealistic.

TABLE 14.5   Enrollment Levels in State-Subsidized Coverage Expansions, Fall 1996

State	Access initiative	Enrollment fall '96	Enrollment target	Total uninsured	Enrollment fall '96 as percentage of uninsured	Enrollment target as percentage of uninsured
CA	Access for Infants and Mothers	11,880	59,900	6,518,700	0.2	0.9
CO	Child Health Plan	3,900	39,300	559,400	0.7	7.0
DE	Diamond State Health Plan	7,704	22,400	108,900	7.1	20.6
FL	Florida Healthy Kids	20,000	177,900	2,599,100	0.8	6.8
HI	Hawaii QUEST	44,000	106,500	103,600	42.5	102.8
MA	Medical Security Plan	33,825	183,100	667,500	5.1	27.4
MN	MinnesotaCare	94,614	190,600	370,000	25.6	51.5
NJ	Health Access New Jersey	17,559	587,600	1,106,700	1.6	53.1
NY	Child Health Plus	110,248	228,100	2,748,300	4.0	8.3
OR	Oregon Health Plan	114,289	178,300	397,600	28.7	44.8
PA	Children's Health Insurance Program	50,879	154,000	1,191,600	4.3	12.9
TN	TennCare	287,767	1,095,000	807,200	35.7	135.7
VT	Health Access Plan	3,733	16,700	78,100	4.8	21.4
WA	Basic Health Plan	930,013	3,704,600	17,928,200	5.2	20.7

Source: Alpha Center: Lipson, D., & Schrodel, S. *State Initiatives in Health Care Reform: State-subsidized Insurance Programs for Low-Income People*, 1996.

Finally, there are issues of equity. Experience in the Medicaid program makes it plain that some states are more likely than others to attempt to address access issues. The Aid for Families with Dependent Children (AFDC) income eligibility threshold for a family of three (which determines Medicaid eligibility for adults, except pregnant women) was $1,968 in Alabama in 1996. In New York and California the level was more than 7,000. As the nation moves more toward relying primarily on the states to assure access to care for the needy, it is clear that there will be substantial disparities in who is considered needy and what is required to meet their health care needs.

The Future: Continuing and Emerging Issues

With the demise of the Clinton health plan in 1994, it is apparent that the broad fundamental issues related to access discussed in the preceding sections are likely to continue to confront the health care delivery system in the short and medium term. Large numbers of Americans will remain without coverage, and patients and providers will continue to struggle to cope with the consequences of this reality. However, as the health care environment continues to evolve, three new sets of issues are emerging that will become increasingly important when considering access to health care services as we approach the millennium.

First, within the next 3–5 years, virtually all Medicaid patients (except the elderly in long-term care and some special-needs populations) will be enrolled in managed care. The floodgates that were cracked ajar with the federal 1115 waiver process have now opened wide with passage of the Balanced Budget Act of 1997, which removes most restrictions on mandatory Medicaid managed care enrollment. This transformation has the potential to help reduce some of the indirect barriers to care for Medicaid recipients, but it also raises many new concerns and issues.

On the positive side, capitated payments create strong financial incentives for managed care plans to solve some of the noneconomic or quasi-economic barriers to care described above. To the extent that preventable hospital admissions for conditions such as asthma can be reduced by more timely and effective outpatient management (better patient education on use of inhalers, improved medication regimens, nurse hotlines for care management advice during acute flare-ups, etc.) or by development of a more accessible health care delivery system (longer clinic hours, shorter waits in clinics, child care services on site, in-home visits, etc.), managed care plans have an interest in solving these problems that have historically eluded the fee-for-service world. While there is no compelling evidence yet that major Medicaid managed care players have begun to invest the energy and resources necessary to develop new strategies to address these old problems, new research to monitor how plans respond as Medicaid managed care matures can help policymakers learn whether the promise of these new incentives is realized.

Medicaid managed care also creates new enforcement mechanisms and opportunities for government agencies to assure better access for enrolled patients. For example, some states have instituted policies stating that plans must assure that patients with urgent care needs can obtain an appointment with their primary car provider within a specified period (e.g., 48 hours). Medicaid patients have historically adapted to long wait times for appointments at some clinics and outpatient departments (60 days or more in many cases) by using emergency rooms for routine care or by tuning to Medicaid mills for much of their care. Medicaid agencies often had no effective means to compel providers to be more responsive because of the logistical problems of monitoring a huge number of care sites and the difficulties inherent in penalizing providers who were often already in financial distress and who were critical to assuring some modicum of access in low-income communities. Moreover, because patients often used multiple providers, it was not possible to hold any single provider responsible for patient care. When a newborn failed to receive the requisite schedule of well-baby care visits or appropriate immunizations, it was not always clear who should be held accountable.

In a managed care environment, a single entity (the plan) is responsible for each patient. Regulators can more effectively monitor the performance of the smaller number of plans (e.g., using mock patients attempting schedule appointments with the plan's providers by telephone, monitoring disenrollment rates, and tracking performance indicators for immunizations, well-baby visits, or follow-up after hospitalization) and have a realistic enforcement mechanism to assure accountability: closing enrollment for new patients or denying reenrollment of current patients. Noncomplying plans can be forced to expand capacity or improve performance of their primary care providers or face serious loss of revenue. Again, the potential may exceed the reality. Accordingly, a critical issue for the future concerns the extent and effectiveness of government oversight of Medicaid managed care. The explosion of Medicaid managed care is happening at a time of overall government cutbacks, and it will be critical to examine whether and how public agencies adapt to this new environment.

Medicaid managed care also presents a serious risk of creating a whole new set of barriers to care for low-income patients. The confusion associated with the enrollment process will undoubtedly have negative consequences. For example, many patients may enroll in plans not realizing that they will be required to change providers, perhaps requiring unrealistic travel times to new care sites, and certainly disrupting continuity of current utilization patterns. Other problems are likely to emerge as well. Aggressive entrepreneurial plans may enroll more patients than their primary care network can adequately serve. New providers brought in by managed care plans may underestimate the special needs of Medicaid populations. Requirements that patients use a gate-keeping primary care practitioner may discourage needed care among patients who have difficulty adapting to the new rules. And of course, the most serious concern relates to the new set of incentives for providers: provision of less care can mean higher profits or a bigger margin. Although barriers to care may ultimately lead to increased morbidity and costly hospitalization for some patients, in the short run, low or no utilization of primary care services may be highly profitable. As patients churn on and off Medicaid and from one plan to another, some plans may find no financial advantage in improving access for many of their patients. Therefore, it is critical that policymakers have a capacity to monitor these developments carefully and to learn more about how these new incentives are affecting utilization and outcomes.

The second set of emerging issues relates to the consequences of the changing health care marketplace. With the growth of managed care (in commercial, Medicare, and Medicaid markets) and the strengthening of market forces in the health care sector, the ability of traditional safety net providers to survive, as discussed above, remains in some doubt. The consequences of their failure are likely to be most dire for the uninsured, especially among immigrant populations, who will find increasing difficulty to take advantage of public programs to provide health insurance coverage. Whereas the market-clearing effect of competition may help reduce system-wide overcapacity, the impact on patients dependent on these vulnerable providers may be serious. A critical issue in the next decade will be how well the imperative to reduce unneeded beds and services is balanced by efforts to assure the availability of resources to these vulnerable populations. Will we allow these safety-net providers to fail? What will be the consequences of such failures for other providers, who begin to see more uninsured patients in their emergency rooms and outpatient departments?

Finally, as efforts to cope with access problems continue to devolve to states and localities, it will become critical to more fully understand the impact and limits of incremental reforms at these levels. With the new funds available from the Balanced Budget Act of 1997, what are the most effective means of expanding coverage for children? How should insurance coverage be balanced with support/ subsidies to providers for direct services to the uninsured? What about uninsured adults (who use substantially more health resources than children do)? As other innovations are attempted at the state and local level, sorting out the balance between what is politically feasible (programs for children and pregnant women) and where limited funds might be invested most effectively (adult immigrant populations, substance abuse programs, safety net providers, etc.) will undoubtedly be a major challenge. Disparities among states and localities will also emerge as some move forward while others remain intransigent, and it will be important to monitor the extent and effect of these differences.

Clearly, serious access problems will remain for many millions of Americans for the foreseeable future. The ultimate issue is when these problems will reemerge as a major national policy concern and whether national policymakers will yet again fail to find a politically viable and financially affordable strategy to assure universal access to needed care.

Mini-Case Study

You are the governor of a midsized industrial state. You have just read this chapter and have decided you want to take on the "health reform/health care access"

Mini-Case Study *(cont.)*

issue. How would you proceed? How would you staff the effort? Who are the stakeholders? How would you obtain input from stakeholders? How would you limit inappropriate influence by stakeholders? What is the likely nature of the problem in your state? What is the realistic range of solutions/reforms that might be considered? What is the likelihood of meaningful reform?

Discussion Questions

1. Who are the uninsured and what does this tell us about the nature of the problem?
2. What are the implications of characteristics of the uninsured on efforts to expand coverage?
3. Who is responsible for reducing noneconomic and quasi-economic barriers to timely and effective health care?
4. What are the costs of barriers to access and how are these costs financed in the current health care delivery system?
5. What were the critical factors in the failure of the Clinton Health Plan? What are the prospects for meaningful reform in the immediate future?

References

Allen, D., & Kamradt, J., "Relationship of Infant Mortality to the Availability of Obstetrical Care in Indiana," *Journal of Family Practice, 33*, 609, 1991.

American Medical Association Enterprise Information Base [ama-assn.org], October 1996.

Ayanian, J. Z., Kohlker, B. B., Toshi, A., & Epstein, A. M., "The Relationship between Health Insurance Coverage and Clinical Outcomes among Women with Breast Cancer," *New England Journal of Medicine, 329*, 326, 1993.

Berk, M. L., Bernstein, A. B., & Taylor, A. K., "The Use and Availability of Medical Care in Health Manpower Shortage Areas," *Inquiry, 20*, 369, 1983.

Billings, J., Anderson, G., & Newman, L., "Recent Findings on Preventable Hospitalizations," *Health Affairs*, Fall, 239, 1996.

Billings, J., Mijanovich, T., Blank, A., *Barriers to Care for Patients with Preventable Hospital Admissions*. New York: United Hospital Fund, 1997.

Billings, J., & Teicholz, N., "Uninsured Patients in the District of Columbia," *Health Affairs*, Winter, 158, 1990.

Billings, J., Zeitel, L., Lukomnik, J., Carey, T. S., Blank, A. S., & Newman, L., "Impact of Socioeconomic Status on Hospital Use in New York City," *Health Affairs*, Spring, 162, 1993.

Bindman, A., Grumbach, K., Osmond, D., Komaromy, M., Vranizan, K., Lurie, N., & Billings, J., "Preventable Hospitalizations and Access to Health Care," *Journal of the American Medical Association, 274*, 305, 1995.

Blendon, R. J., Benson, J. M., Brodie, M., Altman, D. E., Rowland, D., Newan, P., et al., "Voters and Health Care in the 1996 Election," *Journal of the American Medical Association, 277*, 1253, 1997.

Blendon, R. J., Brodie, M., & Benson, J., "What Happened to Americans' Support for the Clinton Health Plan?" *Health Affairs*, Summer, 7, 1995.

Bodheimer, T., "Underinsurance in America," *New England Journal of Medicine, 327*, 274, 1992.

Braveman, P., Bennett, T., Lewis, L., Egerter, S., & Showstack, J., "Access to Prenatal Care Following Major Medicaid Medical Eligibility Expansions," *Journal of the American Medical Association, 269*, 1285, 1993.

Braveman, P., Egerter, S., Bennett, T., & Showstack, J., "Differences in Hospital Resource Allocation among Sick Newborns According to Insurance Coverage," *Journal of the American Medical Association, 266*, 3300, 1991.

Braveman, P. A., Oliva, G., Miller, M. G., Reiter, R., & Egerter, S., "Adverse Outcomes and Lack of Health Insurance among Newborns in an Eight-County Area of California, 1982–1986," *New England Journal of Medicine, 321*, 508, 1989.

Brook, R. H., Ware, J. E., Rogers, W. H., Keeler, E. B., Davies, A. R., Donald, C. A., et al., "Does Free Care Improve Adult's Health?" *New England Journal of Medicine, 309*, 1426, 1983.

Carlisle, D. M., Leake, B. D., Brook, R. H., & Shapiro, M. F., "The Effect of Race and Ethnicity on the Use of Selected Health Care Procedures: A Comparison of South Central Los Angeles and the Remainder of Los Angeles County," *Journal of Health Care for the Poor and Underserved, 7*, 308, 1996.

Chesney, A. P., Chavira, J. A., Hall, R. P., & Gary, H. E., "Barriers to Medical Care of Mexican-Americans: The Role of Social Class, Acculturation, and Social Isolation," *Medical Care, 20*, 883, 1982.

Cohen, J. W., "Medicaid Policy and the Substitution of Hospital Outpatient Care for Physician Care," *Health Services Research, 24*(1), 33, 1989.

Cooper, R. A., "Perspectives on the Physician Workforce to the Year 2020," *Journal of the American Medical Association, 274*, 1534, 1995.

Cotton, P., "Examples Abound of Gaps in Medical Knowledge Because of Groups Excluded from Scientific Study," *Journal of the American Medical Association, 263*, 1051, 1990a.

Cotton, P., "Is There Still Too Much Extrapolation from Data on Middle-aged White Men?" *Journal of the American Medical Association, 263*, 1049, 1990b.

Council on Ethical and Judicial Affairs, American Medical Association, "Black-White Disparities in Health Care," *Journal of the American Medical Association, 263*, 2344, 1990.

Council on Ethical and Judicial Affairs, American Medical Association, "Gender Disparities in Clinical Decision Making," *Journal of the American Medical Association, 266*, 559, 1991.

Council on Scientific Affairs, American Medical Association, "Hispanic Health in the United States," *Journal of the American Medical Association, 265*, 248, 1991.

Employee Benefit Research Institute (EBRI). "Trends in Health Insurance Coverage," *EBRI Issues Brief, 185,* May 1997.

Franks, P., Clancy, C. M., & Gold, M. R., "Health Insurance and Mortality: Evidence from a National Cohort," *Journal of the American Medical Association, 270,* 737, 1993.

Friedman, E., "Money Isn't Everything: Nonfinancial Barriers to Access," *Journal of the American Medical Association, 271,* 1535, 1994.

Gaston, R. S., Ayres, I., Dooley, L. G., & Diethelm, A. G., "Racial Equity in Renal Transplantation: The Disparate Impact of HLA-Based Allocation," *Journal of the American Medical Association, 270,* 1352, 1993.

Grumbach, K., Vranizan, K., & Bindman, A. B., "Physician Supply and Access to Care in Urban Communities," *Health Affairs, 16*(1), 71, 1997.

Grumbach, K., et al., *The Problems of Shortages of Physicians and Other Health Professionals in Urban Areas.* San Francisco: University of California–San Francisco, Center for the Health Professions, 1995.

Guendelman, S., & Schwalbe, J., "Medical Care Utilization by Hispanic Children: How Does It Differ from Black and White Peers?" *Medical Care, 24,* 925, 1986.

Hadley, J., Steinberg, E. P., & Feder, J., "Comparison of Uninsured and Privately Insured Hospital Patients: Conditions on Admission, Resource Use, and Outcome," *Journal of the American Medical Association, 265,* 374, 1991.

Held, P. J., Pauly, M. V., Bovberg, R. R., & Saltvatierra, O., "Access to Kidney Transplantation," *Archives of Internal Medicine, 148,* 2594, 1988.

Henshaw, S. K., "Factors Hindering Access to Abortion Services," *Family Planning Perspectives, 27*(2), 54, 1995.

Jacobson, P. D., Merritt, R., & Bartlett, L., "California Health Care Delivery: A Competitive Model?" in *State Health Reform Initiatives: Progress and Promise.* Baltimore: Health Care Financing Administration, 1994

Johnson, P. A., Lee, T. H., Cook, E. F., Rovan, G. W., & Goldman, L., "Effect of Race on the Presentation and Management of Patients with Acute Chest Pain," *Annals of Internal Medicine, 118,* 593, 1993.

Kindig, D. A., & Ricketts, T. C., "Determining Adequacy of Physicians and Nurses for Rural Populations: Background and Strategy," *Journal of Rural Health, 7*(Suppl.), 313, 1991.

Kirsch, I., Jungeblut, A., Jenkins, L., & Kolstad, A., *Adult Literacy in America: A First Look at the Results of the National Adult Literacy Survey.* Washington, DC: National Center for Education Statistics, U.S. Department of Education, 1993.

Kjellstrand, C. M., "Age, Sex, and Race Inequality in Renal Transplantation," *Archives of Internal Medicine, 148,* 1305, 1988.

Lantz, P. M., Weigers, M. E., & House, J. S., "Education and Income Differentials in Breast Cancer and Cervical Cancer Screening," *Medical Care, 35,* 219, 1997.

Lieu, T. A., Newacheck, P. W., & McManus, M. A., "Race, Ethnicity, and Access to Ambulatory Care among US Adolescents," *American Journal of Public Health, 83,* 960, 1993.

Lipson, D. J., & Schrodel, S. P., *State Initiatives in Health Care Reform: State-Subsidized Insurance Programs for Low-Income People.* Washington, DC: Alpha Center, 1996.

Lohr, K. N., Brook, R. H., Kamberg, C. J., Goldberg, G. A., Leibowitz, A., Kessey, J., et al., "Use of Medical Care in the Rand Health Insurance Experiment: Diagnosis- and Service-Specific Analysis in a Randomized Controlled Trial," *Medical Care, 24*(Suppl.), 1, 1986.

Lurie, N., Manning, W. G., Peterson, C., Goldberg, G. A., Phelps, C. A., & Lillard, L., "Preventive Care: Do We Practice What We Preach?" *American Journal of Public Health, 77,* 801, 1987.

Lurie, N., Slater, J., McGovern, P., Ekstrum, J., Quam, L., & Margolis, K., "Preventive Care for Women: Does the Sex of the Physician Matter?" *New England Journal of Medicine, 329,* 478, 1993.

Lurie, N., Ward, N. B., Shapiro, M. F., Gallego, C., Vaghaiwalla, R., & Brook, R. H., "Special Report: Termination of Medi-Cal Benefits: A Follow-Up Study One Year Later," *New England Journal of Medicine, 314,* 1266, 1986.

Markides, K. S., Levin, J. S., & Ray, L. A., "Determinants of Physician Utilization among Mexican Americans," *Medical Care, 23,* 236, 1985.

Marks, G., Solis, J., Richardson, J. L., & Shelton, D., "Health Behavior of Elderly Hispanic Women: Does Cultural Assimilation Make a Difference?" *American Journal of Public Health, 77,* 1315, 1987.

Mathews, S., Ribar, D., & Wilhelm, M., "The Effects of Economic Conditions and Access to Reproductive Health Services on State Abortion Rates and Birthrates," *Family Planning Perspectives, 29*(2), 52, 1997.

Millman, M. (Ed.), *Access to Health Care in America.* Washington, DC: National Academy Press, Institute of Medicine, 1993.

Mitchell, J. B., & McCormack, L. A., "Access to Family Planning Services: Relationship with Unintended Pregnancies and Prenatal Outcomes," *Journal of Health Care for the Poor and Underserved, 8*(2), 141, 1997.

Nesbitt, T., Connell, F. A., Hart, L. G., & Rosenblatt, R. A., "Access to Obstetric Care in Rural Areas: Effect on Birth Outcomes," *American Journal of Public Health, 80,* 814, 1990.

Newacheck, P. W., "Characteristics of Children with High and Low Usage of Physician Services," *Medical Care, 30*(1), 30, 1992.

Newacheck, P. W., & Halfon, N., "The Association between Mother's and Children's Use of Physician Services," *Medical Care, 24*(1), 30, 1986.

Orr, S. T., Charney, E., & Straus, J., "Use of Health Services by Black Children According to Payment Mechanism," *Medical Care, 26,* 939, 1988.

Politzer, R. M., Harris, D. L., Gaston, M. H., & Mullan, F., "Primary Care Physician Supply and the Medically Underserved," *Journal of the American Medical Association, 266,* 104, 1991.

Riley, A. W., Finney, J. W., & Mellits, E. D., "Determinants of Children's Health Care Use," *Medical Care, 31,* 767, 1993.

Rosenblatt, R. A., Mattis, R., & Hart L. G., "Abortions in Rural Idaho: Physicians' Attitudes and Practices," *American Journal of Public Health, 85,* 1423, 1995.

Schoen, C., Lyons, B., Rowland, D., Davis, K., & Puleo, E., "Insurance Matters for Low Income Adults: Results from a Five State Survey," *Health Affairs, 16*(5), 163, 1997.

Short, P. F., & Banthin, J. S., "New Estimates of the Underinsured Younger than 65 Years," *Journal of the American Medical Association, 274,* 1302, 1995.

Short, P. F., & Lefkowitz, D. C., "Encouraging Preventive Services for Low-Income Children: The Effect of Expanding Medicaid," *Medical Care, 30,* 766, 1992.

Solis, J. M., Marks, G., Garcia, M., & Shelton, D., "Acculturation, Access to Care, and Use of Preventive Services by Hispanics: Findings from HHANES 1982–84," *American Journal of Public Health, 80*(Suppl.), 11, 1990.

Todd, K. H., Lee, T., & Hoffman, J. R., "The Effect of Ethnicity of Physician Estimates of Pain Severity in Patients with Isolated Extremity Trauma," *Journal of the American Medical Association, 271,* 925, 1994.

Todd, K. H., Samaroo, N., & Hoffman, J. R., "Ethnicity as a Risk Factor for Inadequate Emergency Department Analgesia," *Journal of the American Medical Association, 269,* 1537, 1993.

Udvarhelyi, I. S., Gatsonis, C., Epstein, A. M., Pashos, C. L., Newhouse, J. P., & McNeil, B. J., "Acute Myocardial Infarction in the Medicare Population," *Journal of the American Medical Association, 268,* 2530, 1992.

U.S. Census Bureau, *Current Population Survey,* March 1997.

U.S. House of Representatives, Committee on Wage and Means, *1996 Greenbook: Overview of Entitlement Programs* (15th ed.). Washington, DC: U.S. Government Printing Office, 1996.

Weiss, B. D., "Illiteracy among Medicaid Recipients and Its Relation to Health Care Costs," *Journal of Health Care for the Poor and Underserved, 5*(2), 99, 1994.

Weissman, J., & Epstein, A. M., "Case Mix and Resource Utilization by Uninsured Hospital Patients in the Boston Metropolitan Area," *Journal of the American Medical Association, 261,* 3572, 1989.

Weissman, J., Gatsonis, C., & Epstein, A., "Rates of Avoidable Hospitalizations by Insurance Status in Massachusetts and Maryland," *Journal of the American Medical Association, 268,* 2388–2394, 1992.

Wells, C. K., & Feinstein, A. R., "Detection Bias in the Diagnostic Pursuit of Lung Cancer," *American Journal of Epidemiology, 128,* 1016, 1988.

Wells, K. B., Golding, J. M., Hough, R. L., Burnam, M. A., & Karno, M., "Acculturation and the Probability of Use of Health Services by Mexican Americans," *Health Services Research, 24*(2), 237, 1989.

Wenneker, M. B., & Epstein, A. M., "Racial Inequalities in the Use of Procedures for Patients with Ischemic Heart Disease in Massachusetts," *Journal of the American Medical Association, 261,* 253, 1989.

Williams, M. V., Parker, R. M., Baker, D. W., Parikh, N. S., Pitkin, K., Coates, W. C., & Nurss, J. R., "Inadequate Functional Health Literacy among Patients at Two Public Hospitals," *Journal of the American Medical Association, 274,* 1677, 1995.

Whittle, J., Conigliaro, J., Good, C., & Lofgren, R. P., "Racial Differences in the Use of Cardiovascular Procedures in the Department of Veterans Affairs Medical System," *New England Journal of Medicine, 329,* 627, 1993.

Yergan, J., Flood, A. B., Diehr, P., & LoGerfo, J. P., "Relationship Between Patient Source of Payment and the Intensity of Hospital Services," *Medical Care, 26,* 1111, 1988.

15

Health Care Cost Containment: Reflections and Future Directions

Kenneth E. Thorpe

Learning Objectives

1. Understand the factors that contribute to the growth in health care costs.
2. Describe the approaches employed by Medicare, Medicaid, and the private sector to control the growth in costs.
3. Analyze the historic and recent performance of these cost-containment strategies.

Topical Outline

Factors accounting for health care expenditure growth
    Demand-side distortions
    Supply-side factors
Efforts to control rising health care costs: The early experience
    Limits on hospital inputs
    Regulating the utilization of medical care
    Hospital rate setting, 1969–1982
    The process of cost reductions
Efforts to control health care costs (1983–present)
    Role of private payers

Key Words: **Prospective payment, diagnosis-related group, managed care, point of service, preferred provider, hospital rate setting.**

Despite vigorous efforts to control health care costs, health care expenditures continue to rise at rates exceeding general inflation. In 1995 health care accounted for 13.6% of our gross national product (GNP), compared to 12.1% just 4 years earlier (Health Care Financing Administration, 1997; Levit, Lazenby, & Sivarajan, 1994). The sustained rise in health care expenditures has raised a number of concerns. First, public expenditures for health care account for a substantial portion of the federal budget. Thus, recent efforts to reduce the size of the federal budget deficit (estimated at approximately $50 billion in 1997) have focused attention on publicly financed health care programs. Second, though the growth in private health spending has moderated, it is still rising faster than overall inflation. Health insurance spending per insured worker increased 2.2% above the growth in inflation between 1992 and 1995 (derived from Foster Higgins, 1995). Higher growth in health insurance premiums, it is thought, is a contributing factor accounting for the recent sluggish growth in wages.

The continued escalation in health care costs suggests that efforts by third-party payers to lower cost growth have achieved mixed results. Although some payers, in particular those with private insurance, have reduced the growth in expenditures over time, spending by others has remained stable or has increased, leaving the overall rate of growth in health care relatively unchanged. The factors accounting for the sustained increase in health care costs, the effects of recent public and private sector attempts to control this growth, and an assessment of the future direction of health care cost-containment serve as the focus of this chapter.

Factors Accounting for Health Care Expenditure Growth

The United States currently spends $1 trillion on health care (Levit et al., 1997). This represents a 7.4% rise between 1994 and 1997 alone, a $69 billion increase. In its simplest construction, total spending equals price times the quantity of services. This reflects four major factors: general economy-wide inflation, inflation specific to the health care industry (over and above general rates of inflation), population growth, and changes in the nature and intensity of health care delivery. The relative contributions of these factors to yearly changes in health care costs are discussed below. It should be noted, however, that there is some debate over our ability to decompose the elements accounting for health spending growth. Aaron (1994), for instance, notes that we cannot directly measure the quantity of services produced. Moreover, Aaron, along with other economists, is quite skeptical about our ability to distinguish health-sector-specific increases in prices from overall inflation. The decomposition presented below should keep those important caveats in mind.

Approximately 40% of the yearly rise in health care spending is traced to general inflation. This includes inflation in the price of inputs used in the delivery of medical care (e.g., electricity, material, etc.). Another 36% of the yearly increase is traced to growth in prices in the health sector above the general rate of inflation. The remainder, 24%, is traced to growth in the population, changes in its composition (age/sex) and increases in the intensity of care delivered (Levit et al., 1994). Two factors commonly thought responsible for the rise in health care costs are the rapid spread of comprehensive health insurance (traced to demand-side distortions) and technological change (a supply-side issue). These factors and their interrelationships are explored below.

Demand-Side Distortions

Economists have traditionally identified the spread of health insurance as a primary cause for health care cost growth (Pauly, 1986). The rapid increase in availability of health insurance has generated continued increases in demand for health care, in terms of both volume and perceived quality. The rapid increase in the scope (type of health care insured) and comprehensiveness (the proportion of a health care bill paid by a third party) of health insurance during the 1960s and 1970s has been traced to the tax treatment of health benefits (Manning et al., 1987). In particular, employer contributions for health insurance benefits are exempt from federal and state income taxation. With employer health benefit contributions exceeding $200 billion in 1999, this exemption translated into a $76 billion loss in taxes (Office of Management and Budget, 1998). The tax treatment subsidizes the marginal dollar of fringe benefits employees receive from employers relative to other forms of compensation (e.g., wages), therefore increasing the demand for health insurance relative to other goods.

The tax treatment of health insurance benefits has two consequences. First, individuals purchase more insurance than they would without the tax subsidy. Second, more extensive health insurance results in higher health care spending. With respect to insurance, the tax laws encourage individuals to purchase less preventive care and to insure against marginal risks. More comprehensive policies with few cost-sharing obligations also lead to higher spending. The magnitude of the additional expenditures is substantial. An experimental study, conducted by the Rand Corporation, examined the impact of insurance on health care spending. Their results indicate that the use of services responds to the level of cost sharing. In short, per capita expenditures in plans with no cost sharing were approximately 33% greater than in plans with a 95% coinsurance obligation (Manning et al., 1987). Moreover, relative to a free-care plan, per capita spending among those enrolled in plans with 25% coinsurance was approximately 15% lower. Lower expenditures did not result in measurable reductions in patient health status. For example, for an average individual enrolled in the plan, the Rand study did not detect significant differences in health status across insurance plans during the 3-year tracking period. These findings suggest that low coinsurance obligations result in higher rates of utilization with few measurable short-run health benefits.

Supply-Side Factors

Imperfect information and cost-increasing technological changes represent two supply-side factors that distinguish the health care industry from more "competitive" markets. These factors, in conjunction with the demand-side distortions noted above, also have contributed to the real changes in medical care prices as well as intensity of medical care over time.

Imperfection Information. Potential consumers of medical care have imperfect information concerning its price and quality. High search costs and extensive health insurance coverage reduce the potential net benefits of searching for lower-cost providers. The importance of search costs and their impact on medical care prices have received much attention. The "increasing monopoly" thesis, outlined by Pauly and Satterthwaite (1981), consists of two observations. First, consumer information concerning physicians and other providers decreases with higher numbers of providers. Second, if the search for providers is more difficult, consumers are less price-sensitive, and physicians have more discretion in increasing fees. Thus, according to this thesis, growth in the per capita number of physicians would result in higher prices.

Even with extensive price shopping by consumers, comprehensive health insurance coverage reduces any potential savings resulting from identifying low-cost providers. Thus, both high search costs and extensive health insurance coverage dilute the incentives for consumers to engage in vigorous price shopping.

Further complicating the consumer's task is the lack of information concerning provider quality. Measuring the quality of care provided by individual physicians or hospitals has traditionally been very difficult. Although we have witnessed an explosion of medical outcomes research over the past 10 years, the development of outcome-based measures remains in its infancy. Instead, consumers often have used proxies such as the physician's board certification or a hospital's teaching affiliation as a signal for higher quality. As a result, higher perceived quality is also associated with higher fees and costs. At issue is whether these higher fees and prices reflect unobserved quality differences. Thus, price competition among providers will continue to be limited until consumers are able to compare both price and quality differences accurately.

Despite the informational problems facing consumers, hospitals and physicians do compete. However, the features of the health care delivery system noted above have encouraged competition in perceptions of quality rather than price. This includes both inadequate information on price and quality differences and the pervasiveness of first-dollar health insurance coverage. Thus, instead of competing on a price basis to attract patients, hospitals have competed to attract physicians (and through them patients). Hospitals in more concentrated (competitive) markets attempt to attract physicians through specific capital investments. These capital investments include the latest technologies, a broad range of clinical services, and other amenities. Because new technology increases service intensity, quality competition is quite costly. Whether the additional service intensity translates into better health outcomes remains at issue.

That hospitals have traditionally pursued competition in quality, rather than in price, has been the subject of numerous empirical investigations. The results generally lead to the conclusion that, other factors held constant, hospitals in more competitive markets produce more services and have significantly higher costs (Robinson & Luft, 1988). Although these results generally held through the mid-1980s, efforts by state governments and other payers to encourage price competition have altered the behavior of hospitals. The more recent roles of competition and market structure are discussed below.

Technological Change. The demand-side distortions noted above, combined with traditional "nonprice" competition among providers, have created an environment for rapid adoption and diffusion of new technologies. These technologies generally fall into three categories: replacing accepted medical practices (e.g., hip replacement techniques and coronary artery bypass surgery), new therapies (e.g., liver, heart, and other organ transplants; new classes of drugs), and new imaging devices (e.g., magnetic resonance imaging). Without question, many of these new technologies clearly extend years of active life to many who would have died even 25 years ago. The downside is that many of the new technologies have large price tags.

Although international comparisons of health care delivery systems often raise more questions than they answer, some studies have attempted to document the role of technology in increasing health care costs (Aaron & Schwartz, 1984). Based on their analysis of the U.S. and British health care systems, Aaron and Schwartz conclude that per capita health care costs would fall 10% if U.S. physicians used 10 key technologies (e.g., hip replacement, computed tomography, intensive care units) and intensive care at (population-adjusted) rates similar to those of their British counterparts. Their analysis did not detect significant differences in health status resulting from the less intensive use of these technologies.

The critical role assumed by technological change (discussed above as increased service intensity) in rising health care costs has generated a growing volume of research focused on practice patterns and the appropriateness of medical procedures. This research has been spurred by international comparisons as well as by large geographic variations in practice patterns documented domestically. One early pioneer of this type of study, John Wennberg, noted magnitude differences in rates of specific procedures completed by physicians. Fourfold differences in hysterectomy rates, prostatectomies, tonsillectomies, and other common surgical procedures were discovered within and between states (Wennberg, 1984). Subsequent research indicates that these variations are not related to underlying differences in patient characteristics but rather to physician's practice patterns. These large variations among common procedures have resulted in a significant body of research aimed at examining the "appropriateness" of these differences (Wennberg, 1996).

Researchers at the Rand Corporation also have been active in examining the appropriateness of various practice patterns. Their studies of four surgical procedures—coronary artery bypass surgery (CABG), carotid endarterectomy, coronary angioplasty, and upper gastrointestinal endoscopy—examined the magnitude of unnecessary procedures and hospitalizations. With respect to CABG, the Rand researchers judged that 44% of the procedures examined were performed for inappropriate reasons (Chassin, 1987). Some 17% of coronary angiographies, used to diagnose blockages in heart arteries, were deemed inappropriate, as were a similar volume of gastrointestinal endoscopies. Eliminating inappropriate surgery would result in continued savings of billions of dollars per year. Although the precise magnitude of the savings remains speculative, if the rates of inappropriate use found in these procedures are extrapolated, reducing unnecessary use could reduce health care spending by over $50 billion per year.

Private health plans, the federal government, drug makers, and large employers have attempted to further the work on "appropriateness." The federal government, under the sponsorship of the Agency for Health Care Policy and Research (AHCPR) has examined several areas of medical practice and produced a number of specific guidelines designed to help physicians practice the best quality medicine. Moreover, the concept of appropriateness has generated a new nongovernmental industry that attempts to "manage" the process of care, known as "disease management." Here vendors have developed specific protocols for treating specific medical conditions such as asthma, diabetes, and cancer among others. As disease management is in its formative stage, it is too early to detect its impact on practice.

More recent analyses (Schwartz, 1994) outline the flood of new technologies that will come on-line over the next 10 to 15 years. These include new classes of pharmaceuticals that will treat persons with the acquired immune deficiency syndrome (AIDS) and a range of additional autoimmune diseases, advances in molecular and cell biology that could change clinical medicine fundamentally, and advances in genetics. These new technologies are, in the short run, likely to place persistent pressure on the growth in health care spending. It remains to be seen whether the "march of science" will result in slower or higher growth in spending in the longer run.

Efforts to Control Rising Health Care Costs: The Early Experience

This section summarizes previous and current efforts by third-party payers to control health care costs. We focus specifically on hospital cost containment, the area that has attracted most of our cost-control efforts.

Historically, third-party payers have implemented four distinct methods of cost control: control over the inputs used by hospitals, control over hospital admitting practices, limits on hospital payment, and the development of alternative (i.e., competitive) delivery systems. During the 1970s, public payers most actively pursued these cost-containment activities. By the mid-1980s, private payers as well had adopted many of the cost-control techniques discussed below.

Limits on Hospital Inputs

Historically, efforts to control the use of inputs by hospitals have focused on capital expenditure decisions. Government has assumed a major role in initially financing and subsequently limiting hospital capital expansion for more than 40 years. The initial role of the government in health planning was to facilitate expansion of the hospital industry. In this capacity, the Hospital Survey and Construction (Hill-Burton) Act of 1946 supplied federal funds to underwrite new hospital construction. These funds were allocated to states according to population and state per capita income levels to redress a perceived shortage and maldistribution of hospital beds. Using some simple bed-to-population guidelines, local health planners allocated the funds to expand the nation's hospital bed supply.

In light of the rapid growth in the capacity of the hospital sector, health planning efforts have recently focused on limiting future hospital capital expansions. Although some voluntary efforts preceded it, the most comprehensive planning efforts commenced in 1974 with the National Health Planning and Resource Development Act. This act provided federal funding for local health systems agencies (HSA) and state health planning and development agencies. The health planning act developed because of growing concern over rising hospital costs increasingly linked to facility (both physical plant and technology) duplication. Thus, a primary role of the HSAs was to develop planning recommendations for specific hospital investments exceeding some dollar threshold (often $100,000). Based on the work of the local HSA, a certificate of need (CON) was usually issued at the state level granting permission to spend capital. Although health planning agencies reached their peak during the 1970s, HSAs were generally phased out during the mid-1980s.

In practice, state CON programs differed in both structure and organizational goals. There were four characteristics thought to be related to their potential effectiveness (i.e., their stringency): (1) the program's orientation (i.e., planning/redistribution or cost containment), (2) locus of decision making (state or local), (3) the scope of formalized review standards, and (4) extent of an appeals process exemption.

Early evaluations of the ability of the CON process to control were quick to question the cost-containment capabilities of the program. Although the CON process appeared initially to reduce the growth rate in the number of hospital beds, it was accompanied by a larger rise in total assets per bed (Salkever & Bice, 1976). Moreover, even those CON programs that, *ex ante*, appeared more restrictive had little impact on total capital expenditures (Joskow, 1981). These results suggest that hospitals merely substituted another form of capital investment "unconstrained" by planning requirements for beds.

Other studies examining the effectiveness of the CON process focused on the diffusion of specific technologies. Those examining the role of the planning process in slowing the diffusion of potentially "duplicative" technologies (e.g., computerized tomography [CT]) and expensive new technologies (e.g., new surgical techniques) into hospitals were also negative (Sloan, Valvona, & Perrin, 1986). Although the CON process may have achieved other objectives, containing capital expenditures and total health care spending were not among them. Although the growing interest in competition among health plans and hospitals was a factor, the inability of the CON process to achieve its fundamental goal—slower rates of capital expansion and overall cost growth—ultimately led to its decline.

Regulating the Utilization of Medical Care

This section focuses on public-sector efforts to limit the utilization of hospital services. More recent attempts by the private sector to manage the course of a patient's treatment are addressed below. Efforts to prevent unnecessary and low-quality care delivered to publicly insured patients commenced in 1972 with the advent of professional standard review organizations (PSROs). The goals of the PSRO program, albeit quite broadly defined, were to "promote the effective, efficient, and economical delivery of health care services of proper quality." Thus, the language in the enacting legislation included both cost-containment and quality-enhancement goals. The lack of clear direction in the program's goals likely contributed to the inability of most PSROs to focus their efforts effectively. In practice, PSROs focused primarily on Medicare and Medicaid beneficiaries, although some anticipated a broader spillover to privately insured patients. Despite the broad range of goals articulated under the original act, most PSROs attempted to reduce the length of stay among the Medicare population.

Evaluations of the PSRO program showed that it produced mixed results. On average, the PSROs appeared to reduce total days of hospitalization among Medicare patients by 1.5% (Congressional Budget Office, 1981). PSROs appear to have reduced total days through reductions in length of stay rather than by preventing admissions. Although some studies suggest that the PSRO program produced some public sector savings, these costs appear to have been shifted to other payers (Congressional Budget Office, 1981). The impact of the program on the Medicaid population remains unknown. However, Medicare savings (through reduced utilization) were nearly offset by the administrative costs of the program. Viewed more broadly, the Congressional Budget Office researchers found that savings to the Medicare program were offset by increases in charges (and expenditures) by private payers. Hence, when administrative costs and charges in total health care expenditures were examined, the PSROs appeared less effective.

The PSROs were replaced with peer review organizations (PRO) in 1984. The PROs differ from their predecessor, the PSRO, in that PRO contracts are awarded in a competitive bidding process, based in part on the bidder's projected and/or demonstrated ability to achieve specific utilization goals. These goals are developed through negotiations with the Health Care Financing Administration (HCFA) and relate to five objectives (Office of Technology Assessment, 1981, Appendix G): (1) to reduce unnecessary hospital readmissions; (2) to assure the provision of adequate care, that, if not given, would cause serious complications; (3) to reduce the risk of mortality associated with specific procedures and conditions; (4) to reduce unnecessary surgery; and (5) to reduce avoidable postoperative or other complications. Negotiations between a PRO and the HCFA define specific performance markers (e.g., reduce readmissions resulting from substandard care by 20% used to evaluate the effectiveness of each PRO).

Starting in 1989, PROs assumed an extended set of responsibilities beyond hospital care, including review of outpatient procedures, home health care, and care provided to military personnel and their families. By 1993, however, the program's effectiveness was in question, especially given its $300 million annual price tag. Starting that year, PROs began adopting a new strategy called the Health Care Quality Improvement Initiative. Under this initiative, PROs shifted their focus from identifying individual clinical errors to helping providers improve the mainstream of medical care. The PROs use statistical quality controls to examine variations in both the processes and the outcomes of care. They then share this information with hospitals and physicians and work with them to interpret and apply the findings.

Hospital Rate Setting (1969–1982)

Attempts to limit payment rates to hospitals represents a third cost-containment strategy. Between 1969 and 1974, 15 states introduced some form of hospital rate setting program (Coelen & Sullivan, 1981). Although similar in their objectives, these programs differed with respect to a number of key design features, including the unit of payment, the scope of revenue covered (i.e., the number of payers and proportion of total revenue included), and a variety of design issues defining the actual prospectivity of the payments. These technical design features largely determined the restrictiveness of the rate-setting rules and ultimately their effectiveness. A brief description of these programs and their impact on reducing hospital expenditures follows.

Hospital rate setting generally refers to some form of prospective payment (i.e., the determination of payment rates prior to services rendered) by third-party payers. Methods actually used to define the payment rates are, in practice, quite complex. The essential elements include a base year and a trend factor. For example, Medicaid and Blue Cross payments to New York hospitals during 1982 were calculated by using a 1981 base year, increased each year by an allowable trend factor. In this case, actual payment rates to hospitals are effectively divorced from individual hospital spending decisions. Thus, the degree of prospectivity built into the rate-setting system depends on the frequency in which the base year is moved. More stringent or restrictive rate-setting programs (such as the New York State program) move the base year infrequently. The trend factor used to define allowable revenue increases is also critical in determining the ability of rate-setting programs to control cost growth. The allowable trend factor could differ by multiple percentage points depending on key design decisions. For instance, trend factors may or may not include allowances for technological change. Moreover, allowed increases in wages may reflect more general wage trends or focus specifically on changes in the health care sector. Beyond these basic elements, most rate-setting programs differ with respect to the unit of payment (e.g., per diem, per case), who sets the rates (e.g., a separate rate-setting authority), and the extent to which historic (base year) costs are subjected to efficiency screens. These efficiency screens often compare each hospital's inpatient costs (after a variety of adjustments) to the mean or median within the state. In more restrictive programs, costs above the mean are disallowed and not recognized in developing the base year for subsequent payment. In contrast, less restrictive programs effectively pass through all historic costs into the base.

Although state rate-setting programs differed with respect to a variety of important design issues, they also shared some common characteristics. First, rate-setting programs generally determined rates of payment prospectively. Second, the prospective rates generally applied only to inpatient operating expenses, leaving physician fees, direct medical education spending, capital, and outpatient expenses unregulated. There were also differences among the states. For example, three of them—New Jersey, Maryland, and New York—established regulated per diem rates of payment. Elsewhere, rate setting focused on department revenue or total revenue caps. The number of payers within each state participating in the rate-setting program also varied. Prior to 1980 the rate setting program in one state, Maryland, included all third-party payers. Programs in other states were more limited. Most programs included Medicaid and Blue Cross plans, although some, such as Indiana and Kentucky, covered only Blue Cross plans.

An impressive volume of research has examined the impact of state rate setting on hospital costs (Eby & Cohodes, 1985). The research generally concludes that state rate-setting programs reduced hospital costs, although the effects varied across states. During the 1970s cost growth per day and admission was 2% to 3% lower in states with rate-setting programs. The empirical results also suggest that rate setting reduced hospital expenditures over the long run by 10% to 20% (Sloan, 1983). There is less compelling evidence, however, that rate-setting programs reduced the growth in per capita health care spending. If true, this suggests that any reductions in inpatient hospital costs were offset by similar increases in unregulated sources of revenue. These findings are similar to the experience with PSROs discussed above as well as the CON experience with capital expenditures.

Although implementation of rate-setting programs reduces cost growth on average, program performance has varied widely across states. These effects have ranged from none to reductions exceeding 6% per year (Coelen & Sullivan,

1981). Much of the variation across programs stems from important design issues that define payment levels. Key design issues identified by previous studies as associated with their effectiveness include frequency in which the base year is moved, scope of revenue covered, number of payers included, and the construction of the trend factor (Thorpe & Phelps, 1990).

The Process of Cost Reductions

Effective rate-setting programs provide incentives for hospitals to adjust their "behavior" across many dimensions. Most notably, rate-setting programs provide incentives for hospitals to reduce the service intensity of medical care. In an earlier section, increased service intensity was identified as a major factor accounting for real increases in yearly health care costs. Reductions in service intensity are possible through lower staffing levels, a less expensive mix of personnel (e.g., the substitution of licensed practical nurses for registered nurses), slower adoption of new technology, or all of the above. The early literature on rate setting found evidence of adjustment across all dimensions (Cromwell & Kanak, 1982).

More effective rate-setting programs reduced costs by limiting the inputs (most notably technology) used to produce medical care. Hospitals in rate-setting states adopted new technologies at slower rates. Among the diffusion patterns examined were such major expense items as intensive care units, open-heart surgery, coronary artery surgery, obesity surgery, and burn care units (Romeo, Wagner, & Lee, 1984). Moreover, other technologies, most notably imaging devices such as the computerized axial tomography (CAT) scanner, were adopted by hospitals at a slower pace in rate-setting states.

Rate setting also resulted in reduced hospital payroll expenses per patient day (Kidder & Sullivan, 1982). These "productivity" increases were achieved through both reductions in staff per adjusted day and changes in the mix of personnel. In some instances, particularly in teaching hospitals, administrators reduced their ancillary staff component, including intravenous and phlebotomy teams, messenger/transporters, and clerks, among others. Their tasks were generally absorbed by resident physicians, nurses, or both.

Although rate-setting programs during the 1970s achieved some of their goals, some dysfunctional side effects were evident. Rate-setting programs that focused solely on the day of care often led to increases in the average length of a hospital stay (Sloan, 1984). In some cases, average hospital occupancy rates also increased. As a result, per capita days of care remained relatively stable after the implementation of rate-setting programs, blunting the full cost-containment potential. As noted earlier, the first rate-setting programs appeared less effective in reducing per capita health care spending. This led many observers to speculate that hospitals merely shifted their fixed costs to other, unregulated payers (often termed cost shifting) or unregulated sources of revenue (e.g, outpatient care) (Eby & Cohodes, 1985). The ability of hospital administrators to escape the full regulatory potential of the rate-setting laws created increased demand for alternative cost-containment strategies. Sharp increases in charges to unregulated payers—who were largely commercial health insurers—created growing allegations that they bore the burden of any cost savings enjoyed by regulated (generally, government) payers (Sloan & Becker, 1984). The growing differential between "costs" reimbursed by regulated payers and "charges" to unregulated payers raised concerns about the overall effectiveness and equity of rate-setting programs. These concerns were largely responsible for the subsequent generation of rate-setting programs, competitive bidding schemes, and alternative delivery systems described below.

Efforts to Control Health Care Costs (1983–Present)

Informed by the early experience with hospital rate setting, attempts to control rising health care costs changed in four important aspects during the mid-1980s. First, private payers and employers increased their efforts to develop cost-containment programs. Second, state governments and Medicare experimented with new approaches to hospital rate setting. Third, both the public and private sectors created incentives for hospitals to compete on the basis of price, rather than other dimensions. Finally, the cost-containment debate was extended to physician payment in addition to institutional payment reforms.

Role of Private Payers

Perhaps the most important story over the past 5 years with respect to health care spending has been the slower growth in private health insurance spending. During this time employers have become increasingly vigilant in their efforts to control their expenditures; the evidence indicates that these efforts have achieved some level of success.

Facing sharply rising health insurance premiums during the early 1980s, private payers extended their efforts to control health care costs (particularly hospital costs) in three important directions. First, private payers and employers increased efforts to "manage" the utilization of health care. Second, dissatisfied with the ability of private health insurance carriers to control costs, a growing number of employers decided to "self-insure." Third, using their purchasing power for leverage, private payers increasingly negotiated rates of payment with health care providers.

Growth in Managed Care

Managed care is a term applied to a wide variety of health plans (see also chapter 11). In its most general formulation, the managed care plans link patients with primary care physicians for care. Health plans providing care under this rubric may be entirely or partially capitated. Perhaps the best known form of managed care organization is the health maintenance organization (HMO).

During the early 1980s the HMO concept assumed a prominent role in the health care delivery system. The key features of the HMO concept include (1) serving a defined population voluntarily enrolled in the plan, (2) the assumption of contractual responsibility and financial risk by the plan to provide a stated range of services, and (3) the payment of a fixed annual or monthly payment by the enrollee independent of the actual use of services (Luft, 1981). The intent of the HMO concept was to shift some financial risk to providers (rather than to patients under various cost-sharing schemes). Risk shifting would, in theory, create incentives for the plan to provide appropriate levels of medical care in general and preventive care in particular. Payment of a fixed annual fee also limited the ability of providers to thwart the intent of the cost controls through shifting costs to unregulated payers or costs.

Enrollment in HMOs grew rapidly during the 1980s and the 1990s, increasing to over 50 million (over 17% of the population) by 1995 (InterStudy, 1995). Point-of-service (POS) plans and preferred provider organizations (PPOs) are also making impressive enrollment gains. In fact, managed care in its various forms has become the dominant insurance vehicle in the United States. Overall, 75% of employees were enrolled in HMOs, PPOs, or POS plans in 1993, up from 55% in 1992 (KPMG, Peat Marwick, 1996). The interest of corporate America in managed care plans is not without merit. Several studies have documented the wide variation in medical practice patterns, many of which result in costly and inappropriate patterns of medical care. However, estimates of the magnitude of this inappropriate use vary widely.

Among the most popular of the managed-care options is the HMO. The spectacular growth in HMO enrollment noted above was enhanced by their well-documented ability to reduce total health expenditures. Early, nonexperimental experience placed the magnitude of these cost savings between 20% and 40%, compared to those enrolled in more traditional health care plans (Luft, 1981). More recent studies have estimated that HMOs reduce the use of services by 20% compared to traditional health plans (Congressional Budget Office, 1995). As such plans also negotiate price discounts, the overall reduction in spending is even larger. Though these studies have used statistical methods that attempt to estimate spending in HMOs and traditional plans among populations "randomly" assigned to such plans, such selection in practice is not likely. Thus, there is residual concern that some portion of the estimated savings linked to HMOs may in fact simply reflect the enrollment of healthier patients in such plans.

Evidence from the Rand Health Insurance Experiment (HIE) provided insight into the selection issue. Using an experimentally controlled population, the HIE found that, compared to a free, fee-for-service plan, HMOs reduced total expenditures by 29% (Manning et al., 1985). The magnitude of these reductions was impressive, similar to those observed under a 95% coinsurance rate. Thus, the experimental results indicated that HMOs did not require favorable selection to achieve their large apparent cost savings. Remaining at issue, however, is whether these savings represent one-time or continued reductions in health care spending. One early comparison of premium growth among traditional plans with that of HMOs found little difference in rates of increase (Newhouse, Schwartz, Williams, & Witsberger, 1985). If these results are valid, they suggest that HMO savings, although substantial, may be transitory.

Spurred by the studies documenting their effectiveness, selected aspects of HMOs, such as a second surgical opinion, preauthorization of selected hospital admissions, concurrent review, and outpatient surgery and testing requirements, assumed standard roles in many health plans (Jensen, Morrisey, & Marcus, 1987). In some cases, immediate reductions in health care spending resulted. Although evaluations of the cost savings traced to private-sector utilization programs are rare, one study provided some early insight. For the large private health insurer examined, hospital utilization review (which included preadmission certification and on-site and concurrent review) reduced admissions 12.3%, inpatient spending 11.9%, and total per capita expenditures 8.3% (Feldstein, Wickizer, & Wheeler, 1988). More recent studies have confirmed these earlier results (Zwanziger & Melnick, 1996).

In addition to avoiding state benefit mandates, there are other incentives for companies to self-insure. For instance, self-insured funds are not subject to state premium taxes or to laws governing capital and financial reserve requirements. Moreover, self-insured funds do not contribute to state "risk pools," designed to finance insurance for high-risk, low-income individuals through state taxes. Growth in the number of self-insured plans is also symptomatic of the longer-term trend away from "community"-rated plans and toward "experience" rating. Built into traditional group health insurance premiums are costs stemming from uncompensated care, insurance company profits, and cross-subsidies of high-cost policyholders. The rising number of uninsured individuals and uncompensated care has accounted for a portion of the yearly increases in health insurance premiums. Firms that self-insure avoid these additional costs, which are built into a typical group health insurance premium. In this sense, self-insuring eliminates any cross-subsidies included in health insurance premiums. However, the move to self-insuring also transfers all (or in some cases most) of the financial risk of catastrophic cases from private insurers to firms.

Despite the benefits accruing to firms that self-insure, the comparative ability of such plans to contain costs remains unproved. One study compared the level and rate of increase in costs among self-insured, commercial, and Blue Cross plans. The results found no significant differences in expenditures across plans between 1981 and 1985 (Jensen & Gabel, 1988). Moreover, firms self-insuring during this period actually experienced sharper increases in health care spending compared to commercial and Blue Cross plans. Although our experience with self-insured plans is relatively new, their ability to significantly reduce cost growth relative to more traditional payers appears questionable. Though few recent studies have directly compared health insurance premiums between insured and self-insured firms, one recent examination found few significant differences in premiums (Acs, Long, Marquis, & Short, 1996).

Point-of-Service Products

Another important trend is the growing popularity of POS plans. These hybrid plans combine key features of HMO and traditional indemnity products. Enrollees are permitted to choose at the point of service whether to use the plan's provider network or seek care from nonnetwork physicians. Typically, in-panel physicians are paid on a capitated or discounted-fee basis, and out-of-panel physicians receive traditional fee-for-service reimbursement.

From the consumer's perspective, free choice of providers is a major selling point for POS plans. However, the reimbursement provisions of these plans are designed to dissuade enrollees from exercising the out-of-network option. Most enrollees in open-ended products pay coinsurance in the 30% range and deductibles of up to $300 for use of out-of-network providers, whereas services provided in-network are subject to minimal co-payments (KPMG, 1996). These financial differentials effectively deter out-of-network care. Strongly encouraging, but not requiring, use of in-network physicians, POS plans aim to reap the benefits of tightly managed care while bypassing its least popular feature, that is, restricted consumer choice.

Growth in PPOs

Finally, private payers and self-insured firms have increasingly used their purchasing power to negotiate payment rates with providers. Under a PPO arrangement, private payers negotiate a discounted rate with selected physicians and hospitals, often guaranteeing the provider a specified volume of business. For hospitals suffering from low occupancy rate (generally in California, Colorado, and Florida), the arrangements are quite attractive. The number of PPOs increased from

115 in 1984 to 1,036 in 1992. More than 57 million individuals are eligible to join a PPO offered through their or a family member's employer.

Although the sponsorships, form, and incentives found in PPOs differ widely, today's PPOs share four common characteristics:

1. PPOs represent an organized network of providers (e.g., hospitals, physicians) available to provide care.
2. Patients enter the PPO network through financial incentives in their benefits, a physician gatekeeper, or both.
3. PPOs negotiate discounts from providers from prevailing market payment rates.
4. PPOs include a variety of managed-care elements, usually including physician gatekeepers, utilization review, and second-opinion programs.

The early PPOs focused on negotiating reduced rates of payment to both hospitals and physicians. Little attention was directed toward including checks on utilization. As a result, early experience with PPOs provided mixed results. Although unit costs fell, the volume of services often increased, reducing the success of the ventures. More recently, insurers have developed hybrid programs incorporating utilization-control features along with negotiated payments. The utilization-control features in these hybrid plans are similar to those found in most HMOs. A central feature of these plans is the use of a "gatekeeper" primary care physician. The primary care physician in essence manages the patient referral process. Most hybrid plans include financial incentives for the gatekeeper to monitor utilization by setting specific targets for hospital admissions, total hospital days, and outpatient surgery. Because these hybrid plans are so new, few empirical analyses have assessed their impact on health care expenditures. One recent study, however, examined the impact of a PPO for a large western company. The study found no discernible difference in spending among those enrolled in the PPO compared to other employees. Whether these results will generalize to other settings remains unknown.

Innovations in Hospital Rate Setting—Growth in Diagnosis-Related Group Payment Systems

Perhaps the most important change in hospital rate setting during the 1980s was Medicare's shift from a retrospective cost-based program to a prospectively determined payment based on diagnosis-related groups (DRGs). Under this system, hospitals are paid a preestablished amount per case treated, with payment rates varying by type of case. The DRGs measure hospital output by originally classifying patients into 23 major diagnostic categories (MDCs), based on major body systems. The MDCs are divided further into more than 470 diagnostic groups based on the patient's diagnosis or surgical procedure used and on age, sex, and other clinical information. Three aspects of this approach differ from Medicare's previous payment methodology. First, the payments are determined in advance and are fixed. Second, the unit of payment changed from per day to per admission. Finally, payment rates were eventually divorced from each hospital's own cost experience.

The new payment scheme implemented by Medicare applies only to inpatient, operating costs. Excluded are payments for physicians' services (discussed below), capital (which Medicare continues to reimburse at levels slightly below interest and depreciation expenses), direct medical education (e.g., salaries for attending physicians and residents), and outpatient and emergency departments. Not all hospitals were included in Medicare's case payment system. Some specialty hospitals, such as children's, long-term-care, rehabilitation, and psychiatric hospitals, were exempt. Also exempt were four states (New York, Massachusetts, Maryland, and New Jersey) receiving waivers from the HCFA to develop their own experimental payment programs. However, by 1993, only Maryland had retained its waiver.

Payment that an individual hospital receives for treating Medicare patients in a given DRG depends on the DRG's "cost" weight (i.e., its cost relative to an average Medicare admission) multiplied by a "standardized" average cost for all Medicare patients. The standardization process includes adjustments for interhospital differences in wages, teaching status, and amount of care provided to low-income patients. Different rates are also set for urban and rural hospitals. In addition, payment amounts to hospitals are adjusted each year by a "trend factor," consisting of a measure of the price of goods and services purchased by hospitals and a discretionary adjustment factor to account for changes in new technology and productivity.

The original plans called for a gradual phase-in of the case payment system over 3 years. In the first year (1984), 75% of a hospital's per-case payments were to be based on its own cost experience. This level gradually declined over time; by 1988 payment rates (known as prices) to hospitals were based on national standardized average costs per admission. Movement to a pricing system divorced payment rates from each hospital's costs.

The Impact of the Medicare DRG Program: The Early Years

Medicare's experience with the DRG system has produced mixed results. Initially, hospitals responded quite dramatically to the altered incentives created by the DRG payment system. The payment of a fixed price per admission provided hospitals clear incentives to reduce costs. Any savings stemming from these reductions could be retained by the hospital. The new opportunity to earn short-term profits resulted in impressive changes during the early years of the program. In its first year (federal fiscal year 1984) inpatient expenditures declined as the number of full-time equivalent (FTE) employees fell 2.3%, reversing the trend of earlier years. Although lengths of stay among the elderly had been falling for years, the DRG program accelerated the decline. Finally, total admissions fell 2.6% during the first year of the DRG program, again reversing a long trend toward increased admissions.

Falling lengths of stay, admissions, and employment levels resulted in slower hospital expenditure growth. Total Medicare inpatient operating costs decreased by 6% during the first year of the program. Inpatient cost per admission increased slightly, by approximately 1.3%, significantly below the 4.7% update in Medicare payments allowed during the first year. With cost growth slower than increases in revenue, hospital operating margins rose sharply. By 1984 it was 11.3%, the highest in nearly two decades (AHA, 1988).

Unfortunately, the expenditure reductions were short-lived. Many of the trends observed in the initial year of the program were reversed in subsequent years. Total Medicare operating costs increased 3% during fiscal year 1985 and 6.5% during 1986 (see Table 15.1). The latter increase was cause for concern, as it exceeded the allowed increase in revenues (e.g., the trend factor) by 6%. Although the factors accounting for the more recent rise in Medicare spending are unknown, hospitals may simply have reinvested large portions of their "profits" back into

TABLE 15.1 Percentage of Change in Medicare Inpatient Expenses, Hospital Staffing, and Hospital Volume, 1980–1987

Year	Medicare inpatient expenses	Total inpatient expenses	Total hospital FTEs[a]	Length of stay	Admissions
1980	—	16.8%	4.7%	−0.1%	6.7%
1981	—	18.4	5.4	−0.1	3.0
1982	—	15.6	3.7	−2.3	4.1
1983	—	9.6	1.4	−4.5	4.7
1984	−4.4%	3.5	−2.3	−7.6	−2.6
1985	3.0	4.1	−2.3	−2.0	−5.2
1986	6.5	7.1	0.3	0.3	−1.2
1987	—	6.1	0.7	1.1	0.4

[a]FTEs, full-time equivalent employees.

Source: American Hospital Association, National Panel Survey; Prospective Payment Assessment Commission, Annual Report to Congress.

hospital operations. If true, this would account for the cost growth bubble observed in fiscal year 1986.

Lengths of stay also increased during 1986 and 1987, although admissions continued to fall. However, since the average acuity of patients admitted to hospitals increased, adjusted (for case mix) lengths of stay did not rise. In contrast to the initial decline, total hospital employment increased during 1986 and 1987. The bulk of the increase occurred in hospital outpatient departments, with employment levels on the inpatient side continuing to fall.

The new DRG payment system also provided strong incentives for hospital administrators to "unbundle" services. This included encouraging physicians to complete tests and procedures outside the hospital (where they are not subject to the payment controls). Moreover, recent changes in medical technology, most notably for surgical procedures, have accelerated the trend toward outpatient care. These incentives and changes in technology resulted in substantial increases in Medicare's spending for outpatient services. For instance, by 1987, Medicare expenditures for outpatient services increased 21%, more than five times the rate of increase observed for inpatient expenditures (Physician Payment Review Commission, 1988). The large increase in outpatient department expenditures blunted the full cost-containment potential of the DRG program.

In addition to the most recent rise in Medicare spending, the DRG program had uneven impacts on hospital expenditure growth. As discussed above, a central element of the new system was the use of predetermined "prices" for hospital payment. These prices were based on national average Medicare costs per discharge standardized for teaching status, share of low-income patients treated, wage rates, and urban/rural location. Because payments were no longer based on historic hospital costs, payments to some hospitals were lower and others higher than the average costs. Hospitals with payment rates set lower than average costs were considered less efficient and were the initial targets of the regulatory program. However, large numbers of hospitals initially benefited financially from the program because payment rates exceeded their average costs.

Use of the pricing methodology led to an uneven response by hospitals to the DRG payment system. On average, total inpatient costs growth was initially attenuated under the DRG system. To a more modest extent, the DRG system reduced the rate of increase in total (both inpatient and outpatient) expenditures through 1986. The reduced growth in costs, however, was generally limited to those hospitals with payment rates set below costs. Among these hospitals, inpatient cost growth was over 4.4 percentage points lower than the overall average (Feder, Hadley, & Zuckerman, 1987). In contrast, compared to the most tightly constrained hospitals, expenditures for hospitals least constrained were some 7% higher. Thus, the redistributive effect of the pricing system limited the full cost-containment potential of the DRG program.

Throughout the 1980s reforms of the DRG system focused on a variety of "technical" adjustments to the payment rates as well as on adjusting the methodology used to reimburse capital expenses. Until 1992, Medicare reimbursed hospitals a percentage (less than 100) for all depreciation and interest spending. Failure to include capital payments in the prospective payment system likely reduced the potential effectiveness of the DRG program. A capital pass-through ensured that hospital spending decisions were insensitive to interest rates or less costly methods of expansion. Moreover, the pass-through also provided incentives for hospitals to inefficiently substitute capital for labor.

In FY 1992, a 10-year phase-in of prospective payment for hospital capital costs began. When fully implemented, Medicare will reimburse capital costs much as it now pays for operating costs under the DRG program. Payment will be based on standardized national average costs per discharge, adjusted for teaching status, share of low-income patients, wage rates, and urban/rural location. (These adjustments are not identical to their operating costs counterparts.)

The Impact of the Medicare DRG Program: The Recent Experience

The second decade of experience with the Medicare DRG program differs sharply from the experience in the 1980s (see Table 15.2). Starting in the late 1980s, both the nominal and real (here adjusted for the percent change in the consumer price index) growth in Medicare inpatient hospital payments and hospitals costs started to decline. By the early 1990s the inflation-adjusted growth in hospital

TABLE 15.2 Percentage of Change in Medicare-Related Hospital Costs and Payments, Federal Fiscal Years 1988–1994

Year	Costs	Payments	Cost Per Case	Payment Per Case	CPI
1988	9.8%	6.7%	9.0%	6.0%	4.1%
1989	10.4%	7.7%	9.3%	6.6%	4.7%
1990	10.5%	8.2%	8.6%	6.3%	5.0%
1991	9.0%	8.0%	6.9%	5.8%	5.1%
1992	7.0%	7.3%	4.9%	5.2%	3.0%
1993	3.5%	5.9%	1.3%	3.6%	3.1%
1994	0.3%	5.2%	−1.3%	3.5%	2.6%

Source: Prospective Payment Assessment Commission, Medicare and the American Health Care System, Report to Congress, June 1996.

costs had declined to approximately 4%. By 1994, the growth in inflation adjusted payments had declined to 2.6%.

The 1990s witnessed another major difference in the interaction between Medicare hospital payments and costs. Throughout the course of the DRG program, payments to hospitals had always increased at a slower rate than hospital costs. However, by 1993, Medicare payments to hospitals started to rise faster than the overall growth in hospital costs. The dramatic slowdown in costs is partially attributed to changes in Medicare payment policies, as well as to changes in medical technology that have redirected a substantial volume of cases to the outpatient setting. Although these trends are important, the most recent reduction in hospital costs appear primarily motivated by the substantial increase in cost-containment pressures applied by the private sector. The demand for cost containment among private payers has generated a reduction overall in the growth of hospital costs.

Although it appears that the growth in Medicare inpatient hospital spending has slowed dramatically, the growth in outpatient hospital spending continues to rise. Unlike payments for inpatient expenses, Medicare currently employs a variety of methods to pay for outpatient services (i.e., laboratory, ambulatory surgery, other diagnostic). Though some of Medicare's payments are prospective in nature (e.g., laboratory services), most are based in large part on reported hospital costs. Thus, Medicare payments for outpatient services generally rise as costs rise. This differs significantly from the inpatient methodology, where the growth in payments and costs is not directly linked. As a result of both changes in technology that have increased the volume of services provided on an outpatient basis and Medicare's current cost-linked payment strategy, Medicare outpatient payments per enrollee increased 8.8% between 1991 and 1993. This compares to an average annual growth of 4.1% per enrollee between 1987 and 1991. In contrast, inpatient hospital payments increased at an average annual rate of 4.8% per enrollee between 1991 and 1993 (Prospective Payment Assessment Commission, 1995).

In addition to the rapid growth in outpatient payments, Medicare faces additional issues with its outpatient payment methodology. Under current law, Medicare beneficiaries face a 20% coinsurance based on hospital outpatient charges, as opposed to payments. Over the past decade, outpatient charges have risen at a faster pace than Medicare payments, imposing an increasing amount of cost sharing on Medicare beneficiaries. For example, during federal fiscal year 1995 Medicare payments for hospital outpatient services totaled $19.4 billion, 37% of which was financed by beneficiary payments (Prospective Payment Assessment Commission, 1995). Several proposals have been advanced to "fix" this beneficiary overpayment. One proposal seeks to have the Secretary of Health and Human Services establish a prospective payment program for outpatient care. Once adopted, beneficiary payments could be based on 20% of the actual payments, rather than charges. The design of such a program will have to embrace the difficult issue of defining the clinically and financially relevant DRG equivalents. Moreover, given the rapid growth in outpatient volume, some incentives to control inappropriate outpatient care will be required.

Growth and Subsequent Decline in All-Payer Rate-Setting Programs

State experiments with innovative hospital rate-setting programs expanded during the 1980s. Until then, most state rate-setting programs set prospective per diem rates for Medicaid and Blue Cross plans. In some cases, commercial payers were also included. However, Medicare payments to hospitals were outside the prospectively determined rates. Beginning in 1977, Maryland obtained a waiver from the HCFA allowing the state to develop its own payment rules for Medicare. This let the state include all sources of third-party inpatient revenue under the state's rate-setting rules. Three other states—New Jersey, Massachusetts, and New York—subsequently obtained Medicare waivers during the early 1980s. Like Maryland, each state included Medicare payments within its historic rate-setting programs.

The genesis of these four all-payer systems was complicated. It included concern over continued escalation in hospital costs within these states as well as issues regarding the equity of payment rates facing private payers. As discussed below, use of the rate-setting process to achieve both cost reductions and distributional objectives distinguished the all-payer approach from previous efforts (Thorpe, 1987). Each state adopting the all-payer approach had previous rate-setting programs covering some portion of inpatient revenues. Although these programs were often successful in reducing cost growth among some payers (and in the case of New York, all payers), costs among unregulated payers continued to climb. Price controls on Medicaid and Blue Cross plans created incentives for hospitals to increase charges, often referred to as cost or charge shifting, to unregulated commercial payers. As a result, the difference between charges and costs for commercial payers escalated rapidly during the late 1970s and early 1980s. Thus, protecting commercial payers against cost shifting assumed an important role for all-payer systems.

Growth in the number of uninsured individuals over this period created another set of pressures. Between 1979 and 1984 the number of individuals without health insurance increased 20%, to more than 34 million individuals (tabulation from the Current Population Survey, 1980, 1985). Growth in the number of individuals without health insurance increased the volume of bad debt and charity care provided by hospitals. For those hospitals unable to recover such costs from commercial payers (through increased charges) or state and local governments (in the case of public hospitals), a serious deterioration of operating margins resulted. Deteriorating hospital financial conditions, combined with the growing number of uninsured patients, created pressures on state governments to provide some financial relief.

The growing demands of the commercial insurance industry to limit legislatively the difference between charges and costs (e.g., the differential), combined with the mounting requirements of hospitals to finance uncompensated care, presented a dilemma. Limiting the size of the differential would eliminate one traditionally passive method of financing a portion of uncompensated care. Thus, some alternative and more explicit financing method would be required. Moreover, the growth in the differential created a common perception that commercial payers were assuming an unfair burden in financing care for the uninsured (Meyer, Johnson, & Sullivan, 1983). Thus, to distribute the costs of uncompensated care more evenly, each state developed some type of uncompensated care pool. Although methods of collecting revenue and distributing it to hospitals differed across states, the burden of financing uncompensated care was more widely distributed.

Finally, experience with the "partial" payer approaches used by most state rate-setting programs during the 1970s provided mixed results. As noted above, cost growth among regulated payers was often attenuated, although per capita cost growth was generally stable. Thus, the all-payer approach was also designed to provide a uniform inpatient revenue cap, reducing the ability of hospitals to escape the intent of the regulatory controls. Although the programs provided a comprehensive inpatient rate cap, payment methods for outpatient services in each state were largely left intact. The four-state all-payer programs described above generally achieved their intended results. Relative to the "unwaivered" states, the all-payer states were able to reduce total cost growth. Inpatient costs per admission were 2 to 3 percentage points lower between 1982 and 1985 in waivered states relative to unwaivered states (Schramm, Renn, & Biles, 1986). More impressive perhaps was the 2-percentage-point reduction in total costs per admission (adjusted for outpatient visits).

Lower cost growth among the all-payer states was achieved through reductions in labor, rather than reduced admissions or length of stay. The number of FTE personnel in the waivered states grew at significantly slower rates than observed elsewhere (Schramm et al., 1986). Thus, the comprehensive regulatory controls appeared to increase the productivity of hospital care. Fewer labor inputs per patient day were also accompanied by slower rates of technological diffusion. As noted in an earlier section, slower adoption rates were especially pronounced in New York. Although growth in hospital personnel in all-payer states proceeded at a significantly slower pace, there were few discernable differences in the changes in average length of stay between the waivered and unwaivered states.

The all-payer states were also successful in limiting the differential between private charges and costs. Each state enacted a statutory limit on the magnitude of each hospital's allowed difference between costs and charges. In New York this reduced the differential from a statewide average of 30% to less than 15% by 1985 (Thorpe, 1987). Similarly, the all-payer program in Massachusetts reduced the magnitude of the differential by 1.4% in its first year and steadily lowered it to approximately 7.5% by 1985. The magnitude of the differential in these states was significantly lower than the national average of 25% (AHA, 1988).

Finally, the regulatory approach adopted by the all-payer states raised a significant volume of revenue to finance hospital uncompensated care. More than $300 million was raised each year in New York and Massachusetts, with similar amounts (relative to total state hospital costs) in the other states. The pool revenues allowed financially strained hospitals to maintain and often increase the volume of care they provided the medically indigent. Moreover, the significant influx of revenues raised by the pools improved the operating margins of many hospitals. In New York, for example, the magnitude of the statewide hospital operating deficit was over $600 million less during the experiment relative to deficits projected without the pools (Thorpe, 1987). Thus, the redistributive goals of the all-payer programs were largely fulfilled.

The success of the all-payer programs in simultaneously reducing cost growth and internally redistributing revenues to fiscally distressed facilities ironically led to their near elimination. Hospitals in each state were quick to compare the expected revenue under their waivered systems with revenues expected under the national DRG program. For instance, the hospital association in New York State projected a $400 million influx of Medicare revenues in 1986 should the state switch from its waivered system to the DRG program. Similar projections of higher revenues flowing to the waivered states also were developed in other states. In partial response to industry interests in switching to the DRG program, New York and Massachusetts did not extend their waivers, thus joining Medicare's DRG payment programs. New Jersey renewed its waiver once, but in 1989 it also joined the Medicare DRG system.

A final payment innovation during the 1980s was the growth in competitive bidding schemes designed to create incentives for providers to compete on a price basis. As discussed in an earlier section, competition among providers in the health care industry has traditionally occurred along nonprice dimensions (e.g., service intensity, technology, and amenities). Those interested in promoting price competition were quick to highlight the shortcomings of the regulatory approach (Enthoven, 1981). According to this school of thought, vigorous price competition among health care plans and providers would provide the only "practical" solution to the health care cost crisis. Some states moved to increase the scope of regulated hospital revenue; others moved to competitive bidding. The California Medi-Cal program implemented the most notable bidding scheme, known as selective contracting, in 1983. Under this program, hospitals would submit price bids to the state contracting "czar" to provide services to Medi-Cal beneficiaries. Except in emergencies, hospitals not receiving contracts could not receive payment from the state. Two other state Medicaid programs followed California's lead: Illinois in 1985 and, most recently, Washington.

The early experience with selective contracting in California has produced favorable results (Melnick & Zwanziger, 1988). In contrast to earlier research results that found higher cost growth in the most competitive markets, the opposite held for California hospitals after the implementation of selective contracting. Between 1983 and 1985, real (adjusted for general inflation) inpatient costs increased an average of 1% for hospitals in less competitive markets, compared to an 11.3% decrease among hospitals in more competitive markets (Melnick & Zwanziger, 1988). In keeping with the empirical results noted above, the state estimated savings exceeding $1 billion during the selective contracting program.

Both the selective contracting program implemented in California and the all-payer rate-setting systems discussed above were able to reduce cost growth. Still at issue is their relative ability to contain costs. Is competitive bidding the salvation or the imposition of more comprehensive and binding rate-setting programs? Recent studies provide at least an initial insight. Based on a national study, all-payer rate regulation reduced cost growth by 16.3% in Massachusetts, 15.4% in Maryland, and 6.3% in New York between 1982 and 1986 relative to a set of control states (Robinson & Luft, 1988). Cost growth in New Jersey was similar to that observed among the control states. In comparison, cost growth among California hospitals using the selective contracting strategy was 10.1% lower compared to states without rate-setting or competitive bidding. Thus, based on these results, it appears that, on average, the more comprehensive rate-setting programs and selective contracting have similar impacts on cost growth. Whether the longer-term performance of these decidedly different approaches is similar requires continued monitoring.

The Managed Care Revolution:
Impact on Private Health Care Spending

Perhaps the most notable change in the structure of health care payments and costs is the dramatic growth in managed care in both the public and private sector. As interest among employers intensified after the demise of President Clinton's health care reform effort to control costs, they relied almost exclusively on managed care as the vehicle to deliver savings. The growth in the percentage of workers enrolled in such plans over 4 years has been impressive (see Table 15.3). As late as 1992, 45% of workers employed in firms with over 200 employees were enrolled in traditional fee-for-service plans. By 1996 only one quarter of

TABLE 15.3 Private Health Care Spending, 1985–1994 (Billions of Dollars)

	Years							Average annual charge		
	1985	1990	1991	1992	1993	1994		1985–90	1990–94	1985–94
Total										
Total private	$282.2	$450.8	$481.9	$520.1	$544.2	$577.7		9.8%	6.4%	8.3%
Business	$108.6	$185.8	$198.2	$215.9	$226.8	$241.3		11.3%	6.8%	9.3%
Household	$160.5	$245.3	$262.2	$281.9	$292.9	$310.1		8.9%	6.0%	7.6%
Nonpatient spending	$13.1	$19.8	$21.5	$22.3	$24.4	$25.9		8.6%	6.9%	7.9%

Source: Cower, Braden, McDonnell, & Sivorajan, 1996.

all workers were enrolled in such plans. The demise of fee-for-service plans was accompanied by a rapid growth in enrollment in POS plans and health maintenance organizations (HMOs). In 1996 one third of workers in these larger firms were enrolled in HMOs, whereas 16% were enrolled in POS plans.

The growth in managed care has not been limited to the private sector. The growth in managed care within the Medicaid program has been the most impressive. As of July 1996, 40% of Medicaid beneficiaries were enrolled in managed care plans. This compares to only 9.5% enrollment in Medicaid managed care in 1991 (Office of Managed Care, Health Care Financing Administration, 1997). By enrolling certain Medicaid beneficiaries into managed care, several states have generated savings that have, in part, been used to expand coverage to the previously uninsured. Though the growth in Medicare managed care has been slower, there is substantial interest by many policymakers to increase the use of managed care within the program to slow the growth in total Medicare spending. As of 1996, an estimated 3.5 million Medicare beneficiaries—approximately 9.1% of total enrollees—were enrolled in managed care plans. This compares to only 3.7% enrollment in managed care plans in 1991 (unpublished data, Health Care Financing Administration, 1996). Though the increased use of managed care appears to have generated substantial savings within the private sector and the Medicaid program, there is considerable debate surrounding the savings (if any) attributed to the use of managed care in the Medicare program. Some studies have suggested that Medicare saves money through managed care enrollment; other studies disagree. The lack of program savings relates, in part, to the formula used by the federal government in setting payment rates to HMOs. Under current law, Medicare pays each HMO 95% of the estimated (after adjusting for age, sex, disability status, and location) costs of providing services to beneficiaries in the fee-for-service sector. There remains substantial suspicion and some empirical documentation that even with these adjustments, healthier patients are enrolling in managed care. As a result, Medicare ends up paying more than they would have paid for the patients had they remained in the fee-for-service part of the program.

Employers have used several means to shift their workers into managed care plans. These include relying on "defined" contributions toward the price of insurance. In general, the premiums associated with managed care plans are lower than fee-for-service plans. Thus, this would increase enrollment in managed care plans relative to fee-for-service plans. Another method used by employers to direct enrollment into managed care plans is to limit their employees' choice of plan options. Among workers employed in firms with over 200 employees, 47% have a choice of only one plan (KPMG, 1996), 24% have a choice of two plans, and the remaining 29% may select among three plans.

The movement of workers into managed care plans has generated impressive reductions in private-sector health care spending (see Table 15.4). For instance, spending by employers on health insurance increased at an average annual rate

TABLE 15.4   Percentage of Change in Private Health Insurance Premiums, 1991–1996

	1991	1992	1993	1994	1995	1996
Total	11.5	10.9	8	4.8	2.1	0.5
By number of employees						
200–999	—	10.6	8.8	4.6	2.8	1.1
1,000–4,999	—	10.3	7.3	5.4	2.2	0.5
5,000+	—	11	8	4.6	1.9	0.3

Source: KPMG, *Health Benefits in 1996*, October 1996.

of 11.3% between 1985 and 1990 but declined to 6.8% during the 1990s. This includes spending growth on active workers (described below) as well as for retirees. The ability of employers to control the growth in spending among these two populations had differed. In general, the growth in spending among active workers has slowed dramatically, whereas the growth in retiree health spending provides few indications of any decline. The growth in household spending (both on health insurance premiums and out-of-pocket) decreased from 8.9% annually between 1985 and 1990 to 6% during the 1990s. More recent data reveal even sharper reductions in spending among active workers (see Table 15.5). Among such workers, the growth in health insurance premiums across all plans has declined steadily since 1991. By 1996 the growth in health insurance premiums decreased to a low of 0.5%.

TABLE 15.5   Percentage of Workers Enrolled in Traditional Fee-For-Service and Managed Care Plans, 1992–1996

Plan Type	Years				
	1992	1993	1994	1995	1996
Traditional fee-for-service	45	42	35	31	26
Point-of-service	8	10	15	18	16
Preferred provider	26	22	25	22	25
Health maintenance organization	22	26	25	29	33

Source: KPMG, *Health Benefits in 1996*, October, 1996.

A major issue in the managed care revolution is whether the impressive reductions in the growth in private health care spending represents a one-time savings as workers shift to managed care plans or whether the savings will be sustained over time. As the movement into lower-cost managed care plans is still in process, it is difficult to distinguish savings from migration into managed care plans from ongoing savings generated among those enrolled in such plans. As the managed care marketplace becomes more saturated in certain areas, it will become easier to isolate these two effects.

Reform of Physician Reimbursement

During much of the 1980s, efforts to reduce health care costs often focused on payments to institutions (especially hospitals), rather than payments for physician and outpatient services and hospital capital. After implementing the DRG system, however, policymakers turned their attention to reforming the way in which Medicare pays physicians. This attention was justified. Between 1975 and 1987, total Medicare expenditures for physicians increased an average of 18% annually (Physician Payment Review Commission, 1988). More recent data show a slight reduction in the growth in nominal spending, but the growth remains high after adjusting for inflation. The Health Care Financing Administration projects that physician payments will rise 11% per year between 1993 and 2005. Also, although expenditures for physician services accounted for less than one quarter of all spending, physicians potentially influenced over 70% of all health care spending.

Medicare's traditional method for reimbursing physicians was based on the "customary, prevailing, and reasonable" (CPR) reimbursement system, a methodology that was typical of the fee-for-service methods used by most third-party payers. Under the CPR method, payments for each service performed were based on the lowest figure for the physician's historic charge, the billed charge, or an average charge of similar physicians in the area. Payment rates were also limited to yearly increases in the Medicare Economic Index. This system was roundly criticized as inflationary and complex. In addition, it provided higher payment rates (relative to costs) for specialists and those performing complex procedures (relative to those performing more cognitive tasks). This structure was frequently cited as influencing physicians' specialty choices. The apparent "surplus" of surgeons and subspecialists projected over the next 20 years has often been traced to this payment system.

Two options were frequently advanced to address both the cost-growth and the specialty-choice issues. The first payment option was to expand the number of physicians paid on a capitated basis. The role of capitation in addressing cost growth was addressed earlier. The second option was a new fee schedule for physicians.

In the 1989 Budget Act, Congress chose the second option. It mandated the implementation of a specific type of fee schedule, called a resource-based relative value scale (RBRVS), starting in 1992. This particular relative-value scale has three components: a measure of total "work" by the physician, an allowance for practice costs, and an allowance for the cost of malpractice insurance. Each service is assigned a given number of relative value units (RVUs). These RVUs are then multiplied by a national conversion factor to determine a dollar amount of payment for that service. As of 1997 the federal government had created three conversion factors: one for surgical services, one for primary care, and the third for other services.

A major objective of the RBRVS was to develop a more equitable method of reimbursing physicians. In contrast to the CPR, two services that require the same amount of work, practice expense, and malpractice expense should be reimbursed at the same level (except for an adjustment to account for different price levels in different geographic areas). This was intended to eliminate the distortive effect that the CPR has on specialty choice and service mix.

In the 1989 Budget Act, Congress also made two other changes to the way that physicians are reimbursed for services they provide to Medicare patients. First, limits were placed on the amounts that physicians could charge patients above a Medicare-approved amount. In 1992 doctors were not allowed to charge more than 20% more than the Medicare-approved amount. From 1993 on, this percentage dropped to 15%.

The final reform was the creation of the Medicare volume performance standard (MVPS). The MVPS is a target rate that Congress sets annually to reflect its view of the appropriate growth rate in Medicare spending for physician services. It is intended to take into account both general cost inflation and acceptable increases in volume and intensity of services provided.

Under the CPR system, payment rates each year were updated by the amount of the Medicare Economic Index (MEI). The MVPS simply adds another layer to this process. After a year has ended, the MVPS rate of increase in spending and the actual rate are compared. If the MVPS is lower than the actual rate of increase (i.e., spending grew at a higher level than Congress considered appropriate), then the next year's increase (normally the MEI) is decreased by the amount of the excess. If the MVPS is higher than the actual rate of spending, then the annual update is increased by the amount of the shortfall.

The new Medicare relative value fee schedule was gradually phased in, 1991 through 1995–96. During this period the basis for paying physicians changed from historic charges to the relative value fee schedule. Though the phase-in had not been completed by 1996, there are some notable changes in both Medicare payments and in the volume and intensity of services provided under the program. Between 1991 and 1993, for instance, Medicare payments per service actually declined 1.1% even while the volume intensity (per encounter) of services increased 3.2% (Physician Payment Review Commission, 1995, 1996). More recent data indicate that payments per service have increased slightly, rising 3.8% between 1994 and 1995 (Physician Payment Review Commission, 1996). The growth in payments per service has risen at a slower rate during the 1990s compared to the 1980s.

Other indications of change in the program concern the growth in service volume and intensity per beneficiary over time. Starting in 1992, the growth in volume and intensity increased 4.2% in that year, 3% in 1993, 4.2% in 1994, and 5.2% in 1995. The growth in volume and intensity of services increased 7.0% in 1990 and 9.8% in 1991 (Physician Payment Review Commission, 1996). The average annual growth in volume and intensity of services between 1986 and 1991 was 7.1%. Though these experiences after the introduction of the relative value scale seem promising, the most recent data reveal a rise in the use of services.

Summary and Conclusions

Our earlier discussion indicated that the fundamental force driving up health care costs was the diffusion of new technologies. Of the estimated sevenfold real increase in health care spending since 1950, new technologies and practice patterns account for up to 90% of the growth (Manning et al., 1987). Innovations in medicine have been nothing short of remarkable. Our capacity to increase average life expectancy and its quality reflect these developments. The growth in transplant capacity, diagnostic imaging, and drugs represents a few of these medical innovations. If this increase in spending had generated commensurate increases in benefits, then the "problem" of health care cost growth would be illusory. In short, that we spend over 12% of our GNP in the health care sector may simply reflect societal preferences to direct limited resources to health rather than to other areas.

At the center of the debate over the growth of health care costs is whether the same level of health could be purchased for less. A growing body of research indicates that substantial savings could be achieved without significant changes in the health of our population. Critical examination of the appropriateness of various medical procedures indicates that health care spending could be reduced by several billion dollars without a deleterious impact on health. At issue is the appropriate intervention to address the underlying problem of health care cost growth in areas where problems remain. These problem areas include the Medicare program, the small group and individual insurance market, and spending in retiree health care services. Whether an expansion of managed care into these sectors can produce savings similar to those observed among workers in larger firms remains an important policy issue.

Mini-Case Study

New York State recently adopted a new hospital payment system that relied on competitive bidding to determine hospital payments, rather than regulation. New York also has over 2 million uninsured residents and the largest group of teaching hospitals in the country. Can competitive bidding and competition coexist with these other key health policy issues facing state policymakers? If so, how?

Discussion Questions

1. Several states adopted rate setting that applied to all third-party payers, yet only Maryland's system has survived. What factors account for the demise in all-payer rate setting in the other states?
2. Compared to fee-to-service medicine, managed care appears to generate significant savings. How does managed care alter the delivery of medicine, and how are these savings achieved?
3. All-payer rate-setting systems were developed to contain the growth in hospital costs, but they also included a broader range of objectives. What were these additional goals, and how can these objectives be met with the demise of rate setting?

References

Aaron, H. J., "Thinking Straight About Medical Costs," *Health Affairs, 13*(5), 7–13, 1994.

Aaron, H., & Schwartz, W., *The Painful Prescription: Rationing Hospital Care*. Washington, DC: The Brookings Institution, 1984.

Acs, G., Long, S., Marquis, S., & Short, P., "Self-Insured Employer Health Plans: Prevalence, Profile, Provisions and Premiums," *Health Affairs,* (Summer), 266–278, 1996.

American Hospital Association, *Hospital Statistics 1988*. Chicago: Author, 1988.

Chassin, M., *Does Inappropriate Use Explain Geographic Variation in the Use of Health Care Services? A Study of Three Procedures* (N-2748). Santa Monica, CA: Rand Corporation.

Coelen, C., & Sullivan, D., "An Analysis of the Effects of Prospective Reimbursement Programs in Hospital Expenditures," *Health Care Financing Review,* (Winter), 1–32, 1981.

Congressional Budget Office, *The Impact of PSRO on Health Care Costs: An Update on the Congressional Budget Office's 1979 Evaluation*. Washington, DC: U.S. Government Printing Office, 1981.

Congressional Budget Office, U.S. Congress, *The Effects of Managed Care and Managed Competition*. Washington, DC: U.S. Government Printing Office, 1995.

Congressional Research Service, *Workmen's Compensation: Role of the Federal Government*. (IB75054). Washington, DC: Library of Congress, 1976.

Cromwell, J., & Kanak, J., "The Effects of Hospital Rate Setting Programs on Volume of Hospital Services," *Health Care Financing Review, 4*(2), 67–88, 1982.

Eby, C., & Cohodes, D., "What Do We Know About Rate Setting?," *Journal of Health Politics, Policy and Law, 10,* 293–327, 1985.

Feder, J., Hadley, J., & Zuckerman, S., "How Did Medicare's Prospective Payment System Affect Hospitals?," *New England Journal of Medicine, 31,* 867–870, 1987.

Feldstein, P., Wickizer, T., & Wheeler, J., "The Effects of Utilization Review Programs on Health Care Use and Expenditures," *New England Journal of Medicine,* (May 19), 1310–1314, 1988.

InterStudy. Excelsior, MN: Author, 1995.

Jensen, G., & Gabel, J., "The Erosion of Purchased Health Insurance," *Inquiry, 25,* 328–343.

Jensen, G., Morrissey, M., & Marcus, J., "Cost Sharing and the Changing Pattern of Employer-Sponsored Health Benefits," *Millbank Memorial Fund Quarterly, 65,* 521, 1987.

Joskow, P., *Controlling Hospital Costs: The Role of Government Regulation.* Boston: MIT Press, 1981.

Kidder, D., & Sullivan, D., "Hospital Payroll Costs, Productivity, and Employment Under Prospective Reimbursement," *Health Care Financing Review, 4*(2), 89–100, 1982.

KPMG, *Health Benefits in 1996.* Tysons Corner, VA: Author, 1996.

Levit, K., Lazenby, H., Braden, B., Cowan, C., Senseninig, A., McDonnell, P., Stiller, J., Won, D., Martin, A., Sivarajan, L., Dunham, E., Long, A., & Stewart, M., "National Health Expenditures, 1996," *Health Care Financing Review, 19*(1), 161–200, 1997.

Levit, K., Lazenby, & Sivarajan, L., "National Health Expenditures, 1993," *Health Care Financing Review, 16,* 247–294, 1994.

Luft, H., *Health Maintenance Organization: Dimensions of Performance.* New York: John Wiley, 1981.

Manning, W. G., Newhouse, J. P., Duan, N., Keeler, E. B., Leibowitz, A., & Marquis, W. D., "Health Insurance and the Demand for Medical Care: Evidence from a Randomized Experiment," *American Economic Review, 77,* 251–277, 1987.

Melnick, G., & Zwanziger, J., "Hospital Behavior Under Government Competition and Cost-Containment Policies," *Journal of the American Medical Association, 260*(18), 2669–2772, 1988.

Meyer, Johnson, & Sullivan, *Passing the Health Care Buck: Who Pays the Hidden Cost?* Washington, DC: American Enterprise Institute, 1983.

Newhouse, J. P., Schwartz, W., Williams, A., & Witsberger, C., "Are Fee-for-Service Costs Increasing Faster Than HMO Costs?," *Medical Care, 23,* 960, 1985.

Office of Management and Budget, *Federal Budget* (p. 48). Washington, DC: U.S. Government Printing Office.

Office of Technology Assessment, *Policy Implications of the CT Scanner: An Update.* Washington, DC: Author, 1981.

Pauly, M., "Taxation, Health Insurance and Market Failure," *Journal of Economic Literature, 24,* 629–675, 1986.

Pauly, M., & Satterwaite, M., "The Pricing of Primary Care Physicians' Services: A Test of the Role of Common Intervention," *Bell Journal of Economics, 12,* 488–506, 1981.

Physician Payment Review Commission, *Annual Report to Congress, 1988.* Washington, DC: U.S. Government Printing Office, 1988.

Physician Payment Review Commission, *Annual Report to Congress, 1995.* Washington, DC: U.S. Government Printing Office, 1995.

Physician Payment Review Commission, *Annual Report to Congress, 1996.* Washington, DC: U.S. Government Printing Office, 1996.

Prospective Payment Assessment Commission, *Medicine and the American Health Care System—Report to Congress.* Washington, DC: U.S. Government Printing Office, 1995.

Robinson, J., & Luft, H., "Competition, Regulation, and Hospital Costs," *Journal of the American Medical Association, 257*(23), 3241–3245, 1988.

Romeo, A., Wagner, J., & Lee, R., "Prospective Reimbursement and the Diffusion of New Technologies in Hospitals," *Journal of Health Economics, 3,* 1–24, 1984.

Salkever, D., & Bice, T., "The Impact of Cost Controls on Hospital Investment," *Milbank Memorial Fund Quarterly, 54,* 185–200, 1976.

Schramm, C., Renn, S., & Bite, B., "New Perspectives in State Rate Setting," *Health Affairs, 5*(3), 22–25, 1986.

Schwartz, W., "In the Pipeline: A Wave of Valuable Technology," *Health Affairs, 13*(3), 70–80, 1994.

Sloan, F., "Hospital Rate Review: A Theory and Empirical Review," *Journal of Health Economics, 3,* 83–86, 1984.

Sloan, F., & Becker, E., "Cross-Subsidies and Payment for Hospital Care," *Journal of Health Politics, Policy and Law,* (Winter), 1984.

Sloan, F., Valvona, J., & Becker, E., "Diffusion of Surgical Technology: An Exploratory Study," *Journal of Health Economics, 5,* 31–40, 1986.

Thorpe, K. E., "Does All-Payer Rate Setting Work? The Case of the New York Prospective Hospital Reimbursement Methodology," *Journal of Health Politics, Policy and Law, 17,* 290–400, 1987.

Thorpe, K. E., "The Health Care System in Transition: Care, Cost and Coverage," *Journal of Health Politics, Policy and Law, 22*(2), 339–362, 1997.

Thorpe, K. E., & Phelps, C., "The Social Role of Not-for-Profit Organizations: Hospital Provision of Charity Care," *Economic Inquiry,* no. 29, 472–484, 1992.

Thorpe, K. E., & Phelps, C. E., "Regulating Intensity and Hospital Cost Growth," *Journal of Health Economics, 9,* 143–166, 1990.

U.S. Bureau of the Census, *Current Population Survey,* Washington, DC: U.S. Government Printing Office, 1980.

U.S. Bureau of the Census, *Current Population Survey,* Washington, DC: U.S. Government Printing Office, 1985.

Wennberg, J., "Dealing with Medical Practice Variations: A Proposal for Action," *Health Affairs,* (Summer), 6–32, 1984.

Wennberg, J., "On the Appropriateness of Small-Area Analysis for Cost Containment," *Health Affairs,* (Winter), 164–167, 1996.

Zwanziger, J., & Melnick, G., "Can Managed Care Plans Control Health Care Costs?," *Health Affairs,* (Summer), 185–199, 1996.

16

Ethics in Health Care Delivery

Paul B. Hofmann

Learning Objectives

After completing this chapter, the reader should be able to:

1. Distinguish between organizational and community priorities.
2. Describe managed care's conflicting incentives.
3. Discuss institutional, staff, and community needs in times of downsizing.
4. Explain current and future challenges related to rationing of medical services.
5. Defend the provision of unlimited care.
6. Define what constitutes ethical behavior.

Topical Outline

Balancing organizational and community priorities
    Representative indictments
    Prevalence of professional hypocrisy
    Illustrations of incompatible institutional and public interests
    Guidelines for serving and competing ethically
Contending with managed care's conflicting incentives
    Bright and dark sides of managed care
    Problems created by demonizing managed care
    Steps to minimize ethical liabilities
Confronting downsizing's painful dimensions
    Common reasons for avoiding timely decisions

Financial and nonfinancial costs of procrastination
Advantages of taking decisive action
Suggestions for demonstrating ethical sensitivity
Recognizing current and future dilemmas of medical rationing
Examples of current rationing
Crucial questions
Relevant ethical principles
Obstacles and opportunities
Supporting the provision of unlimited care
Unlimited care as an ethical imperative
Financial and nonfinancial costs of overtreatment
Methods of effective advocacy for patient values
Promoting ethical behavior
Importance of reconciling individual and organizational obligations
Value of an ethics audit
Requirements of ethical behavior

Key Words: **Autonomy, beneficence, downsizing, ethics audit, justice, managed care, nonmaleficence, moral traces, professional hypocrisy, rationing, rule of rescue, unlimited care.**

Since the relatively recent publication of the last edition of this book, ethical issues surrounding clinical topics appropriately have continued to receive extensive attention in both the popular press and the professional literature. Concerns about organ transplantation, genetic engineering, the Human Genome Project, euthanasia and physician-assisted suicide, medical experimentation, AIDS treatment, abortion, informed consent, confidentiality, medical futility, and a host of other complex subjects provoke legitimate debate and considerable passion. In her superb description of the historical development of bioethics and its various methodologies and principles, as well as many of the topics noted above and others, Seiden (1995) provided an excellent overview of this compelling field. Because she addressed clinical or medical ethics so effectively, this overview will not cover the same issues.

Although clinical ethics has not diminished in either importance or prominence, unprecedented attention is now being focused on organizational ethics in health care. General industry has recognized the discipline of business or management ethics for decades, but it is relatively recently (1995) that the Joint Commission on Accreditation of Healthcare Organizations (JCAHO) formalized standards in this area. Consequently, in contrast to the traditional examination of ethics in health care delivery, this chapter will concentrate on a diverse array of ethical issues that still reflect sensitivity to clinical values while highlighting the debates surrounding organizational behavior, economic pressures, and personal conduct. It is difficult, indeed impossible, to examine these issues with total objectivity. Inevitably, the author's beliefs and values have influenced both the selection of topics and their analysis. Therefore, readers are encouraged to challenge both the author's assertions and those drawn from the literature. Given the subject matter, the preceding chapters are properly more factually oriented than is this one. The very nature of deliberations on ethics will often be affected, usually implicitly rather than explicitly, by an individual's own experience, education, religious background, and similar factors. However, insular thinking can severely compromise sound judgment, so an active exploration and understanding of divergent views will remain the cornerstone of productive ethical discourse. After completing this chapter, the reader should have a deeper appreciation of why ethical dilemmas and controversies frequently have no "right" answers. Nonetheless, he or she should also have an idea about how to rationally approach the solution of ethical problems in health care in the context of one's own value system.

Balancing Organizational and Community Priorities

Representative Indictments

Health care in the United States is primarily crisis oriented, and the national debate over excessive costs, inequitable access and erratic quality will not be resolved in the predictable future. As noted by former Surgeon General Everett Koop (1992), "There is something terribly wrong with a system of health care that spends more and more money each year to provide less and less service for fewer people." Unfortunately, the present environment produces a remarkable array of competing interests that potentially compromise institutional and individual providers and, most important, patients.

Previous chapters have covered the major problems jeopardizing our health care organizations and the health of our communities, but reiterating five of them is still appropriate because each one has inescapable ethical implications.

1. Accelerating costs—since 1965 real wages and salaries (adjusted for inflation) have increased by approximately 7% while the cost of health care benefits has risen 450% (Schaeffer, 1996).
2. Inadequate access—our nation has no health care system; we have a disease care nonsystem, characterized accurately as "a paradox of excess and deprivation" (Enthoven & Kronick, 1989) with over 40 million uninsured.

3. Disparate quality—medication errors, nosocomial infections, and other iatrogenic incidents remain significant problems, as do indefensible variations in medical practice patterns, indicating that the most common surgical procedure in some parts of the country is still a "remunerectomy."
4. Medical arms race—our society's almost overwhelming bias toward technological rather than human intervention carries a huge financial and nonfinancial price tag.
5. Overemphasis on acute care—Americans' apparently insatiable appetite for medical services, in contrast to preventive care and health promotion programs, prompted the observation, "The vast majority of Americans are thoroughly spoiled; they abuse their bodies with too much food, drink, and tobacco, then expect miracle-making medics to make them well again, and if that doesn't work, they sue" (Katz, 1974).

Prevalence of Professional Hypocrisy

There are undeniable pressures on health care organizations to reduce expenses, improve productivity, enhance the quality of services and expand market share. The ultimate purpose is to strengthen and enlarge the organization. At first glance, this purpose seems irrefutably sound and logical, but bigger may not always be better for the community.

As hospitals convert from being revenue-generating centers in a fee-for-service environment to cost centers in a managed care environment, there is only now belated recognition that in many circumstances a patient's admission to the hospital represents a failure of the health care system. Historically, citing the number of hospital beds has been equivalent to politely announcing the CEO's economic worth; eventually, the figure will be identified as a liability.

At least part of the problem can be attributed to health care executives who "find themselves drifting between idealism and pragmatism, outwardly committed to a human service ideal yet conditioned by a survival mentality to favor the bottom line of financial well-being" (Levey & Hill, 1986, p. 226). Although hospital management's obsession with institutional survival may not be surprising, Derzon (1985) has legitimately observed that saying hospitals exist for the purpose of self-preservation is "the ultimate arrogance of an ego-centered organization." Too frequently, hospitals are accurately perceived as more concerned with their own well-being than with the community's.

Most health care organizations have created and disseminated a laudable set of vision, mission, and value statements. Facing unprecedented scrutiny by attorneys general and others, most nonprofit hospitals, which still represent over 80% of the nation's acute care institutions, have revised these statements to reflect an explicit commitment to provide community benefit. Unfortunately, this impressive rhetoric has rarely been matched by programmatic reality. There is commonly a regrettable dichotomy between what an organization espouses and what it actually does. Freed (1992, p. 19) has noted that "many hospitals are rediscovering values but have not yet converted entrenched attitudes and behaviors that publicly contradict these values. The result is a bizarre juxtaposition of conflicting proclamations and practices."

The same criticisms leveled at hospitals are also applicable to other health care organizations. Home health agencies, skilled nursing facilities, ambulatory surgery centers, and other institutional providers, as well as health plans and individual practitioners, have been buffeted by accusations of insensitivity to the public's welfare. For example, the cover story of one publication asked, "Has Managed Care Lost Its Soul?" (Greene, 1997).

Illustrations of Incompatible Institutional and Public Interests

A number of years ago, I asked that a survey include the question, "What do you consider the single most significant ethical problem that you face in your role as a health care executive?" There was remarkable similarity in the kind of responses received. The following three answers capture the conundrum faced by these individuals.

1. "The conflict between individual and societal values and needs versus organizational values and needs."
2. "Having a mission to improve the overall health of the community but being very happy when the hospital is 90% occupied."
3. "Do I do what is right for the community or for my hospital? Usually they are the same, but can the community afford what I think they should have? Or should I deliver what they say they want, but they really don't want to pay for?" (Foubert, 1992).

Despite the ideal goal of always pursuing programs that will first meet the community's needs, differences between an organization's best interests and those of the public are sometimes irreconcilable. Typical institutional priorities usually include maximizing income-generating services and avoiding the creation of programs that might be deficit producing. At one time or another, most health care executives have considered reducing or eliminating services not financially self-sustaining but needed by the community.

Confronting and resolving such difficult resource allocation decisions in an ethically sensitive manner carries both personal and organizational risks. At a time when there is massive excess hospital bed capacity and, in some communities, excess facilities, it is still unlikely to find many hospital executives promoting institutional euthanasia, unless it is for their competitor's organization.

Guidelines for Serving and Competing Ethically

Competition in health care is not inherently harmful. The fundamental ethical imperative is to think as imaginatively about optimizing its virtues as those who, intentionally or unintentionally, seek to pervert them. Five guidelines for serving and competing ethically should be considered.

1.   Establish generic criteria that will guide decision making. For example, every decision should be morally and legally defensible, responsive to the organization's mission and values, and sensitive to the needs of key constituencies, including patients, staff, payers, health plan members, and the community. It is also essential to recognize that the legally defensible nature of an action may not make it ethically acceptable (e.g., discontinuing an immunization program due to inadequate funding).

2.   Apply the criteria consistently. When resources are adequate, when controversy is absent, when there is no sense of great urgency, and when neither ambiguity nor ambivalence exist, decisions may still be hard, but acting ethically when it is merely convenient is hardly sufficient. It is precisely during periods of limited resources, conflicting opinions, severe time constraints, and significant uncertainty that expedient exceptions that violate the criteria are likely to be made and rationalized.

3.   Using the criteria, perform a comprehensive ethics audit of policies, procedures, and activities in areas with particular sensitivity to organizational values and ethics. These areas could include uncompensated care, access to and levels of care; necessity and appropriateness of care; advertising; release of clinical and other data; conflict-of-interest documents; purchasing, contracting, and vendor relations; and joint ventures.

4.   Take formal steps to ensure that the criteria, along with the institution's mission, vision and value statements, are familiar to every staff member. No one individual, such as the CEO, should be the organization's conscience; the broader the dissemination and understanding of these documents, the more likely will be the adherence to their content.

5.   Anticipate and mitigate any potential toxic effects of competitive strategies and tactics. Until and unless the question is asked about the possible adverse impact of these plans, especially on the most politically impotent and most vulnerable members of the community, a genuine moral analysis will be incomplete.

After 2 years of study and four major conferences, the Woodstock Theological Center published *Ethical Considerations in the Business Aspects of Health Care* (1995). This document was unique because it represented a consensus of a diverse group of health care specialists, physicians, nurses, hospital executives, ethicists, policymakers, academic policy analysts, and religious leaders. Three interrelated responsibilities of health professionals were delineated. These included "to attend to the health needs of the individuals in the communities they serve, . . . to administer and use wisely the physical, technological, financial, and human resources available to health care professionals," and to provide for "continued education, research, and scientific advancement so that the quality of care available for patients, and the efficacy and efficiency with which resources are used in that care, can be improved over time" (p. 9). Given the kinds of "issues, dilemmas, pressures, temptations, and constraints" faced by health care professionals, the participants identified the following attitudes and principles as the basis for making ethical decisions:

- compassion and respect for human dignity
- commitment to professional competence
- commitment to a spirit of service
- honesty
- confidentiality
- good stewardship and careful administration

The Woodstock publication also produced a practical checklist of questions that health care providers can pose to themselves as they confront ethical problems that occur in the business aspects of their profession. Consequently, its contents have relevance for each topic covered in this chapter, including the challenging issue of managed care.

Contending with Managed Care's Conflicting Incentives

Bright and Dark Sides of Managed Care

Managed care, in the view of some observers, "has come to the fore in the medical landscape with such rapidity, vigor, and nearly evangelical zeal that startled witnesses to the transformation have reacted with awe and outrage" (Zoloth-Dorfman & Rubin, 1995, p. 339). In the popular rush to criticize health maintenance organizations (HMOs) and other managed care organizations, many of their ethical attributes are ignored or minimized. Indeed, there are clear advantages not only from the purchaser's perspective but also from the viewpoint of providers and patients.

- Purchasers benefit from the lower utilization and cost of health care services. In addition, expenditures are generally more predictable and consistent. Furthermore, managed care has promoted the production of more data on provider performance. Increasingly, providers will be obligated to disclose information on clinical outcomes as well as expenses.
- Institutional providers benefit because there are more powerful incentives available to encourage reductions in (a) the excessive utilization of services and (b) inappropriate variations in medical practice patterns. Primary care physicians have an expanded role and receive more financial recognition for their responsibilities.
- Patients benefit because managed care encourages the provision of more disease prevention and health promotion services. Patients should also be at an advantage through having access to potentially higher quality and more appropriate care as a result of a reduced number of inefficient, unnecessary and previously overpriced medical and hospital services.

Periodically, the value of managed care seems overwhelmed by its dark side. According to an editorial in the *New England Journal of Medicine*, some managed care plans "cut costs by recruiting the healthiest patients, excluding the sickest, rationing care by making it inconvenient to obtain and denying care by a variety of mechanisms" (Kassirer, 1995, p. 50). At a minimum, critics contend that managed care

- provides incentives for limiting legitimately needed services;
- causes anxiety and inconvenience to patients;
- excludes competent providers;
- denies reimbursement for potentially lifesaving treatment;
- generates excessive administrative burdens for practitioners and hospitals;
- restricts patient choice of providers;
- permits nonphysicians to exercise inappropriate influence over medical decisions;
- rewards primary care physicians for referring patients to specialists too often or too rarely, depending upon capitated risk pool configurations;
- creates a variety of other financial conflicts of interest for providers; and
- expects physician gatekeepers to serve as agents of social justice, rather than unequivocal patient advocates. The physician's loyalty could be divided by the patient's individual needs, the needs of all patients served by the system, the health plan's economic directives, and the physician's own self-interests.

Problems Created by Demonizing Managed Care

The invariably emotional content of the managed care debate, with its detractors' list of indictments, usually accompanied by case examples, can easily create the illusion that managed care represents all that is negative about the U.S. health care delivery system. Authors have written about the souls of physicians being at stake (Auerback, 1994), "disposable doctors" because of economic incentives to abuse physician peer review and deselect ones who are generating high costs (Fielder, 1995), patients becoming commodities (Zoloth-Dorfman & Rubin, 1995), and managed care plans encouraging the "ruthless pursuit of economic efficiency" (Chervenak & McCullough, 1995).

Too quickly, however, we forget fee-for-service was no "ethical Garden of Eden" (Enthoven, 1996). Few would deny fee-for-service and charge-based reimbursement have created powerful incentives for overtreatment. This payment system helped produce a demand for medical services that was essentially cost-unconscious. The assertion that managed care provides incentives for undertreatment may be valid, but conveniently leaving the impression that the conventional indemnity form of reimbursement was pure and virtuous does not contribute to a constructive analysis of how to address the ethical concerns associated with managed care.

Steps to Minimize Ethical Liabilities

The Midwest Bioethics Center (1995) has developed an extensive list of health care provider responsibilities, including respecting member rights, disclosing noncovered treatment options, giving priority to clinical and scientific information over financial data, maintaining confidentiality, treating members without regard to reducing the provider's financial exposure or maximizing the provider's financial gain, and speaking out and resisting when unethical practices are being pursued by peers, purchasers, or the plan.

These are only some of the recommendations proposed by a variety of organizations, ethicists, and others. For example, the Institute on Quality of Care and Patterns of Practice, sponsored by the AHA's Hospital Research and Educational Trust, has published a guide for hospitals, *Managing Risks and Quality in Hospital-Related Managed Care* (1991); the AMA's Council on Ethical and Judicial Affairs has issued a report, "Ethical Issues in Managed Care" (1995); the Pew Health Professions Commission has published *Health Professions Education and Managed Care: Challenges and Necessary Responses* (1995); and two Catholic health systems produced *Ethical Guidelines for Managed Care Contract Negotiations* (Eastern Mercy Health System, 1995). These important contributions have been supplemented by constructive suggestions offered by highly respected bioethicists, including Pellegrino (1995) on the resolution of conflicts of interest and Emmanuel (1995) on the need for institutional structures to ensure ethical behavior under managed care.

According to a general overview summarizing the continuing controversy, ethical decision making and managed care aren't mutually exclusive, but "executives are struggling to find a common denominator" (Appleby, 1996). Minimizing managed care's ethical liabilities requires a collaborative effort among all the stakeholders. The most productive efforts will capitalize on previous work and develop creative strategies to engage health plan members as well as the medical and nonmedical professionals who have a vested interest in the outcome of deliberations. To a large degree, the fundamental issue will remain the same as it has been under fee-for-service: how can the needs of individual patients best be met while preserving sufficient resources to provide some minimum level of health service for everyone in the society as a whole?

Confronting Downsizing's Painful Dimensions

Common Reasons for Avoiding Timely Decisions

Despite massive excess hospital bed capacity, predicted to grow even more with declining admissions and shorter lengths of stay, there are four major reasons that steps to reduce staffing are not taken in a timely manner.

1. Procrastination often occurs because budget projections are usually optimistic. Revenue is expected to be higher because admissions may increase and/or the payer mix will improve, or better reimbursement rates will be negotiated. If revenue improves, then one can avoid submitting a proposal for substantial rate increases to cover the next fiscal year's expense and capital budgets.

2. If revenue is accurately predicted, there may be a tendency to overestimate the organization's ability to decrease costs without layoffs. It is assumed that sufficient expenses can be reduced through attrition (not filling some positions when they become open), increased productivity, less consumption of supplies, delaying capital equipment purchases, outsourcing selected services through contract management at a lower cost, deferring or limiting merit pay adjustments, freezing or reducing salaries and benefits, and encouraging early employee retirement.

3. Historically, many organizations have prided themselves on never having laid off employees. The conventional understanding has been that if you are a competent and conscientious staff member and a recipient of consistently good

performance reviews, you can be assured job security. Executives are predictably reluctant to violate an implicit commitment to loyal and capable employees.

4. Taking the initiative to design and implement a program to achieve a significant reduction in staff is difficult and painful. No one is going to be eager about undertaking such a program, nor should they be expected to approach the assignment with enthusiasm. Indeed, it is a task seldom performed without considerable anguish and distress. Consequently, the tendency to delay taking action is rationalized easily because the alternative is so discomforting.

Financial and Nonfinancial Costs of Procrastination

The repercussions of not taking timely action should be self-evident, but because procrastination occurs so often, they deserve reference. First, conditions almost always deteriorate further. Second, since delaying intervention can exacerbate the situation, corrective action, when it does occur, becomes more severe. Third, management credibility is compromised because problems associated with excess staff and expenses cannot be kept secret; employees and physicians are not naive, and management's failure to address the challenge will be recognized. Fourth, some of the best employees may leave—they will be able to find other jobs more easily than marginally competent personnel.

Advantages of Taking Decisive Action

Prompt action, if exercised correctly, should reduce the organization's financial exposure and minimize the number of actual layoffs. Downsizing may demonstrate proper leadership, but it rarely will be applauded by anyone. Nonetheless, taking decisive action can shorten the period of organizational uncertainty and employee anxiety generated by the inevitable rumors, which seem to grow in volume and magnitude when nothing is done. Finally, the likelihood of retaining the institution's best employees is increased if the process proceeds in a timely and orderly manner.

Suggestions for Demonstrating Ethical Sensitivity

Eight suggestions are offered to convey genuine ethical sensitivity in confronting downsizing's painful dimensions.

1. Develop policies and procedures in advance of needing to implement them to mitigate hardship and stress.

2. Demonstrate consistency between formally stated organizational values and those reflected in downsizing and severance policy documents.
3. Provide timely, accurate, clear, and consistent information to the organization.
4. Support employees whose positions have been eliminated through retraining and redeployment if possible.
5. Design appropriate outplacement assistance and severance benefits for laid-off employees.
6. Address frequently underestimated needs of remaining staff by anticipating feelings of loss, anger, and guilt, as well as anxiety about further changes in workload assignments and additional layoffs.
7. Take action to assure that quality of patient care is not compromised before, during, or after downsizing occurs.
8. Consider what types of communication should be provided to external constituencies to retain or regain a positive community image.

Despite good intentions and careful planning, downsizing will never be painless, nor should it be. Although advice is available from various sources (Bell, 1995; Greene, 1996; Hofmann, 1996; Moore, 1995; Yehle, 1995), it is still unusual to find detailed descriptions about actual cases with a candid discussion of what went well and where mistakes were made. Sharing these kinds of insights can be invaluable, and when such disclosures are made (Rudnick, 1995), they deserve sincere praise.

Recognizing Current and Future Dilemmas of Medical Rationing

Examples of Current Rationing

The allocation of resources, the development of a just health care delivery system, and the adjudication of the rights and claims of different competing groups, according to former Hastings Center president Daniel Callahan (1990), "are and will be the important moral problems of the future." However, the debate over rationing should not be over whether or not to ration medical care. Rationing occurs now, usually silently, insidiously, sporadically, and arbitrarily.

There is a deliberate limitation of potentially beneficial services based on a wide array of factors. Dougherty (1991) has provided an excellent, albeit disturbing, overview of how medical care is currently rationed.

It is rationed on the basis of ability to pay in the open market and on the basis of age in the Medicare program. It is rationed on the basis of income, marital status, and the having of dependent children in the Medicaid program. Access to private health insurance is rationed on the basis of employment and by history of illness. Healthcare is rationed on the basis of race and location by the Indian Health Service and on the basis of military service by the Veterans Administration. It is rationed on the basis of insurance status and on the basis of provider charity for those who are medically indigent. Healthcare is rationed on the basis of geography for those in rural America and inner cities. And it is rationed on the basis of luck—bad luck—for the millions of American children born into uninsured families, the majority of which are headed by an adult working full-time. (p. 35)

He could have added that it is also rationed by type of disease and length of disability, as exemplified by Medicare coverage for patients with end-stage renal disease and others who have been disabled for a minimum of 2 years. Former Colorado governor Richard Lamm (1994, p. 59) summarizes the fundamental problem by noting, "We rationed people out of the system by not providing universal coverage."

Although the vast majority of rationing has been unsystematic and seemingly capricious, the Oregon Health Plan has represented a conscious effort to allocate limited resources on a methodical basis. Promoted by John Kitzhaber, a physician and the president of the Oregon Senate who subsequently was elected governor, the 1988 legislation had its origin in discussions initiated by Oregon Health Decisions, a group established in 1981 to address health care's moral and economic issues (Munson, 1992). Under the law, each Medicaid-covered service is ranked according to the cost of the service, the number of people who would be helped by it, and the length of time a patient could be expected to remain healthy after treatment. Implementation of the legislation was extensively delayed because, as a program jointly funded by the states and the federal government, a waiver of certain federal regulations was required to authorize such a significant change. Not until February 1994 was the program actually begun. As expected, by using money saved through limiting Medicaid care to a prioritized list of services, basic medical care was extended to over 100,000 more Oregonians living below the federal poverty level ("Why Rationing Was Right," 1997). Nonetheless, the principal criticism of the rationing plan has not been resolved: it is unfair because medical care is rationed only to the poor, not to everyone (Munson, 1992). And yet some might argue that the poor are not entitled to the same level of health care or the same choices among various options as are those who can afford to pay for more services. Indeed, people who have the financial means will always be able to obtain additional services—if necessary, going outside the system or the country to acquire treatment.

Crucial Questions

Given that health care is, clearly in practice if not in policy, rationed pervasively now, four questions should be addressed to deal with the issue in a more ethical manner. Three of these questions have been identified by Fuchs (1990): Who will ration? Who will be rationed? What will be rationed? The fourth is, how will services be rationed? Each question must be answered, but not in a vacuum. Loewy (1996) properly notes:

> Important as medical care is, it is nonetheless not the most critical problem: in a country in which a third of children (and about half of African American children) are hungry, in which poverty is growing, in which homelessness is rampant, and in which a lack of education stunts many lives, healthcare is an issue that must be seen embedded in these other social ills. (p. 567)

Indeed, it cannot be overemphasized that genetics, the environment, and lifestyle have a far more profound influence on health status than does medical care. Furthermore, the rationing of medical care must be considered in the context of allocating resources among other competing requirements, such as education, crime prevention, housing, national defense, and welfare.

Relevant Ethical Principles

Applying four classic bioethical principles can help ensure implementation of a just and effective public policy on health care rationing. Although these principles are normally considered in making clinical decisions, they have direct relevance to the broader question of how best to allocate limited resources. The significance of each principle will be noted, but perhaps their general utility should be acknowledged; they constitute an initial set of criteria for judging the relative merit of formal rationing proposals. Consequently, proposal proponents and opponents can apply them to test and argue the ethical legitimacy of their respective positions.

Respect for Autonomy. For the debate on rationing to be meaningful, it must be conducted in a way that respects and promotes participant autonomy. Those involved in the rationing debate must be competent and informed, must understand the issues, must enter the debate voluntarily, and must authorize the policymakers to arrive at a position on the topic.

Respect for the autonomy of those affected by rationing decisions makes public education on the issues essential. Without disclosure of the economic pressures and other factors that explain why finite resources cannot accommodate infinite expectations, citizens will neither understand the predicament nor be competent to participate in the decision-making process. Furthermore, given the American form of government, organized, legislatively authorized, legally regulated rationing will not succeed unless it is accepted voluntarily and authorized through the democratic process.

However, although ethical and successful rationing will largely depend on extensive public input, unconditional adherence to the principle of autonomy is unrealistic. Unencumbered individual freedom is unsustainable when limitations are imposed, regardless of how democratically the development and implementation processes are designed. Indeed, unless personal choices are constrained, rationing will not and cannot occur; and unless social goods are distributed more equitably, the common good will not be served. Ultimately, an ethically sensitive rationing system will be overt, reflect broad societal involvement, and promote public understanding and support.

Beneficence. Beneficence can be defined as acting with charity and kindness, but this definition is inadequate. Inherent in the term is an active promotion of actions to benefit others. Also implicit is a duty both to provide benefits and to balance benefits and potential harms. One of the immense difficulties in developing an acceptable rationing system is determining its proper balance. If we cannot decide how to achieve maximum benefits within a clear set of formally accepted goals, true beneficence will be unachievable. Mere rhetoric and commitment to act are not sufficient to satisfy this principle.

Nonmaleficence. The principle of nonmaleficence prohibits doing harm to others. Although the principle appears self-explanatory, rationing leads inevitably to withholding potentially beneficial services (and thus doing harm), so an appreciation for the concept of double effect is especially important. According to Beauchamp and Childress (1989), four conditions must be satisfied for an act with both a good and a bad effect to be justified:

1. The action itself, independent of its consequence, must not be intrinsically wrong; it must be morally good or at least morally neutral.
2. The agent must intend only the good effect and not the bad effect. The bad effect can be foreseen, tolerated, and permitted but must not be intended; it is therefore allowed but not sought.
3. The bad effect must not be a means to the end of bringing about the good effect; that is, the good effect must be achieved directly by the action and not by the way of the bad effect.
4. The good result must outweigh the evil permitted; there must be proportionality or a favorable balance between the good and bad effects of the action.

These four conditions illustrate the most challenging paradox in complying with the principle of nonmaleficence in rationing health care services. Depending on whether one insists that all four be satisfied or places more emphasis on intentionality or proportionality, it is possible to defend or criticize the various decisions involved in rationing. Nonetheless, struggling with the conflict of reconciling competing values and obligations is an inescapable responsibility in designing an allocation process.

Justice. No other principle of bioethics is more relevant to a discussion of rationing than that of justice. Three major theories of justice have been identified:

- egalitarian theories, which emphasize "equal access to the goods in life that every rational person desires (often invoking the material criterion of need as well as equality)";
- libertarian theories, which stress "rights to social and economic liberty (invoking fair procedures and systems rather than substantive outcomes)"; and
- utilitarian theories, which emphasize "a mixture of criteria so that public utility is maximized." (Beauchamp & Childress, 1989, p. 265)

An egalitarian form of rationing would demand that both economic and noneconomic barriers to basic health services be eliminated. To the extent access to these services is defined as a right, rather than a privilege, egalitarians would insist that personal income, preexisting conditions, employment status, and other variables no longer influence availability of care to those in need.

In contrast, libertarians would view almost any form of rationing with deep reservations if there were significant restrictions on individual prerogatives. Personal freedom, economic efficiency, and an unfettered marketplace would be considered central elements of a libertarian approach to rationing. At a minimum, justice would require agreement among those whose resources were subject to redistribution to benefit the common good.

The utilitarian model has dominated the traditional decision-making process. However, although it advocates the greatest good for the greatest number, it does not guide the distribution of resources. Distribution not only should reflect fairness, it should also consider the legacy of previous inequities. Consequently, justice mandates a close examination of the "moral traces" remaining from past practices of discrimination.

Any dispassionate analysis of how resources have been allocated historically must conclude that such moral traces are ubiquitous. This assessment is consistent with Werhane's (1990) assertion that

> a form of economic egoism has corrupted the health care system, replacing the caring and professional models with that of competing self-interests, encouraging greed, confusing professional interests with profit, depersonalizing patient relationships, diluting benevolence and charity with a concern for economic viability, and thus excluding those who cannot afford health care from the system. (p. 8)

Obstacles and Opportunities

The largest obstacle to the institution of organized health care rationing to replace the random rationing we have presently is the absence of political will. Even raising the issue is considered politically unhealthy, primarily because there is a denial of the need to ration by society at large. This denial is grounded in the naive assumption that savings achieved by reducing excessive administrative costs, unnecessary surgery, defensive medicine, inappropriate variations (geographic and otherwise) in medical practice patterns, and unhealthy behavior will be more than adequate to cover the cost of providing comprehensive medical services to everyone. However, all these efforts combined will not be enough to fund every American's almost insatiable appetite for medical care.

Physicians themselves constitute another barrier. Understandably, as emphasized by Veatch (1991), they view themselves as patient advocates and resent any attempt to force them to perform as conscious de facto rationing agents, even though many are implicitly performing this function now. But Veatch (1986, p. 38) goes a step further by indicating that asking physicians to be cost-conscious would be expecting them to abandon their central commitment to their patients. He says such a request is tantamount to having physicians remove the Hippocratic oath from their waiting room walls and replace it with a sign that reads, "Warning all ye who enter here. I will generally work for your rights and welfare, but if benefits to you are marginal and costs are great, I will abandon you to protect society." This position is interpreted as extreme by some commentators who believe physicians have an important contribution to make to the allocation process (Callahan, 1991; Hitt, 1991; Hofmann, 1991).

Ironically, the opportunity to initiate rationing may be easier as part of a public policy process in contrast to rationing by health care providers. Policymakers have the "luxury" of constructing programs for people who are largely anonymous and invisible. Consequently, it is less painful to deal with statistics rather than identified lives. Lantos (1996) is particularly effective in illustrating this point.

> The present system is unjust in many ways. Resources are devoted to one patient which do little good, while they could go to many other patients and do more good. We are drawn to the identifiable patient, and make exorbitant expenditures to save individuals but cannot make investments that are statistically wiser. We make analogies to the sailor lost at sea or the child who falls down a well, arguing that in such cases, no expense should be saved. And yet, as medicine goes today, hundreds are lost at sea everyday. We are all going to fall down wells. (p. 491)

The Oregon Health Plan has succeeded, at least in part, because the rationing decisions have been at a policy level, which is largely impersonal and shielded from the plight of specific patients. Regardless of future policy decisions reducing the macro-allocation of resources, actions by individual clinicians complicate adherence to such policies; the "rule of rescue" will always dictate a moral response to the imminence of death by rescuing the patient (Jonsen, 1986). As Loewy (1996) acknowledges, "Physicians who are told that they must hew to their obligation to do all they can for their particular patient but are also told that they must simultaneously conserve communal resources are being given a set of internally contradictory instructions" (p. 566). Reconciling these disparate positions will remain central to confronting this complex ethical dilemma. Because we are dealing with conflicting values, duties, and obligations, absolute certainty about the most virtuous course of action becomes especially elusive.

Supporting the Provision of Unlimited Care

Unlimited Care as an Ethical Imperative

Because it is generally conceded that resources are finite, few people believe we can afford to provide unlimited care. We must realize, however, that there is a difference between unlimited care and unlimited treatment. This difference is not simply a semantic quibble. Health care professionals can be criticized for caring too little for patients and treating too much. Real caring often means choosing not to perform invasive diagnostic and therapeutic procedures that extend the dying process instead of improving life (Danforth, 1996). However, the challenge is made even more complicated by the difficulty of determining what constitutes futile treatment. Even the meaning of *futility* is exceptionally controversial and value-laden (Schneiderman & Jecker, 1995; Truog, Brett, & Frader, 1992). Thanks in part to Americans' love affair with technology, death is now viewed as optional—something that can be prevented or delayed indefinitely with the proper medical procedure. Bresnahan (1989) warned against finding ourselves "carried along toward moral disaster by the impersonal momentum of our noble discoveries."

Some patients now increasingly fear becoming the victims of technology rather than its beneficiaries. Because death has become so "medicalized," assisted suicide has gained unprecedented attention (Bennahum, 1996; Capron, 1996; Koch, 1996), and it is not only physicians whose roles are being examined but also those of nurses (Asch, 1996). Regardless of one's personal view of this complex issue, there is increasing agreement that the needs of terminally ill patients for supportive care are not met adequately. Despite the passage of the Patient Self-Determination Act in 1990, there is well-documented evidence that advance directives, such as a living will and/or durable power of attorney for health care, are frequently ignored (Wenger et al., 1996). Consequently, perhaps nothing less than a fundamental change in this country's culture of dying may be required (O'Connell, 1996).

Financial and Nonfinancial Costs of Overtreatment

Indisputably, the costs of overtreatment are both financial and nonfinancial. The ramifications of this quandary have been eloquently described by Bayer (1984).

> The advance of modern medicine in the past two decades has forced on society a set of dilemmas that until recently might have been relegated to fantasy. Now, lives of those who would have been given up for lost are saved. Babies so premature or defective that death would have been the certain end of very brief lives can be treated. And older persons whose vital organs fail can be kept alive with the assistance of mechanical devices or through the transplantation of donated body parts. Yet, the advances of medical technology and knowledge come at a moment when the finitude of resources has become an undeniable reality. Here, then, is the ultimate irony. Now that medical prospects are virtually limitless, resources are not. (p. 22)

More than 10 years ago, over $7 billion in Medicare funds were being consumed annually on terminally ill patients who were within 40 days of death ("Society Urged," 1987), but who is qualified to judge which patients should have received less treatment? The debate has no predictable conclusion, and an exploration of the topic's ethical dimensions will find no simple solutions. Although Americans will remain uncomfortable about examining decisions near the end of life, one notable advantage of the "death with dignity" movement is the greater level and intensity of public discourse. For example, the popularity of *How We Die: Reflections on Life's Final Chapter* (Nuland, 1994) indicates that death, once largely suppressed as a topic, has become an acceptable, albeit still painful, subject for conversation.

Methods of Effective Advocacy for Patient Values

With relatively few exceptions, there is one bioethical principle that should dominate a discussion of promoting unlimited care. Autonomy not only permits but mandates that priority be given to the patient's values. Here the emphasis is properly placed on the wishes of the individual patient, not those of the family nor those of the physician or nurses. In situations where patients are no longer capable of participating actively in decisions affecting their care, the unintentional problems created by countertransference should not be underestimated. This occurs when individual health care providers identify with their patients, assume that they share the same values, and believe that they, as "professionals," know what is in the patients' best interests (Rogers, Field, & Kunkel, 1995).

To guide hospitals in allocating institutional resources in an ethically sensitive manner that also protects patient values, 10 steps have been suggested (Hofmann, 1992):

1. Recognize the strengths and weaknesses of advance directives. Special consideration should be given to asking patients how strictly they want their directives followed and what factors should be evaluated in making treatment decisions.
2. Minimize intervention by the legal system. There is general agreement that decisions should be made closest to the bedside to best reflect the patient's preferences.
3. Reexamine intensive care unit admission and discharge policies. Although the JCAHO requires that all special care units have such policies, many physicians will confirm that patients are occasionally admitted to the unit or remain without legitimate clinical justification.
4. Evaluate compliance with the hospital's do-not-resuscitate (DNR) policy. Mandated by the JCAHO, a DNR policy can be invaluable in promoting timely discussions about a patient's or family's preferences in making decisions near the end of life. However, the policy might also identify those circumstances when such a discussion would not be necessary or appropriate.
5. Monitor referrals from skilled nursing facilities (SNFs) to the hospital. Periodically, to avoid the process involved in dealing with a terminally ill patient, the patient's family and official agencies, an SNF may unilaterally transfer such a patient to a hospital through the emergency department. Almost without exception, this type of transfer does not benefit the patient and consumes needless resources.
6. Establish a biweekly report of all inpatients whose hospital charges exceed an arbitrary figure, e.g., $50,000 or $100,000. The content should include the patient's name, date of admission, hospital location, attending physician, diagnosis, age, anticipated date of discharge, accumulated charges, and expected reimbursement. This type of report can assist the CEO and medical director in reviewing atypical cases as a supplement to the institution's standard concurrent utilization management activities conducted by other staff.
7. Collaborate closely with and support actively local hospice programs. If the hospital does not sponsor its own program and services are unavailable or inadequate, serious consideration should be given to addressing the need for an appropriate system for providing care to terminally ill patients.
8. Conduct periodic ethical and economic grand rounds. Specific cases should be analyzed at both clinical department meetings and general education programs conducted by the medical staff. The hospital's ethics subcommittee on education can be assigned responsibility for coordinating forums on ethical issues.
9. Capitalize on the advice and assistance available through the institution's ethics committee or ethics consultation service. The American Hospital Association recently updated its 1984 guidelines on ethics committees to reinforce the value and importance of this resource.

10. Involve not only the ethics committee in developing and reviewing major policies affecting decisions near the end of life but also the governing body, which may not be represented on the committee. Given the sensitive and sometimes controversial issues that must be covered by such policies, the knowledge and support of the hospital's trustees could be very helpful. (pp. 234–235)

Promoting Ethical Behavior

Importance of Reconciling Individual and Organizational Obligations

Achieving and maintaining a proper balance of personal and professional commitments is an admittedly difficult but essential prerequisite to coping successfully with omnipresent time constraints. Personal and family needs will always compete with job-related requirements. Inevitably, balancing individual and organizational priorities will create enormous pressures to accommodate competing demands by making compromises. The ultimate objective is to make these compromises without jeopardizing relationships or responsibilities.

It could be argued that pressures in health care organizations are really not so different than in other business. Regardless of one's role, everyone is dealing, to some degree, with competing claims and obligations. Griffith (1993) and Worthley (1997) are among those who discuss some of the unique characteristics of health care requiring special attention. Luthringer (1991) provides a useful perspective by noting:

> The legitimate claims of vulnerable patients, demanding caregivers, harried colleagues, and neglected friends or family are often entangled in a daunting variety of perspectives about how the moral choices between acknowledged duties are to be analyzed. Should the concern be with character or conduct, with rules or responsibilities, with individual needs or uniform treatment, with maximum benefit or minimal coercion? (p. 99)

The high expectations placed on health care professionals, including those that are self-imposed, can exacerbate the challenge to find and sustain a reasonable equilibrium. Professionals are presumed to "lead lives that embody an exemplary system of values and ethics" (American College of Healthcare Executives, 1995). This type of performance standard requires ethical behavior both on and off the job.

There are a variety of personal and organizational warning indicators that can be monitored to detect existing or potential problems. The answers to three sets of questions could suggest when and where remedial action may be necessary (Hofmann, 1994):

1. Am I eating properly, getting adequate rest and sufficient exercise, setting realistic expectations, and fostering supportive interpersonal relationships? Vitality, physical as well as mental, is an undeniable prerequisite and ongoing necessity to sustain an appropriate balance.
2. Am I sensitive to emotional as well as physical warning signs of imbalance—not only in myself but in others? Am I willing to seek assistance? Healthcare organizations should provide access to counseling and other services to assist staff in addressing problems that adversely affect job performance.
3. Do I resolve conflicts quickly? Honesty, commitment, trust, understanding, and accommodation are among the many attributes required to achieve timely conflict resolution. (p. 42)

Value of an Ethics Audit

Performing ethics audits is another strategy to evaluate individual and organizational conformance with ethical standards. Although all health care professionals and their organizations would benefit by conducting an ethics audit, evidence of any of the following developments could reflect a special need:

- allegations regarding conflicts of interest
- increase in employee grievances, resignations, terminations, or wrongful discharge complaints
- deterioration in staff opinion survey results
- rise in patient complaints, incident reports, and legal actions
- adverse articles about the organization
- problems with suppliers and other vendors

There are two types of ethics audits that are appropriate. The first focuses on the individual and the second on the organization. An ethics self-assessment survey should promote personal reflection about a variety of critical ethical issues and, in the process, raise the respondents' sensitivity to the ethical implications of their actions. A well-constructed tool will be designed to evaluate actual behavior as well as intent. Following completion, the respondents should have a comprehensive understanding of areas where they are on strong ethical ground and other areas where they may want to examine the bases for their responses. Such a self-assessment document has been developed by the American College of Healthcare Executives (1997).

An organizational ethics audit, like the "Integrity Audit" created by White (1990), serves several purposes. These include

- providing a profile of specific ethical strengths and weaknesses;
- constructing a baseline measure for use in determining progress over time;
- measuring actual practices against established norms; and
- comparing the organization's profile with composite data from firms with reputations for integrity and success.

In recognition that hospitals are confronting unrelenting and intensifying competitive pressures, the American Hospital Association (AHA; 1997) designed a special assessment tool for hospitals. The purpose was "to reach beyond bioethical, medical and clinical ethics to focus on those business and organizational issues which help forge the vital relationship of trust—between healthcare providers and all those they serve." The five-part document incorporates questions asking about (1) written statements of ethical principles, policies, and procedures; (2) activities such as training programs, employee communications regarding organizational ethics, and formal processes to report inappropriate conduct; (3) committees and positions/offices responsible for ethics matters; (4) ethical obligations to the community and the institution's mission, vision, and values; and (5) significant ethical challenges facing the organization.

The best time to conduct an ethics audit will always be when no apparent crisis exists. In fact, one of the primary objectives of performing an audit is to identify potential difficulties and to address them before they become serious problems. To date, ethics audits in health care organizations have not been common, and there have been no reports on their benefits and costs. The AHA initiative is intended to encourage activity that should produce such reports.

Requirements of Ethical Behavior

As noted previously, behaving ethically when merely convenient is not sufficient. The complex environment in which health care professionals must function almost conspires to force them to take actions that do not allow for careful, reflective thought about the ethical implications of their decisions. As a result, they may cope with misgivings by rationalizing that expediency simply could not accommodate a more deliberative process.

Because ethical decision making is rarely self-evident, at least four traits should be considered in judging someone's actions.

- The first is *ethical consciousness*, which is demonstrated by continuing sensitivity to the ethical consequences of daily actions. Many health care professionals fail to apply consistently their moral convictions to routine as well as nonroutine decisions, and they may not even be aware that their actions have ethical ramifications.

- The second is *ethical competency*. It is not enough to be ethically conscious unless an individual demonstrates an actual understanding of what constitutes ethical behavior. One indication of this trait would be a genuine recognition of the fallacy, "if it's legal, it's ethical."
- The third is *ethical commitment*—"a strong desire to act ethically, to do the right thing, especially when ethics imposes financial, social or psychological costs", (Josephson, 1989, p. 6). Such a commitment suggests ethical behavior is more apparent when the choices are most onerous.
- The fourth is *ethical courage*, exhibited by a willingness to move beyond the desire or intent to take action. Commitment is meaningless unless it is implemented.

The misconception that adherence to legal standards is an adequate test of ethical behavior deserves further elaboration. Walters (1988) writes, "Human beings cannot carry on the ordinary affairs of life in a moral vacuum; they have duties—some of which are legal, others of which are ethical, and some, though not all, of which are both" (pp. 127–128). As a four-word description of ethical behavior, obedience to the unenforceable acknowledges that one can be unethical without violating the law. An eloquent distinction between complying with minimal legal requirements and fulfilling a higher obligation was expressed by Solzhenitsyn (1978) in his remarks to Harvard's graduating class.

A society based on the letter of the law and never reaching any higher, fails to take advantage of the full range of human possibilities. The letter of the law is too cold and formal to have a beneficial influence on society. Whenever the tissue of life is woven of legalistic relationships, this creates an atmosphere of spiritual mediocrity that paralyses [a person's] noblest impulses. (p. 17)

It is also crucial that attention not be devoted exclusively to provocative ethical problems. A philosophy professor (Sommers, 1993) has lamented that students taking college ethics are debating abortion, censorship, euthanasia, and capital punishment while learning almost nothing about decency, honesty, personal responsibility, or honor. She said topics such as hypocrisy, self-deception, cruelty, and selfishness rarely are raised. The traditional concentration of most ethics courses on dilemmas and "hard cases" has fostered, in her view, unintentional attitudes of moral agnosticism and skepticism. By concentrating primarily on controversial issues and problems, the false impression could be left that there are no ethical "truths."

Regardless of the business enterprise, health care professionals rely on relationships based on authority, trust, and integrity. To a large degree, ethical behavior is about each of these and the obligation not to abuse or corrupt them.

Conclusions

Given the volatile and frenetic nature of today's competitive health care environment, the number and magnitude of ethical issues will certainly continue to grow. Because Americans' expectations of what medical science can deliver are frequently unrealistic, they are rarely satisfied. The innumerable political, cultural, and financial influences on the configuration of these services will, and should, stir passionate debate about the most appropriate alignment of resources to address this demand.

Formal and informal interest groups will promote their causes with varying degrees of effectiveness. Usually, such advocates have the advantage of taking no responsibility for identifying a better alternative. By passionately arguing their case, they can claim the "ethical superiority of the uninvolved" (Pastin, 1986). Nonetheless, real ethical dilemmas usually have no "right" answers. Thus, it is unrealistic to presume that the ideal solution will always be found if the search is prolonged. The struggle demands not a blind application of moral precepts but an approach permitting people to reach decisions that reflect compassion, respect justice, and recognize human fallibility.

Mini-Case Study

Faced with declining patient days and lower reimbursement rates, you are considering a variety of options to improve the hospital's net income by $1 million. Because all other reasonable steps have been taken to increase revenue and reduce expenses, none of the remaining alternatives is attractive. Among the possibilities are the following:

- Eliminate the obstetrical service.
- Close the hospital-sponsored community clinic.
- Delay the previously approved project to renovate and expand an inadequate intensive care unit.

Each option certainly has significant implications for both the institution and its constituents. Assuming one of the alternatives must be selected, how would you design a decision-making process to maximize the likelihood of an ethical resolution?

Discussion Questions

1. What are some examples of incompatible institutional and public interests, and what steps could assist a health care organization to compete in an ethical manner?

2. What ethical problems have been encountered in the movement toward managed care, and how might these problems be addressed?
3. How can a health care organization demonstrate ethical sensitivity before, during, and after downsizing?
4. What type of health care rationing occurs now, and how can bioethical principles contribute to a just policy?
5. How can unlimited care, as contrasted with unlimited treatment, be promoted to better serve patients and society?
6. What are individual and organizational ethics audits, and how can they encourage ethical behavior?

References

American College of Healthcare Executives, *Code of Ethics*. Chicago: Author, 1995.

American College of Healthcare Executives, "Ethics Self-Assessment," *Healthcare Executive, 12*(2), 45–49, 1997.

American Hospital Association, *AHA's Organizational Ethics Initiative*. Chicago: Author, 1997.

American Medical Association, Council on Ethical and Judicial Affairs, "Ethical Issues in Managed Care," *Journal of the American Medical Association, 273*, 330–335, 1995.

Appleby, C., "Managed Care's True Values," *Hospitals and Health Networks, 70*(13), 20–26, 1996.

Asch, D., "The Role of Critical Care Nurses in Euthanasia and Assisted Suicide," *New England Journal of Medicine, 334*, 1374–1379, 1996.

Auerback, M., "Will Managed Care Alter the Art and Soul of Medicine?" *Western Journal of Medicine, 160*, 269–272, 1994.

Bayer, R., "Prometheus Meets Malthus," *Business and Health, 1*(8), 22–25, 1984.

Beauchamp, T., & Childress, J., *Principles of Biomedical Ethics*. New York: Oxford Press, 1989.

Bell, C., "Advice for Easing the Pain of Layoffs," *Modern Healthcare, 25*(2), 27, 1995.

Bennahum, D., "Encounters with Death," *Cambridge Quarterly of Healthcare Ethics, 5*(1), 7–9, 1996.

Bresnahan, J., "Letter to the Editor," *Health Progress, 70*(4), 9, 14, 1989.

Callahan, D., "Rationing Medical Progress: The Way to Affordable Health Care," *New England Journal of Medicine, 322*, 1810–1813, 1990.

Callahan, D., "Setting Policy: The Need for Full Participation," *Frontiers of Health Services Management, 8*(1), 34–36, 1991.

Capron, A., "Legalizing Physician-Aided Death," *Cambridge Quarterly of Healthcare Ethics, 5*(1), 10–23, 1996.

Chervenak, F., & McCullough, L., "Managed Care and the New Medical Paternalism," *Journal of Clinical Ethics, 6*, 320–323, 1995.

Danforth, J., "Quality of Life Is the Issue in Care for Terminally Ill," *Modern Healthcare, 26*(36), 49, 1996.

Derzon, R., *Second Annual Roger G. Larson Memorial Lecture*, presented at the American Hospital Association annual convention, Chicago, July 29, 1985.

Dougherty, C., "Ethical Problems in Healthcare Rationing," *Health Progress, 72*(8), 32–39, 1991.

Eastern Mercy Health System and Mercy Health System Shared Corporate Ethics Committee, *Ethical Guidelines for Managed Care Contract Negotiations*. Radnor, PA: Eastern Mercy Health System, 1995.

Emanuel, E., "Medical Ethics in the Era of Managed Care: The Need for Institutional Structures Instead of Principles for Individual Cases," *Journal of Clinical Ethics, 6*, 335–338, 1995.

Enthoven, A., *The Clash between Economics and Ethics in the Context of Managed Care*. Paper presented at seminar sponsored by Stanford University Center for Biomedical Ethics, Palo Alto, CA, May 1, 1996.

Enthoven, A., & Kronick, R., "A Consumer-Choice Health Plan for the 90s," *New England Journal of Medicine, 320*, 29–37, 1989.

Fielder, J., "Disposable Doctors: Economic Incentives to Abuse Physician Peer Review," *Journal of Clinical Ethics, 6*, 327–332, 1995.

Foubert, P. (Ed.), *Ethical Leadership in Health Care Management: Reflections of Paul B. Hofmann*. Charlottesville, VA: Ibis, 1992.

Freed, D., "The Long Distance Administrator," *Health Management Quarterly, 14*(4), 17–20, 1992.

Fuchs, V., "The Health Sector's Share of the Gross National Product," *Science, 247*, 534–547, 1990.

Greene, J., "Retooling without Layoffs," *Modern Healthcare, 26*(9), 76–82, 1996.

Greene, J., "Has Managed Care Lost Its Soul?" *Hospitals and Health Networks, 71*(10), 36–42, 1997.

Griffith, J., *The Moral Challenges of Health Care Management*. Ann Arbor, MI: Health Administration Press, 1993.

Hitt, D., "Ethical Roles Can Exist Only in an Ethical System," *Frontiers of Health Services Management, 8*(1), 37–42, 1991.

Hofmann, P., "Ethical Decision-Making Requires Greater Collaboration between Administrators and Clinicians," *Frontiers of Health Services Management, 8*(1), 31– 33, 1991.

Hofmann, P., "Decisions near the End of Life: Resource Allocation Implications for Hospitals," *Cambridge Quarterly of Healthcare Ethics, 1*, 229–337, 1992.

Hofmann, P., "Healthcare Management and Ethics: Balancing Professional and Personal Priorities," *Healthcare Executive, 9*(3), 42, 1994.

Hofmann, P., "Healthcare Management and Ethics: The Ethics of Downsizing," *Healthcare Executive, 11*(1), 46, 1996.

Institute on Quality of Care and Patterns of Practice, *Managing Risks and Quality in Hospital-Related Managed Care: A Guide for Hospitals*. Chicago: American Hospital Association, 1991.

Jonsen, A., "Bentham in a Box: Technology Assessment and Health Care Allocation," *Law, Medicine and Health Care, 14*(3–4), 172–174, 1986.

Josephson, M., *Ethical Obligations and Opportunities in Business: Ethical Decision-Making in the Trenches*. Marina del Rey, CA: The Joseph & Edna Josephson Institute for the Advancement of Ethics, 1989.

Kassirer, J., "Managed Care and the Morality of the Marketplace," *New England Journal of Medicine, 333,* 50–52, 1995.

Katz, D., "Blueprint for a New Medical Care Plan," *San Francisco Examiner,* 37, April 4, 1974.

Koch, T., "Living Versus Dying "With Dignity": A New Perspective on the Euthanasia Debate," *Cambridge Quarterly of Healthcare Ethics, 5*(1), 50–61, 1996.

Koop, E., *Keynote Address,* presented at the American Hospital Association annual convention, Denver, CO, July 27, 1992.

Lamm, R., "Healthcare Heresies," *Healthcare Forum Journal, 37*(4), 45, 46, 59–61, 1994.

Lantos, J., "Seeking Justice for Priscilla," *Cambridge Quarterly of Healthcare Ethics, 5,* 485–492, 1996.

Levey, S., & Hill, J., "Between Survival and Social Responsibility: In Search of an Ethical Balance," *Journal of Health Administration Education, 4*(2), 225–231, 1986.

Loewy, E., "Society, Physicians and Ethics Committees: Incorporating Ideas of Justice into Patient Care Decisions," *Cambridge Quarterly of Healthcare Ethics, 5,* 559–569, 1996.

Luthringer, G., "The Ethics of Ordinary Time," *Nutrition in Clinical Practice, 6*(3), 99–105, 1991.

Midwest Bioethics Center, *Ethical Issues in Managed Care: Guidelines for Clinicians and Recommendations to Accrediting Organizations.* Kansas City, MO: Author, 1995.

Moore, J., "Reengineering Comes at a Psychic Cost," *Modern Healthcare, 25*(50), 58, 1995.

Munson, R., *Intervention and Reflection: Basic Issues in Medical Ethics* (4th ed.). Belmont, CA: Wadsworth Publishing, 1992.

Nuland, S., *How We Die: Reflections on Life's Final Chapter.* New York: Knopf, 1994.

O'Connell, L., "Changing the Culture of Dying," *Health Progress, 77*(6), 16–20, 1996.

Pastin, M., *The Hard Problems of Management: Gaining the Ethics Edge.* San Francisco: Jossey-Bass, 1986.

Pellegrino, E., "Interests, Obligations, and Justice: Some Notes toward an Ethic of Managed Care," *Journal of Clinical Ethics, 6,* 312–317, 1995.

Pew Health Professions Commission, *Health Professions Education and Managed Care: Challenges and Necessary Responses.* San Francisco: UCSF Center for the Health Professions, 1995.

Rogers, C., Field, H., & Kunkel, E., "Countertransference Issues in Termination of Life Support in Acute Quadriplegia," *Psychosomatics, 36,* 305–309, 1995.

Rudnick, J., "Hospital Layoffs: One Facility's Experience with a Work Force Reduction," *Health Progress, 76*(7), 26–29, 1995.

Schaeffer, L., "Promoting Cost Containment and Quality in Health Care," *UC Berkeley Public Health, 5*(1), 7, 1996.

Schneiderman, L., & Jecker, N., *Wrong Medicine.* Baltimore: Johns Hopkins University Press, 1995.

Seiden, D., "Health Care Ethics," in A. Kovner (Ed.), *Jonas's Health Care Delivery in the U.S.* (5th ed.). New York: Springer Publishing Co., 1995.

"Society Urged to Address Growing Costs of Medical Care for Terminally Ill," *American Medical News, 30*(9), 91, 1987.

Solzhenitsyn, A., *A World Split Apart.* New York: Harper & Row, 1978.

Sommers, C., "Teaching the Virtues: A Blueprint for Moral Education," *Chicago Tribune Magazine,* September 12, 1993.

Truog, R., Brett, A., & Frader, J., "The Problem with Futility," *New England Journal of Medicine, 326,* 1560–1564, 1992.

Veatch, R., "DRGs and the Ethical Reallocation of Resources," *Hastings Center Report, 16*(3), 32–40, 1986.

Veatch, R., "Allocating Health Resources Ethically: New Roles for Administrators and Clinicians," *Frontiers of Health Services Management, 8*(1), 3–29, 1991.

Walters, K., "Ethics and Responsibility," in N. Wright (Ed.), *Papers on the Ethics of Administration.* Provo, UT: Brigham Young University, 1988.

Wenger, N., Oye, R., Desbiens, N., Phillips, R., Teno, J., Connors, A., Liv, H., Zemsky, M., & Kussin, P., "The Stability of DNR Orders on Hospital Readmission," *Journal of Clinical Ethics, 7*(1), 48–54, 1996.

Werhane, P., "The Ethics of Health Care as a Business," *Business and Professional Ethics Journal, 9*(3–4), 7–20, 1990.

White, J., "The Integrity Audit: A Means of Assessing and Improving Organizational Ethics in America," in *Proceedings of the First Annual Conference on Ethics in America.* Long Beach: California State University Extension Services, 1990.

"Why Rationing Was Right for Oregon," *Hospitals and Health Networks, 71*(3), 64, 66, 1997.

Woodstock Theological Center, *Ethical Considerations in the Business Aspects of Health Care.* Washington, DC: Georgetown University Press, 1995.

Worthley, J., *The Ethics of the Ordinary in Healthcare: Concepts and Cases.* Chicago: Health Administration Press, 1997.

Yehle, L., "How to Succeed in Business without Laying Off Employees," *Trustee, 48*(2), 21, 1995.

Zoloth-Dorfman, L., & Rubin, S., "The Patient as Commodity: Managed Care and the Question of Ethics," *Journal of Clinical Ethics, 6,* 339–357, 1995.

IV

FUTURES

Part IV of *Health Care Delivery in the United States* (*HCDUS*) is concerned with the future of health care, how we can predict the future, and how current trends make probable particular futures over the next several years. Knickman outlines some of the values and limitations of forecasting and reviews a past forecast made by Kovner in the "Futures" chapter of the fifth edition of *HDCUS*, written 4 or 5 years ago (most of Kovner's forecasts, other than a prediction of national health insurance, have largely come to pass). Knickman then presents his own views of key drivers of change in the late 1990s. These include the economic and political preferences of consumers, the demographic changes in the age and ethnic shifts of the population, and the growing understanding that behavior drives health outcomes more than provision of medical care. Knickman outlines the areas where he believes change may be the most striking in the coming years: an increase in health care resources being provided to the elderly and the chronically ill; advances in molecular genetics and a range of technical innovations; market change with the growth of investor-owned health care organizations, outpatient services and the reduction in patient services; changes in Medicare either to create incentives for elders to join managed care organizations or to turn Medicare into a fixed-benefit program where each beneficiary receives a dollar amount of coverage in the form of a voucher, which then can be used to purchase whatever type of insurance a person desires; the growth of capacity to collect, process, categorize, and access health and treatment information; and an emphasis on health promotion to improve health maintenance.

A glossary, a guide to sources of data, and indices follow Part IV.

17

Futures

James R. Knickman

Learning Objectives

1. Explain the importance of thinking about the future for management and policy.
2. Describe different approaches to forecasting the future.
3. Analyze what social factors drive change in the health care system.
4. Predict what changes are likely to be most important to the future of health care.

Topical Outline

Introduction to the idea of forecasting and approaches to forecasting
Review of a past forecast
Description of the key drivers of change in the late 1990s
  Preferences and ideology of people
  Aging and ethnic changes in the population
  Growing importance of behavior in determining health status
A review of changes in the coming years that will be most striking
  Services for the elderly and chronically ill
  Advances in molecular genetics and associated technological change
  Health system market change
  The organization of the Medicare program
  Information technology

Key Words: Forecasting, Delphi method, drivers of change, aging of the population, behavioral risk factors, molecular genetics, technological change, market change, fixed-benefit programs, information technology, health promotion.

Imagine the future: I wake up, take off my overnight monitor (connected to a health information virtual computer that tracks 300 aspects of my health status, including a list of specialized self-chosen health goals). I lean over to the monitor, make a few key strokes, and quickly get key information on how my 105-year-old mother—who lives 800 miles away—did overnight and get a forecast about how she will feel during the coming day. As I get in my car to commute to work, I am comforted by its advanced anticollision system that makes life-threatening accidents a concern of the past. I do find the many billboards advertising health-enhancing services of every stripe a general nuisance and source of visual pollution. My grandchildren cannot believe my stories of how physicians used to work in small groups or by themselves and how there were thousands of hospitals each operating on its own rather than as a part of the four national chains of health plans that now compete vigorously in the health care market.

Will the future really look like this? Although it is tough to know what the specifics of tomorrow's health system will look like, it is an important exercise to think about the future and spend time forecasting what might be, what could be, and what forces will shape the future. The 16 chapters that precede this one look very closely at key parts of the health environment, explaining the current status of the health system and key issues currently facing the health system. Understanding the present and being knowledgeable about the past are the first steps in predicting the future and shaping the future.

Many readers of this book are beginning careers in the health care field; they will play key roles in shaping the future and should recognize the importance of taking time periodically to think about where the health system is headed and what levers are available to make it head in a desired direction. The saying goes: "If you don't know where you are going, you might wind up somewhere else."[1]

Exercises in forecasting have many practical values. Most important, forecasting is a crucial step in strategic planning. In the public sector and the private sector, deciding where to focus attention depends on a sense of future trends and prospects. What new products must be designed? How large should a new hospital be? How many elderly will use Medicare services 20 years from now? Questions like these guide current actions, and some approach to forecasting is crucial to give tentative answers to these questions.

Forecasting also forces us to look at history. In essence, every approach to forecasting attempts to look at patterns of past trends to make predictions about future trends. In this sense, "history is a vast early warning system."[2] Looking

---

[1]This famous quote is from Yogi Berra. Not all pundits agree with his logic, however. Albert Einstein said: "I never think of the future. It comes soon enough." And Euripides is quoted: "What we look for does not come to pass. God finds a way for what none foresaw." These quotes are from Fitzhenry (1993).

[2]Norman Cousins as quoted in Fitzhenry (1993).

at and studying what caused what in the past often is the approach for devising innovations and new solutions to current problems. Epidemiologists, for example, use the natural patterns of past behavior and events to sort out what behaviors, environmental factors, and interventions seem to lead to good and bad health outcomes (McMahon & Pugh, 1970). This type of analysis then leads to ideas for how to improve health outcomes. Most social scientists use the same basic approach in studying how the health system works and how it can be improved.

Finally, a value of forecasting is that it gives us a reference point in the future to assess our past logic. Four years ago (in early 1994), Anthony Kovner prepared a chapter on "Futures" as the capstone to the last edition of this volume (Kovner, 1995). Reading the chapter in 1998 provides useful information about how we thought about health care dynamics 4 years ago and about how our logic has evolved in just 4 years. As discussed later in this chapter, some of Kovner's 1994 forecasts are happening and some are not, but a real value of his earlier paper when read today is that it allows us to sharpen our analytic abilities to pursue the always important task of linking causes to effects.

There are varied methods to make forecasts. Economists, for example, have developed highly quantitative approaches for analyzing data from the past to make forecasts of future economic events (Granger, 1989). This approach generally involves collecting time series data from the past on a series of economic variables, then developing theories about how each variable influences the others, then testing these theories with data from the past, and finally using statistical techniques to estimate how the variables will change in the future based on the estimated relationships of how they changed in the past. The economic approach works only when extensive empirical data are available, and even in these cases the approach is far from perfect as a forecasting technique and most useful for forecasts of the near future (Berndt, 1991).

The Delphi method, which is a more qualitative approach to forecasting, obtains expert opinion in a systematic manner with an end goal of achieving consensus. Delphi administrators poll experts about their forecasts of the future with a self-administered questionnaire. Participants complete three or four rounds of questionnaires, but after each round, results are tabulated and disseminated to the group. The group completes a Delphi when it reaches a convergence of opinion (Fink, Kosecoff, Chassin, & Brook, 1984).

The Delphi method overcomes geographic barriers that plague many consensus-building exercises. Flexibility represents another strength of the Delphi method as it easily applies to health and medicine, as well as to war and weapons systems and to all levels of decision making. The fact that reliability, as well as required work, increases as the number of rounds and experts increases sets limitations on the utility of the Delphi method. Problems of questionnaire design and expert identification also inhibit the Delphi method.

A third, least scientific, approach to forecasting is to rely on nationally recognized leaders in a field to apply their experience about the past and the dynamics of the present to make predictions about the future. This is the approach used on Sunday morning television and the approach used by many magazines and trade journals. In addition, almost every article in a journal like *Health Affairs* ends with expert authors assessing what the analyses presented in their papers imply for the future. Thus, forecasting is a natural part of most analysis and comment by experts. It is often the ultimate reason for undertaking an analysis.

The approach to looking at the future employed in this paper is of the third variety. I hope to draw on the wide literature contributed by experts analyzing the present to predict the future and to present my interpretation and inferences of what current patterns in the health system suggest for the future. My analysis of "Futures" is shaped by my vantage point—working at a philanthropy that supports efforts to improve the health and health care of the American public. I have the privilege of interacting with many experts in the health field who use our foundation's resources to try to shape the future so that Americans can live in better health and have health care services as accessible and responsive to their needs as possible.

A Review of a Past Forecast

Kovner, in his 1994 paper, made five concrete predictions about the future (a bold exercise), and it is useful to consider how well these forecasts held up:

Prediction 1: There will be national health insurance. Kovner believed that the strong political priority of the Clinton administration would overcome Americans' preferences for pluralism and diversity and their distrust of government.

This prediction clearly has not come true as of 1998, and we no longer seem headed in this direction. In fact, it seems that Americans' distrust of government did overwhelm the Clinton political priority. Opponents of reform were quite successful in heightening public concerns that mandatory insurance with extensive government mandates and regulations could usher in a health care system that gave each person less freedom to select providers and to control the type of coverage and care they receive.

Ironically, many of the feared changes in the health care market have proceeded even in the absence of a national health insurance system A current concern is that we are going to have less ability to choose providers and coverage but will continue to live with the fear of periodic episodes of no insurance due to inherent problems of employer-based insurance. And large numbers of Americans will continue to be uninsured for extended periods of time.

Prediction 2: Fewer larger groups of health care providers will compete for capped purchaser dollars in increasingly organized local markets.

This prediction seems to be on target although the pace of consolidation in the health care system and the pace of capitation has been uneven in different markets across the country. A new version of this prediction is that consolidation and capitation will continue to grow, but each local market will end up at a different point along the consolidation and capitation continuum (Ginsburg, 1996).

Prediction 3: Consumers will use less medical care per capita on an age-adjusted basis.

Again, this prediction seems to be working out at least over the past 3-year period. Inpatient admissions continue to decrease in most areas of the country although average hospital stays have stabilized lately. Use of physicians and specialists—age-adjusted—also continues to decrease slowly as the forces of capitation and managed care increase.

Prediction 4: Governmental regulation will increase regarding cost, quality, and access to health care, and the federal government will supersede state government on these matters.

The verdict is still out on this prediction. There have been efforts at micro-regulation, such as standards for minimum stays after normal deliveries, that are quick reactions to managed care horror stories. And many states are passing comprehensive managed care regulation packages. However, one part of this prediction is not panning out; it seems clear that states will take the lead in regulation over the foreseeable future. The Kovner prediction of a growing federal role was dependent on the unfulfilled prediction of national health insurance.

Prediction 5: The power of physicians to shape and benefit from decision making in health care will diminish.

Again, the verdict is still out on this prediction. Managers and health plans clearly have imposed themselves between physicians and patients over the past 10 years. However, physicians are still reacting to the changing market, and we are nowhere near equilibrium in terms of control over medical decision making. In some areas of the country, physician groups are beginning to compete directly with health plans to regain control of decision making. Interestingly, even when physician groups take control, individual physicians may continue to live in a highly managed environment: physicians as managers and gatekeepers may not act very differently from nonphysician managers.

Overall, the Kovner predictions of 1994 did rather well. They indicate how many issues stay the same even as change occurs. Debates about the role of physicians, the role of regulation, and the prospects for consolidation and utilization control are as active in 1998 as they were in 1994. In the area of insurance coverage, the debate has changed from a focus on universal coverage to a focus on incremental reforms (such as portability rules for coverage) and extended coverage for specific subgroups of the population (such as children and individuals aged 55 to 64).

Key Drivers of Change in the Late 1990s

It is often difficult to know for sure that a given period—as it is happening—is one of rapid change, but the 1990s surely have a reputation of being a time of fundamental change in how we organize and deliver health care and how we think about "maintaining health." As change seems to occur all around, it often is difficult to distinguish drivers of change (the topic of this section) and key aspects of change itself (the topic of the next section). At the core of the dynamics shaping change, however, there seem to be three fundamental forces:

- the preferences of consumers (in economic-speak) or the ideology of the citizenry (in political science-speak);
- the demographic change in the American population shaped both by aging and ethnic shifts in the general population; and
- the growing understanding that behavior drives health outcomes more than health services.

Preferences and Ideology of People

We often talk in 1998 about market forces as a key driving influence in health care right now, but in fact, the current flurry of system change is derivative of the preferences and ideology of the public. Over the past few years, Americans have made clear the preferences and ideology that characterize the majority of the voting population.

Perhaps most striking is the ongoing distrust that Americans place in their governments, especially the federal government. The majority of Americans remain convinced that the federal government cannot be trusted to sponsor or manage large social programs. In 1964, when the American National Election Study first asked about public trust, three fourths (76%) of Americans said they trusted the federal government to do the right thing always or most of the time. This figure declined through the 1970s to a low point of 25% in 1980. This low level of public trust in the government continued through 1995 according to the *Washington Post*/Kaiser/Harvard survey (Blendon et al., 1998).

Of course, not all Americans view the government the same. Hispanic and African Americans, who look to the federal government to redress racial and ethnic inequalities, express higher than average trust. Those with lower incomes, as well as young adults, also view the government as more trustworthy than does the average American. However, deviations remain small; according to the 1995 *Washington Post*/Kaiser/Harvard survey, only about one third of each of these groups believed the federal government does the right thing always or most of the time.

Although political scientists often cite reactions to the conduct of the Vietnam War and to the lack of success of the social programs of the 1960s as the core source of American distrust of government (Nye, 1998), the impact of the high periods of inflation in the economy during the late 1970s and early 1980s and the large federal budget deficits also seem important in shaping Americans' attitudes about the role of government in key parts of the economy. Whether or not Americans' reactions to government efforts of the past are justified, their reactions sharply curtail health system interventions that involve large public sector roles.

Perhaps related to this economic history, as well as the slow economic growth during the 1985–1995 period, Americans were fundamentally price-conscious in the 1990s. This price consciousness partly drives the movement toward managed care in that Americans will choose lower priced insurance options as long as those options have acceptable quality standards. In a recent survey of consumers in 15 communities around the country, concerns about the costs of health care consistently outranked concerns about the potential "evils" of managed care in each community (Knickman, Hughes, Taylor, Binns, & Lyons, 1996).

One other strong preference of Americans that will shape change over the next few years is the importance they place on "choice" in any health care system. Americans are accustomed to being able to pick and choose from various options when making purchases in almost every part of the economy. The ability to "exit" from service systems that they do not like will continue to be a strong preference among consumers, and market changes will have to take this into account.

Aging and Ethnic Changes in the Population

The continued aging of the American population will command significant attention among health care providers and policymakers over the next 30 years. Approximately 47% of all hospital admissions currently are made by Americans over 65, who account for just 13% of the population. The number of people over 65 will double in the next 25 years, thus driving up demand for many types of health care, especially care focused on chronic illnesses and support services for the frail elderly. The population growth rates are most dramatic for the eldest of the old, who are among the very highest users of health and support services.

Even if managed care leads to dramatic decreases in the use of health care, person by person, the aging of the population should make health care and supportive services (e.g., home care and assisted living) an important growth industry in the United States. The style of health care and the sensitivity of the system to the special concerns of the elderly will have to evolve. All of this growth will take place while informal support systems continue to shrink. The number of adults aged 21 to 65—the main cadre of informal caregivers—will decrease from 12.5 per elderly person over age 75 in 1980 to 6.5 per elder in 2025 (U.S. Census Bureau, 1992).

An interesting possibility, of course, is that we will find ways of diverting some personal energies and social resources away from children and toward elders. An important statistic, not often cited in relationship to the growing burdens of an aging society, is that the share of the population who needs support services because they are young will shrink as the elderly share increases. In 1995 there were two children for each person over age 65, but this number will shrink to just 1.18 by 2030 (Francese, 1995).

A second key population shift whose effect is more difficult to predict is the growing ethnic diversity of Americans. By 2060 it is expected that a majority of Americans will be ethnic minorities (U.S. Census Bureau, 1992). Although the non-Hispanic Caucasian population will increase from 191 million in 1992 to 208 million in 2029 and then begin to shrink to 202 million by 2050, the number of African Americans in the population will increase from 32 million in 1992 to 62 million in 2050, and Latino numbers will increase from 24 million to 81 million. In addition, Asians and Pacific Islanders will increase in population from 9 million in 1992 to 41 million in 2050 (Brownson & Kreuter, 1997; U.S. Census Bureau, 1992).

The impacts of this ethnic transformation of America on health care requirements depend crucially on how quickly the growing ethnic groups assimilate into the economic mainstream of American life. Currently, the African American population and Latino population have greater than average health care needs, principally related to lower incomes and the associated stresses on health-related behaviors. If population growth occurs mostly among the low-income part of the American population and if wealth continues to be distributed as skewedly as in the 1990s, we can expect growing demands for health care and public health services.

Even if ethnic America does better economically in the future and has health status patterns closer to overall averages, health care will have to respond to diversity in the style of medicine that will be demanded by growing ethnic populations. It is clear that ethnic minorities prefer services delivered by providers who understand their culture and preferably match their ethnicity. Creating a more diverse health care workforce will be a key challenge facing the health system of the 21st century.

Health and Behavior

Increasingly, Americans are understanding that the real determinants of health have little to do with the trillion dollars we currently invest in the health care system each year but have more to do with the way we lead our lives and the environment we live in. It has been estimated that about half of all deaths in the United States could be attributed to both behavioral and environmental factors, including use of alcohol, tobacco, and other drugs; diet; activity patterns; microbial and toxic agents; firearms; sexual behavior; and motor vehicles (McGinnis & Foege, 1993). The most prominent contributors to these deaths include tobacco, diet, activity patterns, and alcohol (Figure 17.1).

Despite the established linkages between behavioral risk factors and subsequent morbidity and mortality, only about 3% of total health care expenditures in the United States is spent on well care, including preventive care (CDC, 1994). This investment pales compared to the $425 billion in direct health care costs for persons with chronic conditions in the United States (Hoffman, Rice, & Sung, 1996).

An understanding that lifestyles and behavior must change in order to improve population health status should translate into growing demands for public health activities that attack environmental factors associated with health problems and for behavioral health care that attempts to improve the way individuals act to maintain their own health. The Robert Wood Johnson Foundation, for example, is investing in efforts to get managed care providers to institutionalize (or implement) state-of-the-art behavioral interventions to assist patients to stop smoking

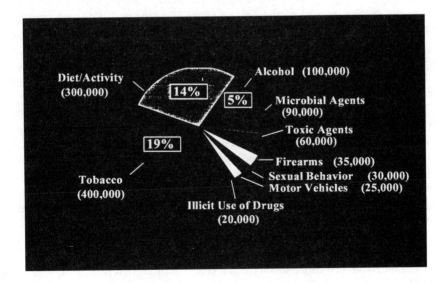

FIGURE 17.1   Actual causes of death in the United States, 1990.

Source: McGinnis & Fooge (1993).

or reduce their risky drinking practices. Similarly, we recognize that improved health outcomes are much more likely to occur if cities can rethink how they intervene in the lives of low-income children than if we expand the number of cardiac catherization laboratories in a city.

A focus on behavior as a key determinant of health problems could lead to more attention for research to improve intervention aimed at helping individuals change behaviors that involve health threats. It also supports the trend toward capitated payments for populations that reward providers and health systems that head off the need for expensive health care interventions by intervening early enough in the onset of chronic health problems to prevent costly disease complications and flare-ups. A number of managed care organizations have successfully demonstrated cost-effective approaches to behavioral risk factor management, but it is clear that additional incentives that encourage investments in preventive care are needed (CDC, 1995).

Areas Where Change May Be Most Striking in Coming Years

Serving the Elderly and the Chronically Ill

The aging of the population will refocus the health system so that its primary concerns revolve around chronic disease management, geriatrics as a medical specialty, and the general field of services for the frail. This transformation will occur slowly and steadily over the next 30 to 50 years, but the contrast in what preoccupies the medical and service fields now and in the future will be striking.

The prospects of positive change in this area are strong. On the medical care side, large analytic investments are well under way to experiment with two quite different but interrelated changes in the service system. First, more sophisticated ways of paying managed care organizations for the care they deliver to the chronically ill are being designed and tested. Second, physicians and other providers are testing new approaches to better manage the way care is delivered to the chronically ill, with central emphasis on the principles of primary, secondary, and tertiary prevention (Mausner & Kramer, 1985). When economic incentives imbedded in payment systems change so that managed care plans are rewarded for enrolling and providing better care for the chronically ill, we should expect widespread implementation of some of the current experiments in chronic disease management.

To date, managed care plans have had perverse incentives relative to services for the chronically ill. Because plans tend to get paid much less than actual costs for the care of each chronically ill person enrolled (and reciprocally much more than actual costs for nonchronically ill enrollees), the natural incentive of a plan is to avoid enrolling the chronically ill through various selection strategies. And there surely are no strong incentives to provide innovative care for the chronically ill so that it will attract greater numbers from this population to a given health plan. The incentives will reverse if risk-adjusted payments can be made more sophisticated and more closely match payments to the expected costs of a person with a chronic illness.

Increasingly, Americans are recognizing that the quality of a managed care plan should be judged by how well it takes care of life-threatening medical episodes (such as care after a heart attack or a serious malignancy) and how well it takes care of chronic diseases. It is medical care that accompanies these serious health threats that is most important to Americans. Thus, in deciding whether to remain in a specific health plan, increasing numbers of people will judge not how well they are taken care of when basically in good health but in how well their friends and relatives who have chronic illnesses and life-threatening problems are cared for. This new mind-set also will help to refocus the attention of managed care plans on the care they provide to the chronically ill.

There also are good prospects for better integration of services directed at both the medical problems of the chronically ill and the social support needs of this population. In the past, health insurance tended to pay only for acute medical services, and most individuals had to use out-of-pocket funds to pay for services such as home care, nursing home care, and assistance with chores. For the poor and for those who became poor because of the high costs of these support services, government would pay for many support services through the Medicaid program and other state and local initiatives. Unfortunately, the two very different financial approaches to covering medical versus support services ignore important interrelationships that jointly determine the needs for these services. Without coordinated planning and recognition that unmet needs in the support area often can lead to severe medical setbacks, the chronically ill have not received cost-effective care that maximizes health outcomes and functioning.

Prospects are changing for better integration of services, partly because of interests of state governments in better coordinating resources coming from Medicare (which mostly focuses on medical care) and Medicaid (which pays for many more support services). Arizona, Tennessee, Oregon, and Minnesota have taken early leads in experimenting with better integration of Medicare and Medicaid funds for the chronically ill (Bonnyman, 1996; McCall, Wrightson, Paringer, & Trapnell, 1994). Other states are moving in similar directions.

Ironically, integration of services is likely to happen more quickly for the poor and near poor than for the wealthy and middle class, who are less likely to be eligible for Medicaid services. However, with the steady but slow growth of private long-term care insurance and with an emerging new wave of financing approaches to prefund long-term care needs, the experience that managed care plans gain on service integration for the population dually eligible for both Medicare and Medicaid can later be applied to the broader population. The final aspect of change related to the chronically ill is the likely emergence of a new industry catering to the various needs of an aging population. The next Microsoft or McDonald's will likely be in the area of services for the elderly. New approaches to assisted living will be in great demand, new approaches for management of retirement resources will be in demand, and approaches for "one-stop shopping" to get medical, support, and lifestyle services in a trusted, easy environment will be desired by the quickly aging population. It is difficult to predict exactly what a new service sector will look like, but it will involve large resources and likely will be led by private corporations.

Advances in Molecular Genetics and a Range of Technological Innovations

Currently, the federal government is funding one of the largest targeted research efforts since the project to create an atomic bomb. This time, however, the investment is directed at health as opposed to defense, with a focus on mapping each of the human genes. This effort is one of basic science directed at a better understanding of our human genetic makeup, and the exact payoffs of this effort in terms of medical knowledge will not be known for some time, but the likely implications for health and medical care are immense.

Perhaps the most dramatic advance in the genetics field in terms of foreshadowing future possibilities is the successful cloning of a sheep in 1996 by a team of applied genetists in Scotland (Kolata, 1997). The methods used are claimed to be applicable, eventually, for human cloning, which raises a host of ethical concerns that must be dealt with in the early part of the 21st century.

Genetics research, however, will lead to an even broader range of medical interventions and prevention possibilities for dealing with many medical problems. These advances likely will make us a healthier population—at least in terms of morbidity and mortality associated with many traditional diseases. The advances also will transform the methods of medical providers and the ways that medical providers spend their time. Many of the efforts that currently take time and energy will be avoided because of better prevention efforts, but new technology will make new medical interventions possible. Constant retraining of medical providers will be more important than it is currently.

Most predictions about the future of new technology and medical interventions suggest that they will add to our health care cost bill. Economists currently are studying exactly how and why different sectors of the technology industry invest in cost-increasing versus cost-reducing technologies. With the spread of managed care and capitated payments, there should be increased investments in cost-reducing technologies than in the past 20 years (Weisbrod, 1991). An optimistic prediction is that there will be a better balance in the introduction of new technologies, with cost-decreasing inventions and strategies somewhat compensating for cost-increasing inventions. What will be essential are better social mechanisms for deciding which of the cost-increasing technologies that emerge in fact enhance quality of life and thus are worth investing in. Americans will continue to be willing to pay for quality-enhancing technologies even if they cost more.

One potential negative side effect of increased knowledge and know-how will be the overuse of testing and medical interventions. Few diagnostic tests are error-free, and to the extent that new tests lead to a fair number of false positives (i.e., indicating a problem when none in fact exists), expensive, unnecessary treatments may be done and people's quality of life may be affected by unnecessary health concerns. An added fear is that some of the genetic testing will identify problems or the likelihood of future problems for which nothing can be done. Again, knowledge of this sort could actually have significant negative impacts on psychological well-being. We may be headed toward a world where we have too much information for our own good.

Market Change

Perhaps the easiest change to predict is a persistent transformation in the way health care is organized, financed, and delivered. Although change started slowly but steadily in a market-oriented direction as early as 1980, the pace of change has been particularly fast since the demise of the Clinton health plan in 1994. Both the prospect and failure of government-led reform seems to have opened the door for industry-led reform, employer-led reform, and Wall Street–led reform.

The Robert Wood Johnson Foundation (RWJF) is supporting a range of efforts to study the changing market and its implications for consumers through its health-tracking initiative (Ginsburg, Hughes, & Knickman, 1995). Through surveys of families, employers, and physicians, as well as frequent site visits, researchers are tracking exactly how change is unfolding in 60 different communities around the country, with in-depth analysis of 12 communities.

Early findings support the obvious sense of the importance and scale of change occurring in the health system. Of individuals covered by employer insurance plans, 74% are in some form of managed care, including 33% who are in formal HMOs with capitated arrangements (KPMG, 1996). According to preliminary findings from the 1996–1997 RWJF community tracking surveys, dramatic shifts away from traditional plans toward managed care have occurred over the past 4 years for firms of all sizes, with only about 20% of small-firm (1–24) employees in indemnity coverage in 1997, compared to 47% in 1993. Physicians are also reporting striking changes in the way they deliver medical care (e.g., increases in the scope of care provided by primary care physicians over the past 2 years have been perceived by roughly 30% of primary care physicians (PCPs) and 50% of specialists) and in the way they relate to patients, with more than 90% of PCPs reporting that they act as "gatekeepers." And more than one in five physicians do not agree that they have the freedom to make clinical decisions to meet their patients' needs.

The delivery system is changing in many ways at the same time. Investor-owned health systems continue to grow and vie with nonprofit models for dominance in both the hospital sector and the health plan sector. For example, enrollments in for-profit health maintenance organizations (HMOs) grew 23% in 1995, compared to an 8% growth for nonprofit HMOs. The number of investor-owned hospitals has been growing slowly but still represents just 7% of all beds in 1996 (Kertesz, Luft, & Sloane, 1996). However, the influence of investor-owned hospitals in the late 1990s exceeds their actual numbers because they are forcing nonprofit hospitals to act more and more like for-profit providers, being more concerned with efficiency and "retained revenues" than with provision of charity care.

Even more important than ownership is the growth of outpatient services and the reduction in inpatient services. For example, in 1980 there were 215 freestanding outpatient surgery centers, compared to 2,314 in 1995 (Kertesz et al., 1996). Similarly, Medicare expenditures for outpatient services grew from $2 billion to $23 billion over the same period.

How will market change evolve over the coming years? The reactions of consumers to all of the change will be most important to the final outcome. Will consumers be willing to put up with some of the restrictions and inconveniences of managed care? Will they accept changing relationships with their physicians and regulated access to specialists and hospitals?

The newspapers have been filled with horror stories about policies and procedures of HMOs, but surprisingly the early survey data we are collecting from consumers suggest that they have at least a "wait and see" attitude about managed care. Clearly, cost savings are important to their assessment. For example, early findings suggest that 56% of Americans are willing to give up some choice in order to save on health care costs. And despite what they're reading in the headlines, 88% of individuals are somewhat or very satisfied with their health care.

At the same time, we must watch as increasing numbers of individuals report that their access to basic health services has gotten worse over the past 3 years, with one of four families reporting that getting the health care their family needs is becoming harder (twice as many as those who say it's getting easier (12%). Roughly 16% of individuals report access problems. And the number without health insurance coverage remains high, with 14% reporting no coverage in 1997).

One thing that seems certain about the changing system is that the forces of change and the outcomes of change will vary from locality to locality. Enrollment in managed care, the ownership patterns of hospitals and health plans, the approach to managing access to services all vary from market to market, and there seems to be no movement toward one model or one end point. Ginsburg (1996) emphasizes in his assessments of the changing market that local factors dominate the way change plays out in communities. He notes that "communities were not even at different points on a common path, but rather were pursuing completely separate paths, with unique destinations" (p. 15).

Medicare

In thinking about future directions of public policy in the health field, Medicare stands out as the area most liable to face sharp changes in structure. Medicare represents a huge public commitment to health care, with expenditures reaching $180 billion in 1995 and projected to grow—unless changes occur—to $448 billion by 2008 (Congressional Budget Office, 1998).

Perhaps more relevant to prospects for change, Medicare represents a substantial share of federal government expenditures. On the nondefense side of the federal budget, Medicare represented 11% of expenditures in 1996, and the companion Social Security program accounted for an additional 29% of the nondefense budget (U.S. Census Bureau, 1996). To the extent that current concerns about budget deficits continue, Medicare will eventually be subject to even greater cost-cutting attention than it typically faces.

This is not to say that changes in this insurance program for the elderly and disabled will be easy. Any efforts to tamper with the current system will face huge political hurdles because of the popularity of the program and the political power of a growing elderly population.

There are two broad paths that change in Medicare might take. The first is to create incentives for elders to join managed care organizations by increasing the out-of-pocket cost differentials between managed care enrollment and fee-for-service enrollment. Even now, the typical Medicare beneficiary enrolled in an HMO pays far less out of pocket for health-related costs than does a beneficiary enrolled in fee-for-service Medicare (Lamphere, Newman, Langwell, & Sherman, 1997). This has occurred in part because HMOs have received favorable capitated payments from the federal government relative to their actual costs, and the HMOs have used some of this windfall to pay for services that typically would be paid out of pocket (e.g., prescription drugs, eye care, and deductibles).

The second broad path toward change would be to turn Medicare into a fixed-benefit program where each beneficiary receives a dollar amount of coverage in the form of a voucher, which then can be used to purchase whatever type of insurance plan a person desires. If the costs of a specific health plan exceed the fixed Medicare benefit, beneficiaries would have to make up the difference. This approach would cap Medicare commitments and allow the exact amount of the commitment to be determined by the political process over time through debates about how fast the fixed dollar amount would increase.

Either of these paths toward change will escalate the trend toward at least two tiers of medical care access in America. The wealthy will be able to opt out of managed care arrangements or specific managed care restrictions through use of point-of-service options. These options increasingly will let people gain access to services at the best medical centers if the individual pays a significant share of the costs for the specific service. The importance of being able to afford the top tier of medicine could become increasingly significant as new technology allows for expensive but effective interventions.

My sense is that the multitiered approach to Medicare is inevitable because of the alternative: equal access to a lower-amenity, less intensive health care system will be unacceptable to the growing cadre of middle-class and wealthy elderly who will want an ability to spend their accumulated wealth on health-enhancing interventions. This desire, coupled with the continuing reluctance of Americans in the late 20th century to redistribute more of our growing wealth to the needy, leads to a prediction of more striking tiers in Medicare coverage.

Other changes in Medicare are more difficult to predict. How many resources will ultimately be devoted to home health and home care services—many of which improve quality of life but are far removed from actual medical care? How active will the federal government be in regulating the quality of medicine associated with the health plans that manage the care of the elderly? How active will government be in refereeing the conflicts that will continue to grow between providers of care and health plans? How will approaches to care and caring at the end of life be reformed to better reflect the needs and wishes of the elderly? Change in all of these areas is needed, but future leadership at the federal level will shape these changes.

Information

The ability to collect, process, and categorize information is changing faster than any other technology in America. Five years ago, consumers were impressed with the rapid diffusion of scanners in food markets; now they are routine. Today (1997) residents of the East Coast are dazzled by the new ability of toll booths to collect tolls using cassette-sized scanning devices in each automobile's glove compartment; by the time this book is published, this information technology also will have become a routine of the commuter's life.

The effects of new information technologies will be striking in the health care field although, again, the exact path of change is difficult to predict, and actual changes are likely to be more dramatic than any predictions one would make at the current time. Despite the potential for change, an important concern about confidentiality and privacy may inhibit some uses of new information technology. For example, it would be straightforward, with existing technology, to track the use of multiple providers by one individual so that each provider could better coordinate the care being considered. However, privacy concerns have slowed efforts to implement such tracking systems. Privacy concerns even hamper efforts to implement computerized systems to track immunization information for young children.

The privacy concerns, however, are important, and more creativity is needed to meet the demands of consumers for privacy. Some solutions may come from technological advances. Perhaps data systems will be designed so that they are accessible only if a consumer provides a private code, or methods could be designed to limit access for specific providers only to certain information, depending on the need for that information.

Information technology, however, will go far beyond tracking health and health care patterns for individuals. Virtual imaging and related technologies will provide significant new information to help providers identify medical problems and potential solutions to the problems. And this type of information may assist centrally located specialists to care for individuals in remote areas of the country without face-to-face contact (Institute of Medicine, 1996).

Information technology also will provide more self-help information to consumers. Already, the Internet has increased the availability of health-related information dramatically. With time, this type of information will become better cataloged and better designed to provide useful help for individuals concerned with their health.

Passive monitoring systems—perhaps like those described in this chapter's opening paragraph—also could provide "real time" information about emerging health problems with protocols for reacting to this information. The challenge will be to make sure that the deluge of new information improves the quality of our lives rather than complicating our lives and adding to the costs of medical care. As discussed earlier, if increased volumes of information about our health serve mostly to scare us about low-probability adverse events, we could end up worse off rather than better off. And if new information leads to more frequent interventions of questionable efficacy, again we could emerge worse off after the information revolution. This inevitable revolution will call for creative management over the next 20 years.

Health Promotion

The growing awareness that healthy lifestyles have much more impact on long-run health than access to health care should translate into significant change in

Americans' approach to health maintenance.[3] The key areas of focus will likely be on the five lifestyle factors that have been identified as most important to mobility and mortality: smoking, unhealthy diets, sedentary lifestyle, alcohol and drug use, and risky sexual practices (McGinnis & Foege, 1993). The importance of noncompliance with medical regimens also can be added to this list. For example, Leventhal (1984) notes that "people are as likely to quit cigarettes or stick with their diets as they are to adhere to blood pressure treatment." Medical noncompliance has been estimated to result in $100 billion avoidable health care costs, and more than half of the elderly are reported to have compliance problems (Sullivan, Kreling, & Hazlet, 1990).

Why will change occur rapidly in lifestyle factors even though they have been so difficult to alter over the past twenty years? Koop and McDonald (1995) point to two "revolutions" to explain their optimism about improvements in behavioral health: "two revolutions—health system change and the building of the national information infrastructure—are transforming American health care . . . and give us some modest confidence that present-day concepts of what determines health and disease, and our methods of intervening, will be dramatically different in the not too distant future" (p. ix). Health system change creates better incentives of health systems to maintain a population's health through prevention approaches, and information technology, as discussed above, will expand the opportunity to get information about behavior change and self-help to consumers.

The payoffs from human genome research also will play a role in this area. Because few inherited diseases are likely to be candidates for drug or gene therapies in the near future, the identification of risk genotypes boosts the demand for more effective and better-targeted prevention efforts. The next generation of behavior change strategies are likely to be strengthened by advances in understanding the biobehavioral mechanisms linking behavioral risk factors and disease. For instance, advances in brain imagery have led to breakthroughs in understanding the neurological basis of drug addiction. Leshner (1996), for example, notes that "drug addiction is not just 'a lot of drug use,' but a brain disease, that is expressed in behavioral ways and occurs in a social context." This awareness will spawn more effective combined pharmacological and behavior intervention approaches. Similarly, Glanz (1997) notes that research into the psychobiology of fat appetite and the role of metabolic factors as promoters of fat and protein intake, offers intriguing possibilities for new biobehavioral models of food intake.

Besides advances in health behavior change technology resulting from multidisciplinary biobehavioral research into the mechanisms linking health behavior to health outcomes, new theories and models of the dynamics of health behavior

---

[3]I want to acknowledge the strong influence of the work of Tracy Orleans, my colleague, in the arguments presented in this section.

change and population-based health improvement strategies will also increase our capabilities to address behavioral threats to health. New models of health behavior change, based on a "stages of change" model, have provided methods for reaching all members of an at-risk population (e.g., all smokers or sedentary members of a health plan), not just those who are motivated to change their behavior (Prochaska & DiClemente, 1983).

In addition, advances in health behavior change have moved away from a strictly clinical behavior change model toward broader public health and public policy models of prevention. Accordingly, experts increasingly argue that strategies for improving healthy behaviors must focus on three very different intervention points: "downstream" interventions focused on the individual, "midstream" interventions focused on work sites and health providers, and "upstream" interventions that involve public health campaigns to change social perceptions about healthy behaviors and that include macro-level public policies to create incentives for health behavior (McKinlay, 1995). Predictions about how public policy will develop in this area are the most difficult to forecast, especially given America's traditional distrust of government.

Conclusions

In 1994, Kovner (1995, p. 552) concluded that it is important "to predict future directions in the American health care delivery system, not so much because of confidence that they will happen but rather to focus discussion on key issues, the constraints that surround them, and the opportunities for resolving them." This conclusion holds up, and it is hoped that the discussion of "futures" presented here provokes new ideas for improving our efforts to bring about better health for Americans.

Mini-Case Study

Your governor appoints you executive director of a Commission on the Future of Health Care in your state. The commission has 1 year to develop a report outlining predicted changes in the health care field in your state. The purpose of this commission is to advise the governor on key changes in the state's health needs and resources so that he or she might develop public policies to make sure the health system evolves on a positive path.

1. How would you go about doing such a forecast? What methods and approaches would you use?
2. What types of people would you suggest that the governor appoint to the commission? Explain how each could be helpful in the workings of the commission.
3. Outline what you would expect the final commission report to include.

Discussion Questions

1. What are the reasons we spend time and energy trying to forecast what will happen in the future?
2. Discuss the advantages and disadvantages of different approaches for forecasting. When do you think it makes sense to be more technical in approach or less technical in approach?
3. What do you think are key drivers of change in the health care system in the 1990s? Do you disagree with any of the items selected in the paper? Would you add some other factors to the list?
4. What changes in health care do you think will be most significant?
5. Can you think of ways for public policy and private managers to shape some of these future changes in positive ways?
6. Take a specific topic covered in one of the previous chapters of this book. Forecast how that part of the health system is likely to change over the next ten years and explain the drivers of these changes.

References

Berndt, E. R., *The Practice of Econometrics: Classic and Contemporary.* Reading, MA: Addison-Wesley, 1991.

Blendon, R. J., Benson, J. M., Morin, R., Altman, D. E., Brodie, M., Brossard, M., & James, M., "Changing Attitudes in America," in J. S. Nye, Jr., P. D. Zelikow, & D. C. Kindig (Eds.), *Why Americans Mistrust Government.* Cambridge, MA: Harvard University Press, 1998.

Bonnyman, G., Jr., "Stealth Reform: Market-Based Medicaid in Tennessee," *Health Affairs, 15*(2), 306–314, 1996.

Brownson, R. C., & Kreuter, M. W., "Future Trends Affecting Public Health," *Journal of Public Health Management Practice, 3*(2), 49–60, 1997.

Centers for Disease Control, "Medical Care Spending—United States," *MMWR, 43*(32), 581–586, 1994.

Centers for Disease Control, "Prevention and Managed Care: Opportunities for Managed Care Organizations, Purchasers of Health Care, and Public Health Agencies," *MMWR, 44*(RR-4), 1–12, 1995.

Congressional Budget Office, *The Economic and Budget Outlook: Fiscal Years 1999–2008.* Washington, DC: U.S. Government Printing Office, 1998.

Fink, A., Kosecoff, J., Chassin, M., & Brook, R. H., "Consensus Methods: Characteristics and Guidelines for Use," *American Journal of Public Health, 74*, 979–983, 1984.

Fitzhenry, R. I. (Ed.), *The Harper Book of Quotations.* New York: HarperCollins, 1993.

Francese, P., "Americans at Mid-Decade," *American Demographics,* 23–31, February 1995.

Ginsburg, P., "The RWJF Community Snapshots Study: Introduction and Overview," *Health Affairs 15*(2), 7–20, 1996.

Ginsburg, P. B., Hughes, R. G., & Knickman, J. R., "A Robert Wood Johnson Program to Monitor Health System Change," *Health Affairs, 14*(2), 287–289, 1995.

Glanz, K., "Behavioral Research Contributions and Needs in Cancer Prevention and Control: Dietary Change," *Preventive Medicine, 26*(5), S43–S55.

Granger, C., *Forecasting in Business and Economics.* Boston: Academic Press, 1989.

Hoffman, C., Rice, D., & Sung, H-Y., "Persons with Chronic Conditions: Their Prevalence and Cost," *Journal of the American Medical Association, 276,* 1473–1479, 1996.

Institute of Medicine, *Telemedicine: A Guide to Assessing Telecommunications in Health Care.* Washington, DC: National Academy Press, 1996.

Kertesz, L., Lutz, S., & Sloane, T., "Sorting Out the Stories That Mattered," *Modern Health Care, 26*(35), 46–90, 1996.

Knickman, J. R., Hughes, R. G., Taylor, H., Binns, K., & Lyons, M., "Tracking Consumers Reactions to the Changing Health Care System: Early Indicators," *Health Affairs, 15*(3), 21–32, 1996.

Kolata, G., "Scientist Reports First Cloning Ever of Adult Animal," *The New York Times,* February 26, 1997.

Koop, C. E., & McDonald, M. D., "Foreword," in L. M. Harris (Ed.), *Health and the New Media Technologies Transforming Personal and Public Health.* Mahway, NJ: Erlbaum, 1995.

Kovner, A., "Futures," in A. Kovner (Ed.), *Health Care Delivery in the United States* (5th ed.). New York: Springer Publishing Co., 1995.

KPMG, *Health Benefits in 1996.* Washington, DC: Author, 1996.

Lamphere, J., Newman, P., Langwell, K., & Sherman, D., "The Surge in Medicaid Managed Care: An Update," *Health Affairs, 16*(3), 127–133, 1997.

Leventhal, H., Zimmerman, R. A., & Gutmann, M., "Compliance: A Self-Regulation Perspective," in *Handbook of Behavioral Medicine* (pp. 369–436). 1984.

Mausner, J. S., & Kramer, S., *Epidemiology: An Introductory Text.* Philadelphia: W. B. Saunders, 1985.

McCall, N., Wrightson, C. W., Paringer, L., & Trapnell, G., "Managed Medicaid Cost Savings: The Arizona Experience," *Health Affairs, 13*(2), 234–245, 1994.

McGinnis, J. M., & Foege, W. H., "Actual Causes of Death in the United States," *Journal of the American Medical Association, 270,* 2207–2212, 1993.

McKinlay, J. P., "The New Public Health Approach to Improving Physical Activity and Autonomy in Older Population," in E. Heikkinen et al. (Eds.), *Preparation for Aging.* New York: Plenum Press, 1995.

McMahon, B., & Pugh, T. F., *Epidemiology: Principles and Methods.* Boston: Little, Brown, 1970.

Nye, N. S., Jr., *Why Americans Mistrust Government.* Cambridge, MA: Harvard University Press, 1998.

Prochaska, J. O., & DiClemente, C. C., "Stages and Processes of Self-Change of Smoking: Toward an Integrative Model of Change," *Journal of Consulting and Clinical Psychology, 51,* 390–395, 1983.

Sullivan, S. D., Kreling, D. H., & Hazlet, T. K., "Noncompliance with Medication Regimens and Subsequent Hospitalizations: A Literature Analysis and Cost of Hospitalization Estimate," *Journal of Research in Pharmaceutical Economics, 2*(2), 19–33, 1990.

U.S. Census Bureau, "Current Population Reports," *Population Projections of the United States, by Age, Sex, Race, and Hispanic Origin: 1992–2050.* Washington, DC: U.S. Government Printing Office, 1992.

U.S. Census Bureau, *1996 Statistical Abstract.* Washington, DC: U.S. Government Printing Office, 1996.

Weisbrod, B., "The Health Care Quadrilemma: An Essay on Technological Change, Insurance, Quality of Care, and Cost Containment," *Journal of Economic Literature, 29*, 523–552, 1991.

Appendix I

Glossary

Access: A measure of an individual's ability to obtain medical services on a timely geographically and financially acceptable basis. Factors determining ease of access include location of health care facilities, transportation, and hours of operation.

Accountability: Having to give reasons to other stakeholders (such as employees or regulators who have legitimate interests in what and how a person or an organization behaves) for organizational performance.

Accreditation: A voluntary system of institutional or organizational review established by the institutions or organizations themselves in which a quasi-independent body created for the purpose periodically evaluates the work of the subject agencies for quality, using written criteria.

Acute care: Medical care of a limited duration, provided in a hospital or outpatient setting, to treat an injury or short-term illness.

Administrative costs: Nonmedical expenditures incurred by the delivery of health care services, including billing, claims processing, marketing, and overhead.

Adverse selection: Literally, recruiting as members of an MCO or HMO persons who are sicker than the general population; usually used to refer to the common, opposite process of recruiting healthier rather than sicker people.

Alternative delivery system (ADS): A method of providing health care benefits paying for and different from the usual indemnity approach. An example is the HMO.

Ambulatory care: Care provided to a person who is not a bed patient in a health care institution.

American Association of Health Plans (AAHP): The trade organization for managed care organizations (MPOs). It is located in Washington, DC.

Average length of stay (ALOS): There are several approaches to computing ALOS. They all produce similar numbers. The American Hospital Association computes the ALOS by dividing the number of inpatient days by the number of admissions.

AWP (any willing provider): This is a form of state law that requires an MCO to accept any provider willing to meet the terms and conditions in the MCO's contract, whether the MCO wants or needs that provider or not.

Balance billing: An excess fee billed to a patient by a provider, over and above what the insurance plan pays to that provider for a particular service (other than contracted copayments).

Beneficiary: Any person, either a subscriber or a dependent, eligible for service under a health plan contract.

Benefits/benefit package: The services provided (e.g., hospitalization, outpatient care, laboratory tests) to a patient under any given health insurance/HMO plan.

Capitation: A fixed amount of payment per patient, per year, regardless of the volume or cost of services each patient requires.

Carrier: An insurer; an underwriter of risk engaged in providing, paying for, or reimbursing all or part of the cost of health services under insurance policies or contracts, medical or hospital services agreements, membership or subscription contracts, or similar arrangements, in exchange for premiums or other periodic charges.

Carve-out: One or more medical services contracted out by plan providers in a health insurance contract. For example, mental health/substance abuse services may be provided by a separate contracting organization to a health plan.

Case management: According to the Certification of Insurance Rehabilitation Specialists Commission, "Case management is a collaborative process which assesses, plans, implements, coordinates, monitors, and evaluates the options and services required to meet an individual's health needs, using communication and available resources to promote quality, cost-effective outcomes" and "occurs across a continuum of care, addressing ongoing individual needs" rather than being restricted to a single practice setting.

Case manager: An individual who coordinates and oversees other health care workers in finding the most effective methods of caring for specific patients.

Case mix: The spectrum of illnesses and the severity in the case-population of any provider.

Catastrophic health insurance: Covers the costs of very expensive health services, the total of which exceeds the monetary limits of the patient's "regular" plan.

Catchment area: The geographic area from which an organized health service draws its patients.

Certificate of need: A permit to provide new services or construct or renovate a hospital or related facilities, issued by a state government.

Certification: A voluntary system for assuring that individual health care practitioners meet certain standards of education, experience, and examination achievement before they begin practice. Certain certified health professions require periodic re-certification for maintenance of the qualification. Certification systems are established by the professions themselves, usually in the case that the profession is not subject to state licensure.

Clinical nurse practitioner: A nurse with additional training who accepts additional clinical responsibility for medical diagnosis or treatment.

Closed panel: A managed care plan that contracts with physicians on an exclusive basis for services and does not allow those physicians to see patients for another managed care organization.

COBRA: Consolidated Omnibus Budget Reconciliation Act of 1985 (P.L. 99-272), a federal law that requires that all employer-sponsored health plans offer certain employees and their families the opportunity to continue, at their personal expense, health insurance coverage under the group plan for up to 18, 24, or 36 months, depending on the qualifying event, after their coverage normally would have ceased (e.g., due to the death or retirement of the employee, divorce or legal separation, resignation or termination of employment, or bankruptcy of the employer).

Coinsurance: A percentage of a physician's total contracted fee, often 20%, paid directly by the patient rather than the insurance company or HMOs.

Community hospital: A hospital offering short-term (ALOS less than 30 days) general and other special services, owned by groups other than the federal government.

Community rating: A method of determining health insurance premiums based on total experience of subscribers or members within a given geographic area, rather than on the actual health care cost experience of certain subsets of users or potential users (experience rating).

Continuing care retirement communities: A group of facilities for older persons, under common management, in which several levels of accommodation, from independent living apartments to full-service nursing are provided.

Copayment: An out-of-pocket expense paid by an insurance or HMO beneficiary regardless of other insurance provision, invariably a flat fee (e.g., $5 for each ambulatory care visit).

Cost sharing: A provision that requires individuals to cover some part of their medical expenses (e.g., co-payments, coinsurance, deductibles).

Cost shifting: Refers to passing the cost of health care for one population subgroup onto another such group. For example, if the rate one group of health plan enrollees pays for services is less than the actual cost of those services, the difference is made up based on charges higher than cost paid by another group.

Credentialing: The most common use of the term refers to obtaining and reviewing the documentation of professional providers.

Custodial care: Care provided to an individual primarily to support the basic activities of living; may be medical or nonmedical, but the care is not meant to be curative and is often lifelong; rarely covered by group health insurance.

Deductible: An amount an insured patient must pay out of pocket, usually annually on a calendar-year basis, before insurance will cover any costs, exclusive of any copayments or coinsurance.

Deinstitutionalization: The term applied to the gradual and continuing closure of state mental hospitals that has been under way since the mid-1960s which has resulted in the discharge of tens of thousands of mental patients nationally, and the national inability to provide ongoing inpatient mental health care to many patients who would have previously been institutionalized.

Department of Veterans Affairs: The federal government agency responsible for, among other things, running the in- and out-patient veterans' health services.

Dependent: A health insurance beneficiary covered by virtue of a family relationship with a person having a health plan coverage.

Diagnosis-related groups (DRGs): Groups of inpatient discharges with final diagnoses that are similar clinically and in resource consumption; used as a basis of payment by the Medicare program, and as a result, widely accepted by others.

Direct contract model: A managed care health plan that contracts directly with private-practice physicians in the community rather than going through an intermediary (e.g., an open-panel HMO).

Discharge: The National Health Interview Survey defines a hospital discharge as the completion of any continuous period of stay of one night or more in a hospital as an inpatient, not including the period of stay of a well newborn infant.

Discharge planning: A part of the patient management guidelines and the nursing care plan that identifies the expected discharge date of the patient and coordinates the various services necessary to achieve the target.

Disease management: The process of intensively managing a particular disease, such as diabetes, in a particular patient.

Disproportionate share hospital (DSH): A hospital that provides a large amount (or disproportionate share) of uncompensated care and/or care to Medicaid and low-income Medicare beneficiaries.

Dual eligibility: Coverage under two or more insurance plans for the same medical problem, for example, because both spouses work and have medical insurance coverage for the family as a condition of employment.

Emergency department: According to the National Ambulatory Medical Care Survey (NAMCS), a hospital facility for the provision of unscheduled outpatient services to patients whose conditions require immediate care; it is staffed 24 hours a day.

Employee Retirement Income Security Act (ERISA): A 1974 federal law (P.L. 93-406) that set the standards of disclosure for employee benefit plans to ensure workers the right to at least part of their pensions. The law governs most private pensions and other employee benefits and overrides all state laws such as mandatory coverage in health plans of mental health care in their application to self-funded private employer-sponsored health insurance plans.

Encounter: An outpatient or ambulatory visit by a member to a provider.

Enrollment: The process by which an individual becomes a subscriber for himself and/or his dependents for coverage in a health plan. This may be done either through an actual signing up of the individual or by virtue of his collective bargaining agreement on the employer's conditions of employment. The result, therefore, is that the health plan is aware of its entire population of beneficiary eligibles. As a usual practice, it is incumbent on the individual to notify the health plan of any changes in family status that affect the enrollment of dependents.

Entitlements: Government benefits (e.g., Medicare, Medicaid, Social Security, food stamps) that are provided automatically to all qualified individuals and are therefore part of mandatory spending programs.

Ethics: A socially determined set of standards of public behavior that do not have the force of law behind them, but for which there is a societal expectation of compliance by each member.

Experience rating: A method used to determine the cost of health insurance premiums, whereby the cost is based on the previous amount a certain group (e.g., all the employees of a particular organization) paid for medical services.

Family income: For purposes of the National Health Interview Survey and National Health and Nutrition Examination Survey, all people within a household related to each other by blood, marriage, or adoption constitute a family. Family income is the total income received by the members of a family in the 12 months before the interview.

Federal Employee Health Benefits Program (FEHBP): The health plans made available to federal employees as part of their employment benefits.

Federalism: One of the fundamental principles of the U.S. Constitution under which sovereignty, the ultimate generally recognized power of government which may be backed up by the use of force, is shared between the states and the Federal government.

Fee schedule: A listing of accepted fees or established allowances for specified medical procedures as used in health plans, it usually represents the maximum amounts the program will pay to an individual provider or medical group for the specified procedures.

Fee for service (FFS): A billing system in which a health care provider charges a patient a set amount for a specific service.

Food and Drug Administration (FDA): The federal government agency, part of the Department of Health and Human Services, responsible for the regulation of certain devices and pharmaceutical drugs.

Formulary: A list of drugs that a physician may prescribe, usually assembled by a medical staff committee of a hospital or an MCO.

For-profit hospitals: Those owned by private corporations that declare dividends or otherwise distribute profits to individuals. Also called *investor-owned*, they are usually short-term general hospitals.

Gatekeeper: The term has two meanings. Originally, it referred to a primary care/practitioner who coordinated all care received by patients in an attempt to organize both quality and efficiency. In managed care, it refers to primary care practitioner control of the volume of services used by patients in an attempt to minimize expenditures.

Generic drug: A drug that is identical, chemically and pharmacologically, to an original, patented, name-brand drug, produced after the original patent has expired, and usually less expensive than the original. Most MCOs that provide only drug benefits cover generic drugs.

GHAA The former Group Health Association of America, now AAHP.

Governance: The decision-making process of an organization, those who monitor the outside environment, select appropriate alternatives, and negotiate the implementation of those alternatives with others outside the organization.

Group model: An HMO that contracts with a physician medical group to provide health care services to the beneficiaries. The relationship between the HMO and the medical group is generally very close, although there are wide variations in the relative independence of the group from the HMO; a form of closed-panel health plan.

Group practice: As defined by the American Medical Association, it is three or more physicians who deliver patient care, make joint use of equipment and personnel, and divide income by a prearranged formula.

Health Care Financing Administration (HCFA): A part of the U.S. Department of Health and Human Services. In addition to its many other functions, HCFA is the contracting agency for HMOs that seek direct contract/provider status for provision of the Medicare benefits package.

Health department: A unit of state or local government (country or city, generally) that has responsibility primarily for public health services (ranging from infectious disease control to the collection of vital statistics) for a given geographic area. In the modern era, some health departments also provide direct treatment services.

Health maintenance organization (HMO): An HMO is a prepaid health plan delivering comprehensive care to members through designated providers, having a fixed monthly payment for health care services, and requiring members to be in a plan for a specified period of time (usually 1 year). HMO model types are as follows:

- **Group:** An HMO that delivers health services through a physician group that is controlled by the HMO unit or an HMO that contracts with one or more independent group practices to provide health services.
- **Individual practice association (IPA):** An HMO that contracts directly with physicians in independent practice, and/or contracts with one or more associations of physicians in independent practice, and/or contracts with one or more multispecialty group practices. The plan is predominantly organized around solo-single specialty practices.

• **Mixed:** An HMO that combines features of group and IPA. This category was introduced in mid-1990 because HMOs are continually changing and many now combine features of group and IPA plans in a single plan.

Healthplan Employer Data Information Set (HEDIS): Developed by the NCQA with considerable input from the employer community and the managed care community, HEDIS is an ever-evolving set of data reporting standard for MCOs. HEDIS is designed to provide some standardization in performance reporting for financial, utilization, membership, and clinical data so that employers and others can compare performance among plans.

Health services and supplies expenditures: Outlays for goods and services relating directly to patient care plus expenses for administering health insurance programs and government public health activities. This category is equivalent to total national health expenditures minus expenditures for research and construction.

Home health care: Defined by the National Home and Hospice Care Survey as care provided to individuals and families in their place of residence for promoting, maintaining, or restoring health or for minimizing the effects of disability and illness, including terminal illness.

Hospice care: Defined by the National Home and Hospice Care Survey as a program of palliative and supportive care services providing physical, psychological, social, and spiritual care for dying persons, their families, and other loved ones. Hospice services are available in home and inpatient settings.

Hospital: According to the American Hospital Association and National Master Facility Inventory, hospitals are licensed institutions with at least six beds, whose primary function is to provide diagnostic and therapeutic patient services for medical conditions by an organized physician staff, with continuous nursing services under the supervision of registered nurses. Hospitals may be classified by type of service, ownership, size in terms of number of beds, and length of stay.

Hospitalization coverage: A type of insurance that covers most inpatient hospital costs, such as room and board, diagnostic and therapeutic services, care for emergency illnesses or injuries, laboratory and x-ray services, and certain other specified procedures.

Indemnity: Monies paid by an insurer/MCO to a provider, in a predetermined amount in the event of a covered loss by a beneficiary; differs from reimbursement, which provides coverage based on actual expenses incurred. There are fewer restrictions on what a doctor may charge and what an insurer may pay for a treatment under indemnity payment, and generally there are also fewer restrictions on a patient's ability to use specialty services.

Indian Health Service: Part of the U.S. Public Health Service, Department of Health and Human Services, the Indian Health Services provides inpatient and outpatient treatment and certain public health services to members of American Indian tribes and Alaska natives.

Individual practice association (IPA): A grouping of independent private medical practitioners, each remaining in his or her own office, who agree under contact to participate in an HMO-like reimbursement mechanism.

Integrated delivery system (IDS): A group of health care organizations that collectively provide a full range of health-related services from prevention to complex hospital-based treatment in a coordinated fashion to those using the system.

Integration, horizontal: Affiliations among providers of the same type (e.g., a hospital forming relationships with other hospitals).

Integration, vertical: Affiliations among providers of different types (e.g., a hospital, clinic, and nursing home forming an affiliation).

Involuntary treatment: Treatment given to a person for which informed consent is not obtained.

Joint Commission on Accreditation of Healthcare Organizations (JCAHO): A not-for profit, national organization formed by the major health care provider organizations, American College of Physicians, American College of Surgeons, American Hospital Association, American Medical Association, and consumer representatives. The JCAHO provides inspection, quality-assurance services, and accreditation to hospitals and other health care provider organizations.

Limitation of activity: In the National Health Interview Survey limitation of activity refers to a long-term amount of activities associated with age group. Each person identified as having a chronic condition is classified according to the extent to which activities are limited, as follows: persons unable to carry on any major activity and persons limited in the amount or kind of major activity performed.

Long-term care: A general term for a range of services provided to chronically ill, physically infirm (usually elderly) persons and those otherwise unable to take care of themselves, such as physically or mentally disabled patients in a nursing home or home health care setting.

Loss ratio (or medical loss ratio): A term used to describe the proportion of payments made for health services actually spent on the provision of health care. A company with a loss ratio of .85, for instance, spends 85 cents of every premium dollar on health care and the remaining 15 cents on administrative costs, including paperwork, marketing, executive salaries, and profits.

Major medical insurance: A precursor of "catastrophic coverage," it covers costs above a fairly high minimum (usually covered by conventional health insurance) to a very high maximum. It is intended to cover the costs associated with a truly major ("catastrophic") illness or injury.

Managed care: A system of health care delivery that influences or controls utilization of services and costs of services. The degree of influence depends on the model used. For example, a preferred provider organization (PPO) charges the patients lower rates if they use the providers in the PPO. HMOs, on the other hand, may choose not to reimburse for health services received from providers with whom the HMO does not contract. An MCO (managed care organization) has at least a panel of individual practitioners, a hospital or hospitals to which they relate a premium collection/payment system, and a utilization control/quality assurance system.

Managed care organization (MCO): An organization providing medical care under which aspects of the care or the payment for care are "managed," for example, negotiated between payers and providers such as limiting providers of care or discounting payment to providers of care.

Managed health care: A regrettably nebulous term. At the very least, a system of health care delivery that tries to manage the cost of health care, the quality of that health care, and access to that care. Common denominators include a panel of contracted providers that is less than the entire universe of available providers, some type of limitations on benefits to subscribers who use noncontracted providers (unless authorized to do so), and some type of authorization system.

Managed information system (MIS): A computer-based system for codifying and analyzing a wide variety of statistical data, as an aid to management.

Mandated benefits: Benefits that a health plan is required to provide by law. This is generally used to refer to benefits above and beyond routine insurance-type benefits, and it generally applies at the state level (where there is high variability from state to state). Common examples include invitro fertilization, defined days of inpatient mental health or substance abuse treatment, and other special-condition treatments.

Medicaid: A joint federal/state/local program providing some payments for some health services for some individuals whose income and resources are insufficient to pay for their care, governed by Title XIX of the federal Social Security Act and administered by the states. Primarily, it pays for health care for certain poor persons and is the major source of payment for nursing home care of the elderly.

Medical savings account: Accounts similar to individual retirement accounts (IRAs), into which employers and employees can make tax-deferred contributions and from which employees may withdraw funds to pay covered health care expenses.

Medicare: A federal entitlement program of medical and health care coverage for the elderly and disabled and persons with end-stage renal disease, governed by Title XVIII of the federal Social Security Act and consisting of two parts: hospital insurance (part A) and supplementary medical insurance (part B, primarily payments to physicians).

Medigap: Also known as Medicare supplement insurance, it is a type of private insurance coverage that may be purchased by an individual enrolled in Medicare to cover certain needed services such as outpatient prescription drugs, that are not included in Medicare parts A & B.

Mental disorder: A consistent, repetitive disturbance of the normal processes of thought and related actions that can be altered, if at all, only by psychotherapeutic intervention of one sort or another.

Mental health care: Health services provided both to persons with mental disorders and to otherwise healthy persons who need help dealing with both internal and external emotional and psychological problems that interfere with daily living, work, interpersonal relationships, and the achievement of happiness.

National health expenditures: This measure estimates the amount spent for all health services and supplies and health-related research and construction activities consumed in the United States during the calendar year.

NCQA (National Committee on Quality Assurance): A not-for-profit organization performing quality assurance reviews and accreditation for MCOs and HMOs.

Network: An arrangement of several delivery points (i.e., medical group practices affiliated with an MCO, an arrangement of HMOs (either autonomous and separate legal entities or subsidiaries of a larger corporation) using one common insuring mechanism such as Blue Cross/Blue Shield; a broker organization (health plan) that arranges with physician group, carriers, payer agencies, consumer groups, and others for services to be provided to enrollees.

Nonprofit: A term applied to a provider to whom no part of the net earnings accrues or may lawfully accrue to the benefit of any private shareholder or individual; an organization that has received 501-C-3 or 501-C-4 designation by the Internal Revenue Service.

Nursing care: The following definition of nursing care applies to data collected in National Nursing Home Surveys through 1977. Nursing care is the provision of any of the following services; application of dressings or bandages; bowel and bladder retraining; catheterization; enema; full bed bath; hypodermic intramuscular, or intravenous injection; irrigation; nasal feeding; oxygen therapy; and temperature-pulse-respiration or blood pressure measurement.

Nursing home expenditures: These cover care rendered in skilled nursing and intermediate care facilities, including those for the mentally retarded. The costs of long-term care provided by hospitals are excluded.

Office visit: A formal face-to-face contact between the physician and the patient in a health center, office, or hospital outpatient department.

Open enrollment period: A time period, usually annual, during which a covered employee may change plans, that is, if a choice is available. Also, there is a requirement that all possible customers for a particular health insurance plan be accepted for coverage and, once accepted, not be terminated by the insurer due to future claims experience.

Open panel HMO: An MCO that contracts (either directly or indirectly) with private physicians to deliver care in their offices and accepts all credentialed physicians willing to adhere to the HMOs rules and regulations.

Organizational performance: Outputs of an organization such as numbers of services produced, turnover of employees, or satisfaction of customers. Organizational performance is commonly measured in terms of measurable objectives or expectations of stakeholders.

Osteopathic medicine (or "Osteopathy"): A fully licensed approach to medical practice that in addition to pharmaceutical and surgical interventions employs musculo-skeletal manual manipulation and stresses the reinforcement of the body's own healing/recovery powers.

Outlier: A provider that is supplying services at either a rate and/or intensity well above or well below the norm. Under a DRG system of payment, additional per diem payments are made to the hospital for cases requiring a patient to stay in the hospital beyond a threshold length of stay. Such cases are referred to as "long stay outliers."

Overutilization: Use of a health service or services by an individual user or subpopulation of users that exceeds use norms established by a large population of users.

Peer review: Quality assessment of a physician's performance by other physicians, usually within the same geographic area and medical specialty.

Penetration: The percentage of total eligibles in a given geographical area that an MCO is able to enroll.

Per diem payment: A reimbursement rate paid to an institutional provider for each day of health care service provided for a patient.

Personal health care expenditures: These are outlays for goods and services relating directly to patient care. The expenditures in this category are total national health expenditures minus expenditures for research and construction, expenses for administering health insurance programs, and government public health activities.

PHO (Physician-hospital organization): An arrangement that links hospitals and their medical staffs for the purpose of contracting jointly with managed care plans.

Physician: Physicians, through self-reporting, are classified by the American Medical Association and others as licensed doctors of medicine or osteopathy as follows:

- Active (or professionally active) physicians are currently practicing medicine, regardless of the number of hours worked per week.
- Federal physicians are employed by the federal government; nonfederal or civilian physicians are not.
- Office-based physicians spend the plurality of their time working in practices based in private offices.
- Hospital-based physicians spend the plurality of their time as salaried physicians in hospitals.

Physician contact: Defined by the National Health Interview Survey as a consultation with a physician in person or by telephone, for examination, diagnosis, treatment, or advice. The service may be provided by the physician or by another person working under the physician's supervision. Place of contact includes office, hospital outpatient clinics, emergency room, telephone (advice given by a physician in a telephone call), home (any place in which a person was staying at the time a physician was called there), clinics, HMOs, and other places located outside a hospital.

Physician Payment Review Commission (PPRC): Created by Congress to recommend changes in current reimbursement procedures and policies for physicians receiving payments from Medicare. The commission first met in 1986 and prepares an annual report to Congress. Recently combined with Hospital Payment Review Commission.

Point-of-service plan (POS): A managed care plan that offers enrollees the option of receiving services from both participating and nonparticipating providers. The benefits package is designed to encourage the use of participating providers, through higher deductibles and/or partial reimbursement for services provided by nonparticipating providers.

Precertification: Also known as preadmission certification, preadmission review, and pre-cert, it is the process of obtaining authorization from a health insurer or MCO for hospital admissions and for many outpatient procedures. It often involves review against preestablished utilization.

Preexisting condition: A physical and/or mental condition known and treated prior to the issuance of a health insurance or application for a health insurance policy.

Preferred provider organization (PPO): A limited grouping (panel) of providers (doctors and/or hospitals) that agrees to provide health care for subscriber groups for a negotiated, usually discounted, fee and that agrees to utilization review. It differs from an HMO in that it does not establish or run the financing mechanism(s).

Premium: A periodic payment for health insurance.

Prepayment: Paying a flat fee, premium, or rate in advance, for a predetermined set of health care benefits, payments to be made regardless of use.

Primary care: The general health care that people receive for most of their ills and illness on a routine basis. It may be provided by a physician, nurse practitioner, or physician's assistant.

Primary care practitioners: First-contact physicians, regular source of care in family practice, general internal medicine, pediatrics, general obstetrics, gynecology; also nurse practitioners, midwives, and according to some, psychiatrists and emergency care physicians.

Private expenditures: Outlays for services provided or paid for by nongovernmental sources–consumers, insurance companies, private industry, philanthropic, and other non-patient-care sources.

Privileges: Rights applied for annually by physicians and affiliate staff members to perform specified kinds of care in the hospital.

Prospective payment: A system for reimbursing institutional and individual providers of health services using a predetermined, fixed fee/payment per unit of service.

Providers: Those institutions and individuals typically licensed to provide health care services (e.g., hospitals, skilled nursing facilities, physicians, pharmacists).

Public expenditures: Outlays for services provided or paid for by federal, state, and local government agencies or expenditures required by governmental mandate, such as workmen's compensation insurance payments.

Quality assurance: A formal set of activities to assess the quality of health services and to apply corrective measures as indicated.

Quality improvement:

Rate: A measure of some event, disease, or condition in relation to a unit of population, along with some specification of time; the amount of money that a group or individual must pay to the health plan for coverage, usually a monthly fee. Rating refers to the health plan developing those rates.

- **Fertility rate** is the number of live births per 1,000 women of reproductive age, 15–44 years.
- **Infant mortality rate** is calculated by dividing the number of infant deaths during a year by the number of live births reported in the same year. It is expressed as the number of infant deaths per 1,000 live births.
- **Mortality rate** is the number of deaths of children under 28 days of age, per 1,000 live births.

Reinsurance: Secondary insurance purchased by a primary health insurer or MCO to protect itself against the potential high costs of complicated cases.

Relative value system (RVS): A method of evaluating medical services, relative to time needed to provide and complete the service, especially physician services, based on California relative value studies of the 1960s through the 1980s. The federal government changed to an RBRVS (Resource-Based Relative Values Scale) physician payment system in early 1992, with an RVS payment system for physician services provided to Medicare recipients.

Reserves: A fund of money held by a health insurer or an MCO to pay for committed but undelivered health care and to cover such uncertainties as higher hospital utilization levels than expected, overutilization of referrals, accidental catastrophes, and the like.

Resource-Based Relative Value Scale (RBRVS): A fee schedule for Medicare payments to physicians, replacing the prior "usual and customary" fee system. The fees are based on such "resource" factors as physician training, time spent, skill required, practice expenses, and malpractice insurance costs.

Risk: For a health care provider or insurer, the measure of chance of financial loss or the possibility that revenues of the health plan will not be sufficient to cover expenditures incurred in the delivery of contractual services. For individual patients or population groups, risk is the chance of incurring a given disease or negative health condition.

Risk contract: A contract to provide services to beneficiaries under which the health plan receives a fixed monthly payment for enrolled members and then must provide all services on an at-risk basis.

Risk management: Management activities aimed at lowering an organization's legal and financial exposures, especially to lawsuits.

Self-insurance: An employer-based program for providing health insurance coverage for its own employees, financed internally. By self-insuring, firms avoid paying state taxes on health insurance premiums and are largely exempt from state-imposed mandates for benefit packages.

Service area: The region in which a health organization provides access to health services. Service areas may be either contiguous (i.e., they border each other) or noncontiguous (e.g., they do not).

Solo practice: Individual practice of medicine by a physician who does not practice in a group or does not share personnel, facilities, or equipment with other physicians.

Staff model: An HMO that employs providers directly, and those providers see members in the HMO's own facilities; a form of closed-panel HMO.

Stop loss: A form of reinsurance for a health insurer or MCO that provides protection for medical expenses above a certain limit, generally on a year-by-year basis.

Strategic planning: A process reviewing the mission, environmental surveillance, and previous planning decisions used to establish major goals and nonrecurring resource allocation decisions.

Total Quality Management (TQM): Originally developed by W. Edward Deming to study systems and processes, identifies sources of error, waste, organizations, and redundancy; uses input and feedback from all staff and patients to understand and make improvements in current procedures.

Triage: The process of sorting out requests for services by members into time categories, such as those who need to be seen right away, those who can wait a little while, and those whose problems can be handled with advice over the phone.

Underutilization: Use of a health service or services by an individual user or a subpopulation of users that falls below use norms established by a large population of users.

Underwriting: Bearing the risk for something (i.e., a policy is underwritten by an insurance company); also the analysis that is done by a group to determine rates or to determine whether the group should be offered coverage at all.

Utilization: The frequency with which a benefit or service is used (e.g., 3,200 doctor's office visits per 1,000 HMO members per year).

Vertical integration: The affiliation of organizations providing different kinds of service, such as hospital care, ambulatory care, long-term care, and social services.

Volunteers: People who offer their time to a health care organization without pay.

Withhold: A percentage of the payment to the provider held back by the HMO until the cost of referral of hospital services has been determined. Physicians exceeding the amount determined as appropriate by the HMO lose the amount held back. The amount of withhold returned depends on individual utilization by the gatekeeper, referral patterns through the year by the gatekeeper groups of physicians, or the overall plan pool; and financial results of the overall capitated plan.

Workers' compensation: A form of social insurance provided through property-casualty insurers, providing medical benefits and replacement of lost wages that result from injuries or illnesses that arise from the workplace. In turn, the employee cannot normally sue the employer unless true negligence exists.

Wraparound plan: Commonly used to refer to insurance or health plan coverage for copayments and deductibles that are not covered under a member's base plan. This is often used for Medicare.

- Medicare Part A—the hospital insurance (HI) program, covering institutional and home health care for most individuals automatically upon reaching 65 year of age.
- Medicare Part B—the Supplementary Medical Insurance Program, which includes coverage for physicians' and other noninstitutional health care services, for which eligible individuals may enroll on a voluntary basis and for which they must pay a monthly premium.

Years of potential life lost (YPLL): A measure of premature mortality that is calculated over the age range from birth to 65 years of age, using the following age ranges from birth to 65 years of age: under 1 year, 1–14 years, 15–24 years, 25–34 years, 35–44 years, 45–54 years, and 55–64 years. The number of deaths for each age group is multiplied by the years of life lost, calculated as the difference between age 65 years and the midpoint of the age group.

Appendix   II

A Guide to Sources of Data

Steven Jonas and Christine T. Kovner

This appendix is a guide to the principal sources of health and health services data for the United States as of 1997. It contains descriptions of those sources, indicates how frequently each is published, lists the categories of data and other information they contain, and gives the address of the publisher and other ordering information as indicated, all as of 1997.

Almost all federal sources of data are available for purchase through the U.S. Government Printing Office (USGPO or GPO, for short), Superintendent of Documents, Mail Stop: SSOP, Washington, DC 20402-9328; tel. (202) 512-1800, FAX (202) 512-2250. There are local USGPO bookstores and phone ordering centers located in major cities around the United States. They are listed in the federal government section of the blue pages of the respective local telephone directories under "Government Printing Office."

Health data are also available on the Internet. Each department of the U.S. Government has an Internet address, many of which are listed below. In addition, most states and professional organizations also have Internet sites. Some Internet addresses are listed below or use the usual Internet search engines such as Yahoo, Excite, or Lycos to locate other sites. [Access to Federal agencies can be obtained via **http://www.Yahoo.com/Government/Executive_Branch/Departments_ and_agencies**]

Comprehensive Guides to Sources Published Annually

There are two comprehensive guides to sources of data that are published annually. The first appears in the *Statistical Abstract of the United States* (see item 1, below). The most recent edition as of this writing was for 1996, published in

September 1996. Its Appendix I contains an extensive listing of sources of health data (as well as the sources of all other data appearing in the *Statistical Abstract*). Appendix III presents brief descriptions and analyses of the limitations of the major sources of data listed in Appendix I.

The second regularly published comprehensive guide to sources appears in *Health, United States* (see item 7, below). The most recent edition as of this writing was for 1996–97, published in July 1997 (DHHS Publication No. [PHS] 97-1232). Its Appendix I contains very useful, detailed descriptions of all the common health data sources published by the several branches of the federal government, the United Nations, and certain private agencies, ranging from the American Medical Association to the National League for Nursing.

Also, the *AHA Guide*, published annually by the American Hospital Association (see item 10, below), in its Part C lists the major national, international, U.S. government, state and local government, and private "Health Organizations, Agencies, and Providers" with addresses and telephone numbers. Health and health care data can be obtained from many of them. [Access to federal data can be obtained via **http:///www.fedworld.gov**] [Federal agencies: **http://www.Yahoo.com/Government/Executive_Branch/Departments_ and_Agencies**]

Principal Sources of Health and Health Care Data

1. *Statistical Abstract of the United States.* Published annually by the Bureau of the Census, U.S. Department of Commerce, Washington, DC 20233, the *Statistical Abstract* contains a vast collection of tables reporting information and data collected by many different government (and in certain cases nongovernment) agencies. They are accumulated under the following headings: Population; Vital Statistics; Health and Nutrition; Education; Law Enforcement, Courts, and Prisons; Geography and Environment; Parks, Recreation, and Travel; Elections; State and Local Government Finances and Employment; Federal Government Finances and Employment; National Defense and Veterans' Affairs; Social Insurance and Human Services; Labor Force, Employment, and Earnings; Income, Expenditures, and Wealth; Prices; Banking, Finance, and Insurance; Business Enterprise; Communications; Energy; Science; Transportation—Land; Transportation—Air and Water; Agriculture; Natural Resources; Construction and Housing; Manufactures; Domestic Trade and Services; Foreign Commerce and Aid; Outlying Areas [under the jurisdiction of the United States]; Comparative International Statistics; and Industrial Outlook. There are health and health services data of varying kinds reported in many of these categories, although the principal ones are of course found under the headings Population, Vital Statistics, and Health and Nutrition. [To order: **http://www.ntis.gov/yellowbk/1nty292.htm** or **http://www.census.gov/stat_abstract/**]

2. *U.S. Census of Population.* The U.S. Constitution requires that a census be taken every 10 years, at the beginning of each decade. The original purpose of the census was to apportion seats in the House of Representatives. Since it was first taken, the census and the voluminous amount of data it produces—going well beyond a simple count—have come to serve many other purposes. Many reports on the decennial censuses, as well as interim special counts and analyses known as "Current Population Reports" (see item 3, below), are published by the Census Bureau (a part of the U.S. Department of Commerce). A good place to begin is in Section 1 of the *Statistical Abstract.* A good deal of highly detailed information drawn from the decennial national census data is published periodically in hardcover compendia. Also available are special analyses for a wide variety of geographical subdivisions of the country.

Census Bureau publications may be ordered from the USGPO through their comprehensive Census Catalog and Guide (itself available for purchase from the USGPO). Many Census Bureau products are also available through a desktop computer on-line service called CENDATA, as well as in the Compact Disc:Read Only Memory (CD:ROM) format. Electronic product orders may be sent to the U.S. Department of Commerce, Bureau of the Census, P.O. Box 277943, Atlanta, GA 30384-7943, tel. (301) 457-4100, FAX (301) 457-3842.**[http:// www.census.gov]**

3. *Current Population Reports.* In addition to reports from the decennial censuses, on a continuing basis the Census Bureau publishes "Current Population Reports" (CPRs). They present estimates, projections, sample counts, and special studies of selected segments of the population. There are seven series of CPRs: P-20, Population Characteristics; P-23, Special Studies; P-25, Population Estimates and Projections; P-26, Local Population Estimates; P-28, Special Censuses; P-60, Consumer Income; and P-70, Household Economic Studies. Catalogs and information on the content of each series are available directly from the Bureau of the Census, U.S. Department of Commerce, Washington, DC, 20233. Publications may be ordered through the USGPO.

4. *Monthly Vital Statistics Report (MVSR). MVSR* is published by the National Center for Health Statistics (NCHS), Centers for Disease Control and Prevention (CDCP), U.S. Department of Health and Human Services, 6525 Belcrest Road, Hyattsville, MD 20782-2003, tel. (301) 436-8500. The NCHS periodically publishes catalogs of its various publications and electronic data products, available free. The MVSR appears in several sections. "Provisional Data," published monthly, contains the most recent figures for the traditional "vital statistics"—births, marriages, divorces, and deaths. There is a series of *MVSR* supplements that appear on a semiregular basis, containing "Advance Reports" of the "Final Data" for the annually collected vital statistics. There are also reports titled "Advance Data." They present what are called "Vital and Health Statistics" for the health care delivery system, including, for example, results of the

"National Home and Hospice Care Survey," the "National Hospital Ambulatory Medical Care Survey," and the "National Hospital Discharge Survey," as well as the results of special studies and technical information on methodology. All *MVSR* reports may be obtained by annual subscription, through the USGPO. **[http://www.cdc.gov/nchswww/index.htm]**

5. *Vital Statistics of the United States.* These are the full, highly detailed annual reports on vital statistics from the NCHS, the summary versions of which are published in the supplements of the *MVSR*.

6. *Vital and Health Statistics.* These publications of the NCHS, distinct from the "Vital Statistics" reports described in items 4 and 5 above, appear at irregular intervals. As of 1997, there were 14 series, not numbered consecutively. Most of them report data from ongoing studies and surveys that the NCHS carries out. The publication of some data shifts periodically between *Vital and Health Statistics* and *Monthly Vital Statistics Report.* The 14 series of *Vital and Health Statistics* are as follows: Series 1, programs and collection procedures; Series 2, data evaluation and methods research; Series 3, analytical and epidemiological studies; Series 4, documents and committee reports; Series 5, international vital and health statistics reports; Series 6, cognition and survey measurement; Series 10, data from the health interview survey; Series 11, data From the National Health Examination Survey, the National Health and Nutrition Examination Surveys, and the Hispanic Health and Nutrition Examination Survey; Series 13, data on health resources utilization; Series 16, compilations of advance data from vital and health statistics; Series 20, data on mortality; Series 21, data on natality, marriage, and divorce; Series 23, data From the National Survey of Family Growth; Series 24, compilations of data on natality, mortality, marriage, divorce, and induced terminations of pregnancy.

7. *Health, United States. Health, United States* is published annually by the NCHS/CDCP, and available for purchase from the USGPO. A wide variety of health and health care delivery systems data are presented, under the following categories: population, fertility and natality, mortality, determinants of health, utilization of health resources, health care resources, and health care expenditures. *Health, United States* also contains a useful appendix, "Sources and Limitations of Data" (described above), as well as a glossary. It is a boon to students and researchers in health care delivery systems analysis because it provides one-stop shopping for the most important health and health care data.

8. *Morbidity and Mortality Weekly Report (MMWR).* This is a regular publication of the Centers for Disease Control and Prevention of the PHS, USDHHS. It is available by annual subscription from the USGPO. However, following a large subscription price increase in 1982, *MMWR*, in the public domain, has been photocopied and circulated at cost by several organizations, including the Massachusetts Medical Society, P.O. Box 9120, Waltham, MA 02254-9120. In the past, *MMWR* has been concerned primarily with communicable disease

reporting. As of 1997, the numbers by state of reported cases of the following diseases are published weekly: AIDS, chlamydia, *Escherichia coli*, gonorrhea, viral hepatitis, Legionellosis, Lyme disease, malaria, *H. influenzae* (invasive), measles, meningococcal disease, mumps, pertussis, rubella (German measles), primary and secondary syphilis, tuberculosis, and animal rabies. *MMWR* also reports deaths in 122 U.S. cities on a weekly basis. In the late 1990s, equally or perhaps more important each week *MMWR* presented brief reports on special studies of such diverse health topics as alcohol consumption among pregnant and childbearing-age women, human rabies, progress toward global poliomyelitis eradication, rubella and congenital rubella syndrome in the United States, adult blood lead epidemiology and surveillance, Clean Air Month, urban community intervention to prevent Halloween arson, sports-related recurrent brain injuries, a tobacco tax initiative in Oregon, and prevalence of cigarette smoking among secondary school students in Budapest, Hungary. *MMWR* also periodically publishes "Recommendations and Reports" of various governmental and nongovernmental health agencies and organizations, and the results of "CDC Surveillance Summaries."

  9. *Health Care Financing Review.* The *Health Care Financing Review* is a quarterly publication of the Health Care Financing Administration (HCFA), USDHHS, Office of Strategic Planning, 1-A-9 Oak Meadows Building, 7500 Security Boulevard, C3-11-07, Baltimore, MD 21244-1850. tel. (410) 786-6572. It is available by subscription through the USGPO. It annually publishes the official HCFA reports, "National Health Expenditures" and "Health Care Indicators." It also publishes an extensive and wide-ranging series of academic articles, reports, and studies. The emphasis is on Medicare/Medicaid (for which HCFA is directly responsible), but "a broad range of health care financing and delivery issues" are also covered. **[http://www.hcfa.gov/stats/stats.htm]**

  10. *American Hospital Association Guide to the Health Care Field.* This is a two-part publication of the American Hospital Association, One North Franklin, Chicago, Illinois 60606-3401, publication ordering tel. (800) AHA-2626, available for purchase from the AHA. The first part, the *AHA Guide*, as of the late 90s is published biennially. It contains a listing of almost every hospital in the United States by location and gives basic data on size, type, ownership, and services of each one; a listing and brief description of the integrated health care delivery networks; a listing of the multihospital health care systems, and information on the AHA itself. It also contains the comprehensive lists of health and health care organizations referred to in the introductory section of this appendix, above. As of the mid-1990s the *Guide's* second part, *AHA Hospital STAT*, is also published biennially. It contains a great deal of summary descriptive, utilization, and financial data on U.S. hospitals, presented in many different cross-tabulations. The two parts together contain the most detailed data available on hospitals in the United States. **[http://www.aha.org]**

11. *Center for Health Policy Research of the American Medical Association.* The Center, located in AMA National Headquarters, 515 North State Street, Chicago, Illinois 60610, ordering tel. (800) 621-8335 produces a variety of useful data on the physician work force and related subjects. As of 1997, titles appearing on a regular basis included: "Socioeconomic Characteristics of Medical Practice," "Physician Marketplace Statistics," "U.S. Medical Practice," "Physician Marketplace Statistics," "U.S. Medical Licensure Statistics and Current Licensure Requirements," "Physician Characteristics and Distribution in the US," and "Medical Groups in the US." **[http://www.ama-assn.org]**

12. The National League for Nursing provides information on Nursing Education Programs including enrollments. Information about their publications is available from the National League for Nursing, 350 Hudson Street, New York 10014, ordering telephone number: 800-669-1656. Titles appearing on a regular basis are: *State Approved Schools of Nursing* and *Nursing Data Source.* **[http://www.NLN.org]**

Internet Guides

"PBS Understanding and using the Internet"
http://www.pbs.org.uti

"Learn the net"
http://www.learnthenet.com

"The net: user guidelines and Netiquette"
http://www.fau.edu/rinaldi/netiquette.html

"A beginner's guide to effective e-mail"
http://www.webfoot.com/advice/estyle.html

"The unofficial smiley dictionary"
http://www.pix.za/mbs/fun/smiley.htm

"FOLDOC-Free on-line dictionary of computing"
http://wombat.doc.ic.ac.uk

Author Index

Subject Index